SECOND EDITION

IMAGING OF CNS DISEASE
A CT AND MR TEACHING FILE

Imaging of CNS Disease
A CT and MR Teaching File

DOUGLAS H. YOCK, JR., M.D.
Departments of Neuroscience and Radiology
Abbott Northwestern Hospital
Minneapolis, Minnesota

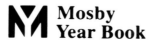

Mosby
Year Book

St. Louis   Baltimore   Boston   Chicago   London   Philadelphia   Sydney   Toronto

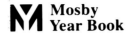
**Mosby
Year Book**

Dedicated to Publishing Excellence

Sponsoring Editor: Anne S. Patterson
Associate Managing Editor, Manuscript Services: Deborah Thorp
Production Project Coordinator: Carol A. Reynolds
Proofroom Supervisor: Barbara Kelly

1 2 3 4 5 6 7 8 9 0 C L P P 95 94 93 92 91

Library of Congress Cataloging-in-Publication Data

Yock, Douglas H.
    Imaging of CNS disease : a CT and MR teaching file / Douglas H.
Yock, Jr. — 2nd ed.
      p.   cm.
    Rev. ed. of: Computed tomography of CNS disease. c1985.
    Includes bibliographical references.
    Includes index.
    ISBN 0-8151-9778-0
    1. Central nervous system—Tomography.   2. Central nervous system—
-Magnetic resonance imaging.   I. Title.
    [DNLM: 1. Central Nervous System Diseases—diagnosis.
2. Diagnosis, Differential. 3. Magnetic Imaging. 4. Tomography,
X-Ray Computed. WL 141 Y54c]
RC349.T65Y63 1991
616.8′04757—dc20
DNLM/DLC
for Library of Congress
                                                    91-6588
                                                    CIP

FOREWORD TO THE SECOND EDITION

The good gets better. The first edition of this book was outstanding; this state-of-the-art second edition improves on perfection. The strengths of the previous text have been maintained and enhanced with the addition of several hundred new cases and the incorporation of magnetic resonance imaging.

Superb MR and CT images of wonderfully educational cases are organized to illustrate all major classes of neuropathology. In clear, concise captions, Dr. Yock gently guides the reader through scan interpretation to expert differential diagnosis and a meaningful contribution to patient management.

This beautiful and delightful book is a "must" for all medical students, residents, practitioners, departments, and institutions that care for patients with neurological disease.

THOMAS P. NAIDICH, M.D.
Director of Neuroradiology
Baptist Hospital of Miami
Clinical Professor of Radiology
University of Miami School of Medicine
Miami, Florida

FOREWORD TO THE FIRST EDITION

The real need for a teaching text in craniospinal CT has now been met. In this unique and wonderful book, Dr. Yock succeeds in teaching and delighting his readers simultaneously. The format is beautiful in its simplicity. On facing pages Dr. Yock provides 4 CT images that illustrate the key features of a common diagnosis or a common differential diagnosis. The patient's age, sex, and chief complaint are printed above each image, so they are known before the image is viewed. Detailed captions are printed below each image to explain what the image shows and how to use it to arrive at the correct diagnosis. By this method the reader is first invited to try his skill in interpreting the scan and history in exactly the fashion required in practice. Thereafter, he or she is gently guided to the correct interpretation of the case by the caption beneath. Often the captions conclude with "pearls" of knowledge or just those statistics the physician must know to function effectively.

As in the best teaching conferences, the companion images are carefully selected to complement each other by illustrating, for example, typical and atypical appearances of the same disease or the strikingly-similar appearances of different disease states. Since the complexity of cases and number of possible diagnoses increase from chapter to chapter, Dr. Yock has carefully interwoven special pages, entitled "Differential Diagnosis," that pair diagnoses from different chapters to help the reader review previous material. Throughout the volume, extensive cross references within the captions lead the reader to page back and forth among the cases to glean additional correlations and insights. By this technique, Dr. Yock expands the reader's appreciation of the range of pathology one must consider in each context, and provides a very close approximation to "instant experience." Selected modern references permit especially interested readers to pursue any particular topic easily.

In a book like this, image quality is paramount. Realizing this, Dr. Yock retrieved all the cases illustrated from the archives of magnetic tape and made new hard copies that accentuate the diagnostic features desired. The final results merit this enormous effort.

This book works very well. By painstaking effort and complete control of organization, Dr. Yock has created a teaching tool which combines the best features of first rate teaching conferences and home study. He has eliminated paragraphs of verbiage and replaced them with concise captions which distill for the readers his broad experience and acumen. This excellent volume will be highly useful to all medical students, to all residents in radiology, neurology, neurosurgery, general surgery and medicine, to all attendings who face increasing numbers of CT scans in their daily practice, and to all those knowledgeable physicians who seek to refresh and extend their understanding of this modality. It properly belongs in the departmental and institutional libraries of all hospitals and medical schools and in the personal libraries of those who practice the neurosciences. Unlike compendiums and reference texts, this book is one to enjoy cover to cover.

THOMAS P. NAIDICH, M.D.
Professor of Radiology
Northwestern University Medical School
Chicago, Illinois

PREFACE

Continuing experience with CT scanning has now been joined by the broad capabilities of magnetic resonance imaging. These advances allow improved recognition of CNS disease and warrant an updated version of the previous teaching file.

Readers of the first edition have requested two features in a revision: (1) "more of the same," and (2) "integration with MR." We have tried to meet both requests by expanding the case collection, adding new illustrated differential diagnoses, and incorporating over 200 selected MR studies. New cases have been concentrated in areas of diagnostic difficulty: pediatric disease, inflammatory and white matter disorders, and spinal canal lesions.

The book is intended to be a representative survey of CNS disease rather than a comprehensive atlas. Anatomical variants are discussed only if they mimic pathology. ENT disease is largely omitted. The chapter on orbital lesions is an overview rather than a complete summary.

MR scans have been liberally included to correlate with CT and to better demonstrate the characteristic features of various neuropathologies. We hope that the book can serve as an introduction to the application of magnetic resonance imaging in the central nervous system. Many direct CT/MR comparisons are presented, but extensive duplication of CT and MR illustrations has been avoided in the interest of brevity. A separate list of MR references is provided at the end of each chapter to help direct further reading.

As in the first edition, the text concentrates on CT and MR interpretation. Comments on clinical presentation, pathophysiology, and therapy are limited. Case histories are intentionally brief.

The "teaching file" format of the first edition has been maintained. Each page features a pair of related scans. Scans have been grouped on facing pages to illustrate comparisons, relationships, or variations. A large number of cross references have been made in an effort to interconnect and reinforce the material. Cases have been purposefully sequenced to build a broadening fund of knowledge. "Differential diagnoses" have been placed to integrate new topics with prior information.

In summary, we have again tried to assemble a teaching collection that is strengthened by cohesion and organization. We hope the result is focused, informative, and fun.

DOUGLAS H. YOCK, JR., M.D.

NOTES TO READERS:
1. Unless otherwise specified, axial and coronal scans are displayed with the patient's right on the reader's left.
2. All MR scans were performed at 1.0T or 1.5T.

ACKNOWLEDGMENTS

The CT and MR studies added to this edition were performed at Abbott Northwestern Hospital in Minneapolis by an outstanding group of skilled technologists. Drs. Stephen Fry, John Steely, and David Tubman shared in the daily supervision of procedures and contributed to the selection of teaching material. Dr. Robert McGeachie of Duluth, Minn., reviewed the manuscript; his careful reading and thoughtful suggestions were greatly appreciated. Dr. Thomas Naidich of Miami kindly agreed to introduce this edition as he did its predecessor; I am again grateful for his help.

Kevin Johnson worked long hours under adverse circumstances to optimally rephotograph images from magnetic tape. Wes Bue efficiently printed the large number of illustrations with unfailing patience and dedication to quality. Deanna Gunderson processed the manuscript with her customary diligence and attention to detail, overcoming a demanding schedule and a change in computer systems.

Gordon Sprenger and Robert Spinner of Abbott Northwestern Hospital have encouraged this specific project as well as supporting the overall development of a strong neuroscience program, from which the following cases have been drawn.

Anne Patterson, Deborah Thorp, and Carol Reynolds of Mosby-Year Book, Inc., provided expert guidance throughout the many stages of production.

Finally, appreciation is due to readers of the first edition who expressed encouragement and an interest in "more of the same." Your comments have played a major role in initiating and sustaining this project.

DOUGLAS H. YOCK, JR., M.D.

CONTENTS

Foreword to the Second Edition   *v*

Foreword to the First Edition   *vii*

Preface   *ix*

Table of Illustrated Differential Diagnoses   *xiv*

1 / Metastases   *1*

2 / Meningiomas   *19*

3 / Gliomas   *41*

4 / Posterior Fossa Tumors   *67*

5 / Pituitary and Suprasellar Tumors   *103*

6 / Other Masses   *135*

7 / Inflammatory and Degenerative Diseases   *161*

8 / Traumatic Lesions   *213*

9 / Infarction and Anoxia   *245*

10 / Vascular Lesions and Hemorrhage   *297*

11 / Hydrocephalus, Cysts, and Developmental Abnormalities   *351*

12 / Orbital Lesions   *397*

13 / Disc Disease and Spondylosis   *425*

14 / Spinal Tumors, Trauma, Inflammation, and Malformation   *453*

Index   *493*

TABLE OF ILLUSTRATED DIFFERENTIAL DIAGNOSES

Cerebral Hemispheres

High attenuation, uniformly-enhancing mass adjacent
  to the falx   24
Well-defined, uniformly enhancing extra-axial mass at the
  skull base   25
Densely calcified mass adjacent to the inner table   36
Cerebral mass with dural attachment   53
Rim-enhancing, deep hemisphere mass with edema   54
Tumor involving the splenium of the corpus
  callosum   55
Cystic neoplasm within the temporal lobe   57
Dense lesion near the foramen of Monro   137
Intensely enhancing midline mass in the pineal
  region   141
Pineal region mass with an eccentric intra-axial
  component   142
Multiple, high-attenuation, enhancing cerebral
  nodules   154
Multiple enhancing cerebral and cerebellar
  nodules   155
Large, thin-walled midhemisphere mass   174
Superficial, rim-enhancing mass with edema   175
Multiple enhancing cerebral nodules   189
Multiple irregular areas of low-attenuation within white
  matter   198
Dense, epidural lesion   227
Multiple, superficial hemorrhagic lesions   234
Multilocular, superficial enhancing mass   242
Vague, low-attenuation in the sylvian region   248
Hemorrhage within a low-attenuation mass   253
Cerebral lesion with complex bands and rims of contrast
  enhancement   256
Low- or mixed-attenuation medial occipital lesion   261
Multiple superficial infarcts   263
Low-attenuation lesions in the basal ganglia   266
The "empty triangle" sign   284
Low-attenuation throughout cerebral white matter
  in an infant   288

Diffuse cerebral low-attenuation and swelling in an
  infant   289
Large lesion with dense, tubular and serpentine contrast
  enhancement   300
Cerebral lesion with extensive calcification   303
Intensely enhancing mass near the vein of Galen   305
Large, midhemispheric intracerebral hematoma   333
Atypical intracerebral hematoma   338, 339
Rim-enhancing mass with central hemorrhage   343

Posterior Fossa and Tentorium

Dural-based, intensely enhancing, extra-axial mass   33
Focally enhancing brain stem mass   69
Fourth ventricular masses in adults   77
Cystic cerebellar tumor with a mural nodule   81
Small, enhancing cerebellar mass   82
Solid, enhancing mass in the cerebellar hemisphere
  of an adult   83
Small, round, dense tissue in the cerebellopontine
  angle   90
Uniformly enhancing, extra-axial posterior fossa
  mass   91
Lesion destroying bone along the floor of the posterior
  fossa   94
Inhomogeneous extra-axial lesion extending from the
  petrous bone   95
Low-attenuation, extra-axial lesion in the cerebellopontine
  angle   147
Thickening and dense enhancement of the
  tentorium   184, 185
Low-attenuation brain stem lesion   271
Low-attenuation cerebellar mass   276
Focal, high-attenuation brain stem lesion   309
Large, enhancing brain stem mass   310
Calcified, enhancing mass at the foramen magnum   322
High attenuation near the dentate nuclei   341
Low-attenuation lesion in the cerebellopontine
  angle   374
Scattered cerebellar calcification   391
Extracranial cyst adjacent to the occipital bone
  in an infant   393

Sella, Parasellar, and Suprasellar Regions

Intensely enhancing, midline suprasellar mass   106, 107
Mixed attenuation, partially enhancing suprasellar
  mass   108
Low-attenuation and superior convexity of pituitary
  tissue   110
Low-attenuation lesion enlarging the pituitary
  gland   111
Midline destructive lesion of the skull base   115
Low-attenuation suprasellar mass with peripheral
  enhancement obstructing the foramina of Monro   120
Low-attenuation nonenhancing suprasellar mass   121
Enhancing mass with suprasellar and intrasellar
  components   123
Calcified suprasellar mass   125

Enhancing parasellar mass causing visual
  symptoms   131
Suprasellar mass with calcification and low
  attenuation   145
Small, midline high-attenuation structure near the anterior
  circle of Willis   321
Uniformly enhancing parasellar mass   323
Mass adjacent to the rostral basilar artery   329
Low-attenuation suprasellar mass   371

Subarachnoid Spaces and Ventricles

Intraventricular and periventricular rim-enhancing
  mass   59
Subependymal tumor spread   62
Pseudoatrophy   205
Wide extracerebral fluid spaces in an elderly
  patient   224
Low attenuation within CSF spaces   240
Large ventricles with peripheral zones of low-attenuation in
  an infant   291
Enhancing subarachnoid spaces with communicating hydro-
  cephalus   316
Large lateral ventricles in a child   354
Developmental abnormality with large supratentorial fluid
  spaces   355
Suprasellar cyst associated with hydrocephalus   356
Low-attenuation lesion within the third ventricle   357
Large lateral ventricles in an elderly patient   363
Low-attenuation lesion extending over the cerebral
  convexity   370
Midline cyst between the lateral ventricles   384
Periventricular calcification in a child   387
Periventricular mass in an adult   390

Orbits

Low-attenuation mass in the superolateral quadrant of the
  orbit   405
Thickened rectus muscles   410
Thickening of the optic nerve   413
Focal high attenuation within the orbit   421

Spine

Epidural density posterior to a vertebral body   433
Epidural mass within the spinal canal   434
Mass within an intervertebral foramen   435
Expansile lesion of the sacral canal   457
"Dumbbell" lesion spanning an intervertebral
  foramen   459
Smoothly marginated bone erosion near a transverse
  foramen   460
Lumbar intradural mass   462
Intrathecal "clumping" of lumbosacral nerve roots   466
Low-attenuation lesion within the sacral canal   467
Flattened shape of the cervical spinal cord   471
Multifocal erosion of vertebral end plates   476

CHAPTER 1

Metastases

METASTASES: SUPERFICIAL LOCATION, HOMOGENEOUS CONTRAST ENHANCEMENT, EDEMA

Case 1

35-year-old woman.

Metastatic Carcinoma of the Breast.

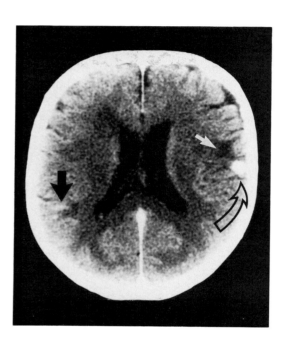

Cerebral metastases are typically found near the junction of gray and white matter *(open arrow)*. This superficial location reflects the high perfusion of cerebral cortex and is comparable to the distribution of hematogenous cerebral infection (see Case 282).

Small metastases usually demonstrate homogeneous contrast enhancement, as in this case. Subtle enhancement of superficial lesions is more apparent on MR scans than on CT studies (due to the absence of masking artifact from the calvarium and the greater sensitivity of MR to minor disruptions of the blood-brain barrier).

On this scan a small amount of edema is seen adjacent to the cortical nodule *(white arrow)*. A suggestion of leptomeningeal carcinomatosis is present over the right hemisphere *(solid black arrow; see Cases 20 and 21)*.

Case 2

71-year-old man.

Metastatic Hypernephroma.

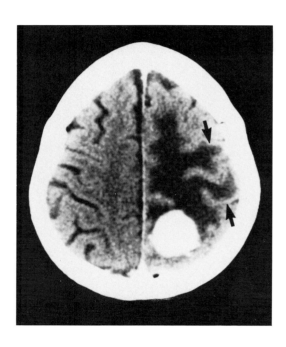

Some large cerebral metastases retain the well-defined, homogeneously enhancing character of small lesions, as seen here. When such masses are near a dural surface, the appearance can closely mimic a meningioma (compare to Cases 29 and 30).

Metastases often provoke cerebral edema, which may be more responsible for symptoms than the tumor itself. In this case, prominent edema extends anteriorly from the mass, including involvement of the precentral and postcentral gyri *(arrows; see Cases 341 and 342 for a review of gyral anatomy at the vertex)*.

Carcinomas of the breast and lung cause the greatest number of cerebral metastases, although melanoma and hypernephroma metastasize to the brain with higher frequency. An intracranial lesion accounts for the initial presentation of carcinoma in about 10% of cases.

METASTASES: MULTIPLE LESIONS, VARIABLE SIZE AND MORPHOLOGY

Case 3

65-year-old man presenting with confusion.

Metastatic Carcinoma of the Lung.

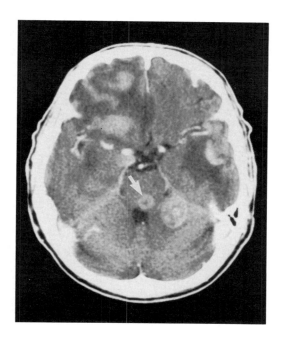

Case 4

52-year-old woman.

Metastatic Hypernephroma.

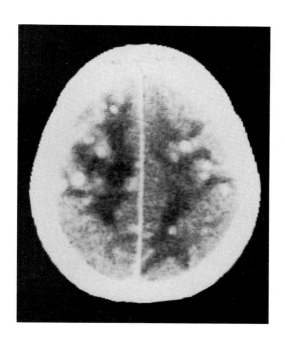

Multiplicity is a hallmark of metastatic disease. The size, shape, enhancement, and edema of individual lesions may vary substantially, as seen here.

Metastases commonly involve the posterior fossa. Brain stem metastases are characteristically well defined, as in this case (*arrow;* see also Case 108). Metastasis is the most common cause for a cerebellar mass in an adult (see Cases 134 and 456).

Occasionally cerebral metastases are remarkably uniform in size and morphology. The majority of the small, enhancing nodules in this case are located near the junction of gray and white matter. Edema associated with the multiple lesions coalesces to involve most of the centrum semiovale.

The differential diagnosis of "innumerable" small, enhancing cerebral nodules includes metastases (see Cases 251 and 308 for other examples), disseminated infection (e.g., cysticercosis as in Case 288, histoplasmosis, tuberculosis), noninfectious inflammatory processes (e.g., sarcoidosis or multiple sclerosis as in Case 307), primary CNS lymphoma (see Case 250), subacute multifocal infarction (as in Case 416), and multiple cavernous angiomas (see Case 510).

Case 5

62-year-old woman.

Metastatic Squamous Cell Carcinoma of the Lung.

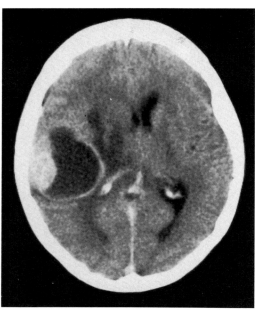

Case 6

40-year-old woman.

Metastatic Carcinoma of the Breast.

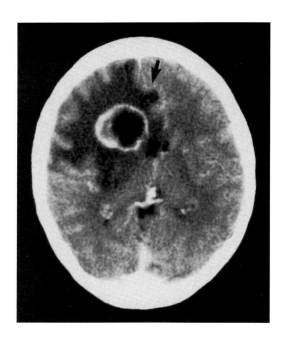

Many large metastases are inhomogeneous, with a rim of contrast enhancement surrounding a nonenhancing center. The enhancing margin of the lesion may be quite smooth and regular as seen here, but an irregular appearance with variable thickness is more characteristic (see Cases 6 and 16). The nonenhancing center within a metastasis (or other tumor) may represent a true cyst, necrosis, or a slowly equilibrating component that may accumulate contrast on later scans.

Large cerebral metastases may grow medially to involve deep hemisphere structures. In this case, the mass approaches the lateral ventricle, and reactive edema is seen within the internal and external capsules.

A "cystic" appearance is often associated with metastatic squamous cell carcinomas, but is also seen in metastatic adenocarcinomas. Solitary metastases of this type may resemble malignant gliomas (see Cases 86 to 89), and the two tumors must often be considered together in differential diagnosis.

Up to 50% of cerebral metastases from pulmonary squamous cell tumors are solitary (compared with about 30% of all intracranial metastases).

Some cerebral metastases are large masses located deep within the cerebral hemispheres. These tumors may demonstrate solid or peripheral enhancement and mimic primary malignant gliomas (see Cases 86 to 89).

The finding of a second lesion in such cases favors the diagnosis of metastases, and a careful search for distant tumor sites is warranted. Delayed scans and/or increased doses of contrast material may clarify ambiguous lesions by demonstrating additional enhancing masses. MR may help to detect or define accompanying lesions.

Rare gliomas are multicentric or may appear to be so (see Case 81), so that the demonstration of multiple masses is not an infallible sign of metastatic neoplasm. Primary CNS lymphoma (see Cases 248 to 250) and inflammatory etiologies (e.g., Case 283) may also cause multiple cerebral nodules.

This case is a good example of subfalcial herniation. The combination of the metastasis and surrounding edema causes prominent frontal mass effect. A large midline shift has developed, with a "step-off" of edematous brain passing beneath the falx (arrow).

METASTASES: HIGH ATTENUATION

Case 7

55-year old woman.
(noncontrast scan)

Metastatic Carcinoma of the Lung.

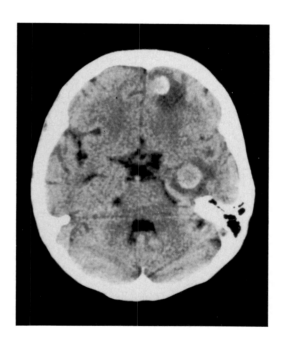

Case 8

58-year-old man.

Metastatic Adenocarcinoma of the Colon.

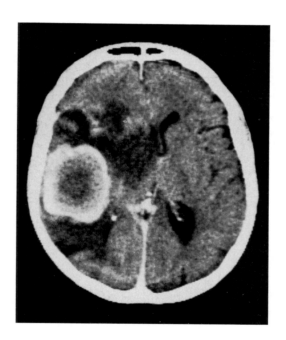

High attenuation values within a metastasis (or any cerebral lesion) may be due to hemorrhage, calcification, and/or dense protein content. Metastases from adenocarcinomas may demonstrate precontrast density in the absence of hemorrhage or macroscopic calcification. This high attenuation is attributable to the tissue density of the tumors and is particularly associated with mucinous carcinomas.

This dense mass was identical in appearance on a precontrast scan. The often unimpressive contrast enhancement of dense metastases may help to distinguish them from meningiomas (see Cases 27 to 30).

Metastases from mucinous adenocarcinomas may also demonstrate an unusual MR appearance, with prominent low signal intensity on T2-weighted images (see Case 14). The high attenuation on CT and the T2-shortening on MR likely reflect the thick, proteinaceous content of these neoplasms.

Case 9

67-year-old man.
(noncontrast scan)

Metastatic Hypernephroma.

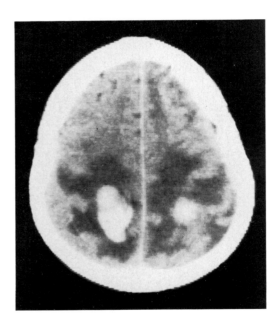

Case 10

72-year-old woman presenting with a "stroke."

Hemorrhage into Metastatic Ovarian Carcinoma.

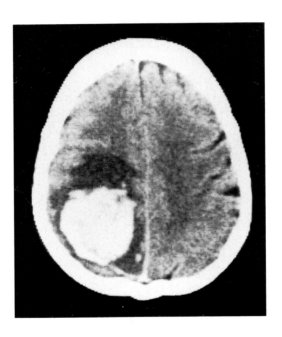

The multiplicity and location of these lesions strongly suggest metastases. The high attenuation values are more dense than mucinous adenocarcinomas and indicate hemorrhage within the nodules. This feature narrows the likely diagnoses to those primary tumors that cause vascular metastases: melanoma, choriocarcinoma, hypernephroma, bronchogenic carcinoma, and occasionally breast carcinoma.

Although hemorrhage into a cerebral metastasis is often the presenting event in metastatic melanoma (see Case 566), a renal or pulmonary neoplasm would be more common in a 67-year-old man. As a result of this scan, a chest x-ray and intravenous pyelogram were recommended, and a previously "silent" hypernephroma was discovered.

A mass is faintly seen within the large parietal hematoma, suggesting hemorrhage into a pre-existing lesion (compare with Cases 94 and 566). The hematoma was evacuated, and metastatic ovarian carcinoma was found.

Hemorrhage into a cerebral neoplasm is one mechanism by which such subacute or chronic lesions may cause acute symptoms ("stroke syndrome"; compare to Case 413). Other mechanisms include the sudden triggering of reactive cerebral edema, ventricular obstruction causing acute hydrocephalus, and critical vascular compression by an enlarging mass. About 5% of "strokes" are found to be the result of an underlying neoplasm.

Case 11A

69-year-old woman presenting with mild
right hemiparesis.
(postcontrast scan)

Metastatic Hypernephroma.

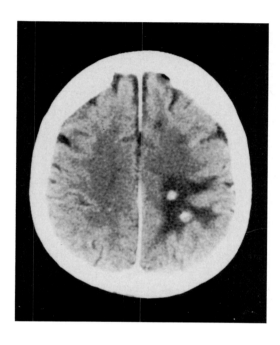

Case 11B

Same patient, 8 days later, now with
dense hemiplegia.
(noncontrast scan)

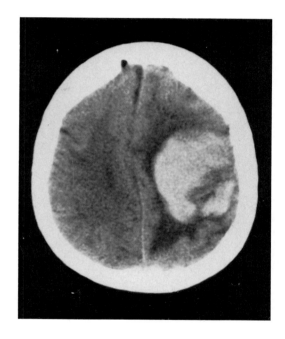

The small enhancing nodules at the vertex of the left hemisphere suggest metastatic disease. A history of prior nephrectomy for renal cell carcinoma was obtained.

Coalescent edema surrounding the nodules is the likely basis for symptoms at this stage.

Interval hemorrhage has occurred at the site of the previously demonstrated metastases. The appearance now resembles Cases 10 or 566, documenting the potentially rapid development of hemorrhage within such lesions. This case also emphasizes the fact that secondary processes in association with cerebral metastases (whether vasogenic edema or intratumoral hemorrhage) may be chiefly responsible for functional impairment.

The differential diagnosis of rapidly worsening hemorrhages near the vertex should include thrombosis of the superior sagittal sinus with venous infarction (see Cases 483 to 486) as well as delayed post-traumatic intracerebral hemorrhage (see Case 380).

MR CORRELATION: METASTASES ON T1-WEIGHTED SCANS

Case 12	**Case 13**
56-year-old man. (sagittal, noncontrast scan; SE 600/17)	67-year-old man. (sagittal, noncontrast scan; SE 600/17)
Metastatic Carcinoma of the Lung.	**Metastatic Hypernephroma.**

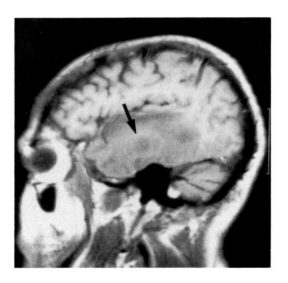 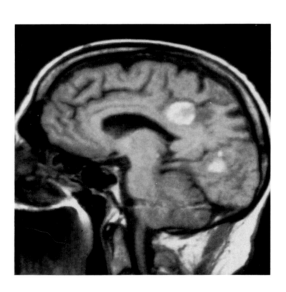

Nonhemorrhagic cerebral metastases usually demonstrate long T1 values on MR scans. Extensive vasogenic edema surrounding the lesion may obscure its margins. In this case, a small metastasis in the temporal lobe is only faintly defined *(arrow)* within a sea of edema.

Metastases may demonstrate T1 shortening on noncontrast scans due to the presence of subacute hemorrhage (see discussion of Cases 560 and 561) or other paramagnetic substances (e.g., melanin). In this case, the high signal intensity of tumor nodules on a T1-weighted scan is due to blood products within vascular metastases from a hypernephroma. MR contrast enhancement within nonhemorrhagic metastases could have an identical appearance (see Case 24B).

There is much less edema bordering these lesions than surrounds the metastasis in Case 12.

MR CORRELATION: METASTASES ON T2-WEIGHTED SCANS

Case 14

58-year-old woman.
(axial, noncontrast scan; SE 2500/90)

Metastatic Carcinoma of the Colon.

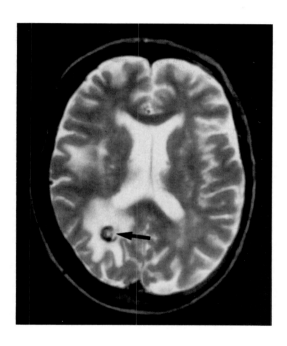

Case 15

39-year-old man.
(axial, noncontrast scan; SE 3000/90)

Metastatic Adenocarcinoma (Unknown Primary).

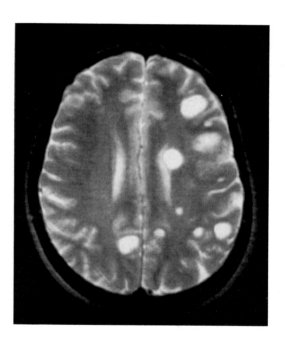

On long TR images the MR appearance of cerebral metastases may be dominated by the high signal intensity of surrounding edema. Most metastases have long T2 values, which may be obscured by this increase in water content within adjacent white matter.

Here an occipital metastasis demonstrates prominent T2-shortening and is clearly defined within the edematous background (arrow; compare to the appearance of the small abscesses in Case 285). T2-shortening may be seen in metastases containing hemorrhage or melanin. The MR detection of such lesions can be enhanced by the use of gradient echo sequences sensitive to local field inhomogeneities associated with blood products.

Low signal intensity on T2-weighted images is also often seen within metastases from adenocarcinoma of the colon. This finding frequently correlates with high CT attenuation, as in Case 8. T2-shortening in such nonhemorrhagic lesions likely reflects the thickly mucinous content of these tumors.

Some cerebral metastases do not incite appreciable edema. MR detection of such lesions depends on their intrinsic signal abnormality or the use of contrast material (see Case 24).

Here the multiple lesions are sharply defined because of long T2 values. (Compare this appearance in a young adult to the CT scans in Cases 250 and 251.)

CALCIFIED METASTASES

Case 16

66-year-old woman.

Metastatic Oat Cell Carcinoma of the Lung (No Previous Treatment).

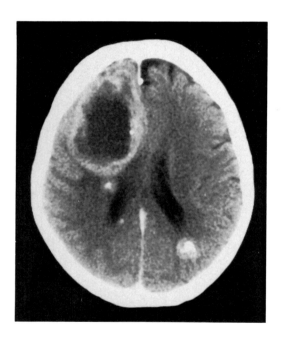

Case 17

76-year-old man, 3 months after radiation therapy for a large parasagittal metastasis from carcinoma of the lung.

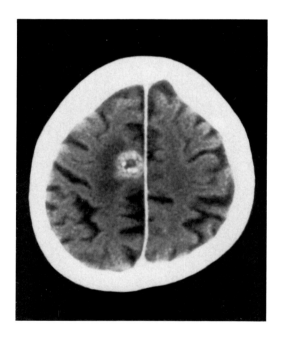

Calcification is occasionally seen in cerebral metastases, either prior to treatment or following therapy. This finding may be attributable to metastases from osteocartilaginous primary neoplasms (e.g., osteosarcoma) or to secondary calcification within metastases of soft tissue origin (e.g., carcinomas of the lung, breast, ovary, and colon). The later may reflect necrosis or metabolic alterations within the lesion, leading to dystrophic deposition of calcium.

Multiple small, calcified metastases can mimic the appearance of inflammatory foci (e.g., cysticercosis) or multiple cavernous hemangiomas (see Case 658 for another example).

The initial scans of this patient demonstrated a noncalcified, parasagittal mass measuring 5 cm in diameter. The metastasis has become substantially smaller after a course of radiation therapy and now demonstrates central calcification.

Chemotherapy and radiation therapy can lead to rapid and dramatic reduction in the size of cerebral metastases, often associated with acquired calcification.

DURAL INVOLVEMENT BY METASTASES

Case 18

79-year-old woman.

Metastatic Carcinoma of the Breast.

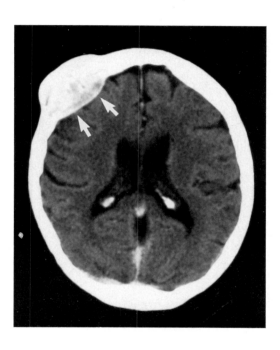

Case 19

74-year-old woman.

Metastatic Carcinoma of the Colon.

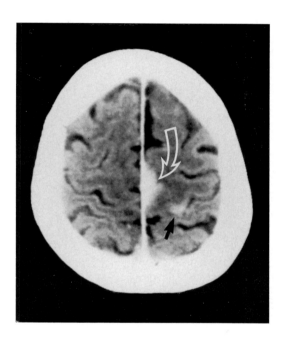

Osseous metastases may extend or enlarge to involve the dura and epidural space, as seen here. Extracranial extension is also present, with a subgaleal mass causing a palpable lump.

In this case the dura appears intact at the medial margin of the lesion *(arrows)*. There is no evidence of underlying cerebral edema or invasion, unlike Case 19.

After radiation therapy the mass resolved and the skull defect recalcified. Such "healing" or sclerosis is commonly seen after treatment of skeletal metastases from carcinomas of the breast.

Metastatic disease may involve the dura primarily, without adjacent calvarial lesions. In this case the dural mass based along the falx *(white arrow)* appears to extend into the adjacent cortex, which demonstrates reactive edema.

The opposite pattern of invasion may also occur: a superficial cerebral metastasis may compress or traverse the subarachnoid space to invade adjacent dura. That is, metastatic involvement of the dura may be a primary process or may reflect extension from either calvarial or cerebral lesions.

Dural-based metastases may present *"en plaque"* or mass-like morphologies, often resembling meningiomas (see Cases 35 and 52). Like meningiomas, such lesions may be associated with reactive changes in adjacent bone and vascular supply from dural arteries.

Leptomeningeal carcinomatosis is also present in this case *(black arrow)*, better seen as Case 20.

Case 20

74-year-old woman (same patient as Case 19).

Metastatic Carcinoma of the Colon.

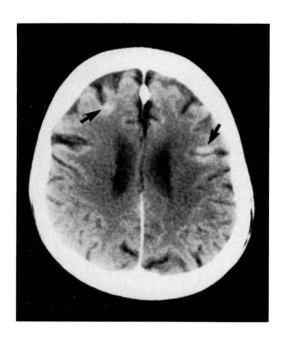

Case 21

76-year-old woman.

Metastatic Carcinoma of the Breast.

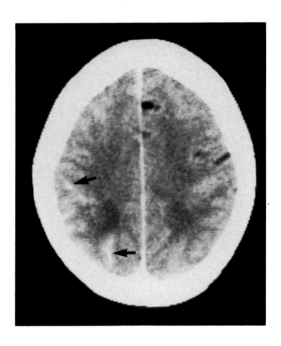

The small areas of abnormal contrast enhancement along the margins of cortical sulci in this case *(arrows)* represent meningeal carcinomatosis.

Meningeal involvement by metastatic solid tumors (especially melanoma and breast carcinoma) is often apparent on CT scans. The detection rate for meningeal lymphoma or leukemia is much lower.

Contrast-enhanced MR is more sensitive than CT scanning for the detection of all forms of meningeal disease, because of (1) the absence of signal or artifact from the adjacent calvarium, (2) a lower threshold for demonstration of contrast enhancement, and (3) multiplanar display.

Focal enhancement at the depth of a sulcus can be a normal finding due to partial volume imaging of a small cortical artery or vein. Meningeal carcinomatosis may also involve the depth of a sulcus (as seen here in the right frontal region), but is usually larger and less well defined than a normal vascular density.

Meningeal metastases may fill cortical sulci focally or diffusely *(arrows)*.

The differential diagnosis of sulcal enhancement includes meningeal tumor (systemic metastasis or seeding of a primary CNS lesion; see Case 121), meningitis (see Cases 258 and 259), the contrast enhancement occurring after subarachnoid hemorrhage (see Case 527), meningeal angioma as in Sturge-Weber syndrome (see Case 340), and superficial enhancement of gyri as in subacute infarction.

Communicating hydrocephalus may develop in association with meningeal carcinomatosis, as with other meningeal pathologies (see Cases 526 and 527).

EPENDYMAL/SUBEPENDYMAL METASTASES

Case 22

70-year-old woman.

Metastatic Carcinoma of the Lung.

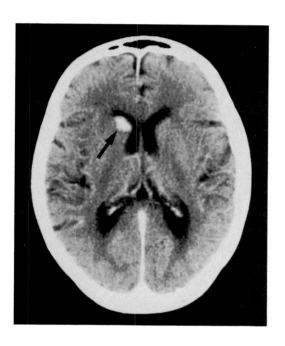

Case 23

62-year-old woman.

Metastatic Oat Cell Carcinoma.

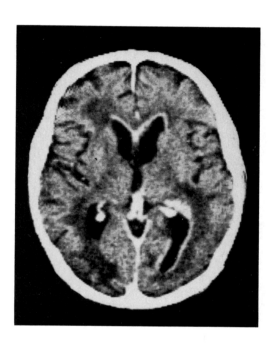

An enhancing mass along the ventricular margin may be due to subependymal metastasis, as in this case (see also Case 656). Tumor cells can arrive at this site hematogenously or through CSF seeding from a metastasis near the cerebral surface.

The differential diagnosis of subependymal masses includes primary CNS neoplasms such as glioma or ependymoma, lymphoma, and giant cell astrocytoma associated with tuberous sclerosis (see Cases 219 and 649). The location would be atypical for intraventricular meningioma (see Case 96) or choroid plexus papilloma (see Case 222).

Intraventricular metastases can also arise from hematogenous seeding of the highly vascular choroid plexus.

The enhancing ventricular margins in this case represent subependymal spread of metastatic small-cell carcinoma of the lung. This occurrence is less common than meningeal carcinomatosis but has been observed with several systemic tumors (e.g., melanoma, carcinomas of the lung and breast).

The differential diagnosis of enhancing ventricular margins also includes ependymal seeding or subependymal spread of gliomas and other primary CNS tumors (see Case 102), primary CNS lymphoma (see Case 244), systemic lymphoma (see Case 103), and inflammatory ventriculitis (see Cases 264 to 267).

Case 24A

51-year-old man.
(axial, noncontrast scan; SE 3000/90)

Metastatic Melanoma.

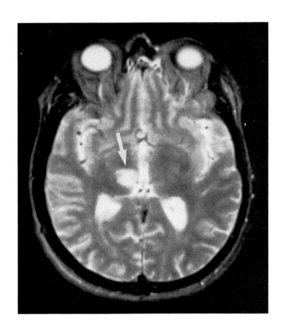

Case 24B

Same patient.
(axial, postcontrast scan; SE 720/17)

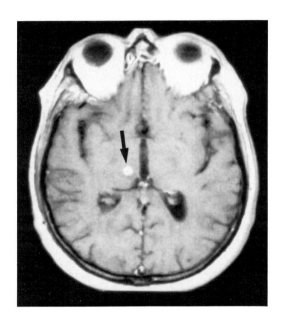

MR is more sensitive than CT to the small amount of edema that may accompany cerebral metastases only a few millimeters in diameter. The improved MR detection of small lesions has demonstrated more frequent occurrence of tiny cortical and deep hemisphere metastases than has been previously noted on CT studies.

In this case, an axial "T2-weighted" image demonstrates an area of focal signal abnormality within the right thalamus *(arrow)*. The appearance is not specific, and differential diagnosis would include "lacunar" infarction as well as an inflammatory focus. Subsequent growth of the lesion and the presence of other masses confirmed the diagnosis in this patient.

Contrast-enhanced MR scans may demonstrate small parenchymal metastases that are not apparent on either contrast-enhanced CT scans or noncontrast MR studies. In this case, the focus of abnormal enhancement in the right thalamus *(arrow)* on the T1-weighted image corresponds to the small area of edema seen prior to contrast in Case 24A. In a different clinical setting the same focal enhancement could represent a subacute infarct or an inflammatory lesion.

Case 25

84-year-old man.
(sagittal, noncontrast scan; SE 600/20)

Metastatic Carcinoma of the Prostate.

Case 26

51-year-old man (same patient as Case 24).
(axial, postcontrast scan; SE 720/17)

Metastatic Melanoma.

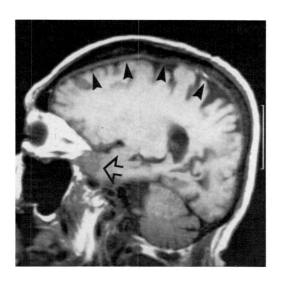

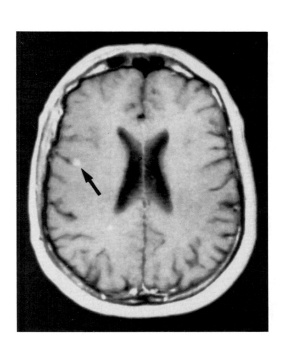

MR scans demonstrate meningeal metastases more effectively than CT. Multiplanar display and the low signal intensity of the calvarium facilitate detection of focal or diffuse dural thickening.

In this case, the convexity dura is uniformly thickened *(arrowheads),* while a dural-based mass has arisen along the sphenoid wing *(open arrow).* Both of these regions enhanced intensely with contrast material.

The signal intensity of the diploic space of the vault is abnormally low on this T1-weighted sequence, reflecting osteoblastic calvarial metastases.

The sensitivity of MR to contrast enhancement combines with the absence of obscuring signal from the neighboring calvarium to highlight subtle superficial lesions, whether cortical or meningeal. As with CT, enhancing meningeal tumor on MR scans may line or fill sulci focally or diffusely with nodular or linear patterns. In this case, a small nodule of subarachnoid tumor is localized to the depth of a sulcus *(arrow).* A tiny parenchymal metastasis is present posterior to the right lateral ventricle.

Melanoma is a common source of leptomeningeal carcinomatosis. Most cases represent metastasis from distant tumors, but primary meningeal melanomatosis may also occur.

REFERENCES: CT

1. Amundsen P., Dugstad G., Syvertsen A.H.: The reliability of computer tomography for the diagnosis and differential diagnosis of meningiomas, gliomas, and brain metastases. *Acta Neurochir. (Wien)* 41:177–190, 1978.
2. Anand A.K., Potts D.G.: Calcified brain metastases: demonstration by computed tomography. *A.J.N.R.* 3:527–529, 1982.
3. Brant-Zawadzki M., Enzmann D.R.: Computed tomographic brain scanning in patients with lymphoma. *Radiology* 129:67–71, 1978.
4. Brown S.B., Brant-Zawadzki M., Eifel P., et al.: CT of irradiated solid tumor metastases to the brain. *Neuroradiology* 23:127–131, 1982.
5. Dearnaley D.P., Kingsley D.P., Husband J.E., et al.: The role of CT of the brain in the investigation of breast cancer patients with suspected intracranial metastases. *Clin. Radiol.* 32:375–382, 1981.
6. Deck M.D., Messina A.V., Sackett J.F.: Computed tomography in metastatic disease of the brain. *Radiology* 119:115–120, 1976.
7. Dubois P.J., Martinez A.J., Myerowitz R.L., et al.: Subependymal and leptomeningeal spread of systemic malignant lymphoma demonstrated by cranial computed tomography. *J. Comput. Assist. Tomogr.* 2:218–221, 1978.
8. Enzmann D.R., Krikorian J., Yorke C., et al.: Computed tomography in leptomeningeal spread of tumor. *J. Comput. Assist. Tomogr.* 2:448–455, 1978.
9. Gaze M.N., Gregor A. Whittle I.R., et al.: Calcified cerebral metastases from cervical carcinoma. *Neuroradiology* 31:291, 1989.
10. Gildersleeve N., Koo A.H., McDonald C.J.: Metastatic tumor presenting as intracerebral hemorrhage. *Radiology* 124:109–112, 1977.
11. Ginaldi S., Wallace S., Shalen P., et al.: Cranial computed tomography of malignant melanoma. *A.J.N.R.* 1:531–535, 1980.
12. Healy J.F., Marshall W.H., Brahme F.J., White F.: CT of intracranial metastases with skull and scalp involvement. *A.J.N.R.* 2:335–338, 1981.
13. Hilal S.K., Chang C.H.: Specificity of computed tomography in the diagnosis of supratentorial neoplasm. *Neuroradiology* 16:537–539, 1978.
14. Holtas S., Cronquist S.: Cranial computed tomography of patients with malignant melanoma. *Neuroradiology* 22:123–127, 1981.
15. Huckman M.S., Ramsey R.G., Shenk G.I.: CT scanning in patients with suspected cerebral metastases. *J. Comput. Assist. Tomogr.* 2:511–512, 1978.
16. Kart B.H., Reddy S.C., Rao G.R., Poveda H.: Choroid plexus metastasis: CT appearance. *J. Comput. Assist. Tomogr.* 10:537–540, 1986.
17. Kelly J.K., Lazo A., Metes J., et al.: Intracerebral hemorrhagic dissemination of acute myelocytic leukemia. *A.J.N.R.* 6:113–114, 1985.
18. Kelly R.B., Mahoney P.D., Johnson J.F.: Calcified carcinoma of the lung and intracerebral metastases. *C.T.* 11:389, 1987.
19. Kingsley D.P., Kendall B.E.: Cranial computed tomography in leukemia. *Neuroradiology* 16:543–546, 1978.
20. Lee Y.-Y., Glass J.P., Geoffray A., Wallace S.: Cranial computed tomographic abnormalities in leptomeningeal metastasis. *A.J.N.R.* 5:559–564, 1984.
21. Lukin R., Tomsick T.A., Chambers A.A.: Lymphoma and leukemia of the central nervous system. *Semin. Roentgenol.* 15:246, 1980.
22. Naheedy M.H., Kido D.I., O'Reilly G.V., et al.: Computed tomography of subdural and epidural metastases. *J. Comput. Assist. Tomogr.* 4:311–313, 1978.
23. Pedersen H., McConnell J., Harwood-Nash D.C., et al.: Computed tomography in intracranial supratentorial metastases in children. *Neuroradiology* 31:19, 1989.
24. Potts G.D., Abbott G.F., Von Sneidern J.V.: National Cancer Institute study: Evaluation of computed tomography in the diagnosis of intracranial neoplasms. III. Metastatic tumors. *Radiology* 136:657–664, 1980.
25. Tarver R.D., Richmond B.D., Klatte E.C.: Cerebral metastasis from lung carcinoma: Neurological and CT correlates. *Radiology* 153:689–692, 1984.
26. Tashiro Y., Kondo A., Aoyama I., et al.: Calcified metastatic brain tumor. *Neurosurgery* 26:1065–1070, 1990.
27. Voorhies R.M., Sundaresan N., Thaler H.T.: The single supratentorial lesion: An evaluation of preoperative diagnostic tests. *J. Neurosurg.* 53:364–368, 1980.
28. Wendling L.R., Cromwell L.D., Latchaw R.E.: Computed tomography of intracerebral leukemic masses. *A.J.R.* 132:217–220, 1979.
29. Zimmerman R.A., Bilaniuk L.T.: Computed tomography of acute intratumoral hemorrhage. *Radiology* 135:355–359, 1980.

REFERENCES: MR

1. Atlas S.W., Grossman R.I., Gomori J.M., et al.: MR imaging of intracranial metastatic melanoma. *J. Comput. Assist. Tomogr.* 11:577–582, 1987.
2. Atlas S.W., Grossman R.I., Gomori J.M., et al.: Hemorrhagic intracranial malignant neoplasms: Spin echo MR imaging. *Radiology* 164:71–78, 1987.
3. Claussen C., Laniado M., Schörner W., et. al.: Gadolinium-DTPA in MRI imaging of glioblastomas and intracranial metastases. *A.J.N.R.* 6:669–674, 1985.
4. Davis P.C., Friedman N.C., Fry S.M., et al.: Leptomeningeal metastasis: MR imaging. *Radiology* 163:449–454, 1987.
5. Destian S., Sze G., Krol G., et al.: MR imaging of hemorrhagic intracranial neoplasms. *A.J.N.R.* 9:1115–1122, 1988.
6. Healy M.E., Hesselink J.R., Press G.A., Middleton M.S.: Increased detection of intracranial metastases with intravenous Gd-DTPA. *Radiology* 165:619–624, 1987.
7. Krol G., Sze G., Malkin M., Walker R.: MR of cranial and spinal meningeal carcinomatosis: Comparison with CT and myelography. *A.J.N.R.* 9:709–714, 1988.
8. Laine F.J., Braun I.F., Jensen M.E., et al.: Perineural tumor extension through the foramen ovale: Evaluation with MR imaging. *Radiology* 174:65–72, 1990.
9. Lee Y.-Y., Tien R.D., Bruner J.M., et al.: Loculated intracranial leptomeningeal metastases: CT and MR characteristics. *A.J.N.R.* 10:1171–1180, 1989.
10. Mathews V.P., Broome D.R., Smith R.R., et al.: Neuroimaging of disseminated germ cell neoplasms. *A.J.N.R.* 11:319–324, 1990.
11. Olsen W.L., Winkler M.L., Ross D.A.: Carcinomatous encephalitis: CT and MR findings. *A.J.N.R.* 8:553–554, 1987.
12. Paako E., Patronas N.J., Schellinger D.: Meningeal Gd-DTPA enhancement in patients with malignancies. *J. Comput. Assist. Tomogr.* 14:542–546, 1990.
13. Phillips M.E., Ryals T.J., Kambhu S.A., et al.: Neoplastic vs. inflammatory meningeal enhancement with Gd-DTPA. *J. Comput. Assist. Tomogr.* 14:536–541, 1990.
14. Russell E.J., Geremia G.K., Johnson C.E., et al.: Multiple cerebral metastases: Detectability with Gd-DTPA-enhanced MR imaging. *Radiology* 165:609–618, 1987.
15. Sze G., Milano E., Johnson C., et al.: Detection of brain metastases: Comparison of contrast-enhanced MR with unenhanced MR and enhanced CT. *A.J.N.R.* 11:785–792, 1990.
16. Sze G., Soletzky S., Bronen R., Krol G.: MR imaging of the cranial meninges with emphasis on contrast enhancement and meningeal carcinomatosis. *A.J.N.R.* 10:965–976, 1989.
17. Sze G., Shin J., Krol G., et al.: Intraparenchymal brain metastases: MR imaging versus contrast-enhanced CT. *Radiology* 168:187–194, 1988.
18. Tyrrell R.L. II, Bundschuh C.V., Modic M.T.: Dural carcinomatosis: MR demonstration. *J. Comput. Assist. Tomogr.* 11:329–332, 1987.
19. West M.S., Russell E.J., Breit R., et al.: Calvarial and skull based metastases: Comparison of nonenhanced and Gd-DTPA-enhanced MR images. *Radiology* 174:85–92, 1990.
20. Woodruff W.W. Jr., Djang W.T., McLendon R.E., et al.: Intracranial malignant melanoma: High-field-strength MR imaging. *Radiology* 165:209–214, 1987.
21. Yousem D.M., Patrone P.M., Grossman R.I.: Leptomeningeal metastasis: MR evaluation. *J. Comput. Assist. Tomogr.* 14:255–261, 1990.

CHAPTER 2

Meningiomas

Case 27

72-year-old man.
(noncontrast scan)

Falx Meningioma.

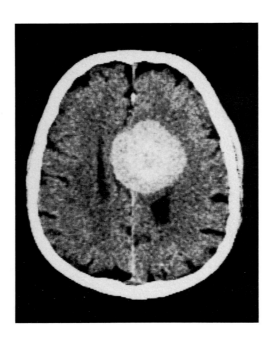

Case 28

84-year-old woman presenting with aphasia
and seizures.
(noncontrast scan)

Sphenoid Wing Meningioma.

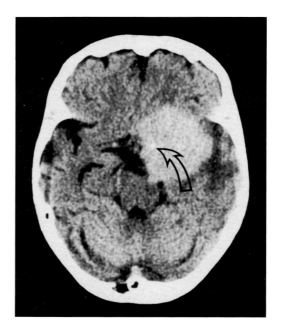

Meningiomas are typically homogeneous, high-attenuation lesions, due to their dense cellularity, fibrous tissue, and/or "psammomatous" calcification. High-resolution scans may show a concentric circular or radial pattern within the tumor, as in this case.

The margins of meningiomas are usually smooth and well defined. Even large tumors may cause relatively little edema and mass effect. This quiescent appearance implies slow growth, with gradual invagination into adjacent parenchyma.

In this case, the tumor is projecting inferiorly to cross beneath the free margin of the falx, as seen in the coronal plane in Case 49.

Meningiomas account for 15% to 20% of intracranial tumors, with the peak age incidence at 45 years and a moderate predominance in women.

The margins of meningiomas are usually well defined, although they may be somewhat lobulated as in this case. Uniform high attenuation throughout the mass is strongly suggestive of the diagnosis, as is the location adjacent to a dural surface.

Occasional meningiomas are low attenuation lesions. Low density values should not exclude this diagnosis if other features (e.g., tissue uniformity, extraaxial location) are suggestive. Prominent contrast enhancement usually clarifies ambiguous cases.

Reactive edema is present in the left temporal lobe correlating with the patient's symptoms. A small amount of edema is also seen within the deformed brain stem.

The small calcification *(arrow)* within the medial portion of tumor represents the atherosclerotic supraclinoid internal carotid artery. Meningiomas frequently surround or "encase" adjacent vessels, and consequent arterial narrowing may be another cause of tumor-related symptoms (see Case 60).

MENINGIOMAS: INTENSE, UNIFORM CONTRAST ENHANCEMENT

Case 29

84-year-old woman (same patient as in Case 28).

Sphenoid Wing Meningioma.

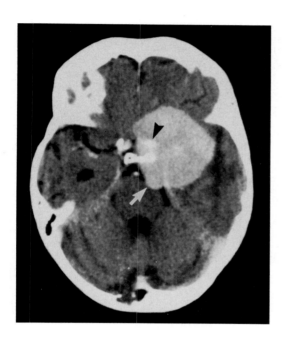

Case 30

61-year-old man.

Bilateral Frontal Convexity Meningiomas.

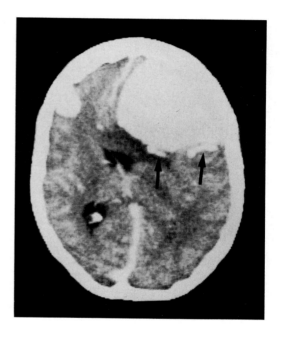

Uniform, intense contrast enhancement is characteristic of meningiomas. The diagnosis of these tumors is based on the combination of homogeneously high precontrast density, uniform contrast enhancement, well-defined margins, and typical location.

Other lesions may have similar precontrast and postcontrast features, including aneurysms, pituitary adenomas, germinomas, medulloblastomas, CNS lymphomas, acoustic schwannomas, and occasionally craniopharyngiomas and colloid cysts.

In this case, the enhancing left supraclinoid internal carotid artery is surrounded by tumor *(black arrow)*. A component of the mass crosses the tentorial margin to deform the brain stem *(white arrow; compare to Cases 50 and 51)*.

Homogeneous contrast enhancement typifies meningiomas of all sizes, as demonstrated here.

The tubular enhancing structures along the posterior margin of the larger meningioma in this case represent draining veins. Prominent vessels are occasionally seen surrounding or within large meningiomas. On spin echo MR scans, such vessels are seen as "flow voids" and may mimic an angiomatous primary tumor (see Cases 33 and 34).

In this patient, the gradual enlargement of the meningioma has caused bowing of the anterior falx. Despite the tumor's slow rate of growth, the ability of the brain to accommodate the enlarging mass has been exceeded. Substantial midline shift is present with deformity and edema of the genu of the corpus callosum.

MR CORRELATION: HOMOGENEOUS SIGNAL INTENSITY AND CONTRAST ENHANCEMENT OF MENINGIOMAS

Case 31

80-year-old man.
(sagittal, noncontrast scan; SE 600/17)

Case 32

44-year-old woman.
(sagittal, postcontrast scan; SE 700/15)

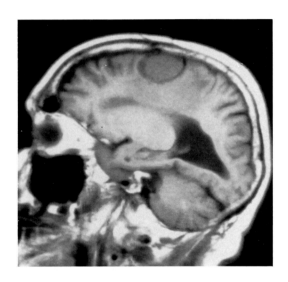

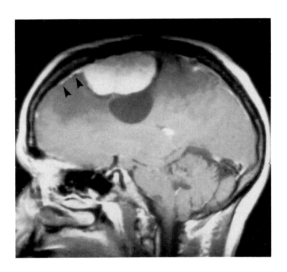

Meningiomas typically demonstrate homogeneous signal intensity on MR scans corresponding to their uniform attenuation values on CT studies. (CT homogeneity is not always correlated with uniform signal intensity on MR; see Case 211.)

These tumors are usually isointense or slightly lower in signal intensity than surrounding brain on T1-weighted images. In this case, the mildly hypointense convexity meningioma is further demarcated from cerebral parenchyma by a thin rim of lower intensity. Many meningiomas demonstrate this "pseudo-capsule," which likely includes components of displaced subarachnoid space and superficial vessels as well as the tumor margin itself.

Inhomogeneity within meningioma tissue on MR scans may be seen secondary to hemorrhage (short T1, variable T2), fat (short T1 and T2), cysts (long T1 and T2), or dense calcification (low signal intensity on all pulse sequences).

Contrast enhancement in meningiomas on MR scans is usually intense and uniform, as expected from CT experience.

A thin layer of dural enhancement extending away from the base of a meningioma is a common MR feature, as seen here (arrows). In some cases such thickening correlates with either "en plaque" extension of tumor or the presence of meningiomatous islands surrounding the main lesion. In other cases dural enhancement near the base of a meningioma represents reactive thickening, without tumor involvement.

A large cyst is present deep to the enhancing tumor in this case. Cystic components may cause an atypical appearance of meningiomas on CT and MR scans (see Case 627).

Case 33

20-year-old man presenting with blurred vision.
(coronal, noncontrast scan; SE 3000/28)

Case 34

24-year-old man.
(coronal, noncontrast scan; SE 600/17)

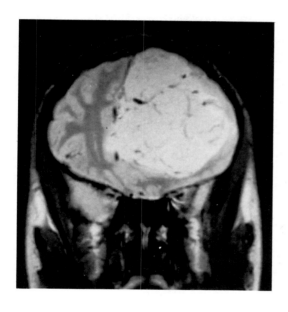

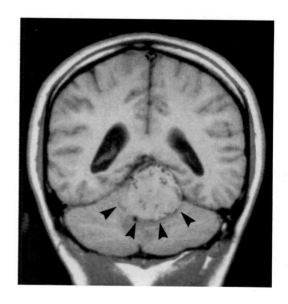

Large vessels surrounding or within a meningioma may be a prominent feature of the CT or MR presentation. Here tubular channels of low signal intensity representing "flow void" are seen throughout the mass, resembling the CT appearance of Case 30.

Meningiomas usually remain homogeneous on MR scans with long TR values. Signal intensity may range from low levels to very high values, as in this case.

The large size of this mass and the lack of surrounding edema attest to the slow growth of the tumor, which has been gradually accommodated by the adjacent brain.

The impressive vascularity of some meningiomas may cause diagnostic confusion on MR scans. In this case, the posterior fossa mass containing multiple vascular channels in a young adult could be assumed to represent a hemangioblastoma. The tumor proved to be a meningioma arising from the tentorium (compare to Case 53).

DIFFERENTIAL DIAGNOSIS:
HIGH-ATTENUATION, UNIFORMLY ENHANCING MASS ADJACENT TO THE FALX

Case 35

60-year-old man.

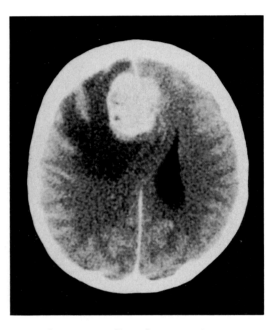

Melanoma (Believed to Be Primary).

Case 36

61-year-old man.
(coronal scan)

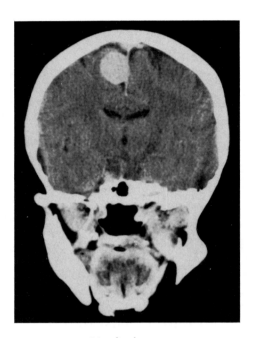

Meningioma.

Metastases may mimic meningiomas because of the shared characteristics of superficial location, well-defined margins, and frequent edema. The correct diagnosis can usually be made by establishing a dural base for a meningioma, versus an intra-axial location for a metastasis. Coronal and sagittal MR scans may be valuable for this purpose.

However, some metastases arise from the dura (see Cases 18 and 19). Alternatively, growth of a superficial cerebral metastasis may secondarily invade the meninges. In either case, the CT appearance may closely resemble a meningioma, particularly if the mass demonstrates increased precontrast attenuation values.

Intracranial melanoma is commonly located near the cerebral surface. Meningeal carcinomatosis or metastatic deposits within the dura are frequent. The precontrast attenuation values of melanomas are often increased due to hemorrhage and/or dense cellularity. The combination of these CT features may mimic meningiomas, as in Case 35. Clues to the correct diagnosis include the lobulated contour of the mass, small cystic or necrotic zones within the lesion, extensive edema, and rapid growth on sequential studies. (However, all of these characteristics can occasionally be seen in meningiomas as well; see Case 45.)

Compare these scans to Cases 84 and 85.

DIFFERENTIAL DIAGNOSIS:
WELL-DEFINED, UNIFORMLY ENHANCING EXTRA-AXIAL MASS AT THE SKULL BASE

Case 37

64-year-old woman.

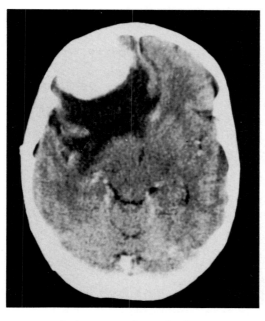

Inferior Frontal Meningioma.

Case 38

3-year-old boy.
(coronal scan)

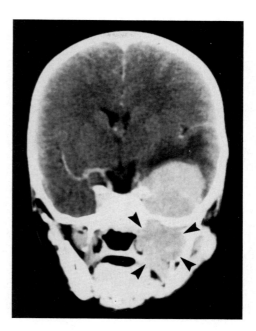

Parapharyngeal Rhabdomyosarcoma With Intracranial Extension.

Malignant neoplasms may present as homogeneous, well-defined extra-axial masses. Such epidural tumors can arise from dural-based metastases (see Cases 18 and 52) or represent direct invasion through the skull base, as in Case 38.

The parapharyngeal component of the rhabdomyosarcoma in Case 38 *(arrows)* is smaller than the intracranial portion of the lesion. Axial scans confined to the brain would demonstrate a middle fossa mass with surrounding edema closely resembling a meningioma.

The differential diagnosis of a transcranial mass near the skull base in a child should also include neuroblastoma and lymphoma. In adults, this occurrence is most commonly due to squamous cell or adenoid cystic carcinoma of the pharynx. Such lesions commonly traverse the skull base by growing along cranial nerves (e.g., through the foramen ovale) as well as by direct invasion of bone.

In Case 37, widespread frontal edema extends to the temporal lobe and is associated with subfalcial herniation (compare to Case 6).

SMALL MENINGIOMAS

Case 39

57-year-old man with decreasing visual acuity
in the left eye.

Case 40

66-year-old woman.
(wide window)

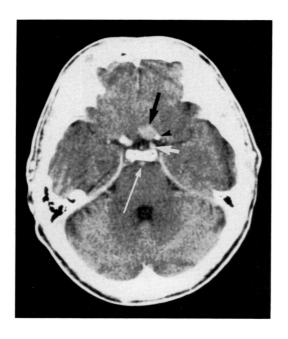

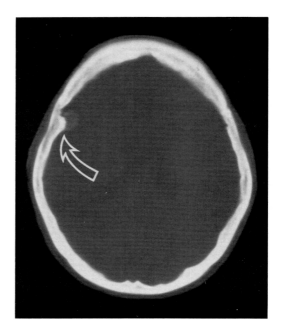

Because of their slow growth, many meningiomas cause no symptoms until the tumor is large. Small meningiomas in a critical location may present much earlier.

This patient's loss of vision is due to a 1 cm meningioma involving the cranial end of the optic canal (*black arrow; see also Case 41*). Adjacent landmarks include the tip of the anterior clinoid process *(black arrowhead)* and the posteriorly displaced supraclinoid internal carotid artery *(short white arrow)*.

The enhancing midline "dot" immediately anterior to the dorsum sella is the pituitary infundibulum. This structure is normally smaller in diameter than the basilar artery, seen posterior to the dorsum *(long white arrow)*.

Small meningiomas can be accompanied and identified by reactive bone changes. In this case, an asymptomatic calcified convexity meningioma is perched on a hyperostotic base (arrow), as is commonly seen in larger lesions (see Cases 56 and 57).

MENINGIOMAS: USE OF MR TO DEFINE ANATOMICAL RELATIONSHIPS

Case 41

57-year-old man with decreasing visual acuity
in the left eye (same patient as Case 39).
(sagittal, postcontrast scan; SE 600/20)

Small Tuberculum Meningioma.

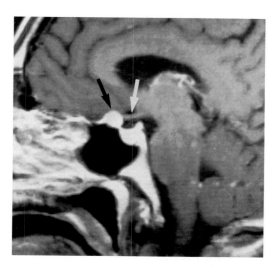

Case 42

31-year-old woman.
(sagittal, postcontrast scan; SE 600/20)

Posterior Convexity Meningioma.

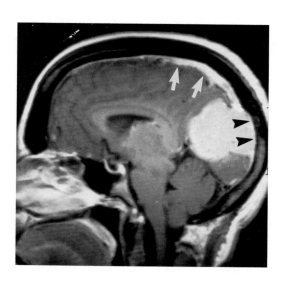

The multiplanar capabilities of MR can help to precisely localize meningiomas with respect to adjacent structures. In this case, a T1-weighted sagittal scan slightly to the left of midline shows a small, enhancing meningioma of the tuberculum sella (black arrow) positioned directly in the course of the left optic nerve (white arrow).

In this case axial CT scans had suggested a tentorial origin for the large meningioma. Coronal and sagittal MR scans corrected this impression by demonstrating a broad tumor base against the occipital inner table (black arrowheads).

Contrast enhancement extending anteriorly from the mass (white arrows) represents stasis in the superior sagittal sinus, which is compressed and/or invaded by the meningioma (see Case 61).

"Waves" or "ripples" of compressed gray and white matter are seen in the cerebral hemisphere anterior to the tumor. Identification of a band of displaced cortex between a superficial mass and distorted white matter establishes the lesion as extra-axial.

ATYPICAL MENINGIOMAS

Case 43

58-year-old man with hemiparesis.

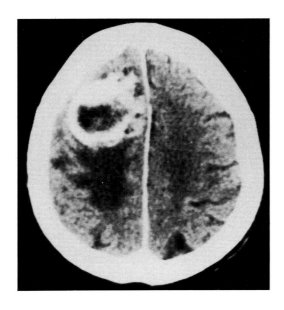

Case 44

44-year-old man.

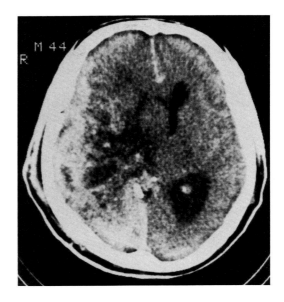

Because the typical appearance of meningiomas is one of the most reliable "stereotypes" on CT, atypical appearances can be confusing. A small number of meningiomas contain or are associated with low-attenuation, nonenhancing areas. These may be due to necrosis, old hemorrhage, cyst formation, or fat within the meningioma tissue, or reflect loculation of adjacent CSF.

The diagnosis is not obscured if these atypical regions are small in proportion to the tumor size. If atypical regions predominate, the possibility of other pathologies (e.g., glioma or metastasis) must be considered.

In this case, the thick rim, central low attenuation, irregular margins, and prominent edema mimic a malignant glioma or metastasis (compare with Cases 5, 6, 70, and 71). Coronal scans may contribute to the diagnosis of such lesions by demonstrating that the mass arises from a dural base. However, superficial gliomas may invade the dura, and dural-based metastases are not uncommon (see Cases 18, 35, 52, and 84).

Occasional meningiomas demonstrate aggressive behavior. Sarcomatous transformation may occur in originally benign lesions, and some histologic varieties (e.g., papillary and "angioblastic" meningiomas) are themselves associated with a tendency toward malignant features.

The tumor in this case was recurrent. It had spread over much of the hemisphere and was found to have invaded deeply into cerebral parenchyma at numerous sites. Pathological examination suggested meningeal sarcoma. (See also Cases 45 and 85).

RAPID GROWTH OF MENINGIOMAS

Case 45A

8-year-old boy, treated for medulloblastoma 4 years earlier with whole-brain radiation (4600R) and chemotherapy (prednisone, vincristine, and CCNU).

Case 45B

Same patient, scanned 10 months later due to rapidly progressive hemiparesis.

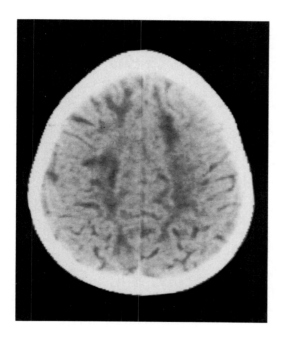

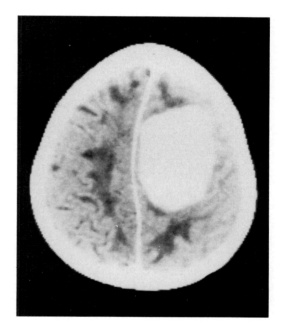

This noncontrast scan was performed to follow white matter changes that had been previously noted. Several regions of abnormal low attenuation are present in the centrum semiovale bilaterally, suggesting disseminated necrotizing leukoencephalopathy (see Case 320). There was no evidence of a mass near the vertex at any level of this study.

A postcontrast scan at the same level as Case 45A now demonstrates a large, uniformly enhancing mass. At surgery, a meningioma over 6 cm in diameter was removed, with meningotheliomatous histology.

Occasional meningiomas demonstrate rapid growth. The tumor in this case likely represents radiation-induced meningioma, a setting in which aggressive tumor behavior is common. Such masses may be multiple and tend to recur after surgery.

Rapid tumor growth of a meningioma developing years after radiation therapy may be mistaken for recurrence of the original CNS neoplasm. The latency period between radiation and the diagnosis of meningioma is often longer than in this case (up to 20 years).

Apparently "routine" meningiomas (with no history of preceding cranial radiation) may also enlarge with surprising speed. In such cases the alternative diagnosis of dural-based metastases (see Cases 19, 35, and 52) must be considered.

Case 46

70-year-old man.

Case 47

75-year-old man being evaluated for dementia.

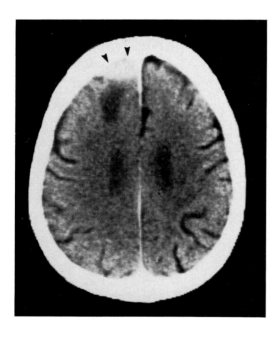

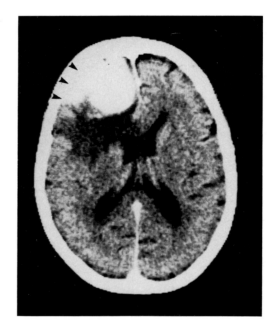

Some meningiomas spread along the inner table as relatively flat sheets of tissue. This "en plaque" morphology may be seen alone or in association with spherical components. The superficial location, homogeneous density, and intense contrast enhancement of the tumor remain characteristic.

This large frontal meningioma has a "comma" shape due to the combination of superficial and plaque-like components. (Compare this configuration with the comma-shaped masses growing around dural margins in Cases 48 and 49.)

Such morphology has been associated with aggressive tumor behavior, a possibility supported here by the extensive reactive edema. (Another CT feature correlated with aggressive meningiomas is abnormal deep venous drainage from the tumor region, suggesting cerebral invasion.)

Ten percent to 20% of patients with dementia are found to have treatable causes for their symptoms. Intracranial masses account for about one fourth of such cases (see Cases 3 and 67 for other examples).

Case 48

52-year-old woman.

Case 49

72-year-old man (same patient as Case 27).
(coronal scan)

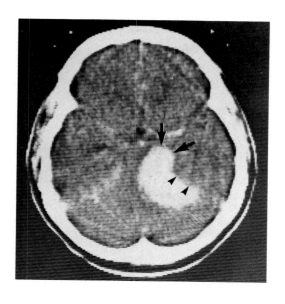

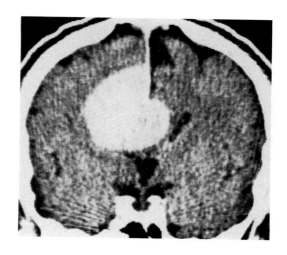

Posterior fossa meningiomas arising from the petrous bone or inferior surface of the tentorium may extend to the incisura. Further growth of the tumor may pass through the tentorial hiatus to accumulate in a parasellar location. While the infratentorial component of the mass retains a straight lateral margin confined by the petrous ridge and tentorium, the middle fossa component is free to assume a spherical shape. The combination of the semilunar and circular components resembles a fat comma.

The lateral tentorial margin similarly shapes the morphology of other adjacent lesions (see Cases 295, 296, 348, 349, 423, 424, 454, and 455).

Falx meningiomas may also develop a "comma" shape. A tumor arising along one side of the falx may grow inferiorly to reach the free margin. The mass may then depress the corpus callosum to cross the midline beneath the falx, as seen in this case. Again, the combination of a semilunar component bounded by a dural surface and a spherical component growing beyond the dural margin produces a "comma" shape.

Coronal CT or MR scans are often useful in the evaluation of falx meningiomas. They may demonstrate (1) the extent of bilateral involvement; (2) the morphology of dependent or exophytic components, as in this case; and (3) possible invasion or compression of the superior sagittal sinus (see Case 61).

Case 50

68-year-old man.

Case 51

49-year-old man with a 4-year history of right facial pain.

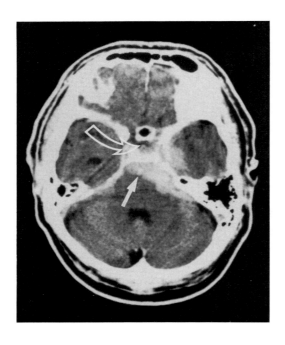

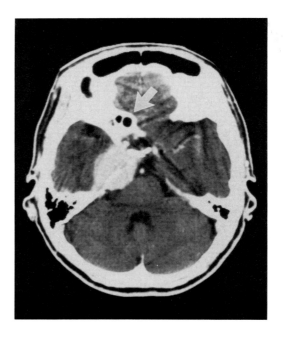

Meningiomas commonly extend across the tentorial hiatus from origins in either the parasellar region or the cerebellopontine angle. The morphology of transtentorial meningiomas may be plaque-like or lobular. The posterior fossa components of such tumors may occupy the prepontine or cerebellopontine angle cisterns, or both as in this case. The middle fossa components of transtentorial meningiomas commonly involve the cavernous sinus and may grow further laterally to displace the temporal lobe.

Here the thick plaque of tumor in the posterior fossa has largely surrounded the basilar artery (solid arrow). A suprasellar component displaces the pituitary infundibulum (open arrow).

The somewhat irregular interface of this mass with adjacent parenchyma resembles Cases 44 and 85, raising the question of aggressive behavior. The differential diagnosis of an irregular, enhancing, extra-axial mass spanning the petrous apex in an adult also includes metastasis and lymphoma.

Some meningiomas are "transtentorial" by virtue of tentorial origin or invasion. Such tumors may extend along the superior and/or inferior surface of the tentorium and are not confined by the tentorial hiatus.

In this case the meningioma has permeated the right side of the tentorium, with well-defined hemispherical components in the posterior fossa and middle fossa. An anterior lobulation of the mass (not shown) extended to the planum sphenoidale, where hyperostosis and "blistering" of the roof of the sphenoid sinus are seen (arrow; see Case 56).

Transtentorial masses are an important cause of facial pain. (Trigeminal neuralgia and atypical facial pain are more commonly due to vascular compression of the fifth cranial nerve; see discussion of Cases 581 and 582.) Other benign lesions that can span the petrous apex with a bilobed configuration are epidermoid cysts (see Cases 236 and 241) and trigeminal schwannomas (see Case 242).

Trigeminal schwannomas may closely mimic the appearance of parasellar or transtentorial meningiomas. The contrast enhancement pattern of large trigeminal schwannomas is often more patchy or inhomogeneous than that of meningiomas, resembling the typical tumor stain at angiography.

DIFFERENTIAL DIAGNOSIS:
DURAL-BASED INTENSELY ENHANCING, EXTRA-AXIAL MASS

Case 52

75-year-old woman presenting with
homonymous hemianopia.
(coronal scan)

Case 53

83-year-old man presenting with syncope.
(coronal scan)

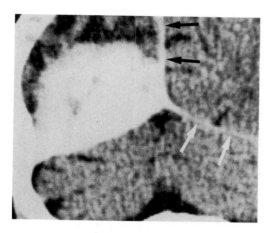

Metastatic Carcinoma of the Breast.

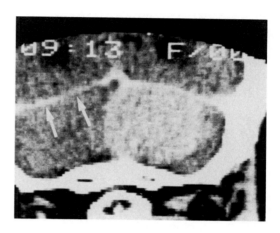

Tentorial Meningioma.

As discussed in Chapter 1, metastases to the skull or dura may produce focal extra-axial masses. Such lesions may closely resemble meningiomas in location, definition, and contrast enhancement. The two types of epidural masses may also be indistinguishable at angiography, with similar dural arterial supply and tumor stains.

The most common tumor to mimic meningioma in this manner is metastatic prostate carcinoma, particularly along the sphenoid wing (see Cases 25, 212, and 552). Melanoma, breast carcinoma, and renal carcinoma can cause similar appearances. Superficial gliomas may invade the dura and occasionally mimic meningioma in other respects as well (see Case 84). Intracranial lymphoma is often dural based (see Case 213) and should be included in the differential diagnosis of "meningioma-like" lesions.

Coronal CT or MR scans are helpful in defining the relationship of lesions to the sloping tentorium *(white arrows)* and posterior falx *(black arrows)*. Tentorial meningiomas may thicken the tentorium (see Case 298) and/or project from its inferior or superior surface. A thickened tentorium may also be seen in cases of meningeal carcinomatosis, chronic basal meningitis, or vascular engorgement (see Cases 297 to 300).

Case 54

79-year-old woman.
(high window level)

Sphenoid Wing Meningioma.

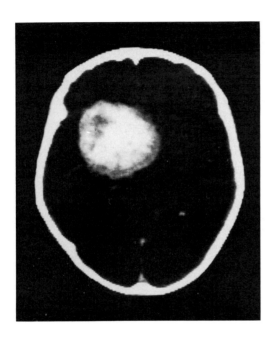

Some meningiomas contain large amounts of dense calcium. Calcification may occupy a portion of the tumor or fill the entire mass, as in this case. Circular and radial components can be seen. (See Case 40 for an example of a small calcified meningioma.)

Case 55

63-year-old woman.
(wide window width, high window level)

"En plaque" Convexity Meningioma.

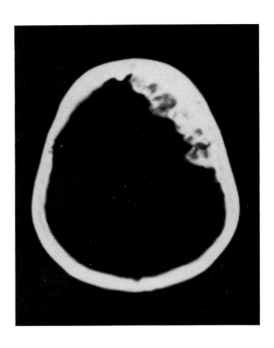

"En plaque" meningiomas may provoke intense calvarial hyperostosis, particularly along the skull base. In such cases it is difficult to judge whether the layer of exuberant calcification is within the tumor or represents hyperostosis of the inner table. Often both components are present.

MENINGIOMAS: ASSOCIATED HYPEROSTOSIS

Case 56

71-year-old woman.
(coronal scan, wide window)

Case 57

75-year-old woman with proptosis.
(wide window)

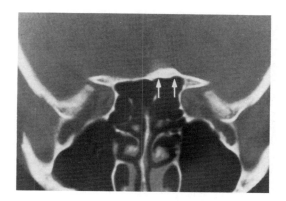

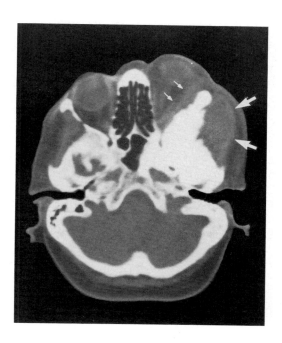

Hyperostosis is frequently seen at the base of meningiomas. This sclerosis may accompany calvarial invasion or be an independent reaction to adjacent tumor.

In this case, the planum sphenoidale is focally thickened *(arrows)* at the attachment of the mass. In addition, tumor-induced remodeling of bone has caused expansion of the sinus toward the meningioma. This "blistering" of the sinus roof is a hallmark of meningiomas arising from the planum sphenoidale or tuberculum sella. (Case 51 illustrates the appearance of "blistering" in the axial plane.)

See Case 40 for another example of localized hyperostosis at the base of a meningioma.

The left sphenoid bone is very dense and greatly thickened due to a meningioma permeating the sphenoid wing (intraosseous meningioma). Sphenoid involvement by sclerosing meningioma may have both orbital and cerebral consequences. This scan demonstrates proptosis primarily resulting from bone deformity. Tumor tissue is seen in the lateral aspect of the orbit *(small arrows)* and extracranially in the infratemporal fossa *(large arrows)*.

The major differential diagnosis for this CT appearance would be fibrous dysplasia of bone, which usually presents in the first decades of life.

DIFFERENTIAL DIAGNOSIS:
DENSELY CALCIFIED MASS ADJACENT TO THE INNER TABLE

Case 58

65-year-old man.

Case 59

58-year-old woman.

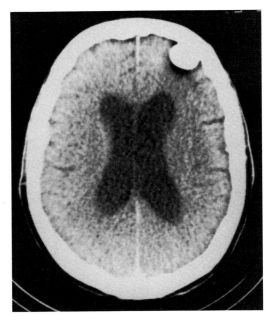

Osteoma.

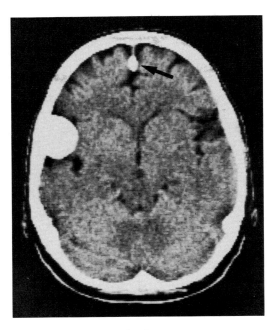

Meningioma.

Densely calcified meningiomas adjacent to the inner table may resemble osteomas. Osteomas are benign bone tumors that may arise from either the inner or outer table of the skull. They typically consist of homogeneous, dense bone with a smooth, hemispherical shape based against the table of origin.

Skull x-rays or routine tomograms may be useful in distinguishing the characteristic "ivory" density of an osteoma from the less uniform calcification of a dense meningioma. Examination of CT scans at wide window widths and high window levels may provide similar differentiation.

In many cases, the two lesions are indistinguishable. Both meningiomas and osteomas may be separated from the adjacent inner table by a thin line of relative lucency.

The small area of calcification associated with the anterior falx in Case 59 (arrow) likely represents dural ossification, which commonly occurs at this site. Such ossified dural plaques often contain central zones of T1-shortening due to lipid material, which can falsely mimic hemorrhage of an enhancing dural lesion on postcontrast MR scans.

MR DEMONSTRATION OF VASCULAR INVOLVEMENT BY MENINGIOMAS

Case 60

70-year-old woman.
(axial, noncontrast scan; SE 2500/28)

Sphenoid Wing Meningioma.

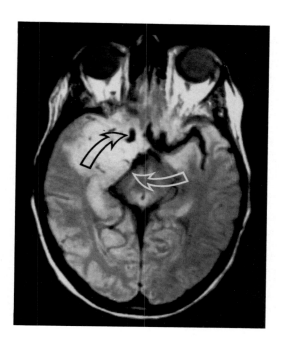

Case 61

57-year-old woman.
(coronal, noncontrast scan; SE 2500/30)

Falx Meningioma.

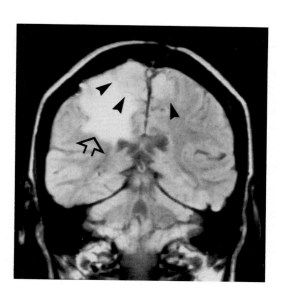

The characteristic absence of signal or "flow void" within cerebral arteries on spin-echo MR sequences helps to define the status of vessels adjacent to tumors. In this case, the relatively isointense parasellar meningioma is seen to surround the supraclinoid internal carotid artery *(black arrow)*. The mass is crossing the tentorial margin to flatten the right side of the midbrain *(white arrow;* compare this scan to the CT appearance of a similar lesion in Case 29).

Encasement of the cavernous segment of the internal carotid artery can be well demonstrated by coronal MR scans, and was also present in this case.

As discussed in prior cases, the coronal plane is useful for evaluating lesions involving the falx or tentorium. Here the relatively isointense signal of meningioma tissue is seen on both sides of the falx *(arrowheads)*. In addition, the expected "flow-void" within the lumen of the superior sagittal sinus has been replaced by tissue with signal intensity matching the adjacent meningioma. This demonstration of tumor invasion and occlusion of a dural sinus can be confirmed by angiographic MR techniques.

The meningioma has triggered marked edema on one side of the falx *(open arrow),* with no edema contralaterally. The mechanisms by which meningiomas incite reactive edema are unclear. Relevant factors probably include the thickness of cortex separating the tumor from underlying white matter and the presence or absence of venous compression. Edema is often a major cause of mass effect and symptomatology.

REFERENCES: CT

1. Alvarez F., Roda J.M., Romero M.P., et al.: Malignant and atypical meningiomas: A reappraisal of clinical, histological, and computed tomographic features. *Neurosurgery* 20:688–694, 1987.
2. Amundsen P., Dugstad G., Syvertsen A.H.: The reliability of computer tomography for the diagnosis and differential diagnosis of meningiomas, gliomas, and brain metastases. *Acta Neurochir. (Wien)* 41:177–190, 1978.
3. Becker D., Norman D., Wilson C.B.: Computerized tomography and pathological correlation in cystic meningiomas. *J. Neurosurg.* 50:103–105, 1979.
4. Claveria L.E., Sutton D., Tress B.M.: The radiological diagnosis of meningiomas: The impact of EMI scanning. *Br. J. Radiol.* 50:15–22, 1977.
5. Dell S., Ganti R., Steinberger A., et al.: Cystic meningiomas: A clinicoradiological study. *J. Neurosurg.* 57:8–13, 1982.
6. Dietemann J.L., Heldt N., Burguet J.L., et al: CT findings in malignant meningiomas. *Neuroradiology* 23:207–209, 1982.
7. Fine M., Brazis P., Palacios E.: Computed tomography of sphenoid wing meningiomas: Tumor location related to distal edema. *Surg. Neurol.* 13:385–397, 1980.
8. Fornari M., Savoiaro M., Morello G., et al.: Meningiomas of the lateral ventricles. *J. Neurosurg.* 54:64–74, 1981.
9. Go D.G., Wilmink J.T., Molenaar W.M.: Peritumoral brain edema associated with meningiomas. *Neurosurgery* 23:175–179, 1988.
10. Helseth A., Helseth E., Unsgaard G.: Primary meningeal melanoma. *Acta Oncol.* 28:103, 1989.
11. Kadis G.N., Mount L.A., Ganti S.R.: The importance of early diagnosis and treatment of meningiomas of the planum sphenoidale and tuberculum sellae: A retrospective study of 105 cases. *Surg. Neurol.* 12:367–371, 1979.
12. Kendall B.E., Pullicino P.: Comparison of consistency of meningiomas and computed tomography appearances. *Neuroradiology* 18:173–176, 1979.
13. Kim K.S., Rogers L.F., Goldblatt D.: CT features of hyperostosing meningioma en plaque. *A.J.N.R.* 8:853–860, 1987.
14. Lippman S.C., Buzaid A.C., Iacono R.P., et al.: Cranial metastases from prostate carcinoma simulating meningioma: Report of two cases and review of the literature. *Neurosurgery* 19:820–23, 1986.
15. Nahser H.C., Grote W., Lohr E., et al.: Multiple meningiomas: Clinical and computed tomographic observations. *Neuroradiology* 21:259–263, 1981.
16. New P.F., Aronow S., Hesselink J.: National Cancer Institute study: Evaluation of computed tomography in the diagnosis of intracranial Neoplasms. IV. Meningiomas. *Radiology* 136:665–675, 1980.
17. New P.F., Hesselink J.R., O'Carroll C.P., et al.: Malignant meningiomas: CT and histologic criteria, including a new CT sign. *A.J.N.R.* 3:267–276, 1982.
18. Parisi G., Tropea R., Giuffrida S., et al.: Cystic meningiomas: Report of seven cases. *J. Neurosurg.* 64:35–38, 1986.
19. Ramos F. Jr., Ba Zeze V., Velut S., et al.: Cystic meningiomas: Practical value of a radiosurgical classification. *J. Neuroradiol.* 14:271, 1987.
20. Rozario R., Adelman L., Prager R.J., et al.: Meningiomas of pineal region and third ventricle. *Neurosurgery* 5:489–495, 1979.
21. Russell E.J., George A.E., Kricheff I.I., et al.: Atypical computed tomographic features of intracranial meningiomas. *Radiology* 135:673–682, 1980.
22. Shapir J., Coblentz C., Melanson D., et al.: New CT finding in aggressive meningioma. *A.J.N.R.* 6:101–102, 1985.
23. Smith H.P., Challa V.R., Moody D.M., et al: Biological features of meningiomas that determine the production of cerebral edema. *Neurosurgery* 8:428–433, 1981.
24. Som P.M., Sacher M., Strenger S.W., et al.: "Benign" metastasizing meningiomas. *A.J.N.R.* 8:127–130, 1987.
25. Stevens J.M., Ruiz J.S., Kendall B.E.: Observations on peritumoural oedema in meningioma. II. Mechanisms of edema production. *Neuroradiology* 25:125–131, 1983.
26. Trittmacher S., Traupe H., Schmid A.: Pre- and postoperative changes in brain tissue surrounding a meningioma. *Neurosurgery* 22:882–885, 1988.
27. Valavanis A., Schubiger D., Hayek J., et al.: CT of meningiomas on the posterior surface of the petrous bone. *Neuroradiology* 22:111–121, 1981.
28. Vassilouthis J., Ambrose J.: Computerized tomography scanning appearances of intracranial meningiomas: An attempt to predict the histological features. *J. Neurosurg.* 50:320–327, 1979.
29. Zagzag G., Gomori J.N., Rappaport Z.H., Shalit, M.N.: Cystic meningioma presenting as a ring lesion. *A.J.N.R.* 7:911–912, 1986.

REFERENCES: MR

1. Aoki S., Barkovich A.J., Nishimura K., et al.: Neurofibromatosis types 1 and 2: Cranial MR findings. *Radiology* 172:527–534, 1989.
2. Breger R.K., Papke R.A., Pojunas K.W., et al.: Benign extra-axial tumors: Contrast enhancement with Gd-DTPA. *Radiology* 163:427–430, 1987.
3. Bydder G.M., Kingsley D.P.E., Brown J., et al.: MR imaging of meningiomas including studies with and without gadolinium-DTPA. *J. Comput. Assist. Tomogr.* 9:690–697, 1985.
4. Curnes J.T.: MR imaging of peripheral intracranial neoplasms: Extra-axial versus intra-axial masses. *J. Comput. Assist. Tomogr.* 11:932–937, 1987.
5. Elster A.D., Challa V.R., Gilbert T.H., et al.: Meningiomas: MR and histopathologic features. *Radiology* 170:857–862, 1989.
6. Haughton V.M., Rimm A.A., Czervionke L.F., et al: Sensitivity of Gd-DTPA-enhanced MR imaging of benign extra-axial tumors. *Radiology* 166:829–834, 1988.
7. Perry R.D., Parker G.D., Hallinan J.H.: CT and MR imaging of fourth ventricular meningiomas. *J. Comput. Assist. Tomogr.* 14:276–280, 1990.
8. Salibi S.S., Nauta H.J.W., Brem H., et al.: Lipomeningioma: report of three cases and review of the literature. *Neurosurgery* 25:122–25, 1989.
9. Spagnoli M.V., Goldberg H.I., Grossman R.I.: Intracranial meningiomas: high-field MR imaging. *Radiology* 161:369–376, 1986.
10. Terasaki K.K., Zee C.-S.: Evolution of central necrosis in a meningioma: CT and MR features. *J. Comput. Assist. Tomogr.* 14:464–466, 1990.
11. Tokumaro A., O'uchi T., Eguchi T., et al.: Prominent meningeal enhancement adjacent to meningioma on Gd-DTPA-enhanced MR images: Histopathologic correlation. *Radiology* 175:431–434, 1990.
12. Wagle V.G., Villemure J.G., Melanson D., et al.: Diagnostic potential of magnetic resonance in cases of foramen magnum meningiomas. *Neurosurgery* 21:622–626, 1987.
13. Wilms G., Lammens M., Marchal G., et al.: Thickening of dura surrounding meningiomas: MR features. *J. Comput. Assist. Tomogr.* 13:763–768, 1989.
14. Zimmerman R.D., Fleming C.A., Saint-Louis L.A., et al.: Magnetic resonance imaging of meningiomas. *A.J.N.R.* 6:149–158, 1985.

CHAPTER 3

Gliomas

LOW-GRADE GLIOMAS: DEEP LOCATION, LOW ATTENUATION, INDISTINCT MARGINS, AND MINIMAL ENHANCEMENT

Case 62	Case 63
18-year-old man presenting with seizures.	34-year-old woman presenting with headaches.

| **Grade 2 Astrocytoma.** | **Grade 2 Astrocytoma.** |

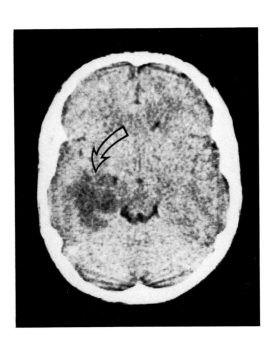 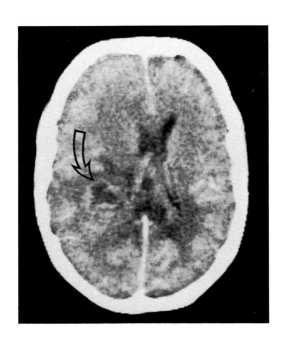

Low-grade gliomas are usually seen as poorly defined areas of low attenuation. Mass effect is variable and contrast enhancement is rarely impressive. The deep temporal lobe is a common location for these lesions in young adults, and the history of seizures is typical for such patients.

Many low-grade gliomas are found in the perisylvian region, where they may mimic recent infarction in the distribution of the middle cerebral artery (see Case 403). The sparing of cortex, indistinct margins, and clinical context of a glioma usually allow distinction from ischemic lesions.

Temporal lobe gliomas may also resemble the appearance of herpes encephalitis (compare this scan to Case 270).

The tumor is seen as a vague area of low attenuation deep within the right cerebral hemisphere. This frequent deep hemisphere location of glial tumors contrasts with the metastases and meningiomas illustrated in Chapters 1 and 2.

Minimal contrast enhancement is seen in this lesion. The more superficial enhancement represents normal vessels within cerebral sulci.

LOW-GRADE GLIOMAS: SUPERFICIAL LOCATION AND WELL-DEFINED MARGINS

Case 64

4-year-old girl with seizures.
(postcontrast scan)

Low-Grade Astrocytoma.

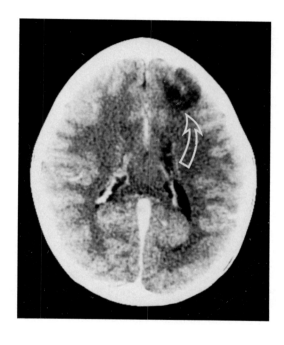

Case 65

25-year-old woman with seizures.
(postcontrast scan)

Low-Grade Astrocytoma.

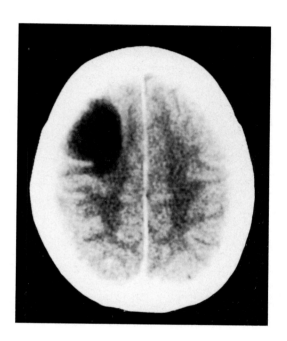

Some low-grade gliomas occur more superficially and demonstrate better definition than the typical lesions illustrated on the previous page. The slow growth of such tumors may cause erosion of the adjacent inner table, as was better demonstrated at bone windows in this case. This feature combines with the absence of contrast enhancement to suggest a long-standing, low-grade lesion.

The low attenuation of a superficial glioma can mimic cerebral infarction, especially when tumor margins are sharply defined as in this case (compare to Case 405). Clues to the correct diagnosis include rounded rather than linear borders of the lesion, relative sparing of the cortical ribbon (best assessed at wide CT windows or by MR), and the absence of an acute clinical event. MR scans often demonstrate a characteristic gyriform morphology within subacute infarctions, which can resolve ambiguous CT appearances (see Cases 400 and 401).

LOW-GRADE GLIOMAS: CALCIFICATION

Case 66

38-year-old man presenting with a first seizure.

Oligodendroglioma.

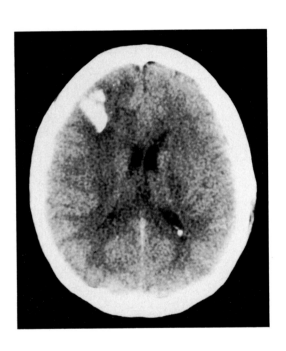

Case 67

39-year-old woman presenting with dementia.

Low-Grade Astrocytoma.

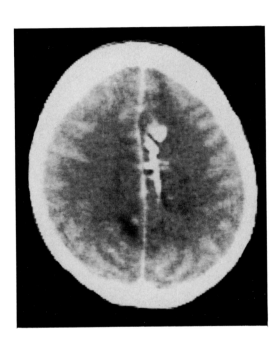

About 10% to 20% of low-grade gliomas contain calcification. Oligodendrogliomas are more frequently calcified than any other glial tumors, with a large majority demonstrating this finding. The frontal lobe location in a young adult as seen here is also characteristic of these tumors.

The CT pattern of tumor calcification is variable and nonspecific. A large "rock"-like calcification could also be seen as the residual of old injury or inflammation ("brain stone"). In this case the parenchyma adjacent to the calcification demonstrates mild low attenuation and mass effect, with slight compression of the frontal horn. These features indicate an active lesion and exclude an old insult (which would be associated with volume loss and lower attenuation values).

The onset of seizures in an adult is a worrisome event. Cerebral masses are detected in approximately 20% of such cases. Seizures are a particularly common symptom of low-grade neoplasms; up to 50% of oligodendrogliomas present in this manner.

The calcification in this glioma is predominantly linear, following the course of the cingulate gyrus superior to the corpus callosum. Vague low-attenuation areas are associated anteriorly and posteriorly.

Despite a lower incidence of calcification in astrocytomas than in oligodendrogliomas, the much greater incidence of the former makes astrocytoma the most common calcified glial tumor.

Low-grade gliomas should be considered in the differential diagnosis of most intracerebral calcifications (see Cases 91, 413, 466, and 501 for other examples). Calcification is less common in high-grade gliomas, except for those representing malignant transformation of low-grade tumors.

CT is highly sensitive to calcification within cerebral lesions, while spin-echo MR scans are not. Even calcifications as dense as these lesions on CT may be inapparent on spin-echo MR images. Gradient echo MR scans emphasizing susceptibility effects can improve the detection of parenchymal calcification.

MR CORRELATION: LOW-GRADE GLIOMAS

Case 68

26-year-old woman with a several-year
history of seizures.
(sagittal, noncontrast scan; SE 600/17)

Oligodendroglioma.

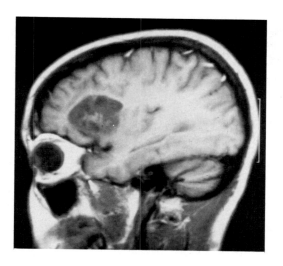

Case 69

28-year-old woman presenting with the
onset of seizures.
(coronal, noncontrast scan; SE 2500/90)

Astrocytoma.

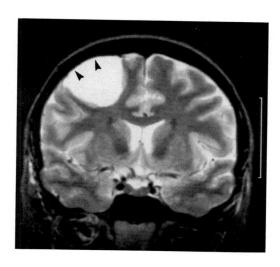

Low-grade gliomas are often better defined on MR scans than on CT studies. The lesions differ more from surrounding white matter in their magnetic relaxation behavior (the basis for contrast in MR) than they do in x-ray attenuation (the basis for contrast in CT). Margins of low-grade gliomas can be surprisingly distinct and smooth on MR examinations, as demonstrated in Cases 68 and 69 (see also Case 104).

Oligodendrogliomas frequently contain coarsely heterogeneous signal intensity, as seen here, while astrocytomas tend to demonstrate more homogeneous prolongation of T1. The mixed intensity of oligodendrogliomas likely reflects the frequent occurrence of calcification, cysts, and hemorrhage in these tumors.

The low-grade astrocytoma in this case is characterized by uniform prolongation of T2 resulting in high signal intensity. Both the presence of the lesion and the definition of its margins are more clearly apparent on MR than would be true on a CT study.

Clues to the long-standing, low grade nature of the tumor include the absence of surrounding edema, the minimal mass effect for the size of the lesion, and subtle erosion of the overlying calvarium (arrowheads).

Coronal MR scans provide excellent visualization of the cerebral convexity and temporal lobes with no degradation by bone artifact (see also Cases 104 and 105).

Case 70

51-year-old woman.

Glioblastoma Multiforme.

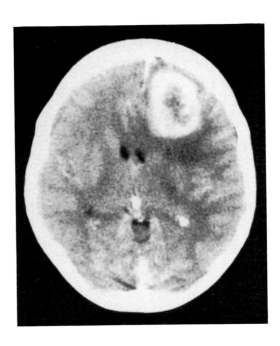

Most high-grade gliomas (Grade 3 or 4 astrocytoma, "ana-plastic astrocytoma," "glioblastoma multiforme," "malignant glioma") demonstrate definite contrast enhancement. The converse is usually true: extensive CT contrast enhancement in a glial tumor suggests a high-grade lesion.

The enhancement commonly consists of a thick, nodular rim surrounding a low-attenuation center of necrosis, cyst, or slowly equilibrating tissue. The central, nonenhancing regions of malignant gliomas vary widely in size and number.

Edema contributes to mass effect in this case, extending into the genu of the corpus callosum and exacerbating subfalcial herniation. It is not possible to separate edema from potential low-attenuation components of tumor. Pathological studies of malignant gliomas often demonstrate tumor cells within the low-attenuation zone of "edema," well beyond the margins of contrast enhancement.

Case 71

45-year-old man presenting with numbness and weakness of the left hand and face.

Glioblastoma Multiforme.

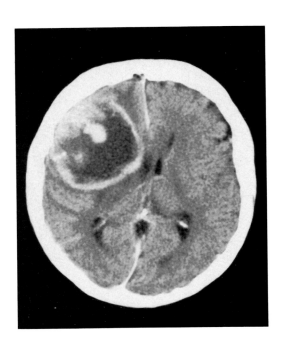

Malignant gliomas may enhance centrally as well as peripherally. The amount of central enhancement may be time dependent, with the low attenuation center of the tumor "filling in" on delayed scans.

Compare the predominantly peripheral enhancement of this glioblastoma with the metastases in Cases 5, 6, and 16. This tumor is transcerebral, extending from the cortical surface to the ventricular margin.

Cavitating gliomas may rupture into the ventricular system with dramatic clinical sequelae (improvement from reduced mass effect or deterioration due to ventricular irritation and obstruction).

Case 72

58-year-old woman presenting with a "stroke."

Glioblastoma Multiforme.

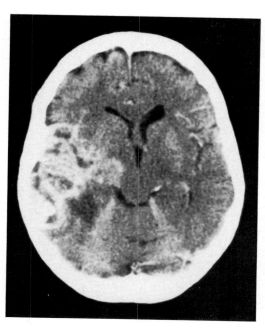

Case 73

65-year-old woman presenting with aphasia and hemiparesis.

Malignant Glioma.

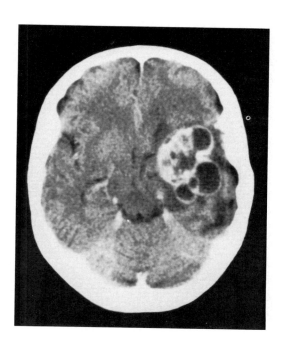

Contrast enhancement in malignant gliomas can be complex and confusing. When tubular or "gyriform" components predominate, as in this case, the appearance may resemble subacute infarction (see Cases 415 and 419) or arteriovenous malformation (see Case 490).

Here the correct diagnosis is suggested by the deep extension of abnormal enhancement, mass effect, and bridging of two major vascular territories (the middle and posterior cerebral artery distributions).

Tumors can present with stroke-like acuity due to hemorrhage, sudden increases in associated edema, obstructive hydrocephalus, or vascular compression.

A variation of the typical rim-enhancing morphology of high-grade gliomas is the occurrence of multiple clustered "rings," as in this case. The multinodular morphology suggests a multilocular cyst, and a complex inflammatory lesion (e.g., fungal abscess; see Cases 277 and 283) could be considered in the differential diagnosis.

Case 74

64-year-old woman with repeated "transient
ischemic attacks."
(postcontrast scan)

Glioblastoma Multiforme.

Case 75

48-year-old man presenting with seizures
and hemiparesis.
(postcontrast scan)

Anaplastic Astrocytoma.

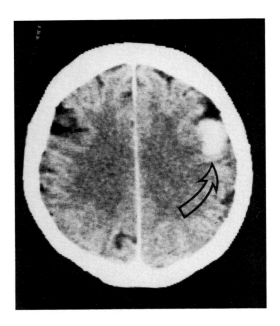

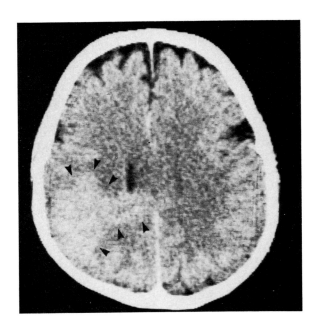

Occasional high-grade gliomas demonstrate homogeneous enhancement and superficial location. This uniformly enhancing lesion resembles a meningioma, but appears to be intra-axial. It had been initially confused with a small, subacute infarction (see Chapter 9). The persistent symptoms and CT enlargement warranted a biopsy, which disclosed a glioblastoma multiforme.

High-grade gliomas may be surprisingly inconspicuous with unusual tissue uniformity. In this case, an area of homogeneous, mildly increased attenuation values is seen in the right parietal lobe (arrowheads). The lesion extends medially to involve the splenium of the corpus callosum.

Case 76

62-year-old woman.
(axial, noncontrast scan; SE 3000/25)

Glioblastoma Multiforme.

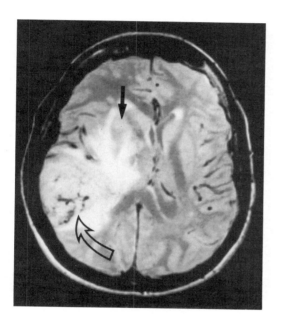

Case 77

6-year-old boy, post shunt for hydrocephalus.
(axial, noncontrast scan; SE 3000/90)

Grade 3 Thalamic Astrocytoma.

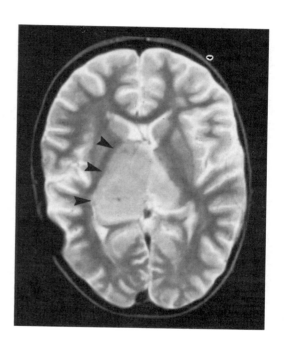

MR scans highlight the reactive edema associated with most malignant gliomas. In this case, high-signal edema deep to the tumor extends through the external and internal capsules, outlining the displaced lenticular nucleus *(solid arrow;* compare to the normal left hemisphere). The mass itself *(open arrow)* is less intense than the surrounding edema.

Large, irregular tumor vessels are seen as low-signal channels within the lesion. This prominent neovascularity suggests a high-grade neoplasm and correlates with the angiographic appearance of malignant gliomas. By contrast, the large vessels seen on MR scans around or within some meningiomas tend to be more regular (compare to Case 33).

The majority of malignant gliomas demonstrate prominent T2 prolongation causing high signal intensity on long TR images, usually associated with high-intensity edema. Occasional anaplastic astrocytomas and glioblastomas remain nearly isointense to normal gray matter and incite little edema.

The latter MR appearance often correlates with precontrast high attenuation on CT scans. Both features may reflect dense cellularity and/or a densely fibrous tumor matrix (compare to Cases 74 and 75). Other tumors that may have a similar appearance on MR scans include primary cerebral lymphoma and germinomas (see Case 230).

GLIOMAS OF THE CORPUS CALLOSUM: "BUTTERFLY" TUMORS

Case 78

74-year-old woman.

Glioblastoma Multiforme.

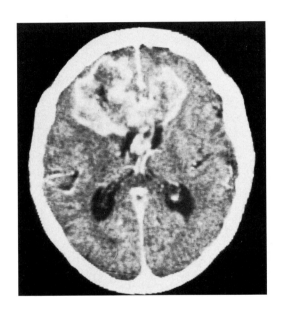

Case 79

50-year-old man presenting with bilateral leg weakness.

Malignant Glioma.

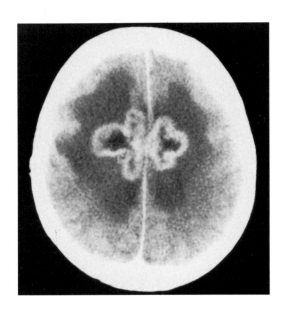

This tumor occupies the genu of the corpus callosum, extending through the minor forceps into both frontal lobes to assume a "butterfly" configuration. The genu of the corpus callosum is thickened, with deformity of the frontal horns and invasion of the septum pellucidum. Septum pellucidum involvement is often a clue to the glial origin of smaller tumors near the foramen of Monro (see Case 218).

Here a "butterfly" glioma extends symmetrically from the corpus callosum into the centrum semiovale of each cerebral hemisphere. Extensive edema is present bilaterally.

Paresis of the lower extremities had led to initial clinical suspicion of spinal cord dysfunction in this case. It is important to remember that parasagittal lesions near the cerebral vertex can also produce bilateral leg symptoms (through compression or invasion of the motor and sensory tracts from the medial portion of the precentral and postcentral gyri).

GLIOMAS OF THE CORPUS CALLOSUM: SOLID TUMORS

Case 80

58-year-old man.
(noncontrast scan)

Malignant Glioma.

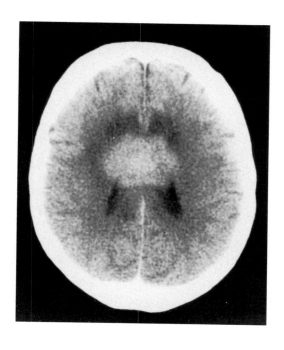

Case 81

60-year-old woman.
(postcontrast scan)

Glioblastoma Multiforme.

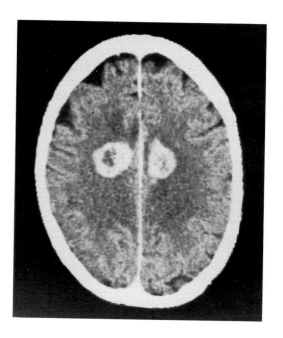

Gliomas of the corpus callosum may grow locally with little hemispheric extension. Here the mass occupies the midline, immediately superior to the lateral ventricles. This location places the lesion within the body of the corpus callosum, which forms the ventricular roof.

The homogeneous precontrast high attenuation seen here is occasionally found in high-grade glial tumors (compare to Cases 74 and 75). This appearance is a more common feature of other malignant neoplasms (e.g., primary CNS lymphoma, germinoma, and medulloblastoma), reflecting dense cellularity and/or a high nuclear-to-cytoplasmic ratio. CNS lymphoma frequently involves the corpus callosum and is a diagnostic consideration in this case.

Coronal CT or MR scans are useful to distinguish an intra-axial tumor of the corpus callosum from a possible meningioma of the falx (compare this scan to Case 27).

A section just above the body of the corpus callosum demonstrates "buds" of solid tumor following callosal radiations into the medial portions of both cerebral hemispheres. The appearance of separate masses on this scan reflects a "U-shaped" tumor with an interhemispheric bridge at the ventricular level.

Multicentric origin of gliomas does occur, but connecting strands of nonenhancing tumor frequently join such apparently discrete nodules. Coronal CT or MR would be helpful to confirm the relationship of these masses to the corpus callosum (see Case 49).

Cases 75 and 89 present examples of gliomas involving the splenium of the corpus callosum.

Case 82

40-year-old man.
(midsagittal, noncontrast scan; SE 600/16)

Astrocytoma within the Corpus Callosum.

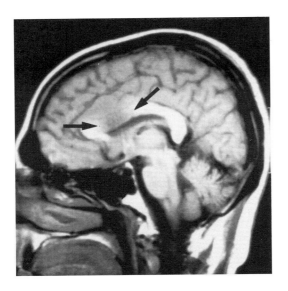

Case 83

26-year-old man presenting with seizures.
(midsagittal, noncontrast scan; SE 600/20)

Oligodendroglioma Deforming the Corpus Callosum.

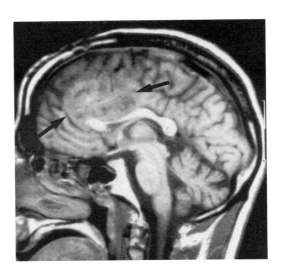

The sagittal display of midline anatomy makes MR valuable in the assessment of gliomas near the corpus callosum. In this case, expansion and abnormally low signal intensity within the anterior body of the corpus callosum (arrows) clearly demonstrate tumor invasion of the commissure itself, in contrast to Case 83.

This medial hemisphere tumor has expanded the cingulate gyrus with marked thinning and depression of the corpus callosum. An axial CT scan through the normal location of the genu and anterior body of the corpus callosum would suggest callosal involvement by tumor, as in Case 82. Coronal and sagittal MR studies can prevent such misdiagnosis by demonstrating anatomical distortions, as in this case.

The excellent visualization of the corpus callosum on sagittal MR scans is also useful in the evaluation of multiple sclerosis (see Case 316) and callosal agenesis (see Case 642).

DIFFERENTIAL DIAGNOSIS:
CEREBRAL MASS WITH DURAL ATTACHMENT

Case 84

66-year-old woman.

Case 85

75-year-old woman.

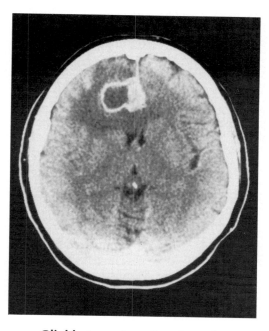

Glioblastoma Invading the Falx.

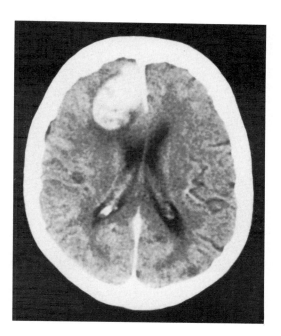

Meningeal Sarcoma Invading the Frontal Lobe.

Malignant gliomas may grow through cerebral cortex to invade adjacent dura, as in Case 84. This association of dural or epidural tumor with a parenchymal mass mimics cerebral invasion by a dural-based metastasis (see Case 35) or meningioma, as in Case 85.

The disproportionate depth of cerebral invasion by the falcine tumor in Case 85 is unusual for meningiomas and suggests an aggressive lesion. The inhomogeneous contrast enhancement and prominent collar of edema also contribute to a "malignant" appearance. The tumor had enlarged dramatically in a 6-month period, and biopsy demonstrated a meningeal sarcoma (compare to Cases 43 to 45).

DIFFERENTIAL DIAGNOSIS:
RIM-ENHANCING, DEEP HEMISPHERE MASS WITH EDEMA

Case 86

59-year-old woman.

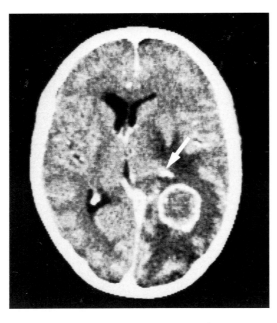

Metastatic Bronchogenic Carcinoma.

Case 87

68-year-old woman.

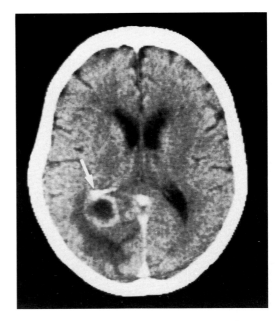

Glioblastoma Multiforme.

The appearance and location of these two lesions are very similar. In each case, the ipsilateral calcified choroid glomus is displaced anteriorly *(arrows)*.

Malignant glioma is the leading possibility when a solitary, peripherally enhancing, deep hemisphere lesion is discovered. However, an unusual metastasis should be included in the differential diagnosis and appropriate evaluation recommended (e.g., chest x-ray).

In immunocompromised patients (e.g., AIDS), primary cerebral lymphoma or an inflammatory mass (e.g., toxoplasmosis) may present a similar appearance.

DIFFERENTIAL DIAGNOSIS:
TUMOR INVOLVING THE SPLENIUM OF THE CORPUS CALLOSUM

Case 88

46-year-old woman.

Case 89

87-year-old woman.

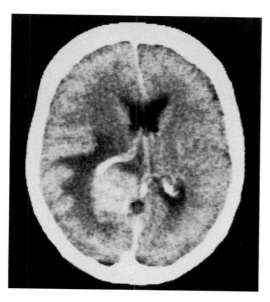

Metastatic Embryonal Cell Carcinoma of the Ovary.

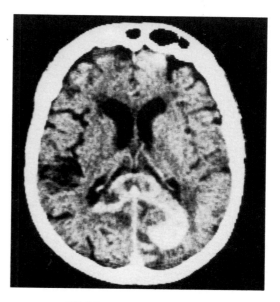

Glioblastoma Multiforme.

Occasional metastases involve the major forceps and splenium of the corpus callosum as in Case 88, strongly resembling a malignant glioma.

The tumor in Case 89 crosses the splenium from one hemisphere to the other, analogous to a "butterfly" glioma of the genu.

Primary CNS lymphoma is a third tumor type that may involve the corpus callosum and should be included in the differential diagnosis.

A number of non-neoplastic disorders can cause abnormal low attenuation and expansion of the corpus callosum resembling a tumor. Among these are multiple sclerosis (see Cases 311 and 312), acute disseminated encephalomyelitis (see Case 317), and progressive multifocal leukoencephalopathy (see Case 321). Machiafava-Bignami syndrome is a rare demyelinating disorder associated with alcohol consumption that frequently involves the corpus callosum.

Case 90

16-year-old man with seizures.

Pleomorphic Xanthoastrocytoma.

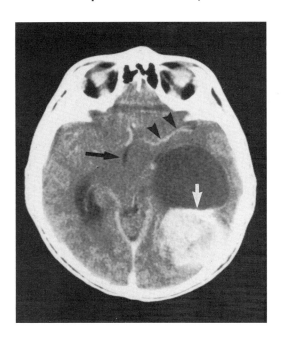

Case 91

28-year-old man.

Cystic Oligodendroglioma.

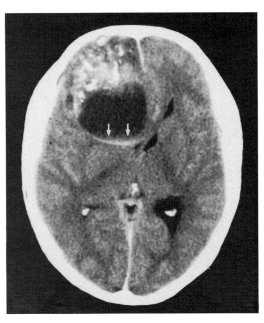

Many low- and high-grade gliomas contain one or more cysts. When a tumor cyst is large and unilocular, palliative drainage may provide symptomatic improvement by reducing mass effect. Aspiration can often be accomplished under CT guidance. Repeated aspiration or continuous drainage may be necessary due to rapid reaccumulation of fluid.

In this case a mass in the temporal lobe of a young patient demonstrates superficial location, calcification *(white arrow)*, and a large cyst. The combination of these features suggests pleomorphic xanthoastrocytoma, a glioma subtype that is often associated with a good prognosis after surgery. Ganglio-gliomas are a second type of primary tumor often occurring in the temporal lobe of young patients and frequently containing cysts and calcification.

The solid, enhancing component of this tumor resembles the mural nodule seen in many cystic cerebellar astrocytomas (see Cases 125 and 126). In the supratentorial compartment, ependymomas may also demonstrate grossly cystic morphology (see Case 98).

Temporal lobe mass effect in this case displaces the middle cerebral artery *(arrowheads)*. Uncal herniation flattens the brain stem and shifts the anterior recesses of the third ventricle *(black arrow)*.

The most reliable CT or MR indication of a truly cystic tumor is the demonstration of a sedimentation level within the lesion. The dense material settling in the dependent portion of a cyst may be cellular debris, hemorrhage, or accumulated contrast material, as in this case *(arrows)*. (See Cases 129, 156, 169, and 179 for other examples of sedimentation levels within cystic tumors.)

In the absence of a sedimentation level, a cyst may be predicted by the homogeneity of its contents. This uniformity may be demonstrated by an image with a narrow window width or by a histogram of attenuation values within the region of interest.

Magnetic resonance imaging is also useful in this assessment. MR scans often identify tissue components of variable intensity within apparently homogeneous, low-attenuation CT lesions. Alternatively, sedimentation levels may be better defined on MR scans than on CT studies.

DIFFERENTIAL DIAGNOSIS:
CYSTIC NEOPLASM WITHIN THE TEMPORAL LOBE

Case 92

26-year-old man.

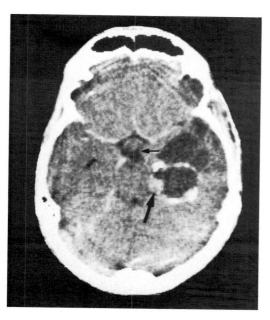

Astrocytoma, Grade 2.

Case 93

69-year-old man.

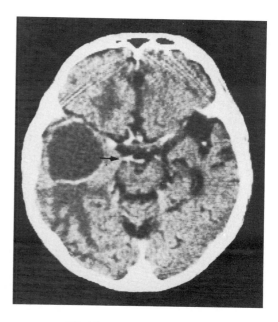

Glioblastoma Multiforme.

The CT features illustrated in Cases 62 to 75 usually distinguish between low-grade and high-grade glial tumors. However, the CT spectrum of malignant gliomas overlaps that of low-grade neoplasms, and occasional tumors have intermediate characteristics.

In Case 92, the extensive calcification and minimal contrast enhancement favor the diagnosis of a long-standing, low-grade mass. The possibility of malignant degeneration is raised when areas of thick contrast enhancement *(large arrow)* are superimposed on otherwise benign features.

The unusually thin and uniform rim of contrast enhancement surrounding the glioma in Case 93 resembles the morphology of a cerebral abscess (see Cases 274 to 279). Some cerebral metastases can present a similar picture (compare to Case 5).

Both of these cases demonstrate medial displacement of the adjacent uncus *(small arrows)*. Both tumors were found to be grossly cystic at surgery.

Case 94

89-year-old woman presenting with a "CVA".
(noncontrast scan)

Malignant Glioma.

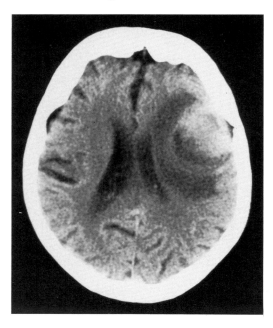

Case 95

65-year-old man presenting with acute
right homonymous hemianopia following
head trauma.
(noncontrast scan)

Glioblastoma Multiforme.

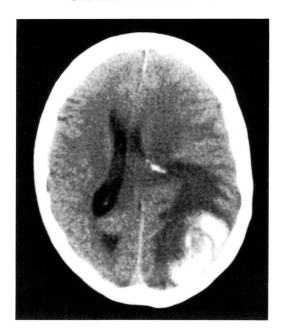

Macroscopic hemorrhage is relatively uncommon in gliomas, occurring in about 5%. Hematomas can account for the acute clinical presentation of both low- and high-grade tumors (see Case 576 for another example).

Malignant gliomas are characterized angiographically by neovascularity, which represents a likely source of bleeding (see Case 76). Among low-grade gliomas, oligodendrogliomas make up a disproportionate share of lesions presenting with gross hemorrhage.

As in the case of hemorrhagic metastases (see Cases 10 and 566), the correct diagnosis depends on looking through or around the blood products to recognize an underlying mass. Extensive edema medial to the lesion in this case would be atypical for an acute, spontaneous hematoma and suggests pre-existing pathology.

Again in this case an acute clinical event is correlated with gross hemorrhage on a CT scan. Although the underlying tumor is less apparent than in Case 94, a number of considerations suggest the correct diagnosis.

The location of the abnormality is atypical for post-traumatic hemorrhage (see Cases 374 to 379). The extensive vasogenic edema throughout the posterior left hemisphere is too prominent to represent a reaction to acute hemorrhage. Similarly, the impressive mass effect exceeds the volume of hemorrhage and implies an underlying lesion. Edema is limited to white matter and does not match the location or morphology of cerebral infarction with secondary hemorrhage (compare to Cases 410 to 412).

DIFFERENTIAL DIAGNOSIS:
INTRAVENTRICULAR AND PERIVENTRICULAR RIM-ENHANCING MASS

Case 96

38-year-old man.

Case 97

60-year-old man.

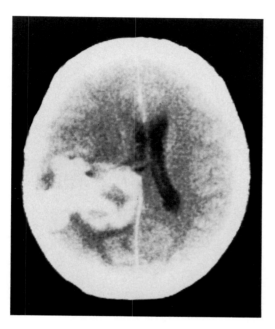

Trigone Meningioma.

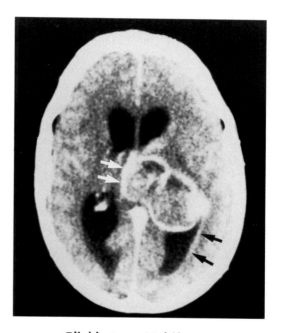

Glioblastoma Multiforme.

In Case 96, the deep hemisphere location, thick-walled contrast enhancement, and occurrence in a young man would make malignant glioma a likely diagnosis. However, the tumor is a meningioma, arising within the trigone of the lateral ventricle and extending into the posterior temporal lobe. One clue to the correct diagnosis is the predominantly smooth, well-defined, intensely enhancing margin of the mass.

Intraventricular meningiomas account for 2% of intracranial meningiomas and most commonly occur within the atrium of the lateral ventricle. The differential diagnosis for an enhancing tumor in this location would include choroid plexus papilloma (see Case 222), ependymoma, metastasis (see Case 22), and vascular malformation. Lateral ventricular choroid plexus papillomas (more commonly seen in children) may invade the cerebral hemisphere and closely resemble the appearance in this case.

In both Cases 96 and 97 the midline shift is smaller than might be expected, because a portion of the tumor bulk has been accommodated within the ventricular chambers. Relatively mild mass effect is characteristic of intraventricular masses, which can enlarge by simply displacing CSF.

The internal cerebral veins are deformed in Case 97 (white arrows). There is a small amount of subependymal tumor extension along the lateral margin of the occipital horn (black arrows; see Case 102).

MR CORRELATION: CYSTIC AND HEMORRHAGIC GLIOMAS

Case 98

4-year-old girl.
(axial, noncontrast scan; SE 2000/90)

Cystic Ependymoma.

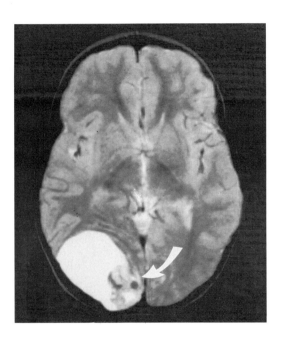

MR may be useful for characterizing cystic components of glial neoplasms. Tumor cysts may be of homogeneous signal intensity or contain sedimentation levels. Intensity values may resemble spinal fluid (e.g., long T1 and T2, as noted in this case) or reflect high protein content or hemorrhage (with associated shortening of T1).

The multiplanar display of MR helps to define the location of mural nodules in cystic gliomas. In this case, a nodular tumor is seen at the medial margin of the lesion (*arrow;* see also Case 126).

Unlike posterior fossa ependymomas, supratentorial ependymomas are often parenchymal (i.e., not related to the ventricular system) and may be grossly cystic, as seen here.

Case 99

89-year-old woman.
(axial, noncontrast scan; SE 2500/90)

Hemorrhagic Glioblastoma.

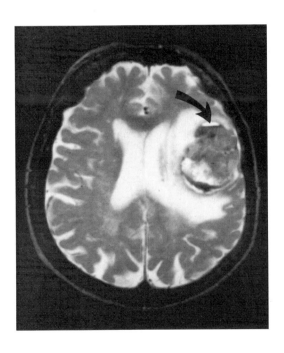

The T1-weighted images in this case demonstrated high signal intensity throughout the left hemisphere mass, compatible with subacute hemorrhage (see Case 13 and discussion of Cases 560 and 561).

The T2-weighted scan seen here shows a heterogeneous lesion of predominantly low intensity, reflecting the presence of blood products. (Compare to the long T2 typically seen in nonhemorrhagic gliomas such as Cases 69 and 76, and to the more homogeneous appearance of spontaneous intracerebral hematomas as in Cases 560 and 561.) A small sedimentation level of blood products is seen at the anterior margin of the tumor *(arrow)*. Marked cerebral edema outlines the medial margin of the mass.

MR CORRELATION: PATTERNS OF CONTRAST ENHANCEMENT IN MALIGNANT GLIOMAS

Case 100

24-year-old woman with seizures.
(coronal, postcontrast scan; SE 1000/20)

Recurrent Grade 3 Astrocytoma.

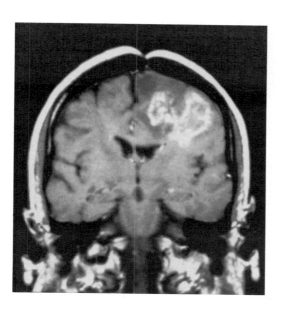

Case 101

61-year-old man.
(sagittal, postcontrast scan; SE 600/20)

Grade 3 Astrocytoma.

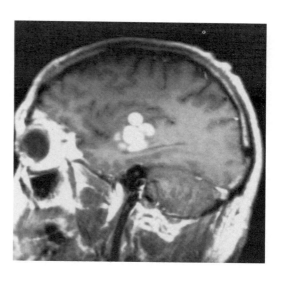

The contrast enhancement of malignant gliomas on MR scans is variable. Many cases demonstrate shaggy rims or irregular fronds of enhancement comparable to CT studies. In this case the extensive, infiltrating pattern of abnormal enhancement suggests a high-grade malignancy.

Occasional high-grade gliomas are associated with unusually well-defined contrast enhancement (analogous to the uniform CT enhancement in Cases 74 and 75).

The homogeneous, circumscribed, nodular appearance of enhancement in this case might suggest low-grade histology (compare to Case 105). Although the irregularity of enhancement patterns on CT and MR generally correlates with the grade of malignancy, individual exceptions are encountered, as seen here.

DIFFERENTIAL DIAGNOSIS:
SUBEPENDYMAL TUMOR SPREAD

Case 102

64-year-old woman.

Case 103

77-year-old man.

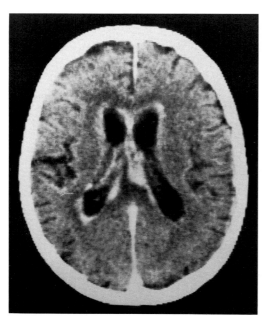

High-Grade Glioma.

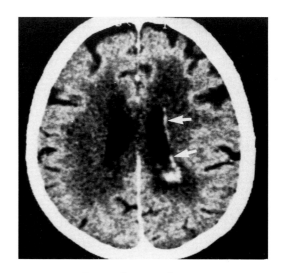

Systemic Lymphoma.

Enhancement along ventricular margins may be due to inflammatory ventriculitis (see Cases 264 to 267) or to subependymal neoplasm. Gliomas and ependymomas are primary considerations in the latter category because of their frequent periventricular location (Case 102; see also Case 97).

Many other tumors can also spread along ventricular surfaces. Metastases from systemic solid tumors (especially oat cell carcinoma of the lung, melanoma, and breast carcinoma; see Case 23), or from other intracranial neoplasms (e.g., medulloblastoma, germinoma) can cause a periventricular "cast" of tumor.

Primary CNS lymphoma (see Case 244) or secondary brain involvement by systemic lymphoma (as in Case 103) may present a similar appearance.

Case 104

23-year-old woman with recent onset
of seizures.
(coronal, noncontrast scan; SE 3000/90)

Grade 2 Astrocytoma.

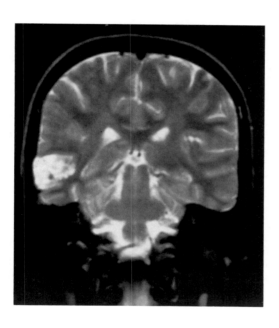

Case 105

37-year-old man with a history of seizures
for several years.
(coronal, postcontrast scan; SE 1000/20)

Grade 2 Astrocytoma.

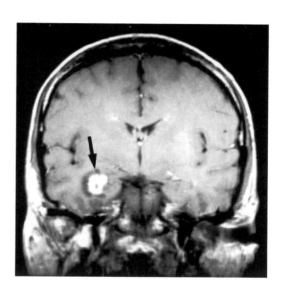

A large number of low-grade gliomas occur in the temporal lobe of young adults, presenting clinically as a seizure disorder. CT is suboptimal for evaluating such patients. The customary axial scans at this level are substantially degraded by artifact from the bony margins of the middle cranial fossa.

Coronal MR scans through the temporal lobe are free from bone-related artifact and provide multiple tangential sections of cerebral surfaces and internal anatomy (e.g., temporal horn, hippocampal formation). These advantages combine with the high tissue contrast of MR to demonstrate temporal lobe pathology much more successfully than CT scanning.

In this case, a low-grade glioma is easily localized within the right temporal lobe. The patient has been seizure free since the tumor was resected.

Lesions in or near the hippocampal formation commonly cause seizures because of the low excitation threshold of neurons in this region. As discussed in Case 104, the medial temporal lobe can be difficult to assess on CT scans. Coronal MR studies are appropriate either as an initial examination or following a negative CT study in such patients.

In this case, a small enhancing glioma is seen near the right hippocampal formation. The presence of contrast enhancement on MR scans of a glioma does not necessarily imply a high-grade lesion, since MR can detect even minor abnormalities of the blood-brain barrier.

Another lesion commonly found in the temporal lobe of young adults with seizures is a cavernous angioma (see Case 517). Such "occult" vascular malformations have a typical MR appearance that includes central T1-shortening on noncontrast images (see Cases 510 to 512).

REFERENCES: CT

1. Afra D., Norman D., Levin V.A.: Cysts in malignant gliomas: Identification by computerized tomography. *J. Neurosurg.* 53:821–825, 1980.
2. Andreou J., George A.E., Wise A., et al.: CT prognostic criteria of survival after malignant glioma surgery. *A.J.N.R.* 4:488–490, 1983.
3. Armington W.G., Osborn A.G., Cubberly D.A., et al.: Supratentorial ependymoma: CT appearance. *Radiology* 157:367–372, 1985.
4. Belender N., Cromwell L.D., Graves D., et al.: Interval appearance of glioblastomas not evident in previous CT examinations. *J. Comput. Assist. Tomogr.* 7:599–603, 1983.
5. Blom R.J.: Pleomorphic xanthoastrocytoma: CT appearance. *J. Comput. Assist. Tomogr.* 12:351, 1988.
6. Braun I.F., Chambers E., Leeds N.E., Zimmerman R.D.: The value of unenhanced scans in differentiating lesions producing ring enhancement. *A.J.N.R.* 3:643–647, 1982.
7. Burger P.C., Dubois P.J., Schold S.C., et al.: Computerized tomographic and pathologic studies of the untreated, quiescent, and recurrent glioblastoma multiforme. *J. Neurosurg.* 58:159–169, 1983.
8. Butler A.R., Horri S.C., Kricheff I.I., et al.: Computed tomography in astrocytomas: A statistical analysis of the parameters of malignancy and the positive contrast-enhanced CT scan. *Radiology* 129:433–439, 1978.
9. Butler A.R., Passalaqua A.M., Berenstein A., Kricheff I.I.: Contrast enhanced CT scan and radionuclide brain scan in supratentorial gliomas. *A.J.R.* 132:607–611, 1979.
10. Centeno R.S., Lee A.A., Winter J., Barba D.: Supratentorial ependymomas: Neuroimaging and clinicopathological correlation. *J. Neurosurg.* 64:209–215, 1986.
11. Demierre B., Stichnoth F.A., Spoerri O.: Intracerebral ganglioglioma. *J. Neurosurg.* 65:177–182, 1986.
12. Dolinskas C.A., Simeone F.A.: CT characteristics of intraventricular oligodendrogliomas. *A.J.N.R.* 8:1077–1082, 1987.
13. Dorne H.L., O'Gorman A.M., Melanson D.: Computed tomography of intracranial gangliogliomas. *A.J.N.R.* 7:281–286, 1986.
14. Geremia G.K., Wollman R., Foust R.: Computed tomography of gliomatosis cerebri. *J. Comput. Assist. Tomogr.* 12:698–701, 1988.
15. Gooding G.A.W., Boggan J.E., Weinstein P.R.: Characterization of intracranial neoplasms by CT and intraoperative sonography. *A.J.N.R.* 5:517–520, 1984.
16. Hasuo K., Fukui M., Tamura S., et al.: Gliomas with dural invasion: computed tomography and angiography. *C.T.* 12:100, 1988.
17. Hasuo K., Fukui M., Tamura S., et al.: Oligodendrogliomas of the lateral ventricle: Computed tomography and angiography. *C.T.* 11:376, 1987.
18. Hoffman W.F., Levin V.A., Wilson C.B.: Evaluation of malignant glioma patients during the post-irradiation period. *J. Neurosurg.* 50:624–628, 1979.
19. Hylton P.D., Reichman O.H.: Clinical manifestation of glioma before computed tomographic appearance: The dilemma of a negative scan. *Neurosurgery* 21:27–32, 1987.
20. Kendall B.E., Jakubowski J., Pullicino P., et al.: Difficulties in diagnosis of supratentorial gliomas by CAT scan. *J. Neurol. Neurosurg. Psychiatry* 42:485–492, 1979.
21. Kieffer S.A., Salibi N.A., Kim R.C., et al.: Multifocal glioblastoma: diagnostic implications. *Radiology* 143:709–710, 1982.
22. Lee Y.-Y., Castillo M., Navert C., Moser R.P.: Computed tomography of gliosarcoma. *A.J.N.R.* 6:527–532, 1985.
23. Lewander R.: Contrast enhancement with time in gliomas. *Acta Radiol. (Diagn.)* 20:689–702, 1979.
24. Lilja A., Bergstom K., Spannare B., et al.: Reliability of computed tomography in assessing histopathological features of malignant supratentorial gliomas. *J. Comput. Assist. Tomogr.* 5:625–636, 1981.
25. Maiuri F., Stella L., Benvenuti D., et al.: Cerebral gliosarcoma: correlation of computed tomographic findings, surgical aspect, pathological features, and prognosis. *Neurosurgery* 26:261–267, 1990.
26. Marks J.E., Gado M.: Serial computed tomography of primary brain tumors following surgery, irradiation, and chemotherapy. *Radiology* 125:119–125, 1977.
27. McGeachie R.E., Gold L.H., Latchaw R.E.: Periventricular spread of tumor demonstrated by computed tomography. *Radiology* 125:407–410, 1977.
28. Murovic J., Turowski K., Wilson C.B., et al.: Computerized tomography in the prognosis of malignant cerebral gliomas. *J. Neurosurgery* 65:799–806, 1986.
29. Pedersen H., Gjerris F., Klinken L.: Malignancy criteria in computed tomography of primary supratentorial tumors in infancy and childhood. *Neuroradiology* 31:24, 1989.
30. Pedersen H., Gjerris F., Klinken L.: Computed tomography of benign supratentorial astrocytomas in infancy and childhood. *Neuroradiology* 21:87–91, 1981.
31. Rao K., Levine H., Itani A., et al.: CT findings in multicentric glioblastoma: Diagnostic-pathologic correlation. *J. Comput. Assist. Tomogr.* 4:187–192, 1980.
32. Russell E.J., Naidich T.P.: The enhancing septal alveal wedge: A septal sign of intra-axial mass. *Neuroradiology* 23:33–40, 1982.
33. Saloman M., Levine H., Rao K.: Value of sequential computed tomography in the multimodality treatment of glioblastoma multiforme. *Neurosurgery* 8:15–19, 1981.
34. Steinhoff H., Lanksch W., Kazner E., et al.: Computed tomography in the diagnosis and differential diagnosis of glioblastomas. *Neuroradiology* 14:193–200, 1977.
35. Stylopoulos L.A., George A.E., de Leon M.J., et al: Longitudinal CT study of parenchymal brain changes in glioma survivors. *A.J.N.R.* 9:517–522, 1988.
36. Tolly T.L., Bruckman J.E., Czarnecki D.J., et al.: Early CT findings after interstitial radiation therapy for primary malignant brain tumors. *A.J.N.R.* 9:1177–1180, 1988.
37. Tomita T., McLone D.G., Naidich T.P.: Mural tumors with cysts in the cerebral hemispheres of children. *Neurosurgery* 19:998–1005, 1986.
38. Van Tassel P., Lee Y.-Y., Bruner J.M.: Synchronous and metachronous malignant glioma: CT findings. *A.J.N.R.* 9:725–732, 1988.
39. Vonofakos D., Marca H., Hacker H.: Oligodendrogliomas: CT patterns with emphasis on features indicating malignancy. *J. Comput. Assist. Tomogr.* 3:783–788, 1979.
40. Wakai S., Andoh Y., Ochiai C., et al.: Postoperative contrast enhancement in brain tumors and intracerebral hematomas: CT study. *J. Comput. Assist. Tomogr.* 14:267–271, 1990.
41. Whittle I.R., Gordon A., Misra B., et al.: Pleomorphic xanthoastrocytoma: Report of four cases. *J. Neurosurg.* 70:463–468, 1989.

REFERENCES: MR

1. Altman N.R.: MR and CT characteristics of gangliocytoma: A rare cause of epilepsy in children. *A.J.N.R.* 9:917–922, 1988.
2. Atlas S.W., Grossman R.I., Gomori J.M., et al.: Hemorrhagic intracranial malignant neoplasms: Spin-echo MR imaging. *Radiology* 164:71–78, 1987.
3. Castillo M., Davis P.C., Takei Y., Hoffman J.C. Jr.: Intracranial ganglioglioma: MR, CT, and clinical findings in 18 patients. *A.J.N.R.* 11:109–114, 1990.
4. Claussen C., Laniado M., Schörner W., et al,: Gadolinium-DTPA in MR imaging of glioblastoma and intracranial metastases. *A.J.N.R.* 6:669–674, 1985.
5. Dean B.L., Drayer B.P., Bird C.R., et al.: Gliomas: Classification with MR imaging. *Radiology* 174:411–416, 1990.
6. Destian S., Sze G., Krol G., et al.: MR imaging of hemorrhagic intracranial neoplasms. *A.J.N.R.* 9:1115–1122, 1988.
7. Earnest F., Kelly P.J., Scheithauer B., et al.: Cerebral astrocytomas: Histopathologic correlation of MR and CT contrast enhancement with stereotactic biopsy. *Radiology* 166:823–828, 1988.
8. Elster A.D., DiPersio D.A.: Cranial postoperative site: Assessment with contrast-enhanced MR imaging. *Radiology* 174:93–98, 1990.
9. Graif M., Bydder G.M., Steiner R.E., et al.: Contrast-enhanced MR imaging of malignant brain tumors. *A.J.N.R.* 6:855–862, 1985.
10. Johnson P.C., Hunt S.J., Drayer B.P.: Human cerebral gliomas: Correlation of postmortem MR imaging and neuropathologic findings. *Radiology* 170:211–218, 1989.
11. Lee B.C.P., Kneeland J.B., Cahill P.T., Deck M.D.F.: MR recognition of supratentorial tumors. *A.J.N.R.* 6:871–878, 1985.
12. Lee Y.-Y., Van Tassel P.: Intracranial oligodendrogliomas: Imaging findings in 35 untreated Cases. *A.J.N.R.* 10:119–128, 1989.
13. Lee Y.-Y., Van Tassel P., Bruner J.M., et al.: Juvenile pilocytic astrocytomas: CT and MR characteristics. *A.J.N.R.* 10:363–370, 1989.
14. Spoto G.P., Press G.A., Hesselink J.R., Solomon M.: Intracranial ependymoma and subependymoma: MR manifestations. *A.J.N.R.* 11:83–92, 1990.

CHAPTER 4

Posterior Fossa Tumors

Case 106

4-year-old boy presenting with ataxia.

Case 107

42-year-old woman.

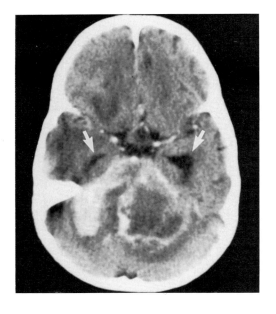

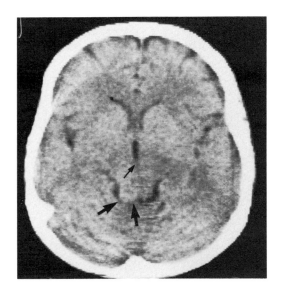

Most brain stem gliomas demonstrate slightly decreased attenuation values on precontrast scans. Some tumors are isodense, and a few show increased attenuation or even gross calcification (see Case 229).

Mass effect depends on tumor size and may be generalized, as seen here, or focal, as in Case 107. In this case the pontine enlargement obliterates adjacent cisterns and effaces the fourth ventricle, causing hydrocephalus *(arrows)*.

The abnormal contrast enhancement seen here is unusually extensive. In other cases, enhancement may be localized (see Case 109), minimal, or absent.

Here peripheral enhancement appears to surround nonenhancing solid tissue. True cysts occur within some brain stem gliomas, allowing palliative decompression (see discussion of Case 90).

Brain stem gliomas may be relatively inconspicuous lesions on CT scans. They often cause early symptoms that lead to evaluation while the tumor is still small. Diagnostic difficulty is increased by the frequent lack of significant attenuation changes and by the common presence of artifacts on scans through the posterior fossa.

Here a small, isodense midbrain tumor fattens the right superior colliculus *(large arrows)* and displaces the posterior portion of the third ventricle *(small arrow)*. Subtle abnormalities of brain stem contour may be highlighted by CT scans performed after subarachnoid contrast material has been injected (see Case 237).

MR offers a better means of detecting small brain stem masses (see Cases 111 and 113). Anatomical details such as the configuration of the quadrigeminal plate are more easily analyzed by multiplanar views, and images are not degraded by bone artifact. Furthermore, the high contrast sensitivity of MR may demonstrate intrinsic lesions causing little or no alteration in the x-ray absorption or contour of the brain stem.

DIFFERENTIAL DIAGNOSIS:
FOCALLY ENHANCING BRAIN STEM MASS

Case 108

55-year-old woman.

Case 109

7-year-old boy.

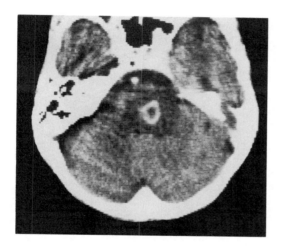

Metastatic Carcinoma of the Breast.

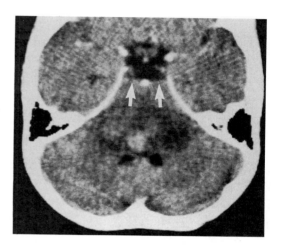

Brain Stem Glioma.

The possibility of metastasis should be considered when brain stem masses are encountered in adults (see also Case 3). The well-defined contrast enhancement in Case 108 contrasts with the typically indistinct margins and vague enhancement of most brain stem gliomas.

Case 109 demonstrates a single nodule of contrast enhancement within a much larger area of abnormal low attenuation (compare the relative amount of enhancement to Case 106). This appearance of an enhancing nodule indenting the floor of the fourth ventricle resembles the morphology of some cavernous angiomas and arteriovenous malformations involving the dorsal brain stem. The characteristic MR appearance of such lesions may aid in the differential diagnosis (see Cases 516 and 517).

The ventral margin of the pons in Case 109 bulges anteriorly on both sides of the basilar artery (*arrows*). Further ventral tumor growth may lead to encasement and posterior displacement of the artery by an exophytic brain stem glioma (see Case 112).

Brain stem infarction or demyelination may cause a combination of low attenuation, mass effect, and vague contrast enhancement resembling a tumor (also see discussion of Cases 446 and 447). Clinical information or follow-up scans will usually establish the diagnosis in such cases.

Rarely, a granuloma (e.g., tuberculosis, sarcoidosis) or an abscess may occupy the brain stem and mimic a neoplasm. Diagnosis in these situations may require biopsy.

MR DEMONSTRATION OF BRAIN STEM GLIOMAS: SAGITTAL T1-WEIGHTED SCANS

Case 110

11-year-old girl.
(sagittal, noncontrast scan; SE 600/17)

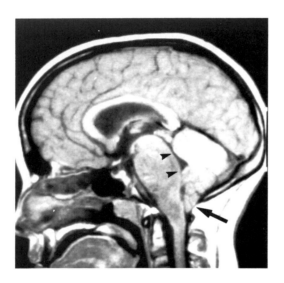

Case 111

10-year-old boy shunted years earlier for hydrocephalus thought to be due to "benign" aqueductal stenosis.
(sagittal, noncontrast scan; SE 600/17)

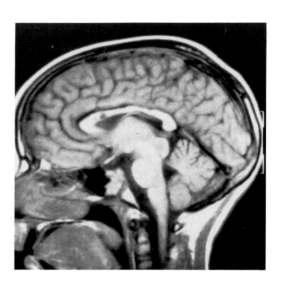

Sagittal MR images with short TRs are valuable for demonstration of brain stem masses. Low-signal CSF in the cisterns of the posterior fossa, aqueduct, and fourth ventricle clearly outlines brain stem morphology.

In this case, the midbrain, pons, and medulla are expanded in anteroposterior diameter (compare to Case 111). The normally linear floor of the fourth ventricle is convex posteriorly (*arrowheads*; prepontine masses can also cause this appearance, as in Case 241A).

In addition, abnormally low signal intensity is present throughout the brain stem, extending caudally through the plane of the foramen magnum to involve the cervical spinal cord. Although many brain stem gliomas demonstrate prolongation of T1 as seen here, other tumors may be isointense on short TR images. High signal intensity within the brain stem on noncontrast T1-weighted images suggests hemorrhage within a tumor or the alternative diagnosis of a vascular malformation (especially cavernous angioma; see Case 516).

The cerebellar tonsils in this case are peg shaped and extend below the plane of the foramen magnum *(arrow),* likely representing a mild Chiari I malformation rather than herniation (compare to Cases 117, 126B, and 624).

As illustrated in Case 107, some brain stem gliomas are focal, low-grade lesions. Many such tumors are relatively isodense on CT scans and isointense on T1-weighted MR images.

In this case, a small glioma expands the midbrain tectum, bulging into the quadrigeminal cistern. (Compare the diameter and morphology of the dorsal midbrain to Case 110.) The localized mass effect of the tumor effaces the aqueduct and accounts for the history of hydrocephalus. "Benign" aqueductal stenosis (see Case 588) should be a diagnosis of exclusion after careful examination of the midbrain, now best performed by MR.

A small area of low signal within the anterior body of the corpus callosum is related to prior shunting. Mucosal thickening is present in the posterior portion of the sphenoid sinus.

MR DEMONSTRATION OF BRAIN STEM GLIOMAS: AXIAL T2-WEIGHTED SCANS

Case 112

9-year-old girl.
(axial, noncontrast scan; SE 3000/50)

Case 113

10-year-old boy (same patient as Case 111).
(axial, noncontrast scan; SE 3000/75)

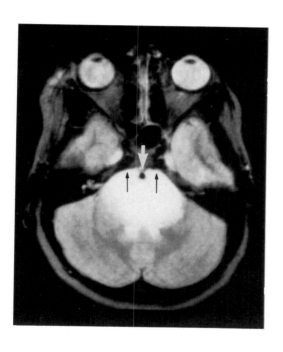

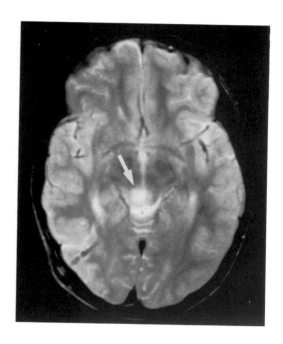

Most brain stem gliomas are readily detected on T2-weighted MR images due to prominent high signal intensity. The tumor in this case (with possible associated edema) diffusely involves and expands the pons. The ventral margin of the fourth ventricle is flattened and posteriorly displaced in a manner similar to Case 110.

High-intensity tumor has grown anteriorly *(black arrows)* to surround the flow-void of the basilar artery *(white arrow)*. The vessel is now circumferentially encased by exophytic glioma (compare to the milder ventral expansion of the brain stem demonstrated in Cases 106 and 109).

Here a localized area of long T2 is seen in the dorsal midbrain, slightly eccentric to the right of the midline. The definite signal abnormality at this site confirms the presence of focal pathology, as suggested on the sagittal T1-weighted image in Case 111.

The appearance is not specific for tumor. For example, a similar lesion within the pons or middle cerebellar peduncle in an adult could represent a plaque of multiple sclerosis (see Case 330) or a metastasis (compare to Case 24A).

MEDULLOBLASTOMAS

Case 114

2-year-old boy presenting with hydrocephalus.
(noncontrast scan after shunting)

Case 115

3-year-old girl presenting with ataxia
and nystagmus.
(postcontrast scan)

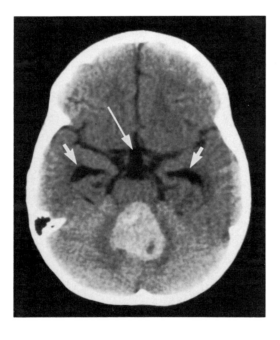

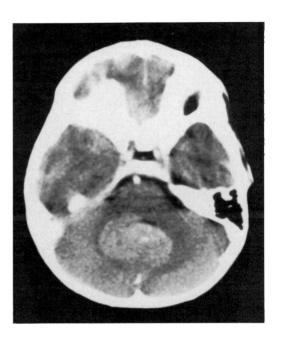

Medulloblastomas are highly cellular tumors arising from primitive cells in the neuroepithelial roof of the fourth ventricle (external granular layer of the inferior medullary velum). Many pathologists classify these neoplasms as "primitive neuroectodermal tumors."

Medulloblastomas usually present as midline masses with homogeneous, mildly increased attenuation. (The degree of precontrast high attenuation in this case is somewhat greater than average.) Calcification and cysts are rarely prominent.

Fourth ventricular obstruction has caused hydrocephalic enlargement of the temporal horns *(short arrows)* and anterior third ventricle *(long arrow),* now decompressed by a shunt.

Medulloblastomas rank with cerebellar astrocytomas as the most common posterior fossa tumors in children.

Contrast enhancement in medulloblastomas is typically uniform and intense. The posterior fossa is often "tight," with compression of the fourth ventricle causing obstructive hydrocephalus.

Medulloblastomas are among the primary CNS neoplasms commonly associated with seeding of the cerebrospinal fluid. (Others include ependymoma, germinoma, and glioma.) For this reason, isodense or enhancing subarachnoid spaces should be noted on initial and follow-up scans in these patients (see Case 121).

Contrast enhancement near the right sphenoid wing in this case may simply represent middle cerebral vasculature accentuated by head tilt (compare to Case 331).

EPENDYMOMAS

Case 116A

5-year-old boy with a history of vomiting
for 2 months and headache for 1 week.
(noncontrast scan)

Case 116B

Same patient.
(postcontrast scan)

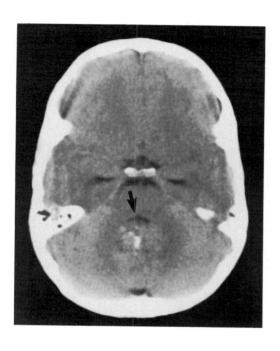

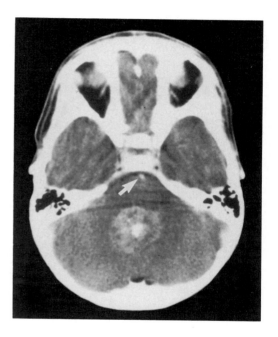

Ependymomas arising from the fourth ventricle are among the posterior fossa masses encountered in children. Their location mimics the more common medulloblastomas, but other CT features usually suggest the correct diagnosis.

Ependymomas are frequently calcified, as seen in this case. They may be inhomogeneous, with mixed attenuation values, sometimes including cysts or hemorrhage. Both calcification and inhomogeneity contrast with the usual appearance of medulloblastomas.

The tumor itself is relatively isodense on this noncontrast scan. A portion of the expanded fourth ventricle *(arrow)* is seen at the anterior margin of the mass (similar to Case 115).

Symptoms of nausea and vomiting may precede the development of overt hydrocephalus in children with fourth ventricular ependymomas, likely due to early involvement of the dorsal brain stem.

The enhancement pattern of ependymomas is usually less homogeneous and intense than that of medulloblastomas. Tumor margins are often irregular and poorly defined, and lobulation is frequent.

In this case the tumor is mildly lobulated with inhomogeneous enhancement. The basilar artery *(arrow)* and pons are displaced anteriorly against the dorsum sellae and clivus.

Although the characteristics discussed above are useful clues to the diagnosis of ependymoma, some of these tumors demonstrate uniform density and enhancement indistinguishable from medulloblastomas. Similarly, some medulloblastomas are heterogeneous and resemble ependymomas. MR may contribute to the differential diagnosis in such cases (see Cases 117 and 118).

Case 117

10-year-old girl.
(sagittal, noncontrast scan; SE 700/16)

Medulloblastoma.

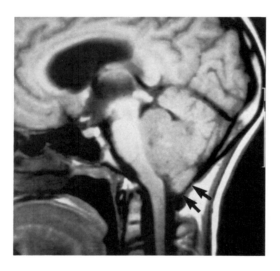

Case 118

23-year-old woman.
(sagittal, noncontrast scan; SE 800/17)

Ependymoma.

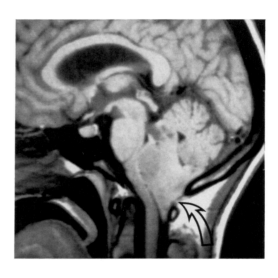

Sagittal T1-weighted MR images clearly define the morphology and extent of fourth ventricular masses (see also Case 162).

Here a medulloblastoma fills and expands the fourth ventricle. The signal intensity of the tumor is homogeneous, correlating with the usually uniform attenuation of these lesions on CT scans. The cerebellar tonsils (arrows) have been displaced through the foramen magnum. The aqueduct has been shortened or "assimilated" into the rostral expansion of the fourth ventricle (compare to Case 110)

In this case the fourth ventricular mass is less homogeneous than Case 117. The zones of low signal intensity within the tumor correlated with calcification on the patient's CT scan.

The lesion has grown caudally through the foramen of Magendie into the vallecula, extending inferiorly as a carpet of tissue dorsal to the cervical spinal cord (arrow). Ependymomas commonly grow out of the fourth ventricle, while medulloblastomas do so less frequently (contrast Cases 117 and 118, but see Case 119).

Another feature potentially distinguishing ependymomas and medulloblastomas on sagittal MR scans is their site of origin or attachment. Medulloblastomas as in Case 117 are often more easily demarcated from the brain stem than from the vermis, where these tumors usually arise (inferior medullary velum). By contrast, fourth ventricular ependymomas as in this case are often more easily separated from the vermis than from the dorsal brain stem, where they are frequently attached at surgery.

Sagittal and coronal MR scans readily document cerebellar tonsillar herniation or extension of tumor through the foramen magnum in cases of posterior fossa masses. (compare to Cases 110, 126, 161, 162, and 624).

LATERAL EXTENSION OR PRESENTATION OF FOURTH VENTRICULAR TUMORS

Case 119

4-year-old boy.
(axial, noncontrast scan; SE 2500/90)

Medulloblastoma.

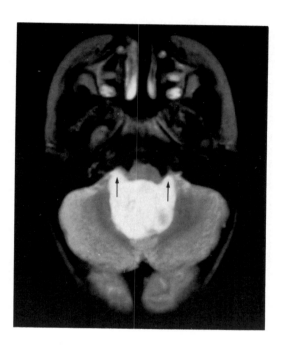

Case 120

5-year-old boy.

Ependymoma.

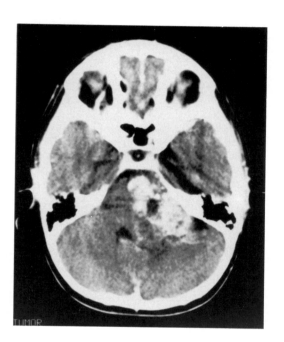

In addition to the caudal extension illustrated in Case 118, fourth ventricular tumors may grow laterally through the foramina of Luschka. The medulloblastoma in this case demonstrates symmetrical extension into the anterolateral recesses of the fourth ventricle *(arrows)*. Further tumor growth could accumulate as masses within the cerebellopontine angles. In extreme cases, cisternal extensions of medulloblastoma or ependymoma may enlarge to surround the brain stem.

The brain stem in this case is severely compressed by the tumor (compare the brain stem diameter to Case 112). The tumor itself demonstrates prominent prolongation of T2, which appears quite homogeneous.

Medulloblastomas may arise in a lateral *intra*-axial location, especially in older patients (see Case 133). Such hemispheric tumors contrast with the occasional lateral *extra*-axial presentation of ependymomas, as seen in Case 120.

Fourth ventricular ependymomas may extend through the foramina of Luschka to accumulate in the cerebellopontine angle. Such growth is commonly more prominent and asymmetrical than is seen with medulloblastomas. In some cases the bulk of the tumor occupies these "secondary" locations.

This large, lobulated, inhomogeneously enhancing extra-axial mass within the cerebellopontine angle cistern was found to be an ependymoma arising from the lateral recess of the fourth ventricle. The body of the fourth ventricle was deformed by mass effect but was surgically free of tumor.

Ependymomas should be considered in the differential diagnosis of a cerebellopontine angle mass in a child. Choroid plexus papilloma, meningioma, schwannoma, and metastasis (e.g., neuroblastoma, lymphoma) are other possibilities, although all are rare. Exophytic extension of a cerebellar astrocytoma may present an appearance similar to this case.

Case 121A

7-year-old boy, 9 months after resection of a fourth ventricular medulloblastoma.

Case 121B

Same patient, 3 months earlier.
(coronal, postcontrast scan; SE 1000/20)

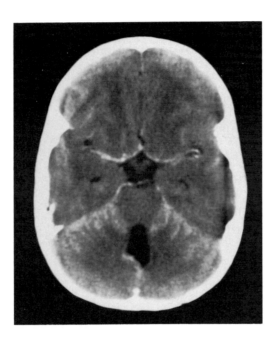

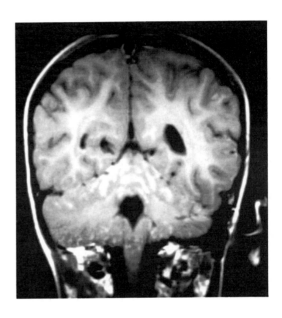

In addition to the caudal or lateral growth of fourth ventricular tumors discussed in Cases 118 to 120, ependymomas and medulloblastomas can spread by "seeding" of CSF spaces. Evidence of such fluid-borne leptomeningeal metastases may be present at the time of diagnosis or develop subsequently, as in this case. Involvement of the spinal canal is common (see Case 778).

Here the sulci between cerebellar folia are symmetrically filled with enhancing meningeal tumor. (Compare this parallel, smoothly curving enhancement pattern to the more irregular appearance of leptomeningeal carcinomatosis within cerebral sulci in Case 21.) A small amount of residual or recurrent tumor also lines the posterior margin of the fourth ventricle.

Subarachnoid seeding is a common form of tumor recurrence for both medulloblastoma and fourth ventricular ependymoma. For this reason, radiation therapy to the entire craniospinal axis and/or chemotherapy are often employed in the initial treatment of these posterior fossa tumors.

In adult patients, the enhancement pattern of leptomeningeal tumor within cerebellar sulci may mimic that of subacute infarction involving the superior cerebellar surface (see Case 455).

Meningeal tumor frequently takes the form of a uniform "coating" or "frosting" on the surface of the brain or spinal cord, as seen here (see also Case 778). Larger nodular components may develop at any location within sulci or cisterns.

In this case, the multiple foci of contrast enhancement apparently "within" cerebellar parenchyma represent cross sections of subarachnoid tumor filling the sulci between folia, as is seen more easily on the axial CT scan of Case 121A.

Meningeal involvement by medulloblastomas, ependymomas, and metastases from other primary CNS or systemic tumors is often most apparent over the superior surface of the cerebellum. Coronal postcontrast MR scans are especially useful in demonstrating such pathology. In this case, coronal MR made the diagnosis at a time when CT was nondiagnostic; subsequent CT scans (Case 121A) demonstrated progressive meningeal disease.

DIFFERENTIAL DIAGNOSIS:
FOURTH VENTRICULAR MASSES IN ADULTS

Case 122

29-year-old man.

Case 123

70-year-old woman.

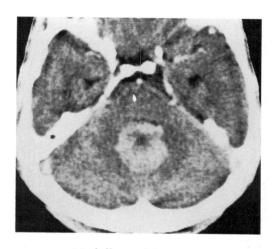

Medullomyoblastoma.

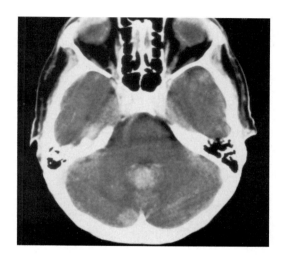

Metastatic Carcinoma of the Lung.

A variety of pathologies can cause masses occupying or bordering the fourth ventricle in adults. Metastases within the brain stem (see Case 108) or cerebellar vermis (as in Case 123) may mimic fourth ventricular tumors.

Medulloblastomas and ependymomas of the fourth ventricle are much less common in adults than in children. Medulloblastomas in adolescents and adults may arise laterally in the cerebellar hemisphere (see Case 133); such "cerebellar sarcomas" often have a fibrotic histologic pattern ("desmoplastic"). Case 122 demonstrates an unusual midline tumor in adult, found to be a malignant variant of medulloblastoma with differentiation toward muscle cells.

The differential diagnosis of a fourth ventricular mass in an adult also includes choroid plexus papilloma (see Case 162), glioma, subependymoma, hemangioblastoma, arteriovenous malformation, rare epidermoid tumors, and inflammatory mass or cyst.

The cerebellar vermis causes a normal indentation along the posterior wall or roof of the fourth ventricle (see Case 109 for an example). The gray matter density and contrast enhancement of the vermis can falsely simulate a mass in this location.

CEREBELLAR ASTROCYTOMAS

Case 124

4-year-old girl presenting with nystagmus.
(postcontrast scan)

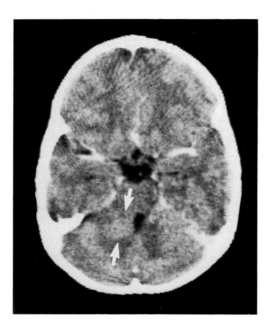

Case 125

5-year-old boy presenting with headache
and papilledema.
(postcontrast scan)

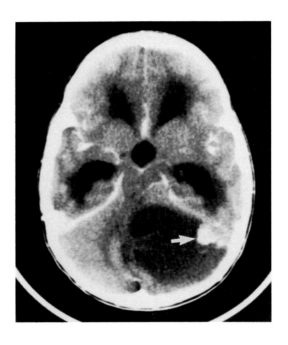

Gliomas of the cerebellum are among the most common posterior fossa tumors in children. These "juvenile cerebellar astrocytomas" often exhibit benign behavior and carry a relatively good prognosis.

The majority of cerebellar astrocytomas are cystic, but solid masses may be seen, as in this case. Low-attenuation tumors sometime prove to be solid lesions with microcystic histology (see Case 161).

Contrast enhancement is variable but usually more prominent than noted here. The lateral compression of the fourth ventricle indicates that the mass has arisen in the brachium pontis or medial cerebellum, in contrast to the midline tumors illustrated in Cases 114 to 118.

Cerebellar astrocytomas may demonstrate an enhancing rim of tissue surrounding the circumference of a cyst. Alternatively, a localized mural nodule may be found along nonenhancing cyst margins, as seen here (arrow).

The cyst may be unilocular or multilocular. Postcontrast MR scans may demonstrate thin, enhancing septations that are inapparent on CT studies. MR scans may also show more extensive enhancement of the cyst wall than is appreciated by CT.

Severe compression of the brain stem is present in this case. (Compare the anteroposterior diameter of the brain stem with that in Cases 106 and 109.) Distortion of the fourth ventricle and aqueduct has caused marked obstructive hydrocephalus, with findings of periventricular edema bordering the distended frontal and temporal horns (see Cases 606 to 608).

CYSTIC CEREBELLAR ASTROCYTOMA MIMICKING DISTENDED FOURTH VENTRICLE

Case 126A

4-year-old girl presenting with hydrocephalus.
(noncontrast scan)

Case 126B

Same patient.
(sagittal, noncontrast scan; SE 700/17)

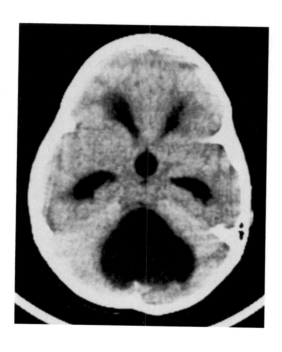

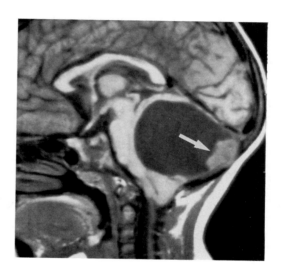

Occasional cerebellar astrocytomas are midline lesions. Solid, enhancing astrocytomas of the vermis may resemble a medulloblastoma or ependymoma. Cystic midline astrocytomas can falsely suggest distention of the fourth ventricle, as in this case. (Such marked enlargement is occasionally seen when the fourth ventricle is "trapped" or "isolated" due to simultaneous outlet obstruction and aqueductal compromise.)

When hydrocephalus is found on CT scans, it is important to carefully examine the third and fourth ventricles to distinguish possible enlargement from an obstructing, low-attenuation lesion (see also Cases 591 to 593).

The postcontrast scan in this case was degraded by motion artifact but did not demonstrate convincing enhancement. As in Case 125, the brain stem is severely compressed by the tumor cyst.

MR is valuable in the evaluation of hydrocephalus and in the assessment of cerebellar masses. Sagittal MR scans define the patency and morphology of the aqueduct and fourth ventricle, demonstrating their relationship to potential midline lesions. Coronal MR (and CT) scans are useful for localizing posterior fossa masses with respect to the fourth ventricle, tentorium, cerebellopontine angles, and foramen magnum (see Cases 52, 53, 129, 130, 162, and 625).

A region of low attenuation resembling CSF on CT studies may demonstrate signal intensity that is different from spinal fluid on an MR examination, as in this case (compare the cyst intensity to the cervical subarachnoid space). In addition, the multiplanar display of MR more easily defines the mural nodule along the posterior margin of this cystic astrocytoma (arrow). (The poorly enhancing mural nodule is seen as a mild indentation along the left posterior border of the tumor cyst on the CT scan in Case 126A.)

This sagittal scan also demonstrates compression of the brain stem (with kinking and occlusion of the aqueduct) and herniation of the cerebellar tonsils.

Case 127

60-year-old man with ataxic gait.

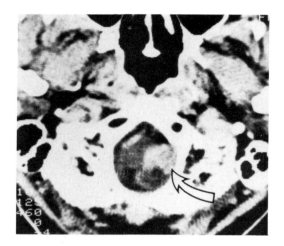

Case 128

45-year-old woman.

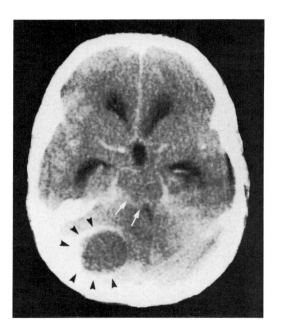

Hemangioblastomas are relatively uncommon tumors of the posterior fossa and spinal cord, usually seen in adults. These masses are often cystic and typically demonstrate an intensely enhancing mural nodule. Hemangioblastomas frequently arise at the pial surface of the cerebellum, as seen here and in Case 128.

Higher scans in this case had disclosed a nonenhancing cerebellar cyst. The associated mural nodule was not apparent until scanning was continued inferiorly through the level of the foramen magnum. The hemangioblastoma nodule *(arrow)* occupies the cerebellar tonsil, displacing the brain stem. (Case 130 presents a coronal scan of this patient.)

Sagittal MR and coronal CT or MR scans are valuable in evaluating the caudal margin of posterior fossa lesions that approach or traverse the foramen magnum (see Cases 149, 150, 161, and 162).

A cystic mass is present in the right cerebellar hemisphere, with a broad crescent of contrast enhancement along the lateral margin *(black arrowheads)*. The fourth ventricle and brain stem are compressed *(white arrows)*, and obstructive hydrocephalus is present.

The differential diagnosis of this mass in an adult would include hemangioblastoma of unusual morphology, cerebellar astrocytoma, metastasis, and atypical lateral medulloblastoma ("cerebellar sarcoma," see Case 133). An angiogram showed the lateral cyst wall to be intensely vascular, and a hemangioblastoma was found at surgery.

In about 20% of cases, cerebellar hemangioblastomas are a manifestation of von Hippel-Lindau disease. This neurocutaneous syndrome may also be associated with retinal angiomas, renal or pancreatic cysts, hypernephromas, pheochromocytomas, and hemangioblastomas of the spinal cord. Funduscopic examination and an IVP (or at least an abdominal x-ray following contrast injection for CT) are warranted when a possible cerebellar hemangioblastoma is discovered.

DIFFERENTIAL DIAGNOSIS:
CYSTIC CEREBELLAR TUMOR WITH A MURAL NODULE

Case 129

31-year-old woman with headache.
(coronal scan)

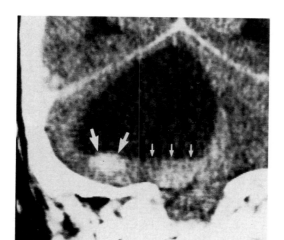

Cystic Cerebellar Astrocytoma.

Case 130

60-year-old man (same patient as Case 127).
(coronal scan)

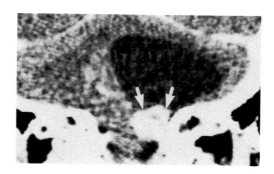

Hemangioblastoma.

Coronal scans define the relationship of the cyst to the mural nodule *(large arrows)* in each case. Case 129 also demonstrates a sedimentation level *(small arrows)*.

The CT appearance of these lesions is indistinguishable, and the diagnoses were made angiographically. The angiogram in Case 129 demonstrated an avascular mass, excluding hemangioblastoma. The angiogram in Case 130 showed the mural nodule to be intensely vascular, which is characteristic of hemangioblastoma. MR can also contribute to this differential diagnosis, since prominent vascular channels are often seen within or surrounding a hemangioblastoma on MR scans.

Angiography or contrast-enhanced MR scans in cases of hemangioblastoma may demonstrate additional small tumors of the cerebellum or cervical spinal cord that are inapparent on CT studies. Multiple hemangioblastomas, particularly involving the brain stem and spinal cord, usually imply von Hippel-Lindau disease.

Case 131

12-year-old girl.

Case 132

39-year-old woman.

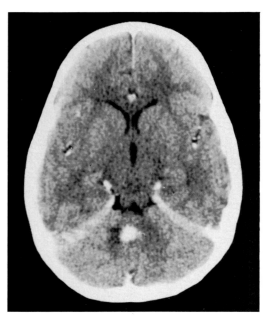

Astrocytoma.

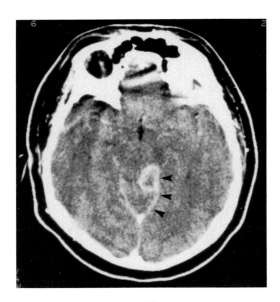

Hemangioblastoma.

Both astrocytomas and hemangioblastomas should be included in the differential diagnosis of focal, enhancing cerebellar lesions. Both tumors can demonstrate solid or peripheral enhancement, as illustrated here and in Cases 124 to 130.

In adults, a cerebellar metastasis is more likely than astrocytoma to mimic hemangioblastoma. The appearance in Case 131 is nonspecific, and a small vascular malformation or inflammatory focus could present a similar morphology.

In Case 132, the location of the lesion medial to the enhancing margin of the tentorium (arrowheads) places it in the posterior fossa. However, it is not clear whether the mass arises from the brain stem, the cerebellum, or the tentorium itself. Coronal and sagittal MR scans demonstrated that the tumor was in fact intra-axial, within the superior vermis. In addition, MR documented prominent vascular channels at the margins of the lesion, suggesting a highly vascular neoplasm. Surgery confirmed a cerebellar hemangioblastoma.

DIFFERENTIAL DIAGNOSIS:
SOLID, ENHANCING MASS IN THE CEREBELLAR HEMISPHERE OF AN ADULT

Case 133

40-year-old man.

Case 134

63-year-old man.

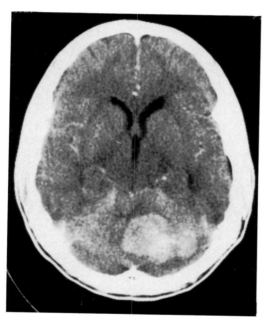

Medulloblastoma.

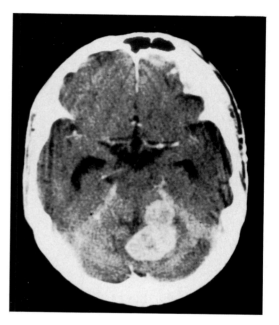

Metastatic Colon Carcinoma.

Medulloblastomas in adults are often hemispheric, as in Case 133. These densely cellular tumors may demonstrate the same homogeneous, precontrast high attenuation and uniform contrast enhancement seen in the fourth ventricular medulloblastomas of children. Hemispheric medulloblastomas are frequently associated with prominent fibrosis and have been called "cerebellar sarcomas."

The uniformly enhancing tumor in Case 133 reached the cerebellar surface adjacent to the tentorium, and a tentorial meningioma (such as Case 53) was also considered in the differential diagnosis. A coronal MR scan demonstrated that the lesion was intra-axial, thereby narrowing the diagnostic possibilities.

Metastasis is the most common etiology for a cerebellar mass in patients beyond young adulthood. Cerebellar metastases may be large, solitary, and solid as in Case 134. A small amount of edema is present medial to the well-defined tumor.

In both Cases 133 and 134, cerebellar mass effect has effaced the quadrigeminal cistern and compresses the dorsal brain stem. Secondary hydrocephalus has developed in Case 134.

A large, solid hemangioblastoma, primary CNS lymphoma, or unusual adult cerebellar astrocytoma could present an appearance similar to these cases.

ACOUSTIC SCHWANNOMAS (NEURINOMAS, "NEUROMAS")

Case 135

75-year-old woman presenting with tinnitus, dizziness, and nausea.

Case 136

24-year-old woman with neurofibromatosis and recent hearing impairment.
(coronal scan)

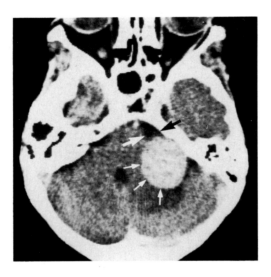

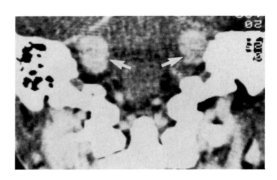

Acoustic schwannomas represent about 10% of primary intracranial tumors and account for the majority of masses in the cerebellopontine angle. They are typically well-defined, uniformly enhancing tumors with smooth, rounded margins. The masses are centered on the midposterior petrous ridge, where they arise near the internal auditory meatus.

Slow growth may allow acoustic schwannomas to gradually invaginate far into the adjacent cerebellum and brain stem (small arrows). However, the extra-axial origin of the mass is usually indicated by contralateral brain stem displacement, causing widening of the ipsilateral cisterns at the margins of the tumor (large arrows; see also Cases 138 and 142).

A small amount of cerebellar edema is seen posterior to the schwannoma.

Here a coronal scan demonstrates well-defined, uniformly enhancing masses arising in the cerebellopontine angles along the midposterior surface of the petrous ridges. Bilateral acoustic schwannomas suggest neurofibromatosis, even if the diagnosis has not been previously apparent.

"Bilateral acoustic neurofibromatosis" (BANF) has now been designated "Type 2 neurofibromatosis" and is clinically and genetically distinct from the more common "Type 1 neurofibromatosis" or von Recklinghausen's disease. In addition to acoustic schwannomas, patients with Type 2 neurofibromatosis may present with multiple cranial meningiomas. Patients with the Type 1 syndrome demonstrate more prominent cutaneous stigmata (e.g., cafe-au-lait spots) and a higher incidence of gliomas, particularly involving the optic pathways (see Cases 689 to 691) and brain stem.

Almost all patients who present with acoustic schwannomas have hearing loss, the presence or absence of which can be of value in the differential diagnosis. On the other hand, less than 5% of patients with unilateral hearing loss are found to have acoustic schwannomas. About three fourths of patients with these tumors experience dysequilibrium and/or tinnitus.

ACOUSTIC SCHWANNOMAS: LOW ATTENUATION AND CYSTS

Case 137

74-year-old man.
(postcontrast scan)

Case 138

70-year-old woman presenting with right facial numbness and a 10-year history of right-sided hearing loss.
(coronal, noncontrast scan; SE 600/17)

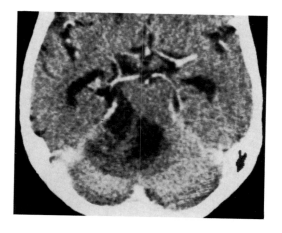

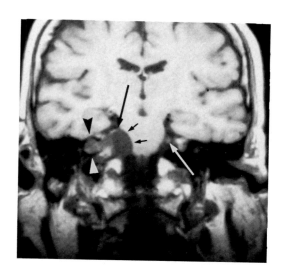

Many acoustic schwannomas have an atypical appearance caused by prominent areas of low attenuation within or adjacent to the tumor. These low-density regions are often cystic, but solid tissue with low attenuation may also occur.

When the bulk of the mass is of low density and nonenhancing, as in this case, the lesion may be confused with an intra-axial tumor extending exophytically into the cerebellopontine angle. Alternatively, a low-attenuation acoustic schwannoma may resemble other low density extra-axial masses (see Cases 239, 626, and 627).

The relationship of the lesion to a widened internal auditory canal may provide the diagnosis. In difficult cases, studies with subarachnoid contrast material can help to separate intra-axial and extra-axial processes. Alternatively, coronal MR scans may be used to identify extra-axial masses adjacent to the brain stem (see Cases 138 and 231).

MR scans are useful in characterizing large cerebellopontine angle masses as well as in detecting small acoustic schwannomas (see Cases 145 and 146).

The solid component of this tumor expands the internal auditory canal (arrowheads) and extends through the porus acusticus. A large cyst is present more medially, deforming the pons (small arrows) and elevating the right fifth cranial nerve (long black arrow; compare to the normal fifth nerve on the left).

Facial numbness due to distortion of the fifth nerve is a common secondary symptom of large acoustic schwannomas.

Case 139

19-year-old woman presenting with hearing loss
and facial numbness.
(wide window)

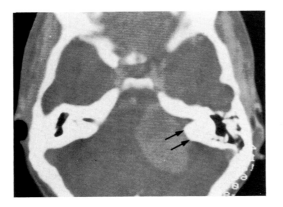

Case 140

69-year-old woman.
(wide window; magnified reconstruction using a
bone algorithm)

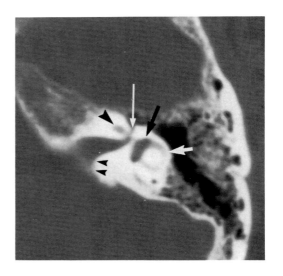

A secondary hallmark of acoustic schwannomas is widening or "flaring" of the internal auditory canal (IAC) from which they arise. The degree of IAC erosion is not necessarily related to the size of the tumor, which may expand exophytically in the adjacent cistern (see Case 145).

In this case, the involved IAC is clearly widened when compared with the contralateral side. The canal is also shortened, due to erosion of the posterior lip of the internal auditory meatus (arrows).

The large cerebellopontine angle mass is faintly seen at this window width and appears centered on the widened internal auditory meatus. This relationship of an enhancing mass to an expanded IAC is useful in distinguishing acoustic schwannomas from meningiomas or aneurysms of the cerebellopontine angle, which rarely cause widening of the canal.

Facial numbness reflects distortion of the fifth cranial nerve by large acoustic schwannomas. The seventh cranial nerve is resistant to compressive dysfunction, and facial paresis rarely accompanies eighth nerve tumors.

Details of anatomy and pathology within the petrous bone are well demonstrated on magnified scans performed with algorithms that emphasize the spatial resolution of high-contrast structures. This scan provides a closer look than Case 139 at the typical bone erosion caused by an acoustic schwannoma. Again, the medial portion of the IAC is widened or "flared," and the posterior lip of the internal auditory meatus is eroded (small black arrowheads) causing shortening of the posterior wall.

Medial "flaring" of the IAC can be a normal variant that is usually bilaterally symmetrical, so comparison to the contralateral petrous bone is warranted in cases of suspected acoustic schwannoma. Care must be taken to examine scans at exactly identical levels on both sides; a difference of a few millimeters in slice location can dramatically alter the apparent morphology of the IAC. Coronal CT or MR scans may be helpful in equivocal cases.

Normal anatomical landmarks visible in this case include the vestibule (black arrow), lateral semicircular canal (short white arrow), a small portion of the cochlea (large black arrowhead), and the facial nerve canal between the IAC and the geniculate ganglion (long white arrow).

Case 141

81-year-old woman with hearing loss.
(intermediate window width)

Case 142

57-year-old woman with hearing loss.
(intermediate window width)

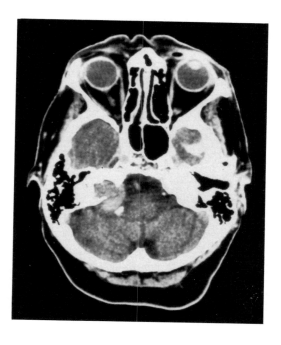

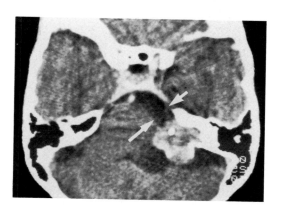

In contrast to the typically smooth widening of the IAC caused by most acoustic schwannomas, some eighth nerve tumors are associated with very irregular erosion of the petrous bone. Such lobulated bone destruction, as in this case, may suggest a more aggressive lesion of the skull base (see Cases 151, 153, 154, and 157). The geographic center of the mass at the IAC and the usual clinical association with long-standing hearing loss support the correct diagnosis.

The expansion of the internal auditory canal caused by this acoustic schwannoma is markedly irregular, matching the lobulated contour of the cisternal mass. The brain stem has been displaced, with prominent widening of the ipsilateral cisterns *(arrows)*. An area of low attenuation medial to the enhancing mass may represent edema and/or a low attenuation component of the tumor.

"Cysts" are frequently seen adjacent to enhancing components of acoustic schwannomas. These fluid collections are often found to be loculations of CSF surrounded by thickened arachnoid membranes rather than tumor cysts enclosed by neoplastic tissue.

Case 143

54-year-old woman with hearing loss.
(decubitus scan with nose to the reader's right)

Case 144

58-year-old man with a 10-year history
of impaired hearing.
(decubitus scan with nose to the reader's right)

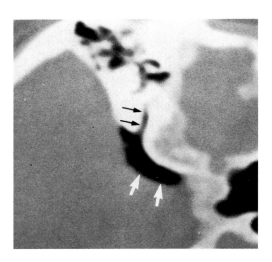

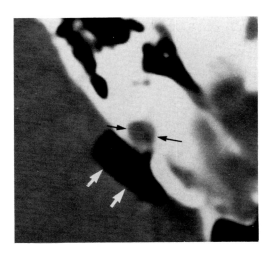

A standard scan may fail to define small acoustic schwannomas, particularly those confined to the internal auditory canal. When initial scans are negative and the clinical suspicion of acoustic schwannoma is strong, the possibility of an intracanalicular tumor is raised.

Such lesions can be better imaged by CT after a few cubic centimeters of gas are injected via a lumbar puncture and maneuvered into the cerebellopontine angle *(white arrows)*. The head is turned to a decubitus position, so that gas in the cistern should rise into the adjacent internal auditory canal. Even small canals will normally fill with gas as in this case *(black arrows)*, thereby excluding an intracanalicular schwannoma. (It is important to image the middle of the IAC with thin sections to avoid the misleading density of partial volume.)

Here the cerebellopontine angle cistern is filled with gas *(white arrows)*. The air fails to enter the widened internal auditory canal *(black arrows)* because it is occupied by a soft tissue mass. The mass was surgically proved to be a small, intracanalicular acoustic schwannoma.

Such tumors may cause more symptoms due to intracanalicular nerve compression than much larger schwannomas growing freely in the cerebellopontine angle.

Contrast-enhanced MR scans provide a less invasive means for detecting intracanalicular acoustic schwannomas, as illustrated in Cases 145 and 146.

USE OF CONTRAST-ENHANCED MR FOR DETECTION OF INTRACANALICULAR ACOUSTIC SCHWANNOMAS

Case 145

67-year-old woman.
(axial, post-contrast scan; SE 600/20)

Case 146

46-year-old man with hearing loss.
(axial, postcontrast scan; SE 600/15)

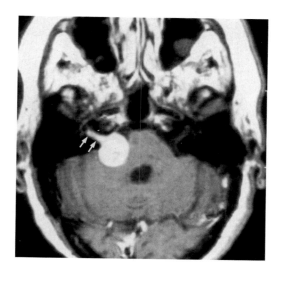

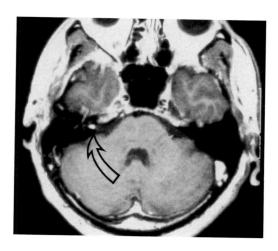

The absence of artifact from the petrous bones on MR scans allows direct visualization of the internal auditory canal. The spinal fluid and neurovascular structures within the canal generate higher signal intensity than the surrounding cortical bone, with an increasingly "bright" appearance as T2-weighting is increased. Intracanalicular components of acoustic schwannomas can sometimes be identified as soft tissue masses within the IAC on noncontrast MR images, but such scans are not reliable for excluding these tumors.

Acoustic schwannomas typically demonstrate intense contrast enhancement on MR exams as on CT studies. The detection of small eighth nerve tumors is an important indication for the use of contrast material in MR procedures. This case demonstrates the common appearance of a bulbous cisternal schwannoma in continuity with a stem or pedicle of enhancement occupying the minimally expanded IAC (arrows). The mass is centered at the internal auditory meatus and has invaginated far into the pons and brachium pontis. Cisternal widening is seen anterior to the lesion.

Contrast-enhanced MR scans can define intracanalicular acoustic schwannomas measuring only a few millimeters in diameter, as in this case (arrow). This technique is less invasive and more reliable than air-contrast CT cisternography as illustrated in Cases 143 and 144.

Contrast enhancement within the IAC on MR studies is not specific for acoustic schwannoma. Hemangiomas or inflammation of the facial nerve can present a similar appearance. Meningeal disease (e.g., carcinomatosis or sarcoidosis) can extend into the IAC with associated abnormal enhancement. Finally, reactive meningeal changes following surgery to remove a schwannoma can lead to intracanalicular enhancement, so postoperative scans must be interpreted cautiously.

DIFFERENTIAL DIAGNOSIS:
SMALL, ROUND, DENSE TISSUE IN THE CEREBELLOPONTINE ANGLE

Case 147

76-year-old woman.
(noncontrast scan)

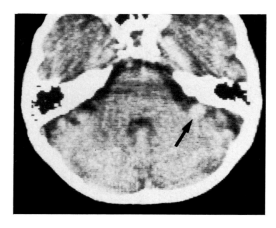

Normal Flocculus.

Case 148

66-year-old man.
(postcontrast scan)

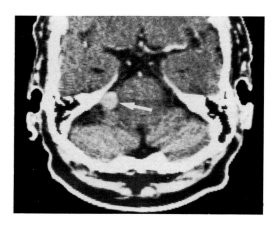

Acoustic Schwannoma.

The flocculus of the cerebellum forms a nodule along its lateral surface near the IAC. When seen in cross section on axial scans, this rounded density (*arrow,* Case 147) may mimic a small acoustic schwannoma.

The flocculus does not enhance as prominently as the usual acoustic schwannoma (Case 148), and there is no associated widening of the IAC. In addition, the location of the flocculus is posterior to the IAC. Coronal CT or MR scans will clarify the anatomy if axial views are confusing.

The "pseudotumor" of the flocculus in the cerebellopontine angle cistern is comparable to the "pseudotumor" of the vermis indenting the posterior fourth ventricle, as discussed in Cases 122 and 123. In both instances a nodular contour of normal anatomy combines with the mildly increased attenuation and contrast enhancement of gray matter to simulate a lesion.

DIFFERENTIAL DIAGNOSIS:
UNIFORMLY ENHANCING, EXTRA-AXIAL POSTERIOR FOSSA MASS

Case 149

76-year-old woman with a 4-month history of
poor balance.
(coronal scan)

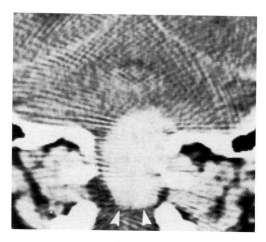

Foramen Magnum Meningioma.

Case 150

75-year-old woman presenting with dizziness
and tinnitus.
(coronal scan)

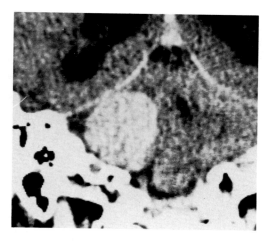

Acoustic Schwannoma.

The CT features of meningiomas and acoustic schwannomas may be very similar. However, most posterior fossa meningiomas are centered above or below the internal auditory meatus, and few are associated with widening of the IAC (or hearing loss). Cerebellopontine angle meningiomas typically have a broader base against the petrous bone than acoustic schwannomas. Meningiomas may also demonstrate precontrast high attenuation, which is unusual in eighth nerve tumors.

Coronal CT or MR views help to define the location of a cerebellopontine angle mass. Coronal scans (and/or sagittal scans or reconstructions) are also valuable for evaluating foramen magnum lesions (see Cases 161 and 162). In Case 149, the meningioma is seen to extend from the posterior fossa through the plane of C1 to the level of C2 *(arrowheads)*.

Aneurysms of the vertebral or basilar arteries may appear as dense, enhancing extra-axial masses. They should be included in this differential diagnosis (see Case 538), along with glomus jugulare tumors (see Case 151) and rare jugular foramen schwannomas and choroid plexus papillomas.

Case 151A

33-year-old woman with tongue weakness.
(wide window)

Case 151B

Same patient.
(postcontrast scan)

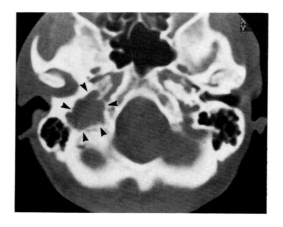

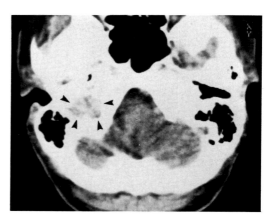

Glomus tumors ("chemodectomas," "paragangliomas") originate from paraganglionic cells in numerous locations, including the carotid sinus ("carotid body tumor"), jugular bulb ("glomus jugulare"), and middle ear ("glomus tympanicum").

Although most of these neoplasms are histologically benign, they may be locally invasive. Associated bone erosion is often irregular and poorly defined, suggesting malignancy. In this case, a large area of bone destruction at the right jugular foramen *(arrowheads)* demonstrates typically indistinct margins.

A large jugular foramen is a common normal variant, particularly on the right side. In association with a prominently enhancing sigmoid sinus, this appearance may simulate a glomus tumor. The bony margins of normally large foramena are usually more smoothly rounded and better defined than the erosive appearance seen with glomus tumors. MR scans often help to evaluate ambiguous cases.

Glomus tumors are highly vascular with prominent contrast enhancement. Here the enhancing mass fills the bone defect demonstrated in Case 151A.

Glomus jugulare tumors may span the skull base, with posterior fossa and extracranial components. Coronal CT scans (or MR studies; see Case 152) provide a useful composite view of these intracranial and extracranial extensions.

A glomus jugulare tumor growing into the cerebellopontine angle may resemble other enhancing extra-axial lesions at this site (e.g., meningioma, acoustic schwannoma, aneurysm; see Cases 149, 150, and 538). However, associated erosion of the jugular foramen usually indicates the diagnosis.

Glomus tumors are multiple in about 3% of spontaneous cases and about 25% of familial cases.

MR CORRELATION: GLOMUS JUGULARE TUMORS

Case 152A

70-year-old woman.
(sagittal, noncontrast scan; SE 800/16)

Case 152B

Same patient.
(coronal, noncontrast scan; SE 1000/16)

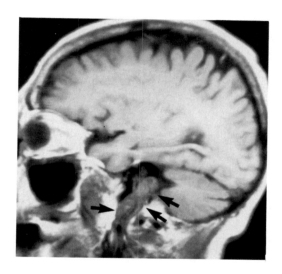

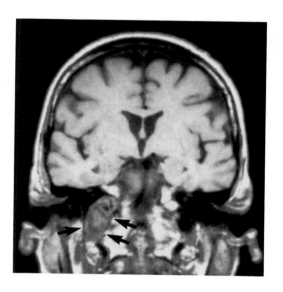

The presence of bone erosion and a mass at the jugular foramen can be difficult to judge on axial CT or MR studies. In such cases, coronal and sagittal MR scans may convincingly demonstrate a tumor while defining its extracranial extension.

The jugular foramen lies along the posterior margin of the midpetrous bone, just posterior and inferior to the internal auditory canal. In this case the region of the foramen is expanded and filled with the intensity of soft tissue rather than the signal void of flowing blood *(arrows)*. The tumor is seen to extend below the skull base, involving the cervical portion of the internal jugular vein.

MR scans performed with motion-refocusing pulse sequences, after contrast injection, or in circumstances of slow jugular flow may normally demonstrate isointense or high signal within the jugular vein, which should not be misinterpreted as evidence of tumor.

The large glomus jugulare tumor spanning the skull base is well demonstrated in coronal projection *(arrows)*. Within the lesion are punctate and tubular areas of low signal intensity, which likely represent flow-related signal loss in prominent vessels of the highly vascular mass. The resultant "salt and pepper" texture of the tumor (which is more prominent on long TR images) may be a helpful clue to the etiology of a jugular foramen lesion, distinguishing glomus tumors from other possibilities such as schwannomas, meningiomas, metastases, or aneurysms.

Angiography in this case demonstrated an intense tissue stain corresponding exactly to the soft tissue mass on these images.

DIFFERENTIAL DIAGNOSIS:
LESION DESTROYING BONE ALONG THE FLOOR OF THE POSTERIOR FOSSA

Case 153

83-year-old woman presenting with occipital headache.

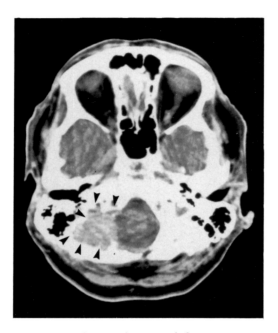

Metastatic Carcinoma of the Breast.

Case 154

79-year-old woman presenting with neck pain, left sixth and seventh cranial nerve palsies, and hyperreflexia.

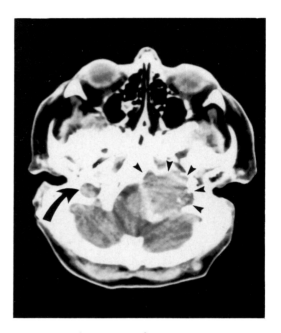

Glomus Jugulare Tumor.

Both of these scans demonstrate soft tissue masses causing aggressive bone destruction at the inferior margin of the posterior fossa. In an elderly patient the possibility of metastasis (as in Case 153) should be considered whenever a lesion is encountered within the skull base. Myeloma and lymphoma should be included in the differential diagnosis. Occasionally direct invasion of the skull base by carcinomas arising in the nasopharynx or parotid gland can cause a similar appearance (see Case 155).

The large glomus jugulare tumor in Case 154 looks nearly as aggressive as the malignancy in Case 153. A clue to the correct diagnosis is the location of the lesion, centered at the expected site of the jugular foramen (compare to the normal contralateral jugular foramen; *curved arrow*). Symptoms in this case are due to compression of the brain stem in addition to distortion of cranial nerves as they pass through the cerebellopontine angle and petrous bone.

Chordoma and chondroma or chondrosarcoma should also be considered as causes of irregular destruction at the skull base. Both lesions more frequently involve the sphenooccipital region (see Cases 157 and 158). Other tumors of bony origin (e.g., osteoblastoma, aneurysmal bone cyst, primary petrous epidermoid tumor, cholesterol granuloma of the petrous apex) usually have a less aggressive appearance than seen in these cases, with smooth margins of well-defined bone erosion (see Cases 156, 160, and 812).

DIFFERENTIAL DIAGNOSIS:
INHOMOGENEOUS EXTRA-AXIAL LESION EXTENDING FROM THE PETROUS BONE

Case 155

68-year-old woman.

Case 156

13-year-old boy.

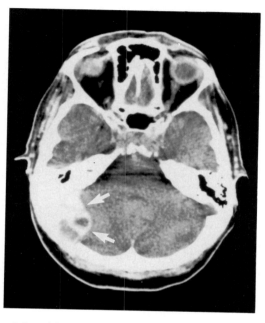

Adenoid Cystic Carcinoma of the Parotid Gland Invading the Skull Base.

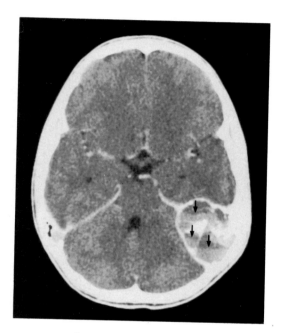

Aneurysmal Bone Cyst.

Benign and malignant tumors of the skull base should be considered in the differential diagnosis of extra-axial lesions in the posterior (or middle) cranial fossa.

In addition to hematogenous metastasis as illustrated in Case 153, the skull base and posterior fossa can be involved by direct extension of carcinoma as in Case 155 (compare to the middle fossa involvement in Case 38). Such extension can reflect direct bony invasion or perineural growth of parapharyngeal neoplasms traversing basal foramina.

The large nonenhancing components of the mass in Case 155 would be unusual for a glomus tumor. Such cystic or necrotic regions are common within malignant neoplasms. The sharp medial definition of the mass *(arrows)* suggests that it remains extradural, which was confirmed at surgery.

Aneurysmal bone cysts are benign lesions that occasionally involve the skull. Their radiographic hallmark is expansion of bone, often with thin residual shells of cortex demonstrating a multiloculated or "bubbly" pattern. The large, blood-filled chambers characteristically found within these lesions are well demonstrated by CT or MR, with sedimentation levels of blood products as seen in Case 156 *(arrows)*.

The aneurysmal bone cyst in Case 156 has expanded superiorly from its petrous origin, bulging into the middle and posterior fossae. The benign, extra-axial nature of the process is suggested by the well-defined margins of expanded bone, dense central calcification, and the absence of reactive edema.

CHORDOMAS

Case 157

24-year-old man.
(wide window)

Clivus Chordoma.

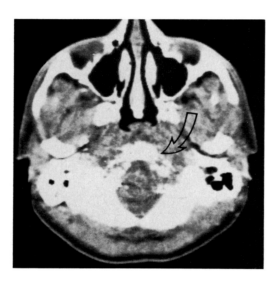

Case 158

24-year-old woman.
(wide window)

Parasellar Chordoma.

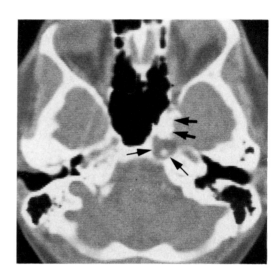

Among the skull base lesions that may involve the posterior fossa are chordomas of the spheno-occipital region. Chordomas arise from remnants of the primitive notochord and are most frequently found in the clivus (35%) or sacrum (50%).

Clivus chordomas may appear as calcified masses projecting intracranially from an intact skull base. Such tumors may mimic a clivus meningioma.

Most chordomas have a more destructive appearance, as illustrated by the permeation in this case. Large soft-tissue components may expand intracranially or into the nasopharynx (see Case 159).

Chordomas may also originate in the parasellar region, appearing as a calcified mass that mimics parasellar meningioma or aneurysm (see Cases 540 and 541). In this case, an area of bone destruction at the petrous apex *(thin arrows)* is associated with dense calcification more anteriorly *(thick arrows)*.

Chondromas are rare tumors of the skull base. Their appearance on CT scans (and skull x-rays) may resemble that of chordoma, with a mixture of lytic and calcified components.

MR CORRELATION: CHORDOMAS

Case 159A

5-year-old girl.
(sagittal, noncontrast scan; SE 700/16)

Case 159B

Same patient.
(axial, noncontrast scan; SE 2500/90)

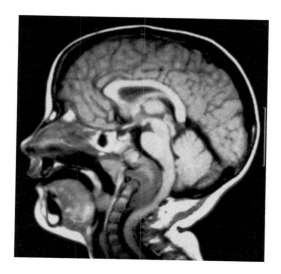

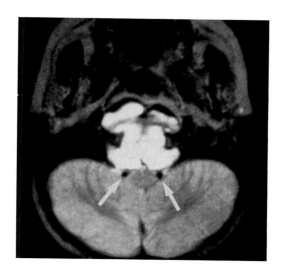

The midsagittal display of MR scans offers excellent visualization of the clivus, pharynx, and foramen magnum, all of which are commonly involved by chordomas of the skull base.

In this case a large soft tissue mass has arisen from the caudal aspect of the clivus. The tumor has grown inferiorly to occupy the ventral two-thirds of the foramen magnum and cervical spinal canal. There is marked posterior displacement and distortion of the cervicomedullary junction.

Prominent nasopharyngeal soft tissue is present. This finding can be a normal variant in children due to hypertrophy of lymphoid structures (i.e., adenoids). Axial scans such as Case 159B help to define components of pharyngeal tumor in cases where the possibility exists.

Occasional chordomas demonstrate short T1 components, presumably reflecting hemorrhage or mucinous content.

Chordomas typically demonstrate very high signal intensity on T2-weighted MR scans due to the long T2 of the tumor matrix. (The "chondroid" subtype of chordomas may have relatively lower signal intensity on long TR images.) Masses are often lobulated and septated, with scalloped margins. The combination of these features in a lesion of the skull base is highly suggestive of chordoma.

In this case the clivus has been completely replaced by tumor, which is symmetrically centered in the midline. The posterior fossa component of the lesion causes posterior displacement of the "flow-voids" within the distal vertebral arteries *(arrows)*. A shallower component of tumor extends anteriorly, causing ventral displacement of overlying nasopharyngeal tissue.

Case 160A

47-year-old man.
(axial, postcontrast scan; SE 600/20)

Primary Epidermoid Cyst.

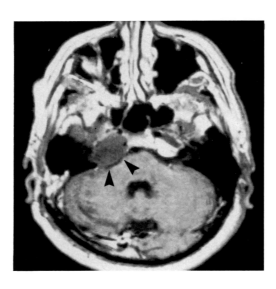

Case 160B

Same patient.
(axial, noncontrast scan; SE 3000/90)

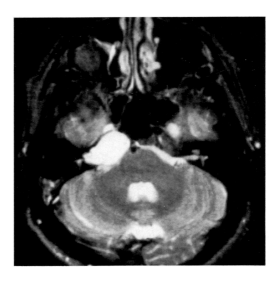

Magnetic resonance imaging is of value in evaluating skull-base lesions involving the IAC, jugular foramen, and clivus (see Cases 145, 152, and 159). In addition, MR can provide important information about pathology near the petrous apex.

A number of tumors arising in the posterior or middle fossa can span and erode the petrous apex, as discussed in Cases 50 and 51. Tumors arising within the petrous bone itself present a different differential diagnosis.

Metastatic disease is an important consideration in adults with pathology at this site. The lack of contrast enhancement (and the well-defined margins of the lesion) argues against metastasis in this case.

Cholesterol "granulomas" or "cholesterol cysts" commonly occur in the petrous bone, arising from chronic hemorrhage into an obstructed air cell. These long-standing, benign lesions are often expansile. They characteristically demonstrate T1-shortening (due to blood products), which is absent in this case.

Schwannomas and meningiomas causing bone erosion at the petrous apex would be expected to demonstrate contrast enhancement.

The correct diagnosis of primary epidermoid cyst is suggested by the appearance of a well-defined, expansile lesion lacking T1-shortening and contrast enhancement.

Like intracranial epidermoid cysts (see Case 241), primary epidermoid lesions of the petrous bone usually demonstrate signal intensity resembling that of CSF. This mass contains uniformly high signal, matching that of spinal fluid.

An eccentric skull base chordoma could present a similar appearance (see Case 159B). Other lesions in the differential diagnosis include schwannoma and mucocele. Aneurysms arising from the petrous segment of the internal carotid artery should also be considered as a cause of bone erosion in this region; such lesions are usually characterized by a combination of "flow void" and laminated thrombus (see Cases 542 to 545).

This lesion extends from the internal auditory canal to Meckel's cave (compare to the normal landmarks on the left). The clinical presentation of such long-standing petrous masses can correspondingly involve cranial nerves 5 through 8.

Case 161

2-year-old girl.
(sagittal, noncontrast scan; SE 700/17)

Astrocytoma of the Medulla and Spinal Cord.

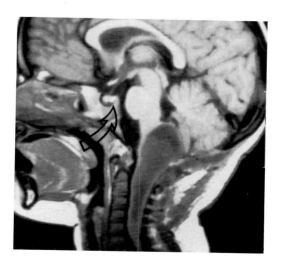

Case 162

46-year-old woman.
(coronal, noncontrast scan; SE 700/16)

Choroid Plexus Papilloma of the Fourth Ventricle.

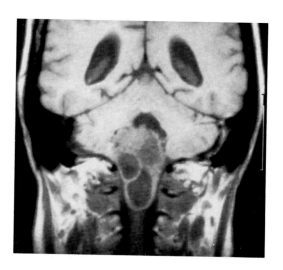

As illustrated by other cases in this chapter, MR exceeds the ability of CT to demonstrate pathology that spans the craniocervical junction. Since many posterior fossa lesions may extend caudally through the foramen magnum, MR has a key role in assessing such patients.

Gliomas of the medulla are often exophytic, laterally or dorsally. The tumor in this case bulges posteriorly into the vallecula, deforming the caudal fourth ventricle. In addition, the mass extends well into the cervical spinal cord, a feature that was poorly demonstrated on CT scans.

The homogeneous signal intensity of the lesion does not imply a cystic tumor. At surgery this astrocytoma was solid with gelatinous consistency.

This case is a good example of the normal "bright spot" in the posterior portion of the sella turcica representing the neurohypophysis (*arrow*; compare to Case 187).

The CT scan in this case had demonstrated a densely calcified mass at the caudal end of the fourth ventricle (see Case 233 for a comparable lesion). Because of artifact from the bony margins of the foramen magnum, no soft tissue or cystic portions of the mass were apparent. There was no evidence of extension below the skull base.

The MR study shows a lesion with two components. The superior half of the tumor deforms the fourth ventricle and correlates with the CT scan. Dense calcification on CT is reflected as a mild reduction in signal intensity on MR.

MR shows the caudal half of the tumor to be a bilocular cyst extending into the cervical spinal canal. This component was inapparent on the patient's CT scan, again demonstrating the superiority of MR for evaluation of lesions involving or traversing the skull base.

REFERENCES: CT

1. Bilaniuk L.T., Zimmerman R.A., Littman P., et al.: Computed tomography of brain stem gliomas in children. *Radiology* 134:89–95, 1980.
2. Bird C.R., Hasso A.N., Drayer B.P., et al.: The cerebellopontine angle and internal auditory canal: Neurovascular anatomy on gas CT cisternograms. *Radiology* 154:667–670, 1985.
3. Braun J., Guilbura J.N., Borovich B., et al.: Occipital aneurysmal bone cyst: CT findings. *J. Comput. Assist. Tomogr.* 11:880–883, 1987.
4. Daniels D.L., Haughton V.M., Williams A.L., et al.: The flocculus in computed tomography. *A.J.N.R.* 2:227–229, 1981.
5. Disbro M.A., Harnsberger H.R., Osborn A.G.: Peripheral facial nerve dysfunction: CT evaluation. *Radiology* 155:659–664, 1985.
6. Dubois P.J., Drayer B.P., Bank W.O., et al.: An evaluation of current diagnostic radiologic modalities in the investigation of acoustic neurilemmoma. *Radiology* 126:173–179, 1978.
7. Duffner P.K., Klein D.M., Cohen M.E.: Calcification in brain stem gliomas. *Neurology* 28:832–834, 1978.
8. Enzmann D.R., Norman D., Levin V., et al.: Computed tomography in the follow-up of medulloblastomas and ependymomas. *Radiology* 128:67–73, 1978.
9. Ganti S.R., Silver A.J., Hilal S.K., et al.: Computed tomography of cerebellar hemangioblastomas. *J. Comput. Assist. Tomogr.* 6:912–919, 1982.
10. Glanz S., Geehr R.B., Duncan C.C., et al.: Metrizamide-enhanced CT for evaluation of brain stem tumors. *A.J.N.R.* 1:31–35, 1980.
11. Hubbard J.L., Scheithauer B.W., Kispert D.B., et al.: Adult cerebellar medulloblastomas: The pathological, radiographic, and clinical disease spectrum. *J. Neurosurg.* 70:536–544, 1989.
12. Johnson D.W.: Air cisternography of the cerebellopontine angle using high resolution computed tomography. *Radiology* 151:401–403, 1984.
13. Kelly W.M., Harsh G.R. IV: CT of petrous carotid aneurysms. *A.J.N.R.* 6:830–832, 1985.
14. Krol G., Sundaresan H., Deck M.: Computed tomography of axial chordomas. *J. Comput. Assist. Tomogr.* 7:286–289, 1983.
15. Latack J.T., Graham M.D., Kemink J.L., Knake J.E.: Giant cholesterol cysts of the petrous apex: Radiologic features. *A.J.N.R.* 6:409–414, 1985.
16. Lee Y.Y., Glass J.P., Van Eys J., Wallace S.: Medulloblastoma in infants and children: Computed tomographic follow-up after treatment. *Radiology* 154:677–682, 1985.
17. Lo W.W.M., Horn K.L., Carberry J.N., et al.: Intratemporal vascular tumors: Evaluation with CT. *Radiology* 159:181–186, 1986.
18. Lo W.W.M., Solti-Bohman L.G., Brackmann D.E., Gruskin P.: Cholesterol granulomas of the petrous apex: CT diagnosis. *Radiology* 153:705–711, 1984.
19. Mawad M.E., Silver A.J., Hilal S.K., et al.: Computed tomography of the brain stem with intrathecal metrazamide. II. Lesions in and around the brain stem. *A.J.N.R.* 4:13–19, 1983.
20. Meyer J.E., Oot R.F., Lindfors K.K.: CT appearance of clival chordomas. *J. Comput. Assist. Tomogr.* 10:34–38, 1986.
21. Möller A., Hatam A., Olivecrona H.: Diagnosis of acoustic neuroma with computed tomography. *Neuroradiology* 17:25–30, 1978.
22. Möller A., Hatam A., Olivecrona H.: The differential diagnosis of pontine angle meningioma and acoustic neuroma with computed tomography. *Neuroradiology* 17:21–23, 1978.
23. Naidich T.P., Lin J.P., Leeds N.E., et al.: Primary tumors and other masses of the cerebellum and fourth ventricle. *Neuroradiology* 14:153–174, 1977.
24. North C., Segall H.D., Stanley P., et al.: Early CT detection of intracranial seeding from medulloblastoma. *A.J.N.R.* 6:11–14, 1985.
25. Phelps P.D., Lloyd E.A.: High resolution air CT meatography: The demonstration of normal and abnormal structures in the cerebellopontine cistern and internal auditory meatus. *Br. J. Radiol.* 55:19–22, 1982.
26. Pinto R.S., Kricheff I.I., Bergeron R.T., et al.: Small acoustic neuromas: Detection by high resolution gas CT cisternography. *A.J.N.R.* 3:283–286, 1982.
27. Sandhu A., Kendall B.: Computed tomography in the management of medulloblastomas. *Neuroradiology* 29:444, 1987.
28. Seeger J.F., Burke D.P., Knake J.E., et al.: Computed tomographic and angiographic evaluation of hemangioblastomas. *Radiology* 138:65–73, 1981.
29. Segall H.D., Zee C.S., Naidich T.P., et al.: Computed tomography in neoplasms of the posterior fossa in children. *Radiol. Clin. North Am.* 20:237–253, 1982.
30. Shaffer K.A.: Computed tomography of the temporal bone. *Radiographics* 1:62–72, 1981.
31. Solti-Bohman L.G., Magaram D.L., Lo W.W., et al.: Gas-CT cisternography for detection of small acoustic nerve tumors. *Radiology* 150:403–407, 1984.
32. Stroink A.R., Hoffman H.J., Hendrick E.B., et al.: Transependymal benign dorsally exophytic brain stem gliomas in children: Diagnosis and treatment recommendations. *Neurosurgery* 20:439–444, 1987.
33. Stroink A.R., Hoffman H.J., Hendrick E.B.: Diagnosis and management of pediatric brain stem gliomas. *J. Neurosurg.* 65:745–750, 1986.
34. Swartz J.D., Zimmerman R.A., Bilaniuk L.T.: Computed tomography of intracranial ependymomas. *Radiology* 143:97–101, 1982.
35. Tanohata K., Maehara T., Aida N., et al.: Computed tomography of intracranial chondroma with emphasis on delayed contrast enhancement. *J. Comput. Assist. Tomogr.* 11:820–823, 1987.
36. Taylor S.: The petrous temporal bone (including the cerebellopontine angle). *Radiol. Clin. North Am.* 20:67–86, 1982.
37. Zee C.S., Segall H.D., Miller C., et al.: Less common CT features of medulloblastoma. *Radiology* 144:97–102, 1982.
38. Zimmerman R.A., Bilaniuk L.T., Pahlajani H.: Spectrum of medulloblastomas demonstrated by computed tomography. *Radiology* 126:137–141, 1978.
39. Zimmerman R.A., Bilaniuk L.T., Bruno L., et al.: Computed tomography of cerebellar astrocytoma. *A.J.R.* 130:929–933, 1980.

REFERENCES: MR

1. Anderson R.E., Laskoff J.M.: Ramsay Hunt syndrome mimicking intracanalicular acoustic neuroma on contrast-enhanced MR. *A.J.N.R.* 11:409, 1990.
2. Barkovich A.J., Wippold F.J., Sherman J.L., Citrin C.M.: Significance of cerebellar tonsillar position on MR. *A.J.N.R.* 7:795–800, 1986.
3. Brown R.V., Sage M.R., Brophy B.P.: CT and MR findings in patients with chordomas of the petrous apex. *A.J.N.R.* 11:121–124, 1990.
4. Byrne J.V., Kendall B.E., Kingsley D.P.E., et al.: Lesions of the brain stem: Assessment by magnetic resonance imaging. *Neuroradiology* 31:129, 1989.
5. Curati W.L., Graif M., Kingsley D.P.E., et al.: Acoustic neuromas: Gd-DTPA enhancement in MR imaging. *Radiology* 158:447–452, 1986.
6. Daniels D.L., Czervionke L.F., Millen S.J., et al.: MR imaging of facial nerve enhancement in Bell's palsy or after temporal bone surgery. *Radiology* 171:807–810, 1989.
7. Daniels D.L., Millen S.J., Meyer G.A., et al.: MR detection of tumor in the internal auditory canal. *A.J.N.R.* 8:249–252, 1987.
8. Elster A.D., Arthur D.W.: Intracranial hemangioblastomas: CT and MR findings. *J. Comput. Assist. Tomogr.* 12:736–739, 1988.
9. Enzmann D.R., O'Donohue J.: Optimizing MR imaging for detecting small tumors in the cerebellopontine angle and internal auditory canals. *A.J.N.R.* 8:99–106, 1987.
10. Filling-Katz M.R., Choyke P.L., Patronaus N.J., et al.: Radiologic screening for von Hippel-Lindau disease: The role of Gd-DTPA-enhanced MR imaging of CNS. *J. Comput. Assist. Tomogr.* 13:743–755, 1989.
11. Gentry L.R., Jacoby C.G., Turski P.A., et al.: Cerebellopontine angle-retromastoid mass lesions: Comparative study of diagnosis with MR imaging and CT. *Radiology* 162:513–520, 1987.
12. Greenberg J.J., Oot R.F., Wismer G.L., et al.: Cholesterol granulomas of the petrous apex: MR and CT evaluation. *A.J.N.R.* 9:1205–1214, 1988.
13. Griffin C., DeLaPaz R., Enzmann D.: MR and CT correlation of cholesterol cysts of the petrous bone. *A.J.N.R.* 8:825–830, 1987.
14. Hutchins L.G., Harnsberger H.R., Hardin C.W., et al.: The radiological assessment of trigeminal neuropathy. *A.J.N.R.* 10:1031–1038, 1989.
15. Lee B.C.P., Kneeland J.B., Walker R.W., et al.: MR imaging of brain stem tumors. *A.J.N.R.* 6:159–164, 1985.
16. Lee S.R., Sanches J., Mark A.S., et al.: Posterior fossa hemangioblastoma: MR imaging. *Radiology* 171:463–468, 1989.
17. Mikhael M.A., Ciric I.S., Wolff A.P.: MR diagnosis of acoustic neuromas. *J. Comput. Assist. Tomogr.* 11:232–235, 1987.
18. Mikhael M.A., Ciric I.S., Wolff A.P.: Differentiation of cerebellopontine angle neuromas and meningiomas with MR imaging. *J. Comput. Assist. Tomogr.* 9:852–856, 1985.
19. New P.F.J., Bachow T.B., Wismer G.L., et al.: MR imaging of acoustic nerve and small acoustic neuromas at 0.6T: Prospective study. *A.J.N.R.* 6:165–170, 1985.
20. Olsen W.L., Dillon W.P., Kelly W.M. et al.: MR imaging of paragangliomas. *A.J.N.R.* 7:1039–1042, 1986.
21. Oot R.F., Melville G.E., New P.F.J., et al.: The role of MR and CT in evaluating clival chordomas and chondrosarcomas. *A.J.N.R.* 9:715–724, 1988.
22. Press G.A., Hesselink J.R.: MR imaging of cerebellopontine angle and internal auditory canal lesions at 1.5T. *A.J.N.R.* 9:241–252, 1988.
23. Raffel C., McComb J.G., Bodner S., Gilles F.E.: Benign brain stem lesions in pediatric patients with neurofibromatosis: Case reports. *Neurosurgery* 25:959–964, 1989.
24. Remley K.B., Coit W.E., Harnsberger H.R., et al.: Pulsatile tinnitus and the vascular tympanic membrane: CT, MR, and angiographic findings. *Radiology* 174:383–390, 1990.
25. Rollins N., Mendelsohn D., Mulne A., et al.: Recurrent medulloblastoma: Frequency of tumor enhancement on Gd-DTPA MR images. *A.J.N.R.* 11:583–588, 1990.
26. Sen C.N., Sekhar L.N., Schramm V.L., et al.: Chordoma and chondrosarcoma of the cranial base: An 8-year experience. *Neurosurgery* 25:931–41, 1989.
27. Sze G., Uichanco L.S., Brant-Zawadzki M., et al.: Chordomas: MR imaging. *Radiology* 166:187–192, 1988.
28. Tien R.D., Dillon W.P.: Herpes trigeminal neuritis and rhombencephalitis on Gd-DTPA-enhanced MR imaging. *A.J.N.R.* 11:413, 1990.
29. Tien R.O., Dillon W.P., Jackler R.K.: Contrast-enhanced MR imaging of the facial nerve in 11 patients with Bell's palsy. *A.J.N.R.* 11:735–741, 1990.
30. Valvassori G.E., Morales F.G., Palacios E., Dobben G.E.: MR of the normal and abnormal internal auditory canal. *A.J.N.R.* 9:115–120, 1988.
31. West M.S., Russell E.J., Breit R., et al.: Calvarial and skull base metastases: Comparison of nonenhanced and Gd-DTPA-enhanced MR images. *Radiology* 174:85–92, 1990.

CHAPTER 5

Pituitary and Suprasellar Tumors

Case 163A

81-year-old man presenting with
hypothyroidism.

Case 163B

Same patient.

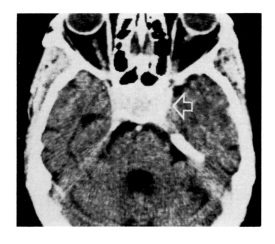

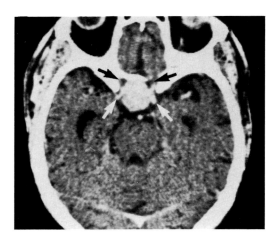

The most reliable CT feature of pituitary adenomas is their origin within the sella turcica. Large adenomas may have confusing suprasellar or parasellar components (see Cases 180 to 182), and enhancement patterns may be variable and nonspecific (see Case 164).

In this case, the sella is moderately enlarged and filled with a uniformly enhancing adenoma. The lateral margins of the tumor merge with contrast density in the cavernous sinuses, which are bowed slightly laterally *(arrow)*.

Pituitary hyperplasia may cause diffuse enlargement of the gland, mimicking an adenoma. This possibility should be considered when a pituitary "mass" is found in appropriate clinical settings (e.g., hypothyroidism, pregnancy).

Another cause of diffuse pituitary enlargement is lymphocytic adenohypophysitis, an idiopathic inflammatory process usually occurring in women during the peripartum period.

A higher scan demonstrates superior extension of the adenoma into the suprasellar cistern. The tumor is centered in the midline, spanning the distance between the supraclinoid internal carotid arteries *(white arrows)*.

The optic nerves pass between the anterior clinoid process and the tumor *(black arrows)*, so that further tumor growth would lead to increasingly compromised visual acuity. Nerve compression or bitemporal hemianopia (from pressure on the optic chiasm) depend both on the tumor size and on the congenitally variable proximity of the optic chiasm to the optic canals.

The well-defined, uniform enhancement of pituitary adenomas may closely resemble other suprasellar lesions (see Cases 165 through 168).

Case 164A

35-year-old asymptomatic volunteer fireman struck on the head; skull x-ray showed a large sella.

Case 164B

Same patient.

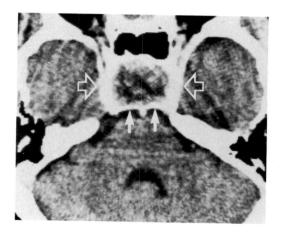

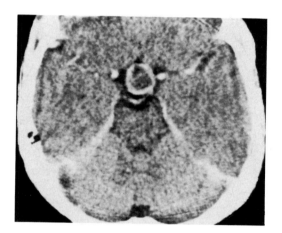

Many pituitary adenomas contain nonenhancing regions representing cysts, hemorrhage, necrosis, or inhomogeneous tissue. Sometimes the entire tumor has this appearance, with only a rim of contrast enhancement.

In this case the sella is enlarged, with the dorsum displaced posteriorly as far as the basilar artery *(solid arrows)*. The lack of central tumor enhancement allows visualization of the cavernous sinuses, which are compressed and bowed laterally *(open arrows)*.

The suprasellar extension of this pituitary adenoma has the same rim-enhancing appearance as the intrasellar component.

Necrosis and hemorrhage are common in pituitary adenomas. MR scans frequently demonstrate blood products within these lesions (see Cases 178 and 179). Acute infarction or hemorrhage may cause rapid swelling of an adenoma, leading to sudden visual and endocrine compromise ("pituitary apoplexy").

Like solid adenomas, rim-enhancing pituitary tumors may resemble other suprasellar lesions (see Cases 169 and 170).

DIFFERENTIAL DIAGNOSIS:
INTENSELY ENHANCING, MIDLINE SUPRASELLAR MASS

Case 165

72-year-old man.

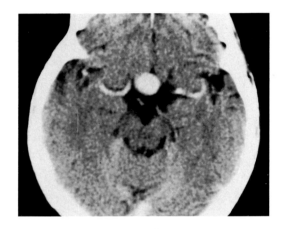

Pituitary Adenoma.

Case 166

58-year-old woman presenting with bitemporal hemianopia.

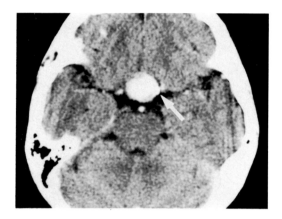

Aneurysm.

Many lesions can present as well-defined, densely enhancing suprasellar masses. In children, chiasmatic/hypothalamic glioma (see Case 201), unusual craniopharyngioma, and rare histiocytosis should be considered when this appearance is encountered. In adolescents or young adults, germinomas are included in the differential diagnosis (see Cases 197 and 198). In adults, the most common mass with these features is a pituitary adenoma, but Cases 166 through 168 illustrate the need for caution.

Suprasellar aneurysms may contain characteristic rim calcifications and variable amounts of intraluminal thrombus. They are often located slightly away from the midline. Aneurysms may be readily documented by digital subtraction angiography or MR (see Cases 542 to 545).

In Case 166 a small calcification at the margin of the lesion *(arrow)* is a clue to its vascular etiology. Nonenhancing tissue elsewhere around the circumference of the mass represents mural thrombus.

Case 167

49-year-old woman presenting with reduced vision and hypogonadism.

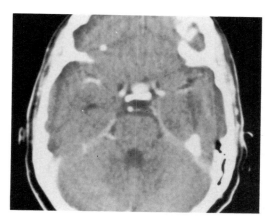

Hypothalamic Glioma.

Case 168

43-year-old woman presenting with decreased visual acuity.

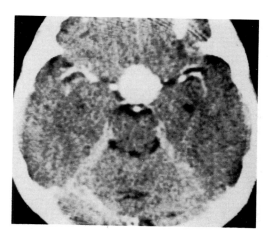

Meningioma.

These cases illustrate two additional pathologies to be considered in the differential diagnosis of enhancing suprasellar lesions. The glioma in Case 167 and the meningioma in Case 168 are indistinguishable from suprasellar extension of a pituitary tumor (see also Cases 551 and 552).

As discussed earlier, expansion of the sella turcica and continuity of suprasellar and intrasellar components are hallmarks of pituitary masses. The absence of these features should suggest an alternative diagnosis. Coronal CT or coronal and sagittal MR scans are valuable for this assessment (see Cases 176, 198, 199, 204, and 205).

Metastasis to the hypothalamus/infundibulum is another enhancing lesion that may present in the suprasellar region, most often seen with primary tumors of the breast and lung. Osseous metastases (e.g., prostate carcinoma) to the anterior clinoid process or sphenoid bone can enlarge to become uniformly enhancing suprasellar masses. Large colloid cysts may extend inferiorly into the suprasellar area, usually with little enhancement (see Cases 216 and 217). Suprasellar inflammatory processes (e.g., sarcoidosis) should also be included in the differential diagnosis.

DIFFERENTIAL DIAGNOSIS:
MIXED-ATTENUATION, PARTIALLY ENHANCING SUPRASELLAR MASS

Case 169

18-year-old man.

Case 170

58-year-old woman presenting with bitemporal hemianopia.

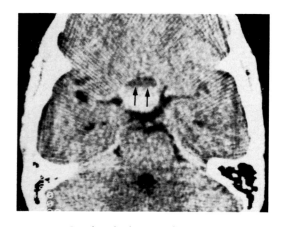

Cystic Pituitary Adenoma.

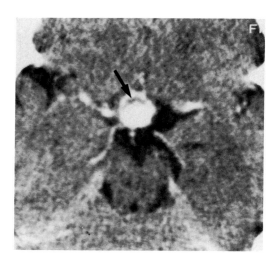

Aneurysm of the Supraclinoid Internal Carotid Artery.

As illustrated in Case 164, the suprasellar extension of pituitary adenomas may be only partially enhancing. The sedimentation level in Case 169 *(arrows)* indicates a truly cystic tumor (compare to Case 179).

The aneurysm in Case 170 contains a small thrombus *(arrow)*, causing enhancement to be inhomogeneous. Greater amounts of intraluminal clot would result in a more prominent appearance of rim enhancement. Such partially thrombosed aneurysms may mimic other suprasellar lesions, including pituitary adenomas and craniopharyngiomas (see Cases 189 and 190).

Hypothalamic glioma belongs in this differential diagnosis as well as that of Cases 165 through 168. Hamartomas of the tuber cinereum usually demonstrate little enhancement and are located more posteriorly than the masses illustrated here. Inflammatory lesions (e.g., sarcoidosis, tuberculosis, sphenoid mucocele) may cause complex suprasellar masses, but other clinical clues are usually present.

MR scans can resolve the CT ambiguity of lesions such as those in Cases 169 and 170. Partially thrombosed aneurysms demonstrate a characteristically laminated pattern of short T1 and short T2 components reflecting the presence of layered blood products (see Cases 543 to 545). Other suprasellar masses may also contain evidence of hemorrhage on MR scans, but the patterns are usually distinguishable from that of an aneurysm (see Cases 205 and 211).

PITUITARY MICROADENOMAS

Case 171A

32-year-old woman presenting with amenorrhea
and galactorrhea.
(coronal, postcontrast scan)

Prolactinoma.

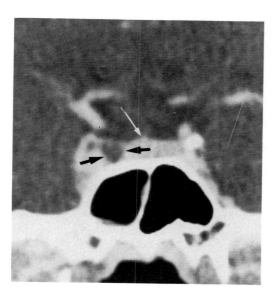

Case 171B

Same patient.
(slightly more posterior scan)

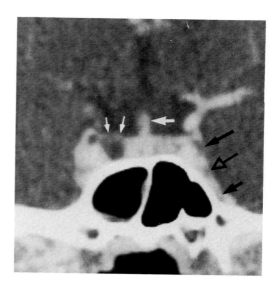

Secreting adenomas of the pituitary may cause significant endocrine symptoms despite small tumor size. (Contrast this case with the nonsecreting adenomas in Cases 180 and 181.) Tumors less than 10 mm in diameter have been termed "microadenomas." Prolactinomas are the most frequent microadenomas to produce clinical symptoms, usually amenorrhea and/or galactorrhea in young women.

Axial scans are often normal in the presence of a microadenoma. Coronal scans performed immediately after a bolus injection of contrast material offer the best CT definition of these tumors. Similar resolution is provided by coronal MR scans.

A microadenoma may be directly imaged as a relatively low-attenuation lesion within the otherwise enhancing pituitary tissue *(black arrows)*. This appearance must be correlated with secondary findings and the clinical presentation, since other low-density regions (e.g., small cysts) are common within the gland.

The lateral location of the tumor in this case is common for prolactinomas. Extension into the cavernous sinus may be associated with very high serum prolactin levels (see Case 177).

Secondary findings of a pituitary microadenoma on coronal scans include increased height of the gland, prominent superior convexity, deviation of the pituitary infundibulum, and focal erosion of the sellar floor. Each of these features can be an isolated normal finding, but their association suggests a responsible mass. Here the small adenoma causes a localized superior bulge *(small white arrows)*, but does not displace the enhancing infundibulum *(large white arrow; compare to Case 173)*.

The superior surface of the pituitary gland may normally be "tented" in the midline at the junction with the infundibulum *(white arrow, Case 171A)*. Occasionally, the entire superior surface of the gland is prominently convex (see Case 172), but the contour is smoothly symmetrical, as opposed to the focal, eccentric deformity in this case. Conversely, microadenomas may be present within glands demonstrating no superior convexity, as is almost true on this scan.

Several cranial nerves are seen in cross section as filling defects within the enhancing cavernous sinus (third nerve, *long black arrow;* fourth and/or sixth nerves, *open black arrow;* fifth nerve, *short black arrow*).

Case 172

18-year-old woman.
(coronal, postcontrast scan)

Case 173

24-year-old woman.
(coronal, postcontrast scan)

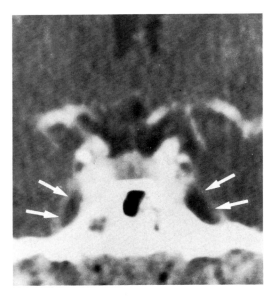

Normal Pituitary Gland.

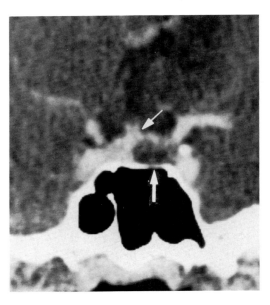

Pituitary Adenoma.

Pituitary enhancement may be less intense than the contrast density of the cavernous sinuses. The gland then appears as a region of relatively low attenuation, as seen in Case 172.

Superior convexity may be a normal feature of pituitary morphology, particularly in young women. In Case 172 the sella is narrow, probably accounting for the relatively tall gland with a prominent superior margin. This normal convexity is smoothly uniform and centered in the midline.

By contrast, the low-density adenoma in Case 173 asymmetrically distorts the superior margin of the gland. In addition, the infundibulum is displaced slightly toward the opposite side *(small white arrow),* and the sella floor is thinned beneath the tumor *(large white arrow).*

Meckel's caves containing the fifth nerve ganglia are well seen within the posterior cavernous sinuses *(arrows)* in Case 172.

DIFFERENTIAL DIAGNOSIS:
LOW-ATTENUATION LESION ENLARGING THE PITUITARY GLAND

Case 174

32-year-old woman.
(coronal, postcontrast scan)

Case 175

55-year-old woman presenting with headaches.
(coronal postcontrast scan)

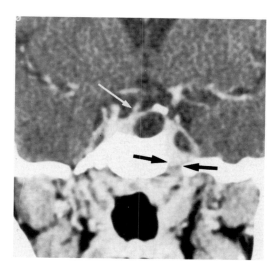

Pituitary Cyst.

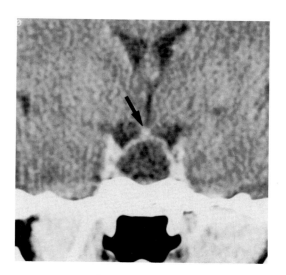

Pituitary Abscess.

Pathologies other than pituitary adenomas may cause low-attenuation masses within the sella turcica. Intrasellar craniopharyngiomas and Rathke pouch cysts may present with this appearance.

The lesion in Case 174 proved to be an incidental cyst. (Calcification at the superior corner of the cyst represents partial volume of the posterior clinoid process, not a calcific rim.) Asymmetrical mass effect causes left-sided bulging of the gland and contralateral displacement of the pituitary infundibulum *(white arrow)*. Smaller pituitary cysts are common and can mimic microadenomas such as Case 171.

Pituitary abscesses may closely resemble a cystic or necrotic adenoma. These lesions often demonstrate a very round shape and a uniformly thin rim of peripheral tissue, as seen in Case 175. The midline mass effect causes symmetrical superior convexity of the gland with flattening and elevation of the enhancing infundibulum *(arrow)*, in contrast to the lateral infundibular displacement in Case 174. Pituitary abscesses may be relatively indolent, and such patients are often not acutely ill.

A small amount of head rotation in Case 174 causes apparent asymmetry of Meckel's caves, which can falsely mimic pathology (see Case 242). The normal foramen ovale is seen on the left in Case 174 *(black arrows)* as a gap in the bony floor of the middle cranial fossa, through which the cavernous sinus communicates with the parapharyngeal region.

Case 176

53-year-old man presenting with bitemporal hemianopia.
(sagittal, noncontrast scan; SE 600/20)

Case 177

36-year-old woman presenting with galactorrhea, amenorrhea, and very high serum prolactin levels.
(coronal, postcontrast scan; SE 650/20)

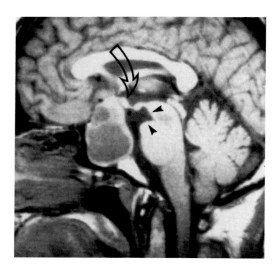

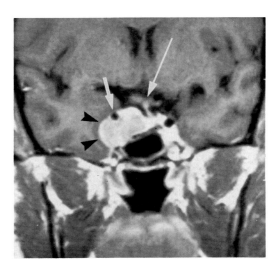

Sagittal MR scans provide excellent visualization of the intrasellar and suprasellar components of pituitary adenomas. Sellar expansion and associated erosion of the skull base are apparent, and deformity of suprasellar structures (e.g., optic chiasm, third ventricle) can be judged.

In this case the sella is grossly expanded. The adenoma bulges into the sphenoid sinus and erodes the clivus. Suprasellar extension of the tumor has elevated and flattened the anterior recesses of the third ventricle and the optic chiasm *(open arrow)*.

Sagittal MR scans are useful for demonstrating subfrontal growth of large adenomas (as in Case 181). Retrosellar extension of suprasellar masses to involve the interpeduncular cistern *(arrowheads)* is also well defined (see Cases 204 and 205).

The adenoma in this case demonstrates large areas of cystic or necrotic degeneration. Axial CT scans through this lesion would resemble Case 164.

Coronal MR scans extend the imaging advantages of coronal CT studies. The pituitary infundibulum, enhancing gland tissue, and cavernous sinuses are well demonstrated, without the CT liabilities of dental artifact, patient motion due to awkward positioning, and oblique scan angles. The optic chiasm, a critical landmark in assessing suprasellar disease, is well-defined by surrounding CSF *(long white arrow)*. The position and caliber of the parasellar internal carotid arteries are established by distinct "flow voids" within the cavernous sinus, in contrast to the poor definition of these vessels on CT studies.

In this case, the right-sided adenoma causes deviation of the infundibulum and erosion of the sellar floor (compare to Cases 173 and 174). The tumor has extended into the right cavernous sinus, which bows laterally *(black arrowheads;* an axial CT scan through this lesion would resemble Case 214).

The cavernous segment of the right internal carotid artery *(short white arrow)* is superiorly displaced and mildly narrowed. Like parasellar meningiomas, pituitary adenomas may be associated with encasement of adjacent arteries.

MR DEMONSTRATION OF HEMORRHAGE IN PITUITARY ADENOMAS

Case 178

35-year-old woman presenting with
bitemporal hemianopia.
(coronal, noncontrast scan; SE 600/17)

Case 179

17-year-old woman.
(axial, noncontrast scan; SE 2500/120)

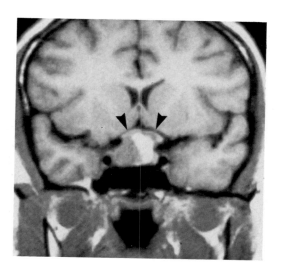

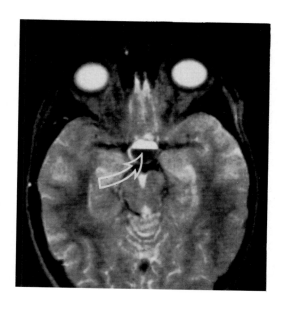

Hemorrhage is common within pituitary adenomas. Acute intratumoral bleeding may cause the sudden clinical presentation of "pituitary apoplexy" (see discussion of Case 164B). More frequently the hemorrhages are small and subclinical.

The sensitivity of MR to the paramagnetic effects of blood products highlights the presence of hemorrhage within tumors. In this case, the high-intensity zone of T1-shortening along the left side of the adenoma is compatible with subacute bleeding. A coronal CT scan of this patient outlined the same region as a "filling defect" within enhancing tumor tissue.

The demonstration of blood products within a pituitary adenoma on MR scans may be incidental. Evidence of hemorrhage does not by itself imply clinical "apoplexy." There was no history of an acute clinical event in this case.

The optic chiasm is stretched over the superior pole of the tumor *(arrowheads)*, accounting for the patient's presentation with bitemporal visual field cuts.

Here the suprasellar extension of a pituitary adenoma is demonstrated to be cystic by virtue of a sedimentation level *(arrow;* compare to Case 169). The marked T2-shortening of the dependent component is characteristic of cystic or necrotic tumors containing blood products (compare to the sedimentation level within the subdural hematoma in Case 361).

Case 180

32-year-old man with a long history of "nasal" voice and a 2-week history of impaired vision.

Case 181

38-year-old man.

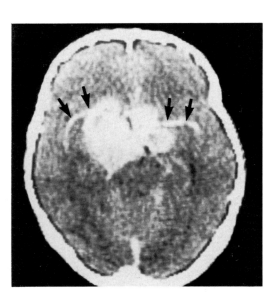

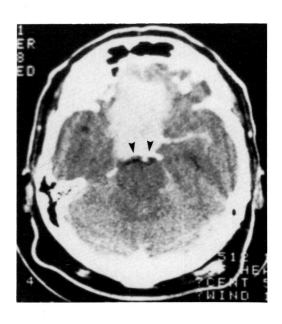

Nonsecreting pituitary adenomas may become very large before compression of the optic chiasm causes symptoms. This huge, lobulated suprasellar mass was accompanied by an equally large extracranial component filling the nasopharynx (and accounting for the history of nasal speech).

At the geographic center of the mass was the faint "ghost" of an expanded sella turcica, a hallmark of intrasellar origin. The diagnosis of giant pituitary adenoma was made and confirmed by biopsy in the pharynx.

The horizontal segments of the middle cerebral arteries are elevated by the suprasellar mass (arrows), which is somewhat restrained by the vessels and grows in lobulations around the vascular grooves. Encasement of basal arteries is characteristic of parasellar meningiomas (see Case 60) but can also be associated with pituitary adenomas (see Case 177).

In this case the large, homogeneously enhancing mass at the floor of the anterior cranial fossa was initially thought to represent a subfrontal meningioma. However, the posterior portion of the lesion occupies the suprasellar region, and the dorsum sella is flattened posteriorly (arrowheads; compare to Cases 163 and 164). For these reasons a sagittal MR scan was obtained demonstrating subfrontal extension of a pituitary adenoma.

Esthesioneuroblastoma or "olfactory neuroblastoma" is a rare midline tumor that can also present as an enhancing subfrontal mass in young patients. The characteristic origin of this neoplasm from the region of the cribriform plate can be demonstrated by coronal CT or MR scans, differentiating such tumors from meningiomas or pituitary adenomas.

DIFFERENTIAL DIAGNOSIS:
MIDLINE DESTRUCTIVE LESION OF THE SKULL BASE

Case 182

55-year-old woman.

Case 183

76-year-old woman.

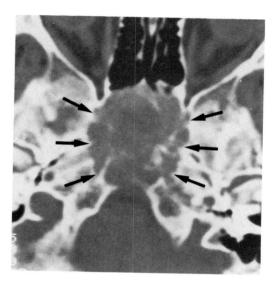

Pituitary Adenoma.

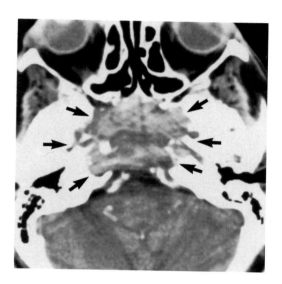

Myeloma.

Some pituitary adenomas grow predominantly inferiorly, filling the sphenoid sinus and eroding through the skull base to reach the nasopharynx. Case 182 demonstrates a large defect in the middle of the sphenoid bone and clivus *(arrows)* due to the inferior extension of a pituitary tumor. Such bone destruction may mimic the skull invasion of a nasopharyngeal neoplasm (see Case 155) or the erosion of a chordoma (see Cases 157 and 159). Aneurysms or pseudoaneurysms of the internal carotid artery should also be remembered as a rare cause of well-defined erosion of the skull base.

Metastasis and myeloma are prime considerations when destructive lesions of the skull base are encountered. The margins of erosion in Case 183 are more permeative and irregular than in Case 182, suggesting an aggressive process and favoring malignancy.

Sagittal and coronal MR scans are valuable for defining the pharyngeal (and intracranial) components of masses involving the skull base (see Case 159 for an example).

Case 184

59-year-old woman with headache, found to
have a large sella on skull films.
(coronal, postcontrast scan)

Case 185

44-year-old woman.
(coronal scan with intrathecal contrast)

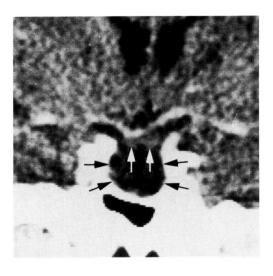

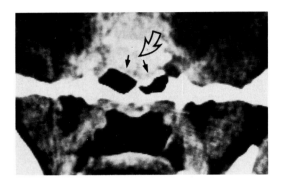

An unusually large aperture in the diaphragma sellae may allow spinal fluid from the suprasellar cistern to extend into the sella. The intrasellar cistern participates in normal CSF pulsations and can cause gradual expansion of the sella, closely resembling the enlargement seen with pituitary adenomas.

This "empty sella syndrome" is often discovered in otherwise healthy, middle-aged, overweight patients (especially women) with vague complaints (especially headache). Associated pituitary dysfunction is rare. Occasional visual symptoms may be caused by prolapse of the optic chiasm, more commonly seen with "secondary" empty sellas following necrosis or removal of pituitary tumors.

In this case the sella is clearly enlarged, with depression of the floor and lateral bowing of the cavernous sinuses *(black arrows)*. The sella is filled with CSF density, and no pituitary tissue is defined. The position of the optic chiasm *(white arrows)* is somewhat low.

A number of low-attenuation lesions can occur within the sella turcica, including some pituitary adenomas, abscesses, cysts, craniopharyngiomas, and dermoid cysts (see Cases 173 through 175). An "empty sella" must be distinguished from these low-density intrasellar masses.

The diagnosis of a true "empty sella" can be made on coronal CT scans if the thin pituitary infundibulum can be seen to traverse the low-density area to reach the pituitary gland at the floor of the sella (see Case 186 for the MR equivalent). The infundibulum is best seen on postcontrast CT studies due to enhancement of the hypophyseal portal venous system.

If this finding cannot be demonstrated, opacification of the subarachnoid spaces with contrast material will determine whether the sellar content is spinal fluid or a low-density lesion. Here contrast fills the enlarged "empty sella," outlining the pituitary infundibulum *(curved, open arrow)* as it extends to the inferiorly flattened pituitary gland *(small arrows)*.

Occasionally a small pituitary adenoma may be found within an otherwise "empty" sella. The latter does not exclude the former, and symptomatic cases of "empty sella" need to be carefully analyzed.

Case 186

20-year-old woman.
(coronal, noncontrast scan; SE 600/20)

"Empty Sella" Syndrome.

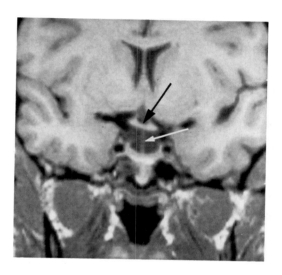

Coronal MR is more reliable and less invasive than CT scans with intrathecal contrast for demonstrating an "empty sella." The anatomy in this case is identical to Case 185: the midline pituitary infundibulum *(white arrow)* traverses the CSF-containing sella to reach a thin rim of pituitary tissue along the sellar floor. The optic chiasm *(black arrow)* is more clearly demonstrated than on coronal CT studies (compare to Case 184) and is slightly "low" on the left.

Case 187

6-year-old boy presenting with small stature.
(sagittal, noncontrast scan; SE 600/20)

Pituitary Dwarfism.

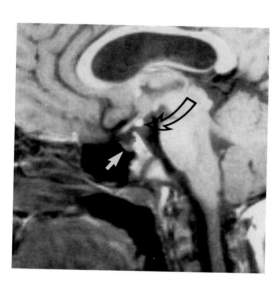

In this case the small adenohypophysis *(solid arrow)* is contained within an equally small sella turcica, indicating congenital pituitary hypoplasia. The pituitary infundibulum is very thin but was faintly visible on the original images.

A "bright spot" of T1-shortening representing the functional neurohypophysis is missing from the sella turcica and is instead demonstrated in an ectopic location at the base of the infundibulum *(open arrow;* compare to the normal appearance of the "bright" neurohypophysis in Case 161). Similar development of an "ectopic posterior pituitary gland" along the floor of the third ventricle can be noted in cases of post-traumatic transection of the pituitary infundibulum. (The infundibulum normally transmits carrier-bound neuropeptide hormones from the hypothalamus to the neurohypophysis.)

CRANIOPHARYNGIOMAS

Case 188

6-year-old girl.
(noncontrast scan)

Case 189

12-year-old boy.
(postcontrast scan)

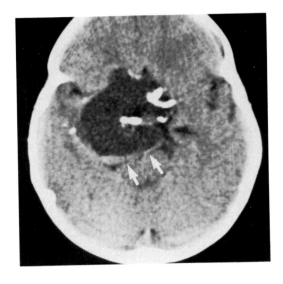

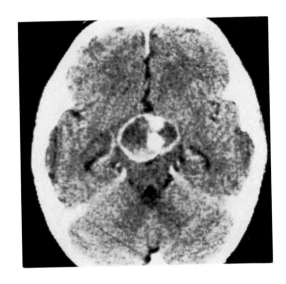

Craniopharyngiomas are typically seen as mixed-attenuation lesions in a suprasellar location. Low-attenuation regions may represent cyst formation or low density tissue. Calcification is characteristic and may take the form of arcs in the periphery of cystic lesions or dense nodules within areas of solid tumor (see Case 202).

Parasellar and retrosellar extension are common (see Case 204). In this case, the tumor occupies the medial portion of the right middle cranial fossa, with a retrosellar component displacing the brain stem posteriorly (*arrows*).

Contrast enhancement in craniopharyngiomas may be minimal or intense. Patterns include homogeneous enhancement of solid tumors and rim enhancement surrounding cystic components. The target appearance in this case resembles a partially thrombosed giant aneurysm (compare to Cases 547 and 549).

Although midline suprasellar location is characteristic of craniopharyngiomas, eccentric tumors are common (see Case 191), and occasional lesions are found within the sella turcica or third ventricle.

ATYPICAL CRANIOPHARYNGIOMAS

Case 190

55-year-old man presenting with diabetes insipidus and bitemporal hemianopia.

Solid Craniopharyngioma.

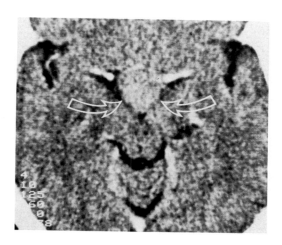

Case 191

15-year-old boy presenting with growth arrest and temporal headaches.

Cystic Craniopharyngioma.

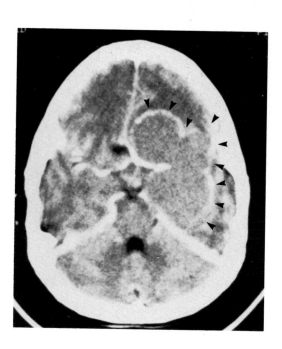

This mass occupies a suprasellar location but lacks other features of craniopharyngiomas. No cyst, calcification, or contrast enhancement is present. The nondescript appearance resembles a low-grade glioma of the hypothalamus or optic chiasm (compare to Case 208), although such tumors are rare in adults. A hamartoma of the tuber cinereum or suprasellar extension of a pituitary adenoma could also be considered in the differential diagnosis for this scan.

About 30% of craniopharyngiomas are found in adults, and about 25% are solid masses.

Cystic craniopharyngiomas do not always present as low-attenuation lesions. Hemorrhage or high protein levels may cause tumor cysts to appear isodense or even hyperdense. The same components may cause prominent T1-shortening on MR scans.

Here a trilobed mass in the frontotemporal region demonstrates calcification and enhancement within rims of tissue surrounding homogeneous, isodense, nonenhancing central material. Despite the high attenuation values, the homogeneity of the lesion suggests a cyst. Scans at lower levels connected the eccentric mass with a small suprasellar component. The combination of rim calcification, central cyst, and relationship to the suprasellar area favors the diagnosis of craniopharyngioma.

Occasional craniopharyngiomas are filled with high-attenuation material mimicking an aneurysm or meningioma on precontrast scans. The lack of central contrast enhancement within cystic craniopharyngiomas aids the differential diagnosis in such cases.

DIFFERENTIAL DIAGNOSIS:
LOW-ATTENUATION SUPRASELLAR MASS WITH PERIPHERAL ENHANCEMENT OBSTRUCTING THE FORAMINA OF MONRO

Case 192

31-year-old woman presenting with rapidly decreasing level of consciousness.

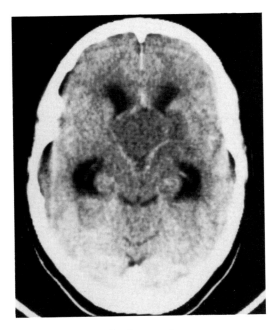

Craniopharyngioma.

Case 193

5-year-old boy presenting with nausea and vomiting.

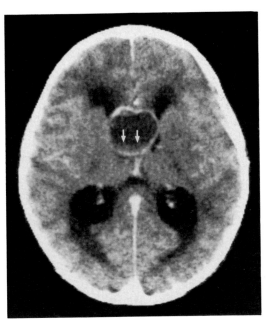

Cystic Astrocytoma of the Septum Pellucidum.

Craniopharyngiomas can enlarge superiorly to obstruct the foramina of Monro and cause hydrocephalus, as in Case 192. The acute clinical presentation in this case resembles the history of patients with sudden ventricular obstruction due to colloid cysts of the third ventricle (see Cases 216 and 217).

The midline location and moderately low attenuation of the mass in Case 192 are consistent with craniopharyngioma. Colloid cysts of the third ventricle are occasionally low-attenuation lesions but rarely reach this size before causing symptoms.

Case 193 demonstrates a similar appearance in a child, with a sedimentation level posteriorly *(arrows)*. The diagnosis of craniopharyngioma had been made at another institution. However, scans at lower levels did not document a suprasellar component of the lesion. For this reason, sagittal and coronal MR studies were performed, demonstrating that the mass was localized within the septum pellucidum. A cystic, Grade 2 astrocytoma was discovered at surgery.

Solid gliomas of the hypothalamus may also present as low-attenuation suprasellar masses (see Cases 209 and 592).

DIFFERENTIAL DIAGNOSIS:
LOW-ATTENUATION NONENHANCING SUPRASELLAR MASS

Case 194

47-year-old woman.

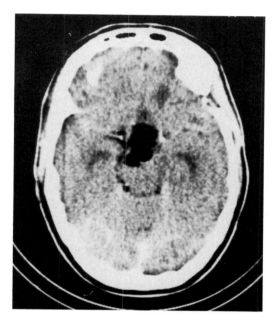

Dermoid Cyst.

Case 195

42-year-old woman.

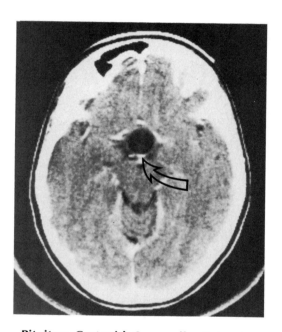

Pituitary Cyst with Suprasellar Extension.

Craniopharyngiomas are one of several low-attenuation extra-axial lesions that may be found in the suprasellar region. Dermoid and epidermoid cysts and arachnoid cysts are frequently located at this site.

Dermoid cysts often contain very low attenuation values due to their lipid content, as in Case 194. These low values contrast with the less extreme low density of most craniopharyngiomas or epidermoid cysts (see Case 621).

Calcification is common in dermoid cysts as well as in craniopharyngiomas (see Cases 232 to 234). The combination of fat content and marginal calcification may also be seen with simple lipomas, but these are less frequent in the suprasellar area.

Case 195 is an unusual example of a simple pituitary cyst extending into the suprasellar region, mimicking a cystic tumor or arachnoid cyst. The focal enhancement along the midposterior rim of the cyst *(arrow)* is the flattened pituitary infundibulum.

Case 196

14-year-old girl.
(noncontrast scan)

Case 197

23-year-old man presenting with reduced
visual acuity.
(coronal, postcontrast scan)

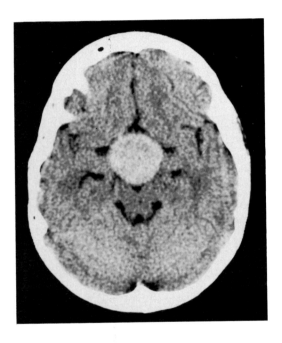

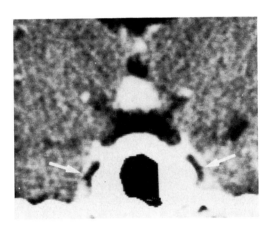

Germinomas are the most common tumors of the pineal region (see Cases 224 and 225). They may also occur in a suprasellar location, where they have been called "ectopic pinealomas." (The term "atypical teratoma" is also used to refer to such germinomas.) Most patients with suprasellar germinomas are teenagers or young adults presenting with diabetes insipidus or visual impairment.

Germinomas are densely cellular and typically demonstrate uniformly increased attenuation values on precontrast CT scans, as seen here. Hemorrhages can occur within these lesions, and the MR appearance may be less homogeneous than the CT picture (see Cases 205 and 211).

Germinomas usually enhance uniformly and intensely, mimicking suprasellar pituitary adenoma, meningioma, or aneurysm (compare this scan with Cases 165 to 168).

Here the coronal view clearly identifies the mass as a midline, suprasellar lesion, separated from the sella by uninvolved cistern. The inferior portion of the third ventricle is compressed by the tumor, while the region of the foramen of Monro is normal (compare with Case 220).

Meckel's caves containing the trigeminal ganglia are seen as filling defects within the cavernous sinuses *(arrows)*.

DIFFERENTIAL DIAGNOSIS:
ENHANCING MASS WITH SUPRASELLAR AND INTRASELLAR COMPONENTS

Case 198

14-year-old girl with poor school performance
due to hypothyroidism and markedly
reduced visual acuity.
(coronal scan)

Case 199

55-year-old man found by an optometrist to
have bilaterally reduced visual acuity.
(coronal scan)

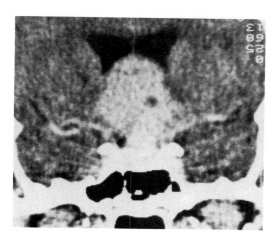

Germinoma.

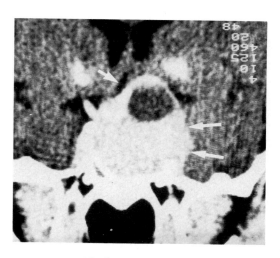

Pituitary Adenoma.

The distinction between a pituitary tumor with suprasellar extension and a suprasellar mass reaching into the sella may be difficult.

Although the enhancing suprasellar mass in Case 198 seems to merge with pituitary enhancement, there is a "waist" and a change in density at the apparent junction. Furthermore, the center of the tumor is suprasellar, and the sella itself is not grossly expanded. The same CT or MR features usually allow the distinction between suprasellar meningiomas and pituitary adenomas.

In Case 199, the marked enlargement of the sella and the broad continuity between the intrasellar and suprasellar components favor a pituitary adenoma. The tumor demonstrates eccentric parasellar and suprasellar growth and contains a large low-density region superiorly. An axial scan through the suprasellar component would appear as a parasagittal, rim-enhancing lesion resembling a thrombus-filled aneurysm or craniopharyngioma.

The "waist" or junction between the intrasellar and suprasellar components of the adenoma on Case 199 is very broad, facilitating transsphenoidal removal of the entire mass. Narrow-waisted pituitary adenomas with a tight diaphragma sellae are more difficult to resect via a transsphenoidal approach.

The germinoma in Case 198 extends superiorly through the region of the third ventricle to deform the inferior portions of the lateral ventricular bodies and obstruct the foramina of Monro (compare to Case 192).

Case 200

3-year-old girl being evaluated for suspected "battered child syndrome." The child's mother was subsequently noted to have multiple cafe-au-lait spots.
(noncontrast scan)

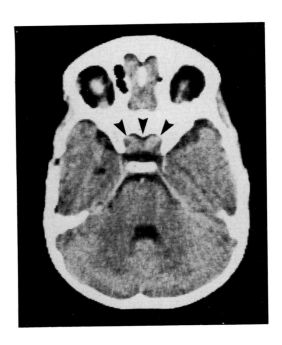

Case 201

5-month-old boy.
(postcontrast scan)

Grade 2 Chiasmal Astrocytoma.

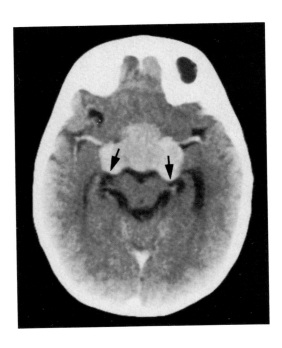

Optic gliomas are a common manifestation of Type 1 neurofibromatosis (see discussion in Case 136; also see Cases 689 to 696). The optic gliomas of neurofibromatosis are typically low-grade lesions, behaving more like hyperplasia than neoplasms. Contrast enhancement in this type of glioma may be minimal.

Erosion and enlargement of the chiasmatic sulcus at the entrance to the optic canals (arrowheads) are hallmarks of masses involving the chiasm and extending toward the optic nerves. These findings may be useful in distinguishing optic gliomas from other suprasellar lesions. Similarly, posterior extension of tumor into the optic tracts favors the diagnosis of chiasmatic glioma.

Sagittal and coronal MR scans provide excellent definition of the optic chiasm. MR is currently the best procedure for evaluating intrinsic or extrinsic lesions in this region (see Cases 206 and 207).

Gliomas of the optic chiasm in patients without neurofibromatosis are more aggressive lesions. Such tumors frequently demonstrate intense, uniform contrast enhancement, as in this case.

Here a transversely oriented midline mass fills the suprasellar cistern. Bilateral lobulations of tumor extend posteriorly into the optic tracts (arrows).

MR scans of optic gliomas often demonstrate signal abnormality extending far posteriorly along the visual pathways, beyond the limits of contrast enhancement.

DIFFERENTIAL DIAGNOSIS:
CALCIFIED SUPRASELLAR MASS

Case 202

58-year-old woman presenting with headache.

Case 203

42-year-old man presenting with decreased visual acuity.

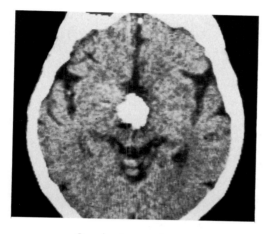

Craniopharyngioma.

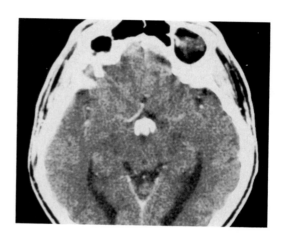

Optic Chiasm Glioma.

Craniopharyngiomas are characterized by suprasellar calcification, which is occasionally dense and solid as in Case 202.

Many other suprasellar lesions may also contain calcium. The calcification of the chiasmal glioma on Case 203 closely resembles that of a solid craniopharyngioma. Cavernous angiomas can occur within and around the optic chiasm and are typically associated with increased attenuation values due to blood products and calcification. Other suprasellar masses containing calcium include aneurysms, dermoid cysts (see Case 234), and occasional meningiomas.

Case 204

45-year-old woman presenting with
impaired vision.
(sagittal, noncontrast scan; SE 600/17)

Craniopharyngioma.

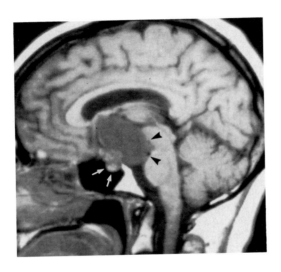

The sagittal plane of MR scans is useful for analyzing the origin and relationships of suprasellar masses. In this case, lack of sellar expansion *(white arrows)* virtually excludes pituitary adenoma as the source of the large suprasellar tumor. The mixed signal intensity of the lesion suggests a partially cystic mass, and prominent retrosellar extension into the interpeduncular region is seen *(black arrowheads)*. These features favor the diagnosis of craniopharyngioma, which was confirmed at surgery.

MR scans of craniopharyngiomas (or their "cousins," the suprasellar Rathke pouch cysts) may demonstrate areas of prominent T1-shortening. Such components reflect the presence of blood products and/or unusual protein content (see Case 191).

Case 205

14-year-old girl presenting with decreased vision and hypothalamic dysfunction (same patient as Cases 196 and 211).
(sagittal, noncontrast scan; SE 600/20)

Germinoma.

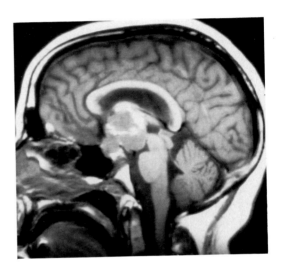

The sagittal MR scan in this case is compatible with craniopharyngioma, which commonly demonstrates T1-shortening and retrosellar extension as seen here. As in Case 204, the center of the mass is clearly suprasellar, arguing against pituitary adenoma (although the lesion does have a small intrasellar extension).

At surgery the tumor was found to be a suprasellar germinoma containing hemorrhage. (Compare to the hemorrhagic pituitary adenoma in Case 178, to the thrombosed basilar artery aneurysm in Case 543, to the coronal CT scan of a comparable germinoma in Case 198, and to an axial MR scan of this patient presented as Case 211.)

Case 206

46-year-old woman (same patient as Case 204, 1 year later). (sagittal, noncontrast scan; SE 600/20)

Case 207

10-year-old girl with Type 1 neurofibromatosis. (coronal, noncontrast scan; SE 600/17)

Optic Glioma.

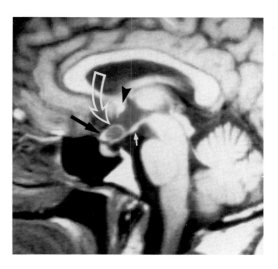

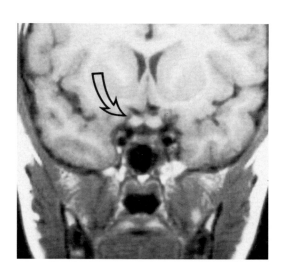

In addition to its role in characterizing large suprasellar lesions as in Cases 204 and 205, MR may be of substantial value in localizing small tumors. Here a very small, cystic recurrence *(large white arrow)* of the craniopharyngioma in Case 204 is demonstrated immediately posterior to the optic chiasm *(black arrow)*.

The tumor had been grossly removed 1 year previously, with no evidence of residual mass on initial postoperative scans. Postsurgical recurrence is a recognized tendency of craniopharyngiomas, and postoperative radiation therapy may be advocated for these "benign" lesions.

Other anatomical details on midsagittal MR images include the anterior commissure *(black arrowhead)* and the mammillary bodies *(small white arrow)*.

Coronal and sagittal MR scans exceed the ability of CT to define the morphology of the optic chiasm. In this case, the chiasm is in normal position but demonstrates diffuse expansion. The bilobed configuration represents thickening of both optic nerves as they join at the chiasm. (Other scans showed thickening of the orbital portion of the optic nerves bilaterally; see Cases 689 to 691.) Comparison of Cases 206 and 207 demonstrates the capacity of MR to distinguish between pathologies within or adjacent to the optic chiasm.

Case 208

5-year-old boy with "gelastic" seizures
(laughing spells).
(coronal, postcontrast scan)

Case 209

16-year-old boy.
(axial, postcontrast scan)

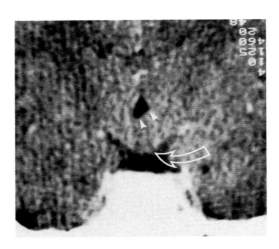

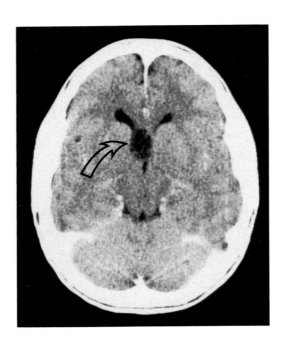

Hypothalamic gliomas rank with optic gliomas and craniopharyngiomas as the most common suprasellar masses in children. Some of these tumors are low-grade lesions demonstrating isodensity and minimal contrast enhancement. Their diagnosis depends on distortions of anatomy caused by displacements of the suprasellar cistern or the anterior third ventricle.

When axial scans are ambiguous in the suprasellar region, coronal CT or MR studies may define a mass by simultaneously demonstrating its interfaces with cistern (large arrow) and ventricle (arrowheads), as in this case. Sagittal MR scans may similarly document deformity of the anterior third ventricle.

A solid, noncalcified, nonenhancing craniopharyngioma would be unusual in a child (see Case 190 for an example in an adult).

Hypothalamic gliomas (especially in children) may present as nonenhancing, low-attenuation lesions. Such masses may grow into the third ventricle to cause obstructive hydrocephalus, with the lesion being falsely assumed to represent ventricular enlargement (see Case 592).

Alternatively, hypothalamic gliomas may present as densely enhancing suprasellar masses. Such lesions resemble optic chiasm gliomas as in Case 201.

It may be difficult or impossible to distinguish between hypothalamic and chiasmatic gliomas on CT scans. Eccentric location (as in these cases) suggests tumor arising along the wall of the third ventricle (i.e., hypothalamus), while erosion of the chiasmatic sulcus as discussed in Case 200 favors a mass originating in the chiasm.

Case 210

4-year-old boy.
(axial, noncontrast scan; SE 3000/45)

Hypothalamic Glioma.

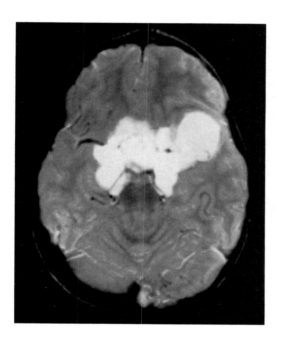

Case 211

14-year-old girl (same patient as
Cases 196 and 205).
(axial, noncontrast scan; SE 2500/90)

Suprasellar Germinoma.

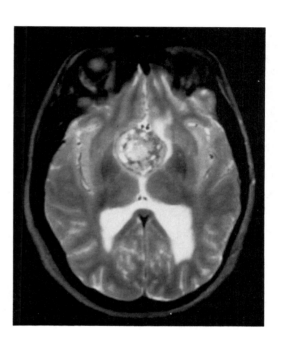

Low-grade gliomas may be better defined on MR scans than on CT studies. Such tumors differ more from surrounding normal brain in magnetic relaxation behavior than they do in x-ray absorption.

The large, lobulated tumor in this case is much more obvious than the lesions of Cases 208 and 209 due to its long T2 values. The morphology of the lesion is indistinguishable from that of a large optic glioma (compare to Case 201). Such distinction is often not meaningful, since bulky tumors arising from either the chiasm or the hypothalamus usually invade the adjacent structures.

Although hypothalamic gliomas are intra-axial tumors, they frequently extend exophytically into basal cisterns as demonstrated here. This behavior may combine with a lobulated morphology to mimic the appearance of craniopharyngiomas.

If the imaging of this case were limited to axial sections as seen here, the possibility of an intra-axial glioma would be strongly considered. The accompanying sagittal scans (presented as Case 205) demonstrate that the hypothalamic lesion instead represents invagination of an extra-axial mass. High-intensity rims of reactive edema are present around the margins of the lesion.

The heterogeneous signal intensity and suprasellar location of this tumor in a young patient suggest craniopharyngioma. Suprasellar germinoma should be remembered as a diagnostic possibility in such cases, occurring most commonly in adolescent girls.

Comparison of the homogeneous CT attenuation of this mass (Case 196) with the heterogeneity of MR signal intensity demonstrates that CT stereotypes do not always correlate with MR appearances.

Case 212

56-year-old man.

Metastatic Prostate Carcinoma Arising from the Anterior Clinoid Process.

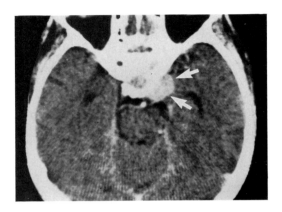

Case 213

67-year-old man.

Systemic Lymphoma Involving the Cavernous Sinus.

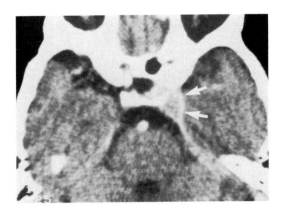

Several sellar and parasellar structures may be involved by metastatic disease. Metastases to the pituitary gland and infundibulum (e.g., breast carcinoma) may mimic the appearance of pituitary adenomas or other suprasellar masses. Metastatic involvement of the sphenoid bone may produce parasellar masses resembling benign lesions such as aneurysms or meningiomas.

In this case, mixed sclerosis and destruction of the anterior clinoid process were seen at wide window widths. Rapid tumor growth confirmed the diagnosis of metastatic disease.

Metastatic involvement of the cavernous sinus may resemble other parasellar masses. An appearance similar to this case could be caused by trigeminal schwannoma (see Case 242), a carotid artery–cavernous sinus fistula (see Case 665), an aneurysm of the internal carotid artery (see Case 540), meningioma (see Case 541), or parasellar inflammatory disease.

Metastatic lymphoma frequently involves the meninges or ventricular surfaces (see Case 103).

DIFFERENTIAL DIAGNOSIS:
ENHANCING PARASELLAR MASS CAUSING VISUAL SYMPTOMS

Case 214

36-year-old woman presenting with the acute onset of painful diplopia.

Case 215

62-year-old woman presenting with decreased vision in the right eye.

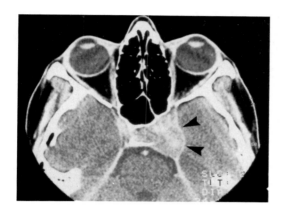

Pituitary Adenoma.

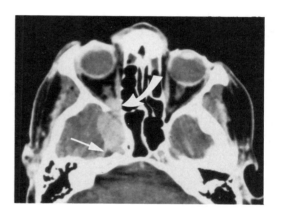

Meningioma.

Lateral extension of a pituitary adenoma may present as a mass involving the cavernous sinus, sometimes with little expansion of the sella itself. The tumor in Case 214 mimics a parasellar meningioma, widening the dural junction between the tentorium and the cavernous sinus. However, the mass does not enhance as intensely as the usual meningioma (compare to Case 215).

As discussed in Case 164B, adenomatous pituitary tissue may undergo spontaneous hemorrhage or infarction. Such an event in a lesion within the cavernous sinus could account for the acute onset of cranial nerve dysfunction, as in Case 214.

The meningioma in Case 215 extends anteriorly to pass through the superior orbital fissure *(curved arrow)*. This component of the tumor compromises the orbital apex and probably accounts for the patient's decreased vision by compression of the optic nerve at this site. The posterior margin of the meningioma has flattened Meckel's cave *(straight arrow)*; identification of this unenlarged structure argues against the alternative diagnosis of trigeminal schwannoma (see Case 242).

Aneurysms of the internal carotid artery are another common cause of an enhancing parasellar mass (see Case 540). Other etiologies include metastases and lymphoma (see Cases 212 and 213), carotid-cavernous fistulae (see Case 665), and inflammatory processes (e.g., Tolosa-Hunt syndrome), and occasional cavernous angiomas.

REFERENCES: CT

1. Ahmadi J., North C.M., Segall H.D., et al.: Cavernous sinus invasion by pituitary adenomas. *A.J.N.R.* 6:893–898, 1985.
2. Banna M., Baker H.L., Houser O.W.: Pituitary and parapituitary tumours on computed tomography. *Br. J. Radiol.* 53:1123–1143, 1980.
3. Bilaniuk L.T., Moshang T., Cara J., et al.: Pituitary enlargement mimicking pituitary tumor. *J. Neurosurg.* 63:39–42, 1985.
4. Braun I.F., Pinto R.S., Epstein F.: Dense cystic craniopharyngiomas. *A.J.N.R.* 3:139–141, 1982.
5. Chambers E.F., Turski P.A., LaMasters D., et al.: Regions of low density in the contrast-enhanced pituitary gland: Normal and pathological processes. *Radiology* 144:109–113, 1982.
6. Constine L.G., Randall S.H., Rubin P., McDonald J.: Craniopharyngiomas: Fluctuation in cyst size following surgery and radiation therapy. *Neurosurgery* 24:53–59, 1989.
7. Daniels D.L., Williams A.L., Thornton R.S., et al.: Differential diagnosis of intrasellar tumors by computed tomography. *Radiology* 141:697–701, 1981.
8. Davis P.C., Hoffman J.C. Jr., Tindall G.T., Braun I.F.: CT—Surgical correlation in pituitary adenomas: Evaluation in 113 patients. *A.J.N.R.* 6:711–716, 1985.
9. Davis P.C., Hoffman J.C. Jr., Tindall G.T., Braun I.F.: Prolactin-secreting pituitary microadenomas: Inaccuracy of high resolution CT imaging. *A.J.N.R.* 5:721–726, 1984.
10. Davis P.C., Hoffman J.C. Jr., Weidenheim K.M.: Large hypothalamic and optic chiasm gliomas in infants: Difficulties in distinction. *A.J.N.R.* 5:579–586, 1984.
11. Diebler C., Ponsot G.: Hamartoma of the tuber cinereum. *Neuroradiology* 25:93–101, 1983.
12. Dietemann J.L., Bonneville J.F., Buchheit F., et al.: CT findings in symptomatic Rathke's cleft cysts of the pituitary gland. *Neuroradiology* 24:263–267, 1983.
13. Dolinskas C.A., Simeone F.A.: Transsphenoidal hypophysectomy: Postsurgical CT findings. *A.J.N.R.* 6:45–50, 1985.
14. Fitz C.T., Wortzman G., Harwood-Nash D.C., et al.: Computed tomography in craniopharyngioma. *Radiology* 127:687–691, 1978.
15. Fletcher W.A., Imes R.K., Hoyt W.F.: Chiasmal gliomas: Appearance and long-term changes demonstrated by computerized tomography. *J. Neurosurg.* 65:154–159, 1986.
16. Floyd J.L., Dorwart R.H., Nelson M.J., et al.: Pituitary hyperplasia secondary to thyroid failure: CT appearance. *A.J.N.R.* 5:469–471, 1984.
17. Gardeur D., Naidich T.P., Metzker J.: CT analysis of intrasellar pituitary adenomas with emphasis on patterns of contrast enhancement. *Neuroradiology* 20:241–247, 1981.
18. Haughton V.M., Rosenbaum A.E., Williams A.L., Drayer B.P.: Recognizing the empty sella by CT: The infundibulum sign. *A.J.N.R.* 1:527–529, 1980.
19. Hemminghytt S., Kalkoff R.K., Daniels D.L., et al.: Computed tomographic study of hormone-secreting microadenomas. *Radiology* 146:65–69, 1983.
20. Inoue Y., Nemoto Y., Fujita K., et al.: Pituitary dwarfism: CT evaluation of the pituitary gland. *Radiology* 159:171–174, 1986.
21. Kaplan H.C., Baker H.L. Jr., Houser O.W. et al.: CT of the sella turcica after transsphenoidal resection of pituitary adenomas. *A.J.N.R.* 6:723–732, 1985.
22. Lin S.R., Bryson M.M., Gobien R., et al.: Radiologic findings of hamartoma of the tuber cinereum and hypothalamus. *Radiology* 127:697–703, 1978.
23. Macpherson P., Anderson D.E.: Radiological differentiation of intrasellar aneurysms from pituitary tumors. *Neuroradiology* 21:177–183, 1981.
24. McGrail K.M., Beyerl B.D., Black P.M., et al.: Lymphocytic adenohypophysitis of pregnancy with complete recovery. *Neurosurgery* 20:791–793, 1987.
25. Numaguchi Y., Kishikawa T., Ikeda J., et al.: Neuroradiological manifestations of suprasellar pituitary adenomas, meningiomas and craniopharyngiomas. *Neuroradiology* 21:67–72, 1981.
26. Okamoto S., Handa H., Yamashita J., et al.: Computed tomography in intra- and suprasellar epithelial cysts (symptomatic Rathke cleft cysts). *A.J.N.R.* 6:515–520, 1985.
27. Peyster R.G., Hoover E.D.: CT of the abnormal pituitary stalk. *A.J.N.R.* 5:49–52, 1984.
28. Post M.J.D., David J.N., Glaser J.S., et al.: Pituitary apoplexy: Diagnosis by computed tomography. *Radiology* 134:665–670, 1980.
29. Post M.J.D., Mendez D., Kline L.B., et al.: Metastatic disease to the cavernous sinus: Clinical syndrome and CT diagnosis. *J. Comput. Assist. Tomogr.* 9:115–120, 1985.
30. Roppolo H.M., Latchaw R.E., Meyer J.D., et al.: Normal pituitary gland. I. Macroscopic anatomy—CT correlation. *A.J.N.R.* 4:927–935, 1983.
31. Roppolo H.M., Latchaw R.E.: Normal pituitary gland. II. Microscopic anatomy—CT correlation. *A.J.N.R.* 4:937–944, 1983.
32. Sage M.R., Chan E.S., Reilly P.L.: The clinical and radiographic features of the empty sella syndrome. *Clin. Radiol.* 31:513–519, 1980.
33. Saris S.C., Patronas N.J., Doppman J.L., et al.: Cushing syndrome: pituitary CT scanning. *Radiology* 162:775–778, 1987.
34. Savoiardo M., Harwood-Nash D.C., Tadmor R., et al.: Gliomas of the intracranial anterior optic pathways in children. *Radiology* 138:601–610, 1981.
35. Suejima T., Takeshita I., Yamamoto H., et al.: Computed tomography of germinomas in basal ganglia and thalamus. *Neuroradiology* 29:366, 1987.
36. Swartz J.D., Russell K.B., Basile B.A., et al.: High resolution computed tomographic appearance of the intrasellar contents in women of childbearing age. *Radiology* 147:115–117, 1983.
37. Swenson S.A., Forbes G.S., Younge B.R., et al.: Radiologic evaluation of tumors of the optic nerve. *A.J.N.R.* 3:319–326, 1982.
38. Syvertsen A., Haughton V.M., Williams A.L., et al.: The computed tomographic appearance of the normal pituitary gland and pituitary microadenomas. *Radiology* 133:385–391, 1979.
39. Takeuchi J., Handa H., Otsuka S., et al.: Neuroradiological aspects of suprasellar germinoma. *Neuroradiology* 17:153–158, 1979.
40. Taylor S.: High resolution computed tomography of the sella. *Radiol. Clin. North Am.* 20:207–236, 1982.
41. Tibbs P.A., Challa V., Mortara R.: Isolated histiocytosis X of the hypothalamus. *J. Neurosurg.* 49:929–934, 1978.
42. Wakai S., Fukushima T., Teramoto A., et al.: Pituitary apoplexy: Its incidence and clinical significance. *J. Neurosurg.* 55:187–193, 1981.
43. Wolpert S.M., Molitch M.E., Goldman J.A., et al.: Size, shape and appearance of the normal female pituitary gland. *A.J.N.R.* 5:263–267, 1984.

REFERENCES: MR

1. Barkovich A.J., Fram E.K., Norman D.: Septo-optic dysplasia: MR imaging. *Radiology* 171:189–192, 1989.
2. Barrai V., Brunelle F., Brauner R., et al.: MRI of hypothalamic hamartomas in children. *Pediat. Radiol.* 18:449, 1988.
3. Beningfield S.J., Bonnici F., Cremin B.J.: Magnetic resonance imaging of hypothalamic hamartomas. *Br. J. Radiol.* 61:1177, 1988.
4. Burton E.M., Ball W.S. Jr., Crone K., Dolan L.M.: Hamartoma of the tuber cinereum: A comparison of MR and CT findings in four cases. *A.J.N.R.* 10:497–502, 1989.
5. Chakares D.W., Curtin A., Ford G.: Magnetic resonance imaging of pituitary and parasellar abnormalities. *Radiol. Clin. North Am.* 27:265–282, 1989.
6. Daniels D.L., Pech P., Mark L., et al.: Magnetic resonance imaging of the cavernous sinus. *A.J.N.R.* 6:187–192, 1985.
7. Davis P.C., Hoffman J.C. Jr., Spencer T., et al.: MR imaging of pituitary adenoma: CT, clinical, and surgical correlation. *A.J.N.R.* 8:107–112, 1987.
8. Doppman J.L., Frank J.A., Dwyer A.J., et al.: Gadolinium-DTPA-enhanced MR imaging of ACTH-secreting microadenomas of the pituitary gland. *J. Comput. Assist. Tomogr.* 12:728–736, 1988.
9. El Gammal T., Brooks B.S., Hoffman W.H.: MR imaging of the ectopic bright signal of posterior pituitary regeneration. *A.J.N.R.* 10:323–328, 1989.
10. Elster A.D., Chen M.V., Williams D. III, Key L.L.: Pituitary gland: MR imaging of physiologic hypertrophy in adolescents. *Radiology* 174:681–686, 1990.
11. Freeman M.P., Kessler R.M., Allen J.H., Price A.C.: Craniopharyngioma: CT and MR imaging in nine cases. *J. Comput. Assist. Tomogr.* 11:810–814, 1987.
12. Fujisawa I., Kikuchi K., Nishimura K., et al.: Transsection of the pituitary stalk: Development of an ectopic posterior lobe assessed with MR imaging. *Radiology* 165:487–490, 1987.
13. Hirsch W.L. Jr., Hryshko F.G., Sekhar L.N., et al.: Comparison of MR imaging, CT, and angiography in the evaluation of the enlarged cavernous sinus. *A.J.N.R.* 9:907–916, 1988.
14. Hutchins W.W., Crues J.V. III, Miya P., Pojunas K.W.: MR demonstration of pituitary hyperplasia and regression after therapy for hypothyroidism. *A.J.N.R.* 11:410, 1990.
15. Karnaze M.G., Sartor K., Winthrop J.D.: Suprasellar lesions: Evaluation with MR imaging. *Radiology* 161:77–82, 1986.
16. Kaufman B., Kaufman B.A., Arafah B., et al.: Large pituitary gland adenomas evaluated with magnetic resonance imaging. *Neurosurgery* 21:540–546, 1987.
17. Kaufman B., Tomsak R.L., Kaufman B.A., et al.: Herniation of the suprasellar visual system and third ventricle into empty sellae: Morphologic and clinical considerations. *A.J.N.R.* 10:65–76, 1989.
18. Kelly W.M., Kucharczyk W., Kucharczyk J., et al.: Posterior pituitary ectopia: An MR feature of pituitary dwarfism. *A.J.N.R.* 9:453–460, 1988.
19. Kucharczyk W., Davis D.O., Kelly W.M., et al.: Pituitary adenomas: High-resolution MR imaging at 1.5T. *Radiology* 161:761–766, 1986.
20. Kucharczyk W., Peck W.W., Kelly W.M., et al.: Rathke cleft cysts: CT, MR imaging, and pathologic features. *Radiology* 165:491–496, 1987.
21. Kulkarni M.V., Lee K.F., McArdle C.B., et al.: 1.5T MR imaging of pituitary microadenomas: Technical considerations and CT correlation. *A.J.N.R.* 9:5–12, 1988.
22. Kyle C.A., Laster R.A., Burton E.M., Sanford R.A.: Subacute pituitary apoplexy: MR and CT appearance. *J. Comput. Assist. Tomogr.* 14:40–44, 1990.
23. Laine F.J., Braun I.F., Jensen M.E., et al.: Perineural tumor extension through the foramen ovale: Evaluation with MR imaging. *Radiology* 174:65–72, 1990.
24. Lee B.C.P., Deck M.D.F.: Sellar and juxtasellar lesion detection with MR. *Radiology* 157:143–148, 1985.
25. Levine S.N., Benzel E.C., Fowler M.R., et al.: Lymphocytic adenohypophysitis: Clinical, radiological, and magnetic resonance imaging characterization. *Neurosurgery* 22:937–941, 1988.
26. Michael A.S., Paige M.L.: MR imaging of intrasellar meningiomas simulating pituitary adenomas. *J. Comput. Assist. Tomogr.* 12:944, 1988.
27. Mikhael M.A., Ciric I.S.: MR imaging of pituitary tumors before and after surgical and/or medical treatment. *J. Comput. Assist. Tomogr.* 12:441–445, 1988.
28. Naheedy M.H., Haag J.R., Azar-Kia B., et al.: MRI and CT of sellar and parasellar disorders. *Radiol. Clin. North Am.* 25:819–848, 1987.
29. Nemoto Y., Inoue Y., Fukuda T., et al.: MR appearance of Rathke's cleft cysts. *Neuroradiology* 30:155, 1988.
30. Newton D.R., Dillon W.P., Norman D., et al.: Gd-DTPA-enhanced MR imaging of pituitary adenomas. *A.J.N.R.* 10:949–954, 1989.
31. Nichols D.A., Laws E.R. Jr., Houser O.W., Abboud C.P.: Comparison of magnetic resonance imaging and computed tomography in the preoperative evaluation of pituitary adenomas. *Neurosurgery* 22:380–385, 1988.
32. Ostrov S.G., Quencer R.M., Hoffman J.C. Jr., et al.: Hemorrhage within pituitary adenomas: How often associated with pituitary apoplexy syndrome? *A.J.N.R.* 10:503–510, 1989.
33. Peck W.W., Dillon W.P., Norman D., et al.: High resolution MR imaging of microadenomas at 1.5T: Experience with Cushing's disease. *A.J.N.R.* 9:1085–1092, 1988.
34. Pigeau I., Sigal R., Halimi P., et al.: MRI features of craniopharyngiomas at 1.5 tesla: A series of 13 cases. *J. Neuroradiol.* 15:276, 1988.
35. Pojunas K.W., Daniels D.L., Williams A.L., Haughton V.M.: MR imaging of prolactin-secreting microadenomas. *A.J.N.R.* 7:209–213, 1986.
36. Pusey E., Kortman K.E., Flannigan B.D., et al.: MR of craniopharyngiomas: Tumor delineation and characterization. *A.J.N.R.* 8:439–444, 1987.
37. Sartor K., Karnaze M.G., Winthrop J.D., et al.: MR imaging in intra-, para-, and retrosellar mass lesions. *Neuroradiology* 29:19, 1987.
38. Scotti G., Yu C.-Y., Dillon W.P., et al.: MR imaging of cavernous sinus involvement by pituitary adenoma. *A.J.N.R.* 9:657–654, 1988.
39. Steiner E., Imhof H., Knosp E.: Gd-DTPA-enhanced high resolution MR imaging of pituitary adenomas. *Radiographics* 9:587–598, 1989.
40. Tien R., Dillon W.P.: MR imaging of cavernous hemangioma of the optic chiasm. *J. Comput. Assist. Tomogr.* 13:1087, 1989.
41. Yeakley J.W., Kulkarni M.V., McArdle C.B., et al.: High resolution MR imaging of juxtasellar meningiomas with CT and angiographic correlation. *A.J.N.R.* 9:279–286, 1988.
42. Young S.C., Grossman R.I., Goldberg H.I., et al.: MR of vascular encasement in parasellar masses: Comparison with angiography and CT. *A.J.N.R.* 9:35–38, 1988.
43. Yousem D.M., Atlas S.W., Grossman R.I., et al.: MR imaging of Tolosa-Hunt syndrome. *A.J.N.R.* 10:1181–1184, 1989.

CHAPTER 6

Other Masses

Case 216

55-year-old man with a history of unexplained
falls while jogging.
(noncontrast scan)

Case 217

41-year-old woman presenting with headache.
(postcontrast scan)

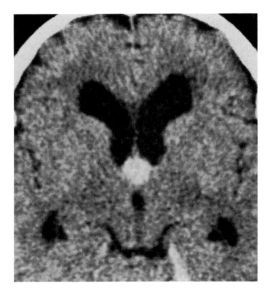

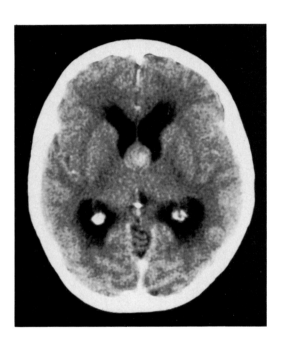

A well-defined, high-attenuation midline mass at the foramina of Monro is highly characteristic of a colloid cyst. This lesion typically arises from the anterior roof of the third ventricle. The mass usually demonstrates precontrast high attenuation due to dense protein content, which may be pathologically gelatinous or caseous.

The strategic position of colloid cysts leads to hydrocephalus as the masses enlarge. The cysts are typically about 1 cm in diameter at the time of diagnosis. (Compare to the much larger size of suprasellar craniopharyngiomas or germinomas obstructing the foramina of Monro as in Cases 192 and 198.)

Some patients experience episodic positional headaches, thought to be due to intermittent ventricular obstruction caused by shifts in position of mobile cysts. (However, similar histories are obtained from patients with large, apparently immobile lesions.)

Colloid cysts are occasionally isodense or low-density lesions. Contrast enhancement is rare but can be seen both peripherally and centrally as in this case. (The precontrast scan had demonstrated uniform isodensity.) Peripheral contrast enhancement associated with colloid cysts on CT or MR scans often reflects a surrounding layer of reactive inflammatory tissue (rather than enhancement of the cyst's epithelium).

The paired columns of the fornix form a normal bulge along the anteromedial margin of the foramen of Monro and should not be confused with an isodense mass (see Case 221).

DIFFERENTIAL DIAGNOSIS:
DENSE LESION NEAR THE FORAMEN OF MONRO

Case 218

58-year-old woman.
(postcontrast scan)

Case 219

13-year-old boy presenting with seizures.
(postcontrast scan)

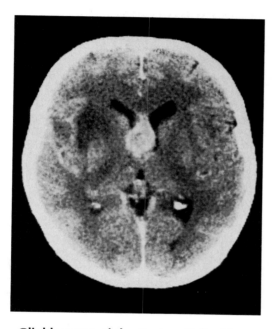

Glioblastoma of the Septum Pellucidum.

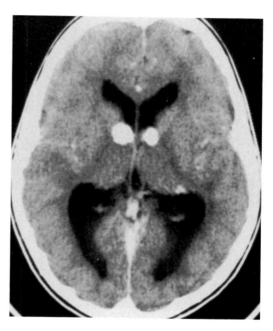

Tuberous Sclerosis.

Colloid cysts are among many dense or enhancing lesions that may occur near the foramen of Monro. Some masses project superiorly from the skull base to reach this level, e.g., suprasellar extension of pituitary adenomas, craniopharyngiomas, aneurysms, or dolichoectatic basilar arteries (see Cases 192, 198, 199, 551, and 552). Other lesions may arise within the third ventricle or frontal horns, e.g., intraventricular meningiomas, choroid plexus tumors or granulomas, or arteriovenous malformations involving the septal, thalamostriate, or internal cerebral veins.

Gliomas are commonly seen near the frontal horns and frequently invade the septum pellucidum, as in Case 218. (Compare this scan to the cystic glioma within the septum pellucidum in Case 193.) Thickening of the septum suggests intra-axial origin of a deep frontal lesion. The finding is most common in gliomas but can also be seen with other pathologies (e.g., primary CNS lymphoma).

Tuberous sclerosis is discussed in Cases 648 to 654. Calcified, subependymal tubers often occur along the lateral margin of the foramen of Monro, as in Case 219 (although they are more frequently unilateral). Subependymal tubers may develop into giant cell astrocytomas, characterized on CT scans by an enlarging and enhancing mass. These tumors may obstruct the foramen of Monro to cause unilateral or bilateral hydrocephalus, but they behave otherwise as low-grade neoplasms.

Case 220

27-year-old man.
(coronal, noncontrast scan; SE 800/16)

Colloid Cyst of the Third Ventricle.

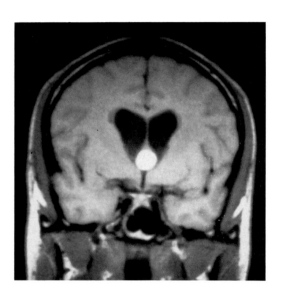

Case 221

13-year-old boy (same patient as Case 219).
(coronal, noncontrast scan; SE 800/17)

Tuberous Sclerosis.

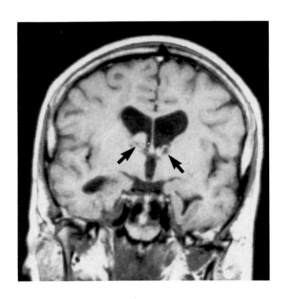

Coronal and sagittal MR scans add anatomical detail and new tissue contrast to the CT evaluation of lesions near the foramen of Monro. The coronal examination in this case precisely localizes the lesion to the junction of the lateral and third ventricles, clearly differentiating it from a suprasellar or hypothalamic mass (compare to Cases 197 to 199).

The signal intensity of colloid cysts on MR scans is as variable as their CT attenuation. The prominent T1-shortening seen in this case is common, but other lesions demonstrate moderately long T1. Similarly, both high and low signal intensity have been observed within colloid cysts on T2-weighted MR scans.

In this case, small masses are apparent along the lateral margins of the foramina of Monro. (The small, paired soft tissue structures in the midline are the normal columns of the fornix.) Their location is characteristic for the subependymal nodules seen in tuberous sclerosis (see discussion in Cases 648 to 654). Components of T1-shortening have been noted in some periventricular tubers.

The foci of low signal intensity within these subependymal nodules represent dense calcification. Comparison of Cases 219 and 221 illustrates a major difference in the presentation of CNS lesions on CT and MR scans: CT scans accentuate calcification, while routine MR pulse sequences minimize it.

CHOROID PLEXUS PAPILLOMAS

Case 222

11-month-old boy with an enlarging head.
(postcontrast scan)

Case 223

68-year-old woman.
(noncontrast scan)

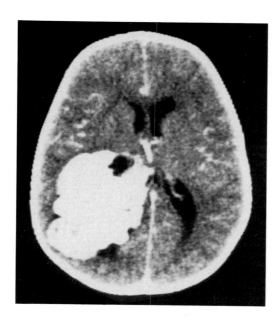

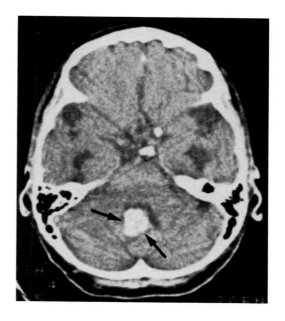

Choroid plexus papillomas are among the intracranial tumors that may be present at birth. They are often associated with hydrocephalus, sometimes due to excessive production of spinal fluid. More commonly, a secondary communicating hydrocephalus develops after repeated tumor hemorrhages with high cerebrospinal fluid loads of protein and cells.

Choroid plexus papillomas in children are most common in the lateral ventricles, particularly on the left. They usually arise from the trigone and are often massive when discovered. Even "benign" papillomas may demonstrate bulky involvement of the adjacent hemisphere, often associated with large cysts. Such aggressive-appearing papillomas can be indistinguishable on CT or MR studies from choroid plexus carcinomas or from malignant ependymomas or gliomas.

Most choroid plexus papillomas demonstrate uniform, mildly increased density on noncontrast scans. Intense, homogeneous contrast enhancement is common. These features may mimic primitive neuroectodermal tumors or intraventricular meningiomas (see Case 96), but the latter are rare in infancy and childhood.

In adults, choroid plexus papillomas occur most commonly in the fourth ventricle, particularly caudally. (See Case 162 for another example as demonstrated by MR.) This location can suggest the diagnosis, with the differential diagnosis including hemangioblastoma, ependymoma, subependymoma, vermian metastasis, unusual glioma, and arteriovenous malformation (see discussion of Cases 122 and 123).

A lateral ventricular tumor in an adult is unlikely to be a choroid plexus papilloma and should suggest meningioma, metastasis, glioma, ependymoma, central neurocytoma, AVM, or an inflammatory lesion (e.g., granuloma, parasitic or fungal mass).

Case 224

22-year-old man presenting with headaches,
nausea, and vomiting.
(postcontrast scan)

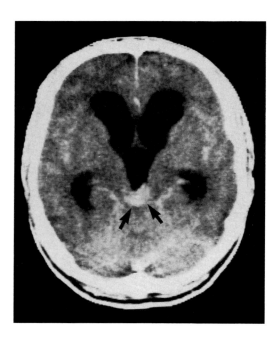

Case 225

11-year-old boy presenting with a 2-week
history of headache and tremors.
(postcontrast scan after shunting)

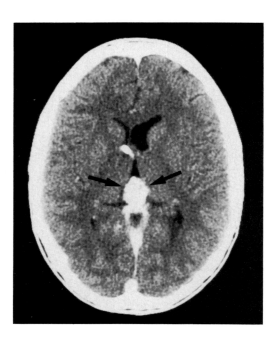

Germ cell tumors form the most common group of pineal masses. Within this category, germinomas are the most frequent pathology. (Other pineal germ cell tumors include teratoma, choriocarcinoma, embryonal cell carcinoma, and endodermal sinus tumor.) Pineal germinomas are common in boys but relatively rare in girls, who more often have suprasellar versions of this tumor (see Cases 196 and 198).

Germinomas (sometimes called "atypical teratomas") usually demonstrate homogeneous high attenuation on precontrast scans and uniform, intense enhancement following contrast injection.

The clinical presentation of pineal tumors is usually due to hydrocephalus from obstruction of the posterior third ventricle and aqueduct, as in this case.

Mixed histology is commonly present in pineal germ cell tumors. Biopsy in this case demonstrated a combination of germinoma and choriocarcinoma.

The characteristic homogeneous enhancement of pineal germinomas may be mimicked by meningiomas of the quadrigeminal plate (see Case 504) or "aneurysms" of the vein of Galen (see Case 505). One clue to the diagnosis can be the tendency of pineal germinomas to grow anteriorly along the walls of the third ventricle (see Case 230), rather than accumulating posteriorly in the quadrigeminal cistern.

Germinomas are usually radiosensitive. Even bulky masses may disappear completely without recurrence after a course of radiation therapy.

However, germinomas are among the primary CNS neoplasms that are associated with CSF seeding causing distant meningeal or ventricular implants. A search for isodense or enhancing cisterns and sulci is therefore appropriate in these cases. Contrast-enhanced MR scans are more sensitive than CT studies for the detection of meningeal dissemination of tumor (see Case 121).

DIFFERENTIAL DIAGNOSIS:
INTENSELY ENHANCING MIDLINE MASS IN THE PINEAL REGION

Case 226

17-year-old boy with behavioral change.

Case 227

17-year-old girl with headaches and paresis of upward gaze.

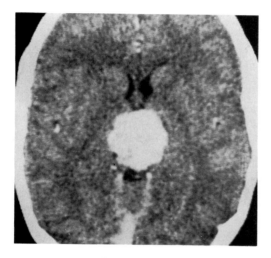

Pineocytoma.

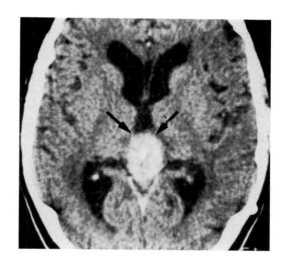

Brain Stem Astrocytoma.

The most common pineal tumors with this general appearance are germinomas, as in Cases 224 and 225.

The rare pineocytoma in Case 226 is a tumor of true pineal cell origin. The margins of pineocytomas are often mildly lobulated, as seen here. The tumor has grown anteriorly to occupy much of the third ventricle. Hydrocephalus is, remarkably, absent.

Gliomas of the brain stem or thalamus may extend into the pineal region to mimic a primary pineal tumor (see also Case 229). In Case 227, the midline mass has displaced the pineal superiorly while obstructing the posterior third ventricle *(arrows)*. More caudal sections demonstrated the mass arising within the midbrain and extending exophytically into the quadrigeminal cistern. Sagittal and coronal MR scans can help to distinguish exophytic brain stem tumors from primary extra-axial masses (see Case 231).

Other lesions in this diagnostic group include subsplenial meningiomas and the so-called "vein of Galen aneurysm" (see Cases 504 and 505).

Paresis of upward gaze as in Case 227 is a component of "Parinaud's syndrome," a pattern of dorsal midbrain dysfunction suggesting pathology in the quadrigeminal region (see also Case 233).

DIFFERENTIAL DIAGNOSIS:
PINEAL REGION MASS WITH AN ECCENTRIC INTRA-AXIAL COMPONENT

Case 228

8-year-old girl with 4-year history of headache
and a 2-week history of nausea, vomiting,
and ataxia.

Case 229

23-year-old woman.

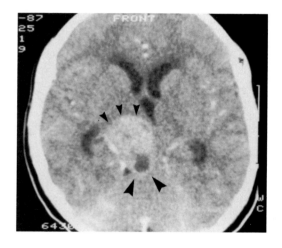

Pineoblastoma.

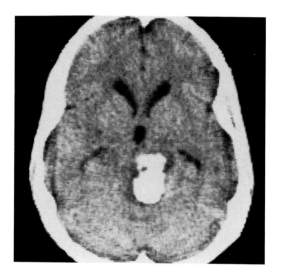

**Astrocytoma of the Thalamus
and Brain Stem.**

Occasionally a pineal tumor invaginates far into adjacent parenchyma. (Compare to the brain stem deformity associated with some acoustic schwannomas, as in Cases 135 and 138.) The lesion in Case 228 was initially thought to represent a thalamic glioma, because the size of the ventral component deforming the third ventricle *(small arrowheads)* exceeds the small dorsal component in the quadrigeminal cistern *(large arrowheads)*. More caudal scans suggested an extra-axial extension of the mass within the right ambient cistern. An MR examination (presented as Case 231) confirmed this impression and supported the diagnosis of a pineal neoplasm.

Pineoblastomas are tumors of true pineal cell origin with less differentiation than pineocytomas such as Case 226. Biopsy in Case 228 demonstrated highly malignant histopathology.

Case 229 represents another example of a glioma involving the pineal region (compare to Case 227). Here a densely calcified astrocytoma obliterates the posterior third ventricle. The eccentricity of the tumor, while occasionally seen in pineal neoplasms such as Case 228, is more typical of intra-axial gliomas. The apparent involvement of the midbrain and thalamus could be confirmed by MR scans. Together, these features suggest an intra-axial neoplasm, which was found at biopsy.

Coarse calcification within an extra-axial mass of the pineal region suggests pineal teratoma or dermoid cyst (see Cases 232 and 234). Both lesions may also contain fat, which is usually more prominent in dermoid cysts.

Case 230

19-year-old man.
(axial, noncontrast scan; SE 3000/90)

Pineal Germinoma.

Case 231

8-year-old girl (same patient as Case 228).
(coronal, noncontrast scan; SE 600/17)

Pineoblastoma.

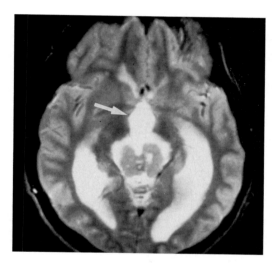

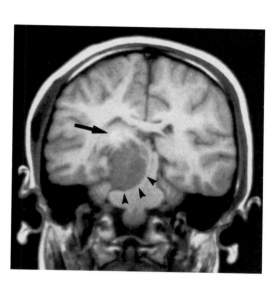

Obstructive hydrocephalus is present in this case, with distention of the third ventricle *(arrow)* and the temporal and occipital horns of the lateral ventricles.

The pineal mass causing the hydrocephalus is centered in the midline. Bilobed anterior extensions of the tumor along the walls of the third ventricle are well outlined by a halo of intense edema. As discussed in Case 225, this pattern of ventral growth is commonly noted with pineal tumors and does not imply an intra-axial lesion of the diencephalon or hypothalamus.

MR provides a second clue to the nature of this tumor by the lesion's relative isointensity (*i.e.*, lack of prolonged T2). This finding is associated with highly cellular tumors and has been noted in germinomas, primary CNS lymphomas, and densely cellular gliomas (compare to Case 77).

In this case the coronal view provided by MR offers key diagnostic information. Contrary to the impression of an intra-axial lesion given on axial CT scans (see Case 228), the MR study demonstrates that the mass lies adjacent to the brain stem, which is displaced and compressed rather than expanded. The superior pole of the lesion invaginates into the thalamus, where a small amount of T1-shortening *(large arrow)* suggests hemorrhage.

The advantages of accentuated tissue contrast and tangential displays of anatomy, as demonstrated in Cases 230 and 231, make MR valuable for evaluating masses of the pineal region.

DERMOID CYSTS

Case 232

61-year-old woman with a history of seizures
since age 19.

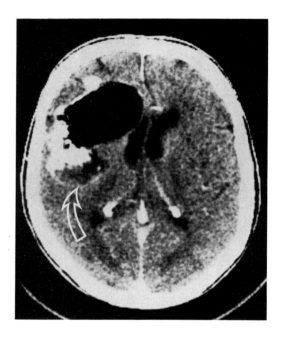

Case 233

38-year-old man with nystagmus and
Parinaud's syndrome.

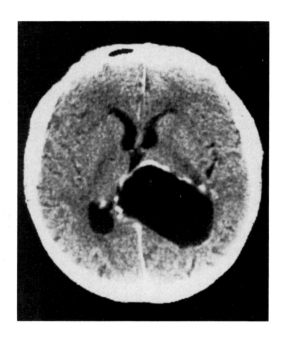

Dermoid tumors or "cysts" are benign masses arising from epithelial cells enclosed intracranially during embryogenesis. In addition to squamous epithelium, dermoid cysts contain mesodermal cells, which may form skin appendages such as hair follicles, sweat glands, and sebaceous glands. Slow proliferation of these tissues leads to gradual accumulation of a pilosebaceous mass, causing the congenital lesions to appear in adulthood.

The CT appearance of dermoid cysts is usually a characteristic combination of central lipid material and dense peripheral calcification. Some regions of the mass may have intermediate attenuation values (as seen posteriorly in this case; *arrow*) due to the presence of hair or other proteinaceous material. Contrast enhancement is rare.

The mass in this case arose from the parasellar region, with large lobulations occupying the anterior and middle cranial fossae.

This dermoid cyst extends from the pineal region to the atrium of the left lateral ventricle. Mass effect is apparent, with mild hydrocephalus due to obstruction of the posterior third ventricle.

The thin rim of calcification surrounding a low attenuation center is typical of dermoid cysts. Teratomas can also demonstrate both lipid material and calcification, but the latter is usually more dense and central within the mass (which may also contain ossified elements).

Epidermoid cysts present a similar low-attenuation appearance but are less frequently calcified. Small lipomas commonly occur in the quadrigeminal cistern, but have very low-density values indicating homogeneous fat content.

Dermoid cysts adjacent to ventricular margins as in Cases 232 and 233 may rupture into the ventricular system. Cases 234 and 394 illustrate the resultant appearance of intraventricular lipid material, seen as tiny black droplets or as "fat/fluid levels" crossing ventricular chambers. Cisternal or ventricular fat/fluid levels may also be associated with some leaking epidermoid cysts and teratomas.

DIFFERENTIAL DIAGNOSIS:
SUPRASELLAR MASS WITH CALCIFICATION AND LOW ATTENUATION

Case 234

60-year-old man.

Case 235

6-year-old girl.

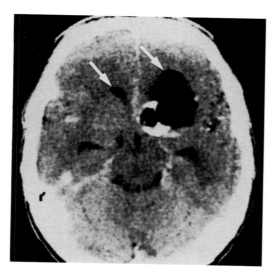

Dermoid Cyst.

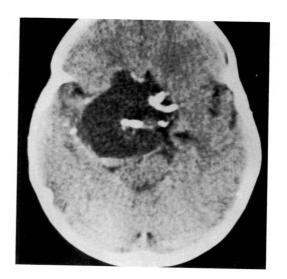

Craniopharyngioma.

Many dermoid cysts are found in the parasellar or suprasellar region. Another common location is the midline of the posterior fossa, either within the fourth ventricle or between the cerebellar hemispheres.

The heavy calcification and low density of a parasellar dermoid cyst may resemble a craniopharyngioma, as in Case 234. The extremely low attenuation of lipid material within dermoid cysts usually distinguishes these lesions from the fluid and debris within craniopharyngiomas. Craniopharyngiomas often contain cholesterol, but the cyst content rarely matches the homogeneous fatty nature of a dermoid cyst.

The tumor in Case 234 has ruptured into the ventricular system, with lipid droplets floating in the frontal horns (arrows). Intraventricular rupture or leakage of fatty material is often clinically silent. Some patients experience a severe chemical meningitis, particularly when the contents of a ruptured cyst extend beyond the ventricles to involve the subarachnoid spaces.

Hypothalamic gliomas may also demonstrate low attenuation (cystic or solid; see Cases 209 and 592) and calcification, resembling these other suprasellar lesions.

EPIDERMOID CYSTS

Case 236

50-year-old woman with tic douloureux and
facial nerve paresis.

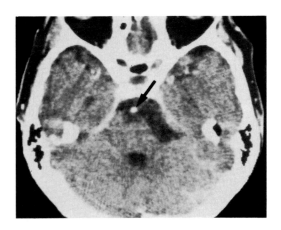

Case 237

52-year-old man with a 3-year history of
memory loss culminating in arrest
for shoplifting.
(scan with intrathecal contrast)

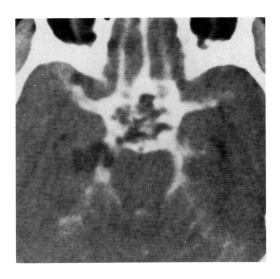

Epidermoid cysts are usually low-attenuation, nonenhancing, extra-axial lesions. The density of the masses represents the average of mixed cholesterol and keratin components. Occasional high-attenuation epidermoids are seen, probably reflecting a preponderance of dense keratin over low-attenuation cholesterol or rare calcification associated with cholesterol esters.

The low density of most epidermoids may resemble arachnoid cysts or cisterns (see also Cases 620, 621, and 626). In this case, the expansion of peripontine cisterns could be mistaken for widened CSF spaces due to brain stem displacement by an extra-axial mass. Narrow window width displays and histogram analysis will usually show an epidermoid cyst to be less homogeneous than a widened cistern. MR may also be useful in distinguishing epidermoid tissue from CSF (see Case 241).

Epidermoid cysts are often soft, extensively infiltrating lesions that surround vessels and cranial nerves. Here a portion of the tumor has insinuated itself between the basilar artery *(arrow)* and the pons. (See Case 241B for the MR equivalent of this appearance.)

As discussed in Case 51, masses involving the medial portion of the cerebellopontine angle and/or posterior cavernous sinus are an important cause of facial pain, as demonstrated by this patient.

The surface of epidermoid cysts is typically papillary or frond-like, resembling a cauliflower. This characteristic irregularity cannot be appreciated when the tumor is surrounded by CSF of similar density.

The addition of subarachnoid contrast material outlines the tumor interstices and provides the diagnosis. This technique is useful for distinguishing epidermoid cysts from arachnoid cysts when a low-density, extra-axial lesion is encountered.

In this case, a routine scan had demonstrated a low-attenuation suprasellar mass splaying the cerebral peduncles and compressing the medial temporal lobes (see Case 621). The intrathecal contrast study outlines the typical irregular surface of an epidermoid cyst.

Normal gyral anatomy is also well demonstrated on such scans. Here the gyrus rectus of the inferior frontal lobe is outlined anterior to the suprasellar cistern. Distortions of the adjacent sulci may be a secondary finding associated with CSF rhinorrhea from the cribriform region (see Cases 391 and 392).

DIFFERENTIAL DIAGNOSIS:
LOW-ATTENUATION, EXTRA-AXIAL LESION IN THE CEREBELLOPONTINE ANGLE

Case 238

74-year-old man.
(noncontrast scan)

Case 239

40-year-old man.
(postcontrast scan)

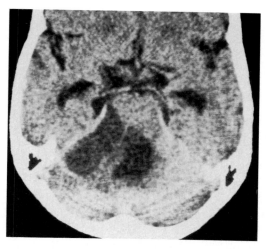

Acoustic Schwannoma.

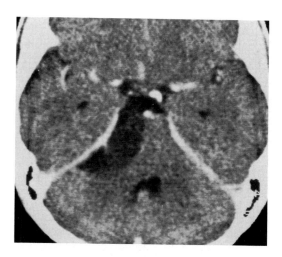

Epidermoid Cyst.

Several low-attenuation lesions may occupy the cerebello-pontine angle. Some acoustic schwannomas contain low-density components, either solid or cystic. Only minimal contrast enhancement occurred in Case 238. (Case 137 presents a postcontrast scan of this patient.)

The cerebellopontine angle is a common location for epidermoid cysts, as seen in Cases 236 and 239.

Arachnoid cysts may also be found at this site and should be included in the differential diagnosis (see Case 626). Rarely a cerebellopontine angle meningioma may be cystic or lipomatous, resembling other low-attenuation extra-axial lesions (see Case 627).

Case 240A

36-year-old woman.
(sagittal, noncontrast scan; SE 600/20)

Case 240B

Same patient.
(axial, noncontrast scan; SE 2500/90)

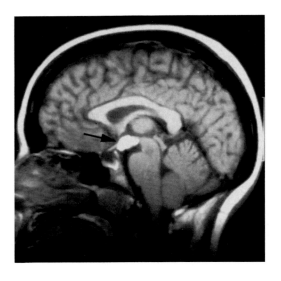

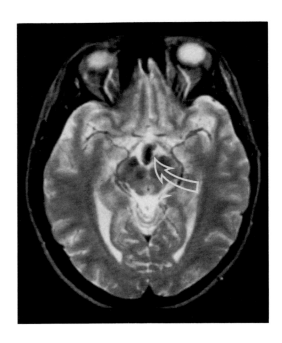

The lipid content of dermoid cysts causes high signal intensity on T1-weighted MR studies. In this case, the suprasellar dermoid mass is much more clearly separated from surrounding CSF than would be true on a CT scan.

The occurrence of T1-shortening within a suprasellar lesion is not specific for dermoid cysts. Craniopharyngiomas, Rathke's pouch cysts, lipomas, hemorrhage into pituitary adenomas, or an "ectopic" neurohypophysis (see Case 187) may present a similar appearance.

Most fat-containing masses demonstrate a relative loss of signal intensity on T2-weighted MR images, as seen here. The dermoid cyst occupying the interpeduncular cistern is now much lower in intensity than surrounding CSF, a reversal of the relationship in Case 240A.

Masses with T1-shortening due to proteinaceous contents (e.g., Rathke's pouch cyst) usually demonstrate higher signal than seen here on T2-weighted scans. Blood products may cause shortening of both T1 and T2 similar to this case, but the morphology of such signal changes is usually characteristic (see Cases 179 and 211).

The MR distinction between lipid material and other causes of T1-shortening within a cerebral lesion can also be based on (1) the presence of chemical shift artifact, or (2) the use of pulse sequences that selectively suppress the signal from water or lipid protons.

MR CORRELATION: EPIDERMOID CYSTS

Case 241A

51-year-old man.
(sagittal, noncontrast scan; SE 550/20)

Case 241B

Same patient.
(axial, noncontrast scan; SE 3000/45)

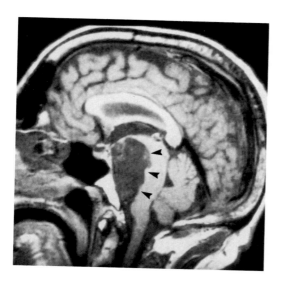

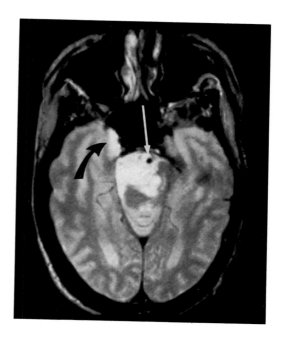

MR scans can usually distinguish epidermoid tumors from other lesions of low attenuation on CT studies, thereby avoiding the need for intrathecal contrast as demonstrated in Case 237.

The signal intensity of most epidermoid cysts remains close to that of CSF on a variety of pulse sequences. However, subtle differences are usually apparent. In this case, the large prepontine lesion is slightly but definitely higher and less homogeneous in intensity than the CSF within the third ventricle.

Some epidermoid cysts demonstrate short T1 values (and associated T2 shortening) resembling dermoid cysts. Such masses usually contain viscous liquid components, rather than lipid material, with high signal intensity on T1-weighted scans due to enhanced relaxation of *water* protons.

MR is also helpful in defining the characteristically lobulated surface of epidermoid cysts. Here the interface between the lesion and the brain stem is notably irregular, a feature that would be distinctly unusual for an arachnoid cyst.

The slow growth of this benign mass has led to impressive displacement and deformity of the brain stem, as well as marked superior bowing of the floor of the third ventricle.

The greatest difference in signal intensity between epidermoid cysts and CSF is often noted on "balanced" spin-echo images obtained with long TR and short TE values. On this "intermediate" sequence the intensity of the prepontine epidermoid cyst is greater than that of CSF in the occipital horns. More importantly, MR suggests the correct diagnosis by clearly demonstrating the lesion's morphology.

The lobulated contour of the mass is apparent, as is the marked deformity of the brain stem. Both of these features are hallmarks of a prepontine epidermoid cyst. Even more characteristic is the manner in which the mass has surrounded the vessels and cranial nerves in the region, insinuating itself between the basilar artery *(white arrow)* and the displaced midbrain (compare to Case 236).

In this case the posterior fossa mass has also grown into Meckel's cave on the left *(black arrow)*. Epidermoid cysts are among the lesions with a tendency to span the petrous apex (see Cases 50 and 51) and among the masses that may be responsible for trigeminal neuralgia.

Case 244

45-year-old man presenting with hemiparesis.
(postcontrast scan)

Case 245

74-year-old woman.
(noncontrast scan)

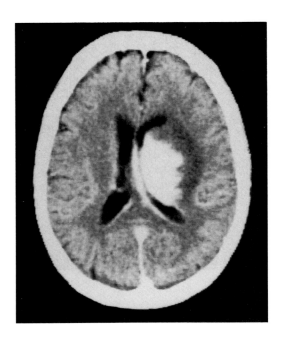

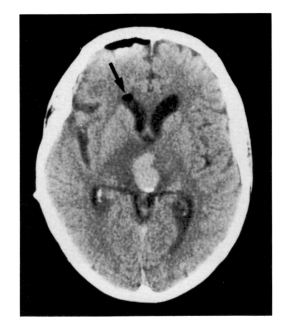

Primary CNS lymphoma ("reticulum cell sarcoma," "microglioma," "immunoblastic lymphoma") usually presents as one or more deep hemisphere masses. Frequent areas of involvement include the basal ganglia, corpus callosum, cerebellar vermis, and periventricular white matter.

The tumor in this case has arisen along the wall of the lateral ventricle. Extensive subependymal spread is apparent (compare to Cases 102 and 103). Contrast enhancement within CNS lymphomas may be solid or peripheral. Intense, uniform enhancement as seen here is common.

CT findings often regress in response to steroid therapy and may wax and wane spontaneously. Clues to the diagnosis include involvement of deep hemisphere structures, multicentricity, steroid response, and a clinical association with immunosuppression (see Cases 247 and 250).

Deep hemisphere masses due to primary CNS lymphoma are often isodense on noncontrast scans. Some lesions demonstrate mildly or definitely increased attenuation values before contrast, as seen here. This finding is typically homogeneous (in patients who do not have acquired immune deficiency syndrome [AIDS]) and likely reflects dense cellularity with a high nuclear-to-cytoplasmic ratio.

The MR scans of such lesions may demonstrate relative isointensity on "T2-weighted" images, similar to germinomas as in Case 230. Other cases of primary CNS lymphoma demonstrate high signal intensity on long TR pulse sequences.

The precontrast density and homogeneous contrast enhancement of masses such as Case 245 can mimic meningiomas or germinomas in appropriate locations. Here the tumor involves the posterior third ventricle, growing anteriorly and inciting adjacent edema in a manner that would suggest a pineal neoplasm in a younger patient (compare to Cases 225 and 230).

The small amount of air over the right frontal lobe and within the right frontal horn (arrow) in this case is due to a recent stereotactic biopsy and illustrates the CT appearance of pneumocephalus.

PRIMARY CNS LYMPHOMA: LOBAR LESIONS

Case 246

58-year-old man presenting with hemiparesis.

Case 247

27-year-old man with AIDS.

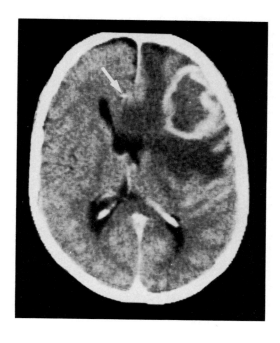

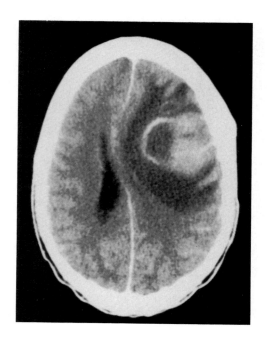

Primary CNS lymphomas can assume a variety of appearances and may mimic other pathologies. This large, rim-enhancing, solitary lesion closely resembles a glioblastoma. Lobar location of primary CNS lymphoma is not unusual.

Primary lymphoma of the CNS is more common than parenchymal involvement by systemic lymphoma, which more typically infiltrates the meninges or ventricular surface (see Case 103).

This case is a good example of subfalcial herniation. The edematous frontal lobe passes beneath the falx and deforms the frontal horns. The pericallosal arteries are markedly displaced (arrow).

Patients with AIDS have a high incidence of primary CNS lymphoma. This diagnosis should be considered (along with toxoplasmosis; see Cases 289 and 290) whenever a cerebral mass is discovered in this setting.

CNS lymphomas in AIDS patients are often inhomogeneous lesions with large areas of central necrosis outlined by peripheral enhancement, as in this case. Deep hemisphere involvement and multiple masses are common, as is the simultaneous presence of inflammatory lesions.

DIFFERENTIAL DIAGNOSIS:
MULTIPLE, HIGH-ATTENUATION, ENHANCING CEREBRAL NODULES

Case 248

61-year-old man.
(noncontrast scan)

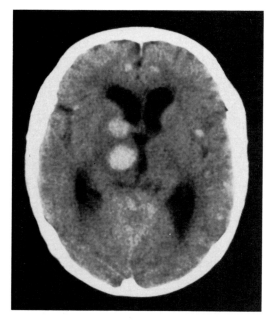

**Leukemia ("Chloromas" or
"Granulocytic Sarcomas").**

Case 249

62-year-old woman.
(postcontrast scan)

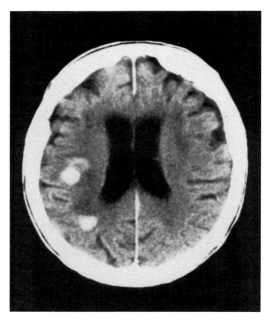

Primary CNS Lymphoma.

Both systemic leukemia and primary CNS lymphoma can cause multiple cerebral nodules with high precontrast attenuation and homogeneous contrast enhancement. The appearance resembles that of cerebral metastases from melanoma or solid tumors with high vascularity (e.g., hypernephroma, choriocarcinoma, bronchogenic carcinoma; see Cases 4, 9, and 308). Both metastatic leukemia and primary CNS lymphoma commonly involve deep hemisphere structures as well as superficial cortical and subcortical sites.

DIFFERENTIAL DIAGNOSIS:
MULTIPLE ENHANCING CEREBRAL AND CEREBELLAR NODULES

Case 250

32-year-old woman with a renal transplant.

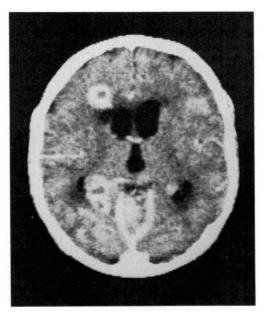

Primary CNS Lymphoma.

Case 251

53-year-old woman from Southeast Asia with fever and pulmonary infiltrates.

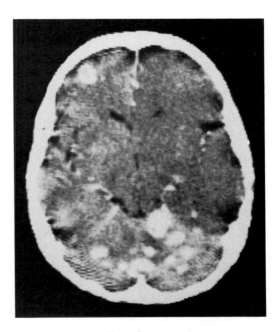

Metastatic Adenocarcinoma.

Multiple, focal, enhancing lesions may be inflammatory (e.g., multiple sclerosis, disseminated infection, neurosarcoidosis), vascular (e.g., multifocal infarctions, hemangiomas), or neoplastic (see Cases 288, 307, 416, and 510). In the latter category, metastases and primary CNS lymphoma are the leading possibilities.

Primary CNS lymphomas are rare in otherwise healthy individuals. They are much more common in patients who are immunosuppressed due to disease (e.g., lymphoma, AIDS) or medication (e.g., transplant regimens).

Infection was a primary consideration in Case 251, but the pulmonary and cerebral lesions proved to represent adenocarcinoma. The CT scan had been performed because of an acute cerebrovascular accident, and the left hemisphere shows slightly decreased attenuation with a conspicuous lack of enhancing metastases.

Case 252

14-year-old girl.

Uremic Encephalopathy.

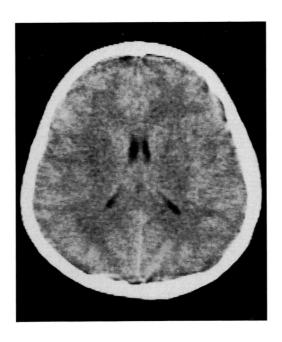

Case 253

35-year-old woman with headaches
and papilledema.

Pseudotumor Cerebri.

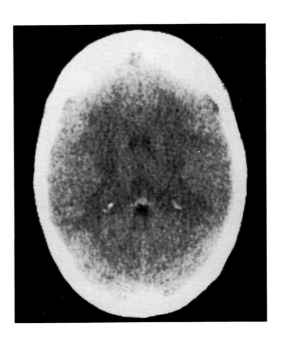

Several categories of diffuse encephalopathy may present with increased intracranial pressure mimicking a mass lesion. In these cases, CT scans may show cerebral swelling with compression of ventricles and sulci.

The differential diagnosis for diffusely swollen hemispheres includes metabolic encephalopathy (e.g., uremia, Reye's syndrome, and hypertensive encephalopathy; see Case 255), pseudotumor cerebri, and superior sagittal sinus thrombosis. Head trauma, anoxia, and encephalitis may present a similar appearance but are usually evident clinically (see Cases 268A, 385, 386, 475, and 476).

The ventricles may normally be quite small in young patients (especially women), and compression may be difficult to judge. In this case, the ventricles are small enough to suggest cerebral swelling. They returned to a normal size following resolution of the patient's uremia.

The syndrome of "benign intracranial hypertension" or "pseudotumor cerebri" may be considered in young patients (especially overweight women) with papilledema and symptoms of elevated intracranial pressure. Apart from a few specific associations (e.g., hypervitaminosis A, tetracycline toxic reaction), the cause of the syndrome is undefined and controversial. It is characterized by the typical clinical picture in the absence of specific intracranial pathology.

In such patients, CT or MR serves the primary purpose of excluding a mass lesion, hydrocephalus, or venous thrombosis. The secondary finding of small ventricles suggesting cerebral swelling (as in this case) is seen in a minority of patients.

Case 254

8-year-old boy.
(noncontrast scan)

Head Trauma.

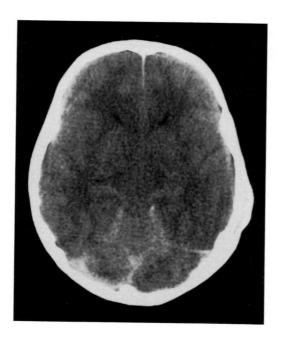

Case 255

53-year-old man presenting with headache.

Malignant Hypertension.

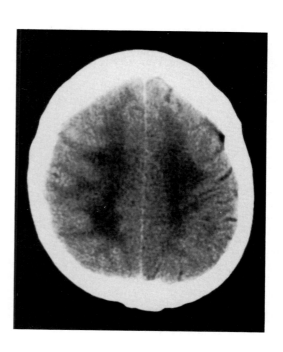

Cerebral swelling is a common result of severe head trauma (see also Cases 385 and 386). Components may include increased intracranial blood volume as well as cerebral edema. The process may be symmetrical, diffuse, and unaccompanied by contusion or hemorrhage. In this case, the cerebral surface is relatively featureless, with poor visualization of sulci and cisterns.

Post-traumatic cerebral swelling may cause secondary injury due to parenchymal herniation and vascular compromise. In this case, bilateral herniation of the uncus and parahippocampal gyrus led to compression of the posterior cerebral arteries against the tentorial margin, with consequent infarction of the occipital lobes (see Case 451 for a follow-up scan of a similar patient).

The dural surfaces and dural sinuses often appear relatively dense on noncontrast scans in cases of head trauma. This density likely represents hyperemia or venous stasis from increased intracranial pressure accentuated by decreased attenuation values of adjacent cerebral parenchyma. True superior sagittal sinus thrombosis should be included in the differential diagnosis of cerebral swelling (see Cases 468 to 472).

Here a noncontrast scan near the vertex demonstrates striking demarcation between gray and white matter. This abnormal definition is due to diffuse white matter edema causing uniformly decreased attenuation values throughout the centrum semiovale.

Such cerebral edema is even more obvious on T2-weighted MR scans as regions of high signal intensity. A similar finding has been noted in women with increased intracranial pressure due to toxemia of pregnancy.

REFERENCES: CT

1. Barsky M.F., Coates R.K., Macdonald D.R.: Computed tomographic features of primary brain lymphoma. *J. Can. Assoc. Radiol.* 40:80, 1989.
2. Berger M.S., Wilson C.B.: Epidermoid cysts of the posterior fossa. *J. Neurosurg.* 62:214–219, 1985.
3. Camacho A., Abernathy C.D., Kelly P.J., Laws E.R. Jr.: Colloid cysts: Experience with the management of 84 cases since the introduction of computed tomography. *Neurosurgery* 24:693–700, 1989.
4. Cecchini A., Pezzotta S., Paoletti P., et al.: Dense dermoids in craniovertebral region. *J. Comput. Assist. Tomogr.* 7:479–483, 1983.
5. Chakeres D.W., LaMasters D.L.: Paragangliomas of the temporal bone: High-resolution CT studies. *Radiology* 150:749–753, 1984.
6. Chambers E.F., Turski P.A., Sobel D., et al.: Radiologic characteristics of primary cerebral neuroblastoma. *Radiology* 139:101–104, 1981.
7. Chang T., Teng M.M.H., Guo W.-Y., Sheng W.-C.: CT of pineal tumors and intracranial germ cell tumors. *A.J.N.R.* 10:1039–1044, 1989.
8. Futrell N.N., Osborn A.G., Cheson B.D.: Pineal region tumors: Computed tomographic-pathologic spectrum. *A.J.N.R.* 2:415–420, 1981.
9. Ganti S.R., Antures J.L., Louis K.M., et al.: Computed tomography in the diagnosis of colloid cysts of the third ventricle. *Radiology* 138:385–391, 1981.
10. Ganti S.R., Hilal S.K., Stein B.M., et al.: CT of pineal region tumors. *A.J.N.R.* 7:97–104, 1986.
11. Gardeur D., Palmieri A., Mashaly R.: Cranial computed tomography in the phakomatoses. *Neuroradiology* 25:293–304, 1983.
12. Goldberg R., Byrd S., Winter J., et al.: Varied appearance of trigeminal neuroma on CT. *A.J.R.* 134:57–90, 1980.
13. Hildenbrand P.G., Gabrielsen T.O., Dorouini-Zis K., et al.: Radiology of primary intracranial yolk-sac (endodermal sinus) tumors. *A.J.N.R.* 4:991–993, 1983.
14. Hinshaw D.B., Ashwal S., Thompson J.R., et al.: Neuroradiology of primitive neuroectodermal tumors. *Neuroradiology* 25:87–92, 1983.
15. Holtas S., Nyman V., Cronqvist S.: Computed tomography of malignant lymphoma of the brain. *Neuroradiology* 26:33–38, 1984.
16. Jack C.R. Jr., O'Neill B.P., Banha P.M., Reese D.F.: Central nervous system lymphoma: Histologic types and CT appearance. *Radiology* 167:211–216, 1988.
17. Jack C.R. Jr., Reese D.F., Scheithauer B.W.: Radiographic findings in 32 cases of primary CNS lymphoma. *A.J.N.R.* 6:899–904, 1985.
18. Jooma R., Kendall B.E.: Diagnosis and management of pineal tumors. *J. Neurosurg.* 58:654–665, 1983.
19. Kaye A.H., Hahn J.F., Kinney S.R., et al.: Jugular foramen schwannomas. *J. Neurosurg.* 60:1045–1053, 1984.
20. Kazner E., Stochdorph O., Wende S., et al.: Intracranial lipoma: Diagnostic and therapeutic considerations. *J. Neurosurg.* 52:234–245, 1980.
21. Kendall B., Reider-Grosswasser I., Valentine A.: Diagnosis of masses presenting within the ventricles on computed tomography. *Neuroradiology* 25:11–22, 1983.
22. Komatsu Y., Shinohara A., Kukita C., et al.: Reversible CT changes in uremic encephalopathy. *A.J.N.R.* 9:215–216, 1988.
23. Laster D.W., Moody D.M., Ball M.R.: Epidermoid tumors with intraventricular and subarachnoid fat. *A.J.R.* 128:504–507, 1977.
24. Latchaw R.E., L'heureux P.R., Young G., et al.: Neuroblastoma presenting as central nervous system disease. *A.J.N.R.* 3:623–630, 1982.
25. Lee Y.-Y., Bruner J.M., Van Tassel P., Libschitz H.I.: Primary central nervous system lymphoma: CT and pathologic correlation. *A.J.N.R.* 7:599–604, 1986.
26. Lo W.M., Solti-Bohman L.G., Lambert P.R.: High resolution CT in the evaluation of glomus tumors of the temporal bone. *Radiology* 150:737–742, 1984.
27. Lukin R., Tomsick T.A., Chambers A.A.: Lymphoma and leukemia of the central nervous system. *Semin. Roentgenol.* 15:256, 1980.
28. McCormick P.C., Bello J.A., Post K.D.: Trigeminal schwannoma: Surgical series of 14 cases with review of the literature. *J. Neurosurg.* 69:850–860, 1988.
29. Mendenhall N.P., Thar T.L., Agee O.F., et al.: Primary lymphoma of the central nervous system: Computerized tomography scan characteristics and treatment results for 12 cases. *Cancer* 52:1993–2000, 1983.
30. Moore T., Ganti S.R., Mawad M.E., Hilal S.K.: CT and angiography of primary extradural juxtasellar tumors. *A.J.N.R.* 6:521–526, 1985.
31. Morrison G., Sobel D.F., Kelly W.M., Norman D.: Intraventricular mass lesions. *Radiology* 153:435–442, 1984.
32. Naheedy M.H., Biller J., Schiffer M., et al.: Toxemia of pregnancy: Cerebral CT findings. *J. Comput. Assist. Tomogr.* 9:497–501, 1986.
33. Neuwelt E.A., Glasberg M., Frenkel E., et al.: Malignant pineal region tumors: A clinico-pathological study. *J. Neurosurg.* 51:597–607, 1979.
34. Palacios E., Gorelick P.B., Gonzalez C.F., et al.: Malignant lymphoma of the nervous system. *J. Comput. Assist. Tomogr.* 6:689–701, 1982.
35. Poon T., Matoso I., Tchertkoff V., et al.: CT features of primary cerebral lymphoma in AIDS and non-AIDS patients. *J. Comput. Assist. Tomogr.* 13:6–9, 1989.
36. Silver A.J., Ganti S.R., Hilal S.K.: Computed tomography of tumors involving the atria of the lateral ventricles. *Radiology* 145:71–78, 1982.
37. Tubman D.E., Frick M.P., Hanto D.W.: Lymphoma after organ transplantation: Radiologic manifestation in the central nervous system, thorax, and abdomen. *Radiology* 149:625–631, 1983.
38. Waldron R.L. II, Abbott D.C., Vellody D.: Computed tomography in preeclampsia-eclampsia syndrome. *A.J.N.R.* 6:442–443, 1985.
39. Weingarten K.L., Zimmerman R.D., Leeds N.E.: Spontaneous regression of intracerebral lymphoma. *Radiology* 149:721–724, 1983.
40. Weingarten K.L., Zimmerman R.D., Pinto R.S., Whelan M.A.: Computed tomographic changes of hypertensive encephalopathy. *A.J.N.R.* 6:395–398, 1985.
41. Yang P.J., Knake J.E., Gabrielson T.O., et al.: Primary and secondary histiocytic lymphoma of the brain: CT features. *Radiology* 154:683–686, 1985.
42. Zimmerman R.A., Bilaniuk L.T.: CT of primary and secondary craniocerebral neuroblastoma. *A.J.N.R.* 1:431–434, 1980.
43. Zimmerman R.A., Bilaniuk L.T., Wood J.H., et al.: Computed tomography of pineal, parapineal, and histologically related tumors. *Radiology* 137:669–677, 1980.

REFERENCES: MR

1. Bolen J.W., Lipper M.H., Caccamo D.: Juxtaventricular central neurocytoma: CT and MR findings. *J. Comput. Assist. Tomogr.* 13:495–497, 1989.
2. Coates T.L., Hinshaw D.B. Jr., Peckman N., et al.: Pediatric choroid plexus neoplasms: MR, CT, and pathologic correlation. *Radiology* 173:81–88, 1989.
3. Gibby W.A., Stecker M.M., Goldberg H.I., et al.: Reversal of white matter edema in hypertensive encephalopathy. *A.J.N.R.* 10:578, 1989.
4. Hahn F.J., Ong E., McComb R.D., et al.: MR imaging of ruptured intracranial dermoid. *J. Comput. Assist. Tomogr.* 10:888–889, 1986.
5. Horowitz B.L., Chari M.V., James R.: MR of intracranial epidermoid tumors: Correlation of in vivo imaging with in vitro C-13 spectroscopy. *A.J.N.R.* 11:299–302, 1990.
6. Kilgore D.P., Strother C.M., Starshak R.J., Haughton V.M.: Pineal germinoma: MR imaging. *Radiology* 158:435–438, 1986.
7. Latack J.T., Kartush J.M., Kemink J.L., et al.: Epidermoidomas of the cerebellopontine angle and temporal bone: CT and MR aspects. *Radiology* 157:361–366, 1985.
8. Lee D.H., Norman D., Newton T.H.: MR imaging of pineal cysts. *J. Comput. Assist. Tomogr.* 11:586–590, 1987.
9. Mamourian A.C., Towfighi J.: Pineal cysts: MR imaging. *A.J.N.R.* 7:1081–1086, 1986.
10. Miyazawa N., Yamazaki H., Wakao T., Nukui H.: Epidermoid tumors of Meckel's cave: Case report and review of the literature. *Neurosurgery* 25:951–954, 1989.
11. Moser F.G., Hilal S.K., Abrams G., et al.: MR imaging of pseudotumor cerebri. *A.J.N.R.* 9:39–46, 1988.
12. Nakagawa H., Iwasaki S., Kichikawa K., et al.: MR imaging of pineocytoma: Report of two cases. *A.J.N.R.* 11:195–198, 1990.
13. Olson J.J., Beck D.W., Crawford S.C., Menezes A.H.: Comparative evaluation of epidermoid tumors with computed tomography and magnetic resonance imaging. *Neurosurgery* 21:357–360, 1987.
14. Pollack I.F., Sekhar L.N., Jannetta P.J., Janecka I.P.: Neurilemomas of the trigeminal nerve. *J. Neurosurg.* 70:737–745, 1989.
15. Rippe D.J., Boyko O.B., Friedman H.S., et al.: Gd-DTPA-enhanced MR imaging of leptomeningeal spread of primary intracranial CNS tumors in children. *A.J.N.R.* 11:329–332, 1990.
16. Roosen N., Gahlen D., Stork W., et al.: Magnetic resonance imaging of colloid cysts of the third ventricle. *Neuroradiology* 29:10, 1987.
17. Savader S.J., Murtagh F.R., Savader B.L., et al.: Magnetic resonance imaging of intracranial epidermoid tumors. *Clin. Radiol.* 40:282, 1989.
18. Schwaighofer B.W., Hesselink J.R., Healy M.E.: MR demonstration of reversible brain abnormalities in eclampsia. *J. Comput. Assist. Tomogr.* 13:310–312, 1989.
19. Schwaighofer B.W., Hesselink J.R., Press G.A., et al.: Primary intracranial CNS lymphoma: MR manifestations. *A.J.N.R.* 10:725–730, 1989.
20. Scotti G., Scialfa G., Colombo N., Landoni L.: MR in the diagnosis of colloid cysts of the third ventricle. *A.J.N.R.* 8:370–372, 1987.
21. Silbergleit T., Junck L., Gebarski S., Hatfield M.K.: Idiopathic intracranial hypertension (pseudotumor cerebri): MR imaging. *Radiology* 170:207–210, 1989.
22. Steffey D.J., De Filipp G.J., Spera T., Gabrielson T.O.: MR imaging of primary epidermoid tumors. *J. Comput. Assist. Tomogr.* 12:438–440, 1988.
23. Stephenson T.F., Spitzer R.M.: MR and CT appearance of ruptured intracranial dermoid tumors. *Comput. Radiol.* 11:249, 1987.
24. Tampieri D., Melanson D., Ethier R.: MR imaging of epidermoid cysts. *A.J.N.R.* 10:351–356, 1989.
25. Tash R.R., Sze G., Leslie D.R.: Trigeminal neuralgia: MR imaging features. *Radiology* 172:767–770, 1989.
26. Vion-Dury J., Vincentelli F., Jiddane M., et al.: MR imaging of epidermoid cysts. *Neuroradiology* 29:333, 1987.
27. Waggenspack G.A., Guinto F.C. Jr.: MR and CT of masses of the anterosuperior third ventricle. *A.J.N.R.* 10:105–110, 1989.
28. Yuh W.T., Wright D.C., Barloon T.J., et al.: MR imaging of primary tumors of the trigeminal nerve and Meckel's cave. *A.J.N.R.* 9:665–670, 1988.

CHAPTER 7

Inflammatory and Degenerative Diseases

Case 256

11-year-old boy.
(noncontrast scan)

Meningococcal Meningitis.

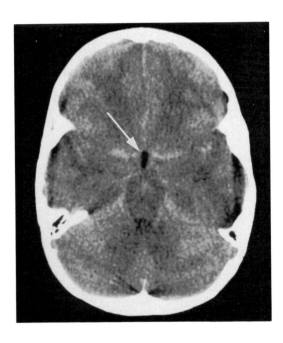

Case 257

1-year-old boy.
(noncontrast scan)

Meningitis due to *Hemophilus influenzae*.

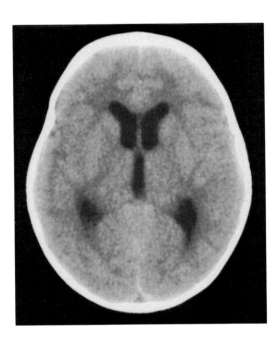

CT scans are frequently negative in the clinical setting of meningitis. In some cases a mild communicating hydrocephalus is the only clue to meningeal pathology.

In other cases exudate and debris may be seen within subarachnoid spaces. Cells, protein, and reactive tissue within sulci and cisterns may raise their attenuation values above those of surrounding brain. The consequent density mimics mild subarachnoid hemorrhage (compare to Cases 520 and 521). High-attenuation cisterns due to meningitis are most often associated with bacterial, fungal, or granulomatous pathogens and are most commonly found near the base of the brain.

In this case the mildly distended anterior recesses of the third ventricle *(arrow)* are outlined by the surrounding density of the suprasellar cistern, indicating associated communicating hydrocephalus.

In this case the increase in subarachnoid attenuation values due to meningitis is not as dramatic as in Case 256. The result is "isodense" subarachnoid spaces, with a featureless cerebral surface. (Compare the region of the tentorial hiatus and superior vermian cistern to Case 195.) The absence of normal sulcal and cisternal contours is an important clue to meningeal pathology, whether generalized as seen here or more localized.

Moderate communicating hydrocephalus due to impaired cisternal circulation of CSF is present in this case. (The degree of ventricular dilatation is not sufficient to explain the obliteration of sulcal markings as an effect of increased intracranial pressure.)

MENINGITIS: SUPERFICIAL ENHANCEMENT

Case 258

7-month-old boy.

Nonspecific Meningitis.

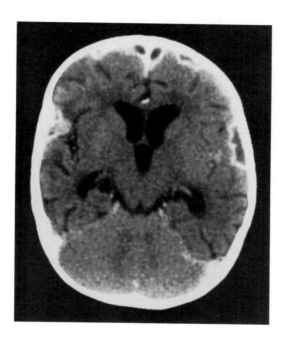

Case 259

1-year-old boy presenting with fever
and right hemiparesis.

Nonspecific Meningitis.

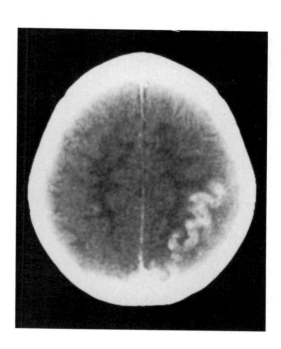

Superficial contrast enhancement may confirm the suspicion of meningitis raised clinically or on noncontrast CT studies. Abnormal enhancement is frequently confined to the meninges, as in this case. Involvement may be generalized or localized. The pattern may be predominantly "dural" (linear, paralleling the calvarium) or "pia-arachnoidal" (with invaginations into cerebral sulci and cisterns).

The nonenhancing fluid collections located between enhancing membranes and the inner table can represent either sterile effusions or loculated subdural or epidural empyemas (see Cases 293 to 296).

Contrast-enhanced MR scans are more sensitive than CT studies in detecting inflammatory meningeal pathology. Sarcoidosis is another cause of meningeal thickening and enhancement, best demonstrated by MR.

The superficial contrast enhancement seen in meningitis may include a cortical component in addition to meningeal involvement.

Here abnormal contrast enhancement is seen in the area of the left intraparietal sulcus. In contrast to Case 258, this enhancement is very localized and demonstrates a "pia-arachnoid" pattern extending into sulci.

Enhancement of cortex lining the sulcus appears to contribute to the postcontrast pattern in this case. Such cortical enhancement reflects reactive inflammation or infarction of the underlying gray matter and correlates with this patient's hemiparesis.

Compare this scan to the more generalized cortical enhancement in Case 261, and to the similar "tram-track" morphology of "gyriform" calcification in Case 340.

Case 260

3-month-old boy with decreased level
of consciousness.

Pneumococcal Meningitis.

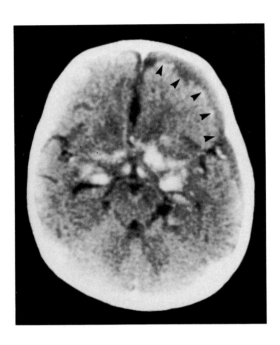

Case 261

6-month-old girl.

Nonspecific Meningitis.

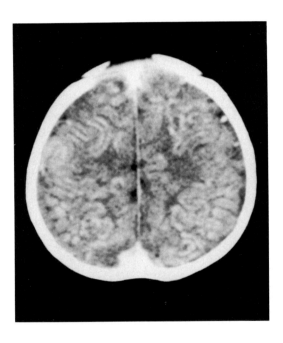

Meningeal inflammation may extend to the cerebral parenchyma, causing localized or generalized cerebritis. In many cases encephalitis and meningitis are concurrent.

The solid, rounded areas of enhancement near the base of the brain in this case proved to represent pneumococcal cerebritis. Basal accumulation of thick exudates in meningitis can spread infection to the inferior surface of the brain. A pattern similar to this scan may also be seen in cases of viral encephalitis, with abnormal enhancement near the hypothalamus. In adults, sarcoidosis may present with basal involvement resembling this appearance.

Another mechanism of parenchymal enhancement associated with meningitis is subacute cerebral infarction, due to spasm or occlusion of arteries traversing the infected subarachnoid space (or to septic thrombophlebitis). Arteritis involving penetrating arteries at the base of the brain could cause an enhancement pattern similar to this case.

The subdural fluid collection over the left frontal region *(arrowheads)* was found to be a sterile effusion. Subdural effusions are common in bacterial meningitis (particularly in cases due to *Hemophilus influenzae;* see Case 293). They may be indistinguishable from subdural empyemas on CT scans (compare to Case 296).

This case of meningitis is associated with diffuse cortical enhancement. Gray matter along the margins of sulci enhances, causing a uniform "tram-track" appearance (compare to Cases 259 and 340). Cortical enhancement may represent reactive hyperemia, direct extension of infection (*i.e.,* cerebritis) and/or secondary infarction.

Compare the "tram-track" or "marginal" pattern of gray matter enhancement in this case to the more solid or "gyriform" enhancement seen in diffuse encephalitis (Case 268B).

MR CORRELATION: MENINGITIS

Case 262

1-year-old girl with nonspecific meningitis.
(axial, noncontrast scan; SE 3000/45)

Case 263

25-year-old Filipino man with tuberculous
meningitis.
(coronal, postcontrast scan; SE 600/15)

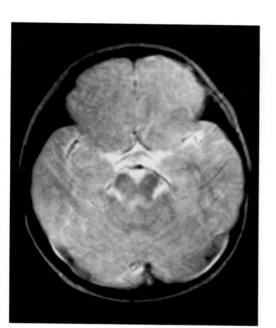

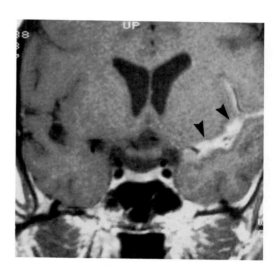

The scan parameters in this case are set in a manner that causes normal CSF to be nearly isointense to brain. The relatively high signal intensity filling the basal cisterns is due to cells and protein within the CSF spaces, confirming the clinical diagnosis of meningitis. This finding is the MR equivalent of increased subarachnoid density on CT scans, as seen in Cases 256 and 257.

Fungal or granulomatous meningitis may localize to a small portion of the subarachnoid space, as illustrated here. Prominent contrast enhancement fills the left sylvian cistern *(arrowheads)*. The normal branches of the middle cerebral artery are seen as filling defects within this "cast."

Cisternal or sulcal enhancement on MR scans is often more easily detected and more extensive than appreciated on CT studies. The absence of masking artifact from the adjacent calvarium, multiplanar display, and higher sensitivity to small amounts of contrast material contribute to the advantage of MR in cases of superficial pathology (see Cases 25 and 26).

Case 264

49-year-old man admitted to the hospital
in a coma.

**Ventriculitis due to Aspergillosis (With
Obstruction of the Foramina of Monro).**

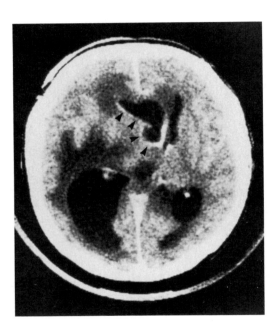

Case 265

2-month-old boy, previously shunted
for hydrocephalus.

Bacterial Ventriculitis.

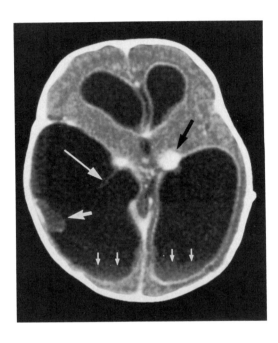

Bacterial, fungal, viral or parasitic infections may involve the ventricular lining. Findings on CT scans in ventriculitis include enhancement of the ependymal or subependymal tissues, as seen surrounding the right frontal horn in this case. Secondary hydrocephalus may be present due to obstructing tissue or septations.

Here, the right foramen of Monro has been compromised to a greater extent than that on the left. The resulting asymmetrical hydrocephalus is associated with unilateral periventricular edema (see Cases 606 to 608) and a marked midline shift (subfalcial herniation).

The ventricle on the side of the mass effect is enlarged rather than compressed. This finding identifies unilateral hydrocephalus as a major component of the lesion and places the inciting process at the foramen of Monro.

Enhancing ventricular margins may also be seen with primary or metastatic tumor (see Cases 22, 23, 102, and 103) and in noninfectious inflammatory disease such as sarcoidosis.

Fungal or viral ventriculitis most commonly occurs in immunosuppressed patients (see Case 267). Bacterial ventriculitis may develop in previously healthy individuals when organisms are introduced through trauma or surgery. In this case, the diffuse ependymitis indicated by enhancement of all ventricular surfaces was associated with previous shunt placement.

Abnormally intense enhancement of the inflamed choroid plexus is also present *(black arrow)*. Subtle sedimentation levels are seen posteriorly in the ventricular trigones *(small arrows; see Case 266)*. The relatively isointense mass adjacent to the margin of the right lateral ventricle *(short white arrow)* probably represents a clump of inflammatory debris.

Septations and loculations within the ventricular chambers are common sequelae of ventriculitis. Here, a portion of a septation is seen within the right ventricular trigone *(long white arrow)*.

VENTRICULITIS: OTHER FEATURES

Case 266

81-year-old woman found unresponsive.
(noncontrast scan)

Meningitis and Ventriculitis.

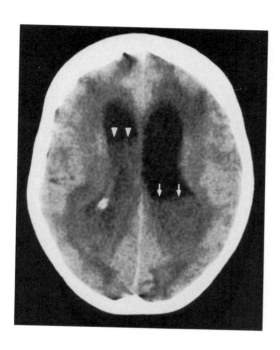

Case 267

49-year-old man with AIDS.
(axial, noncontrast scan; SE 2500/25)

CMV Ventriculitis.

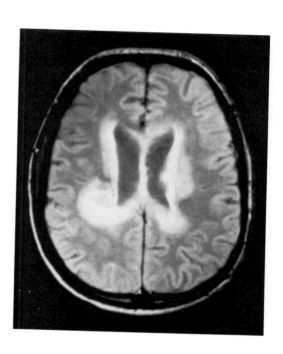

A second important CT finding in ventriculitis is sedimentation of debris within the ventricular system. Here a sedimentation level is apparent in the left lateral ventricle *(arrows)*, representing the intraventricular load of cells and proteinaceous material. A smaller sedimentation level is seen more anteriorly within the right lateral ventricle *(arrowheads)*. Periventricular edema causes prominent low attenuation surrounding the posterior portions of the ventricular bodies.

The visualization of intracranial sedimentation levels requires a period of limited head movement prior to the scan. A patient who is actively shaking his or her head will disperse sediment and make detection more difficult.

More subtle sedimentation levels are present in Case 265. Intraventricular leakage of contrast material from inflamed ependyma or choroid plexus may contribute to the density layering in dependent portions of the ventricular system (or within other cystic structures).

Cytomegalovirus (CMV) is recognized as a cause of intrauterine encephalitis and ventriculitis (see Case 650) but is rarely associated with cerebritis in healthy adults. Patients with AIDS or other immunodeficiency states are susceptible to infection by opportunistic pathogens, and CMV encephalitis and ventriculitis may be encountered in such cases.

The thick rind of subependymal inflammation and edema in ventriculitis is well demonstrated by this "balanced" MR image. (Compare to the periventricular edema in Case 266; to the morphology of subependymal tumor spread in Cases 23, 102, and 103; and to the postcontrast scan of this patient in Case 292.) The inflammatory process is beginning to "bud" or extend away from the ventricular system into the deep white matter of both hemispheres.

Case 268A

2-month-old girl presenting with seizures.
(postcontrast scan)

Herpes Encephalitis (Type 2).

Case 268B

Same patient, 6 days later.
(postcontrast scan)

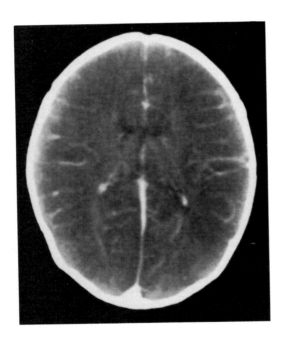

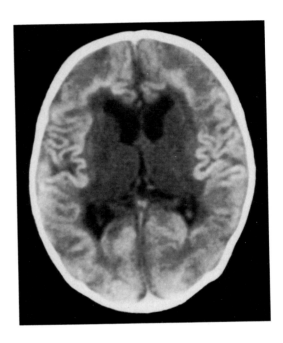

Some cases of viral encephalitis cause focal areas of cerebritis comparable to the appearance in Case 260. A predilection for the base of the brain is often noted.

In other cases a panencephalitis occurs. This is particularly true of neonatal infection with herpes simplex virus Type 2.

This case illustrates the acute phase of herpes encephalitis (see Case 481 for another example). Symmetrical edema and swelling are present throughout the cerebral hemispheres. Gray-white matter discrimination is lost (compare to the appearance of acute anoxia in Cases 464 and 465). Tubular enhancement over the cerebral surface represents normal vessels compressed and highlighted by the swelling and low attenuation of edematous brain. Ventricles are small due to supratentorial mass effect.

The CT appearance in this case has changed dramatically in less than a week. Enlargement of the lateral ventricles reflects early loss of parenchymal volume. Diffuse, gyriform cortical enhancement is now present, distinct from the earlier pattern of compressed vessels within sulci. (The enhancement pattern is also different from the "tram-track" or marginal appearance of cortical enhancement sometimes accompanying meningitis, as in Cases 259 and 261.)

This prominent cortical "stain" may persist for days in the subacute phase of herpes Type 2 encephalitis. (Compare to the contrast enhancement of subacute anoxia in Case 472.) A similar pattern of cortical density on CT (and T2 shortening on MR) may be seen on noncontrast scans in intermediate stages of herpes encephalitis, possibly reflecting hyperemia or early mineralization of damaged gray matter.

Deep hemisphere edema remains, with no differentiation between the basal ganglia and adjacent white matter.

Case 268C

Same patient, 2 months later.
(noncontrast scan)

Case 269

4-month-old boy with a history of neonatal
herpes encephalitis (type 2).

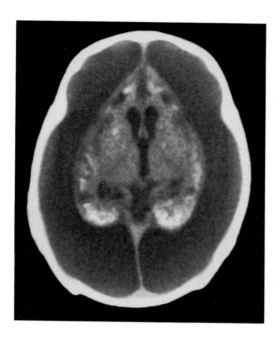

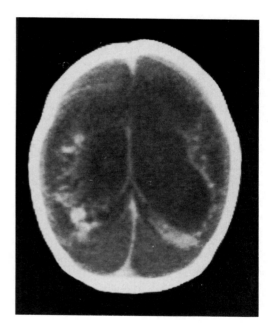

The result of panencephalitis in an infant is usually widespread destruction of cerebral parenchyma, as seen here. The loss of hemisphere volume has caused collapse of the cortical mantle, with secondary development of large subdural fluid collections. Scattered parenchymal calcification and atrophic enlargement of the ventricles indicates that this appearance is the result of a previous insult, rather than representing primary subdural effusions or hygromas.

The rapid evolution in CT pattern from Case 268A to 268C is commonly encountered when widespread viral infection overwhelms the limited reactive capability of the neonatal brain. (Compare to the development of multicystic encephalomalacia as discussed in Case 628.)

It may be difficult to distinguish the acute and chronic effects of cerebritis from the ischemic consequences of associated meningitis and arteritis.

Scans performed after perinatal meningoencephalitis typically demonstrate a combination of patchy encephalomalacia and extensive intracerebral calcification. The pattern is nonspecific and can be seen with many viruses.

The loss of cerebral parenchyma may lead to collapse of the mantle, as in Case 268C, or marked ventricular enlargement, as seen here. Only periventricular fringes of calcified "normal" parenchymal density remain. The "ghost" of cerebral tissue along the margins of enlarged ventricles distinguishes this appearance from hydranencephaly (see Case 587).

Calcification following perinatal encephalitis may develop rapidly (weeks to months) and may include a gyriform cortical pattern resembling Sturge-Weber syndrome (see Case 340). Widespread encephalomalacia may also be caused by perinatal anoxia without infection (see Case 485), but extensive calcification as in this case suggests an infectious insult.

HERPES ENCEPHALITIS (ADULT)

Case 270

37-year-old man with fever and reduced level of consciousness.

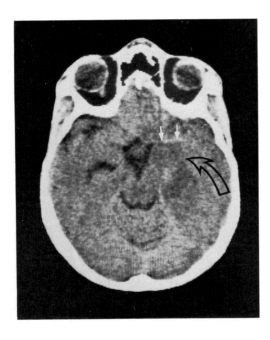

Case 271

36-year-old man scanned 10 days after the onset of symptoms.

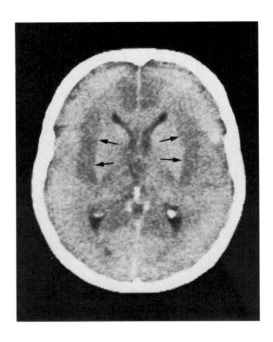

Adult encephalitis due to herpes simplex (Type 1) typically begins in the medial anterior temporal and posteroinferior frontal lobes. Initial CT findings are limited to subtle low attenuation and mass effect. As the disease progresses, patchy hemorrhage and abnormal contrast enhancement are common. (A rare alternative cause of rapidly progressive edema and patchy hemorrhage in the temporal lobe is thrombosis of the transverse sinus with venous infarction.)

The characteristic CT pattern may not develop until the patient has become comatose. Close attention to the frontotemporal regions on early scans often demonstrates mild edema, which can support the clinical diagnosis and/or guide biopsy. MR is more sensitive than CT in detecting early evidence of herpes encephalitis (see Cases 272 and 273).

Involvement is unilateral in this case, with vague, low density and mass effect in the medial left frontotemporal region. (Compare this scan with that of the low-grade glioma in Case 62.) The ipsilateral temporal horn is compressed, and the uncus is swollen and displaced medially. The proximal middle cerebral artery (small arrows) appears relatively dense due to surrounding low attenuation and possible stasis; (compare with Case 480).

In this case involvement is bilateral. Lower sections demonstrated mass effect and poorly defined low attenuation in the medial frontotemporal lobes.

At this level there is symmetrical involvement of the parasagittal frontal lobes and the deep sylvian regions. The striking margination of the lenticular nucleus (arrows) is characteristic of herpes encephalitis. (Occasionally an embolic infarction involving only the cortical distribution of the middle cerebral artery can present a similar appearance within one hemisphere.)

Pyogenic or fungal cerebritis may initially appear as a nonspecific region of low attenuation and swelling similar to that seen in viral encephalitis. Patchy contrast enhancement may occur. Peripheral enhancement may be seen prior to the formation of a true abscess capsule (see discussion of Case 274).

MR CORRELATION: HERPES ENCEPHALITIS

Case 272

60-year-old woman with a 3-day history
of worsening aphasia and memory loss.
(axial, noncontrast scan; SE 2500/90)

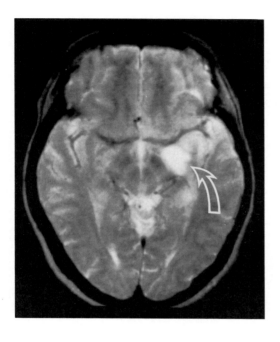

Case 273

35-year-old man presenting with fever and a
2-day history of increasing aphasia.
(axial, noncontrast scan; SE 2500/100)

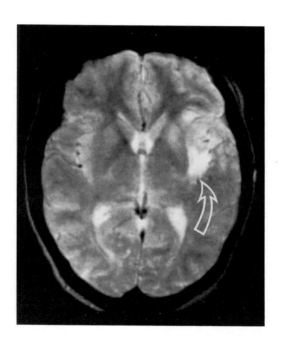

MR is more sensitive than CT to small amounts of cerebral edema. MR also provides axial and coronal views of the temporal lobe that are free of artifacts arising from the bony walls of the middle cranial fossa. For these reasons, MR is able to demonstrate herpes encephalitis at a stage when CT scans are still negative or equivocal.

In this case, the very high signal intensity of the left uncus *(arrow)* is clearly pathological. (Compare to the CT definition of a comparable lesion in Case 270.) Although the appearance is nonspecific, the characteristic location in the medial temporal lobe suggests herpes encephalitis in the appropriate clinical context. The diagnosis was confirmed by biopsy, and the patient made a good recovery on antiviral therapy.

Patchy areas of hemorrhage within the edema of herpes encephalitis may be apparent on MR scans as zones of T1- and/or T2-shortening (see discussion of Cases 560 and 561).

In this case a T2-weighted scan at the level of the basal ganglia demonstrates an area of high signal intensity extending superiorly from the temporal lobe into the hemisphere *(arrow).* Involvement of the insula and white matter lateral to the lenticular nucleus is characteristic of herpes encephalitis (compare to the bilateral involvement in Case 271).

Case 274

34-year-old man presenting with headache and a left visual field cut 3 weeks after extensive dental work.

Case 275

25-year-old man with a 3-week history of headache, lethargy, and "flu," now presenting with hemiparesis.

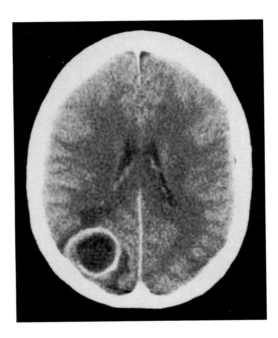

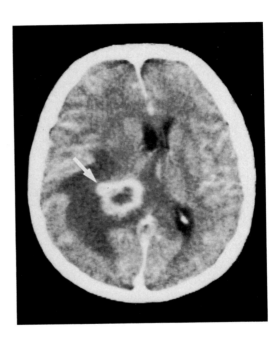

Pyogenic cerebral abscesses typically demonstrate a thin, uniform rim of contrast enhancement surrounding a low attenuation center, as seen here. The usually smooth contour of the enhancing periphery contrasts with the thicker, more irregular margin of most cerebral neoplasms (but see Cases 93 and 278).

The abscess capsule may be visible on noncontrast scans as an isodense band separating the central cavity from surrounding edema. (MR may also demonstrate the capsule of an abscess on noncontrast scans, with the structure often displaying zones of T1- and T2-shortening; see Cases 284 and 285.)

The formation of a true abscess capsule is preceded by a stage of cerebritis that may demonstrate peripheral enhancement. Clues to the lack of an organized capsule include nonvisualization of the capsule on precontrast scans and diffusion of contrast material into the center of the lesion on postcontrast images.

Attenuation values within an abscess are usually higher than CSF density due to the content of cells and protein. Associated edema is often prominent, and additional "daughter" abscesses may be seen near the primary lesion (see Cases 275 and 283).

The enhancing capsule of pyogenic abscesses may occasionally be thick and irregular (see also Case 281). When such lesions are located deep within the hemisphere as in this case, the appearance resembles a malignant glioma or metastasis (compare to Cases 86 and 87).

Clues to the correct diagnosis include the hazy margin of the enhancing capsule, favoring an inflammatory process rather than the edge of a neoplasm. The appearance of a small "bud" or "daughter" lesion along the lateral border of the larger mass (arrow) also suggests the possibility of an abscess with developing "satellite" foci. (This is not a specific feature; some gliomas and metastases demonstrate "buds" of tumor tissue extending from the margin of a large mass.)

Drainage of this lesion yielded staphylococci.

CEREBRAL ABSCESSES IN COMPROMISED HOSTS

Case 276

56-year-old alcoholic man presenting with headaches.

Pyogenic Abscess.

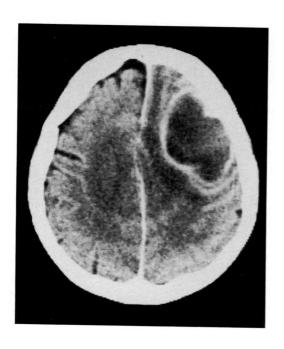

Case 277

47-year-old diabetic man.

Mucormycosis.

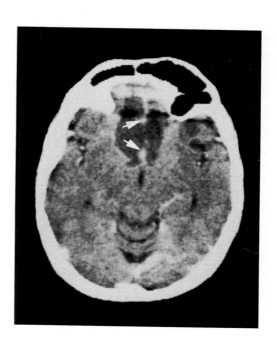

Patients whose immune systems are compromised by debilitation or disease are susceptible to intracranial infection. This possibility should encourage early investigation of symptoms in such cases.

Here a frontal lobe abscess has become very large, with prominent edema and subfalcial herniation at the time of discovery. Although the rim of this abscess is not perfectly circular as in Case 274, its uniform thinness strongly suggests the correct diagnosis.

Fungal abscesses are rare in otherwise healthy individuals. They more commonly occur in immunocompromised hosts and are a feared cerebral complication of diabetes mellitus.

In this case, the infection has crossed the cribriform plate from the ethmoid sinus to the inferior frontal regions. The abscess cavity bridges the interhemispheric fissure to involve both medial frontal lobes. The proximal segments of the anterior cerebral arteries are stretched above the bridging portion of the abscess, serving to restrain its lobulations (arrows; compare with Case 180).

Several fungi (including *Aspergillus* and *Mucor*) have a tendency for vascular invasion. This patient later suffered infarction in the anterior cerebral artery distributions. At postmortem examination the arterial lumens were occluded by hyphae.

Case 278

70-year-old man.

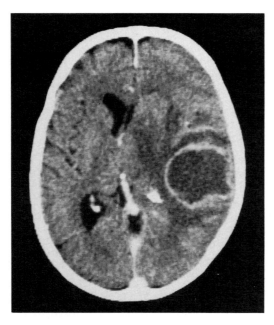

Glioblastoma.

Case 279

4-year-old girl with hypoplastic right heart syndrome treated in infancy by creation of a right-to-left atrial shunt.

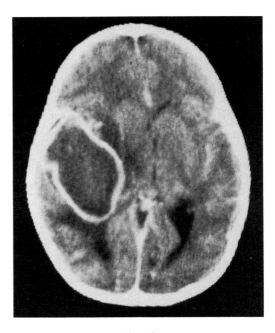

Pyogenic Abscess.

The enhancing rim of some gliomas and metastases may be thin and uniform, resembling an abscess, as in Case 278 (see also Cases 5 and 93). However, an abscess should remain the first diagnostic consideration when a thin-walled cystic lesion is encountered.

Porencephalic cysts can reach similar proportions but lack peripheral enhancement and contain lower density fluid (see Cases 629 to 632). Arachnoid cysts are usually more angular in morphology and are clearly extra-axial (see Cases 614 to 617).

Many abscesses can be aspirated with CT guidance and/or followed to resolution by serial scans during antibiotic therapy. Enhancement of the abscess capsule may persist for weeks or months during successful treatment. In Case 279, aspiration yielded 40 ml of pus containing streptococci and gram-negative anaerobic rods. The abscess disappeared over a 2-month treatment period.

DIFFERENTIAL DIAGNOSIS:
SUPERFICIAL, RIM-ENHANCING MASS WITH EDEMA

Case 280

80-year-old woman.

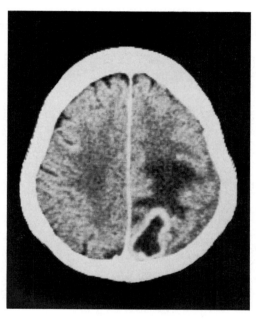

Glioblastoma.

Case 281

28-year-old Asian male immigrant.

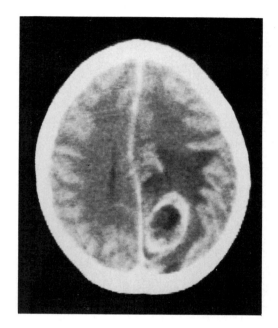

Pyogenic Abscess.

The enhancing rim of some malignant gliomas is fairly uniform and may mimic the capsule of an abscess (see Cases 278 and 279).

Conversely, some pyogenic abscesses (such as in Case 281) develop a relatively thick capsule, which resembles the periphery of a high-grade glioma or metastasis. Fungal abscesses may also demonstrate a thick-walled, loculated, or semisolid morphology (see Case 253).

The relatively poor inflammatory response of deep hemispheric white matter may cause the capsule of an abscess to be less developed along the medial wall than along the superficial margin. When present, this feature may aid in distinguishing an abscess from a neoplasm.

FUNGAL AND OPPORTUNISTIC INFECTIONS

Case 282

64-year-old man with a history of lung resection for histoplasmosis.

Histoplasmoma.

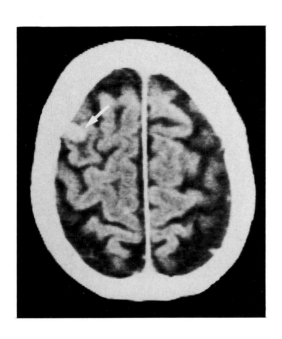

Case 283

76-year-old woman with systemic lymphoma.

Nocardia Brain Abscesses.

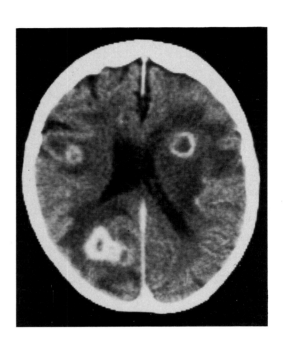

Fungal infections may cause a wide variety of CT abnormalities. The simplest lesions are solitary peripheral granulomas, as seen in this case *(arrow)*. The superficial location, edema, and frequent multiplicity often mimic metastases.

In other cases, a region of fungal cerebritis may evolve to a frank abscess, similar to the development of a pyogenic infection (see Case 277). Fungal meningitis (e.g., coccidiomycosis, histoplasmosis) may present as a densely enhancing process filling the basal cisterns. Ependymal and subependymal infection may also be seen (as in Case 264).

A variety of opportunistic infections may develop in immunosuppressed hosts. Fungal pathogens *(e.g., Aspergillus)* are common in such cases. Cerebral lesions may also be caused by unusual bacteria (e.g., *Nocardia*, as seen here) or mycobacteria. Protozoal infection in the form of toxoplasmosis is frequently observed in AIDS (see Cases 289 and 290).

Nocardial cerebral abscesses are often multiloculated and numerous, as seen above. The possibility of primary CNS lymphoma (see Cases 244 to 250) or progressive multifocal leukoencephalopathy (usually nonenhancing; see Cases 321 to 323) should also be considered when multiple lesions are encountered in an immunodeficient host.

Case 284

34-year-old man (same patient as Case 274).
(sagittal, noncontrast scan; SE 600/17)

Pyogenic Abscess.

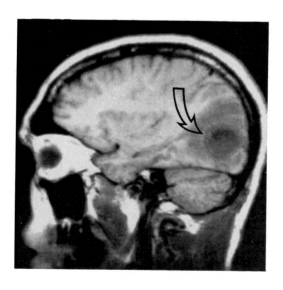

Case 285

14-year-old girl with systemic candidiasis after chemotherapy for disseminated suprasellar germinoma.
(axial, noncontrast scan; SE 2500/90)

Candida Abscesses.

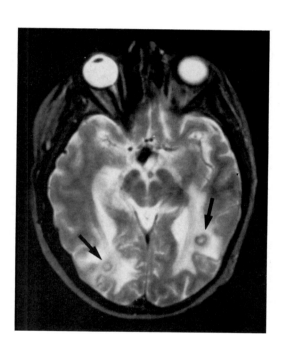

The overall appearance of cerebral abscesses on MR scans is comparable to the CT pattern illustrated in Cases 274 to 277. A central, necrotic cavity, typically demonstrating long T1 and long T2 values. Extensive edema surrounds the lesion, seen as a peripheral zone of markedly reduced signal intensity on this T1-weighted image.

Abscess capsules can be identified as discrete structures on noncontrast MR images. They may be homogeneously isointense or appear to have two concentric layers, one with long T1 values and one with short T1 relaxation times.

Segments of an abscess capsule often demonstrate shortening of both T1 and T2. As a result, the capsule may be seen as a high signal intensity rim on T1-weighted sequences and as a low-intensity rim separating edema from the abscess cavity on T2-weighted series. This behavior does not correlate well with the presence of blood products in the abscess wall, and other etiologies (e.g., the presence of free radicals produced by activated macrophages) are being investigated as sources of paramagnetic effects.

The capsules of cerebral abscesses are usually identifiable as isointense to low-intensity structures on T2-weighted MR scans. They are characteristically round and uniformly thin as on CT studies, defined by the higher signal intensity of the abscess contents and surrounding edema.

In this case, small, fungal abscesses are present in the occipital lobes bilaterally (arrows). The relatively low intensity capsules are outlined by extensive peripheral edema.

A calcified residual mass at the site of the original germinoma is seen in the suprasellar region.

CYSTICERCOSIS

Case 286

24-year-old Mexican woman with seizures.

Parenchymal Cysticercosis.

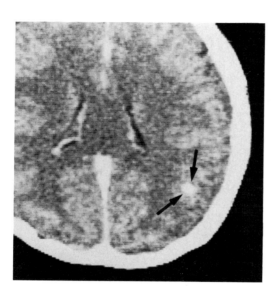

Case 287

17-year-old girl with hydrocephalus.
(scan with intraventricular contrast material)

Intraventricular Cysticercosis.

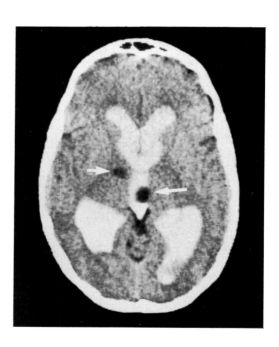

Cysticercosis ranks as the most important parasitic infection of CNS in this hemisphere. The disease occurs when man serves as an intermediate host for the larval form of the pork tapeworm, *Taenia solium.*

The encysting larvae of cysticercosis can cause a wide spectrum of cerebral lesions. Cisternal, ventricular, and parenchymal involvement may be seen separately or in combination. Lesions may be cystic or solid, calcified or enhancing, solitary or multiple.

In this case, a small, calcified parenchymal lesion demonstrates minimal contrast enhancement. Calcification is the final result of the host's response to the death of the larva. This appearance marks the end of the granulomatous phase in cysticercal infection.

Cysts of cysticercosis may be found within the cerebral ventricles, cranial subarachnoid spaces (especially basal cisterns) and spinal canal as well as within brain parenchyma. They may present as solitary lesions or clustered aggregates. Typical parenchymal cysts are approximately 1 cm in diameter, with a small nodule along the perimeter of the cyst representing the scolex of the parasite. "Racemose" cysts are commonly found in the suprasellar, sylvian, or cerebellopontine angle cisterns.

Cysticercosis cysts often blend with surrounding spinal fluid, requiring subarachnoid contrast material for demonstration. In this case, the ganglionic cyst *(small arrow)* was apparent on a routine scan, but the third ventricular lesion *(large arrow)* was not identified until the contrast study. Cysticercosis cysts are among the low-attenuation lesions that can obstruct the ventricular system while remaining hidden within distended ventricles (see also Cases 126, 592, and 593).

CYSTICERCOSIS (CONTINUED)

Case 288A

2-year-old Mexican-American girl presenting
with encephalitis.
(postcontrast scan)

Case 288B

Same patient.
(scan at higher level)

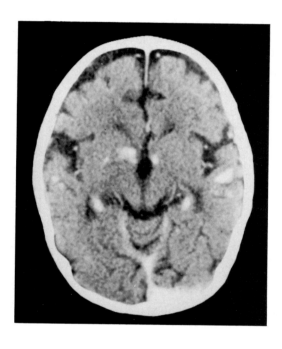

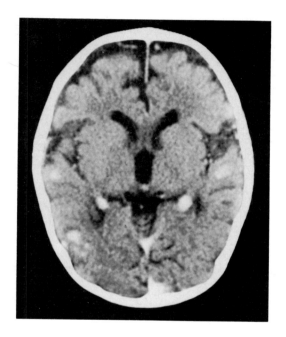

Multiple foci of contrast enhancement are present in this case. Although the hypothalamic lesions near the third ventricle might suggest a viral encephalitis, the presence of scattered superficial enhancement would be unusual. The overall distribution of lesions is more compatible with cysticercosis, which frequently involves all areas of the brain.

This enhancing, granulomatous stage follows the cystic form of parenchymal cysticercosis and usually implies larval death. A solitary lesion in this stage may resemble primary or metastatic tumors.

Another possible etiology for inflammatory lesions near the third ventricle is the extension of basal meningitis into the hypothalamus (see Case 260). Bacterial or fungal pathogens (e.g., cryptococcus) may ascend along prominent Virchow-Robin spaces accompanying penetrating arteries at the base of the brain to present as lesions at the hypothalamic level.

Contrast enhancement is seen when cysticercal larvae have incited a host response. Since living larvae are usually immunologically "invisible" and do not provoke cerebral edema or enhancement, the presence of these features usually implies larval death. In fact, edema and contrast enhancement may be CT correlates of successful treatment in cysticercosis.

Cysticercosis should also be included (along with tuberculosis and other potentially "miliary" infections) in the differential diagnosis of multiple focal enhancing lesions in an adult (see Cases 4, 307, and 308).

TOXOPLASMOSIS

Case 289

48-year-old man with AIDS.

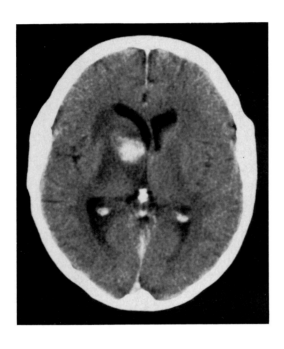

Case 290

30-year-old man with a history of AIDS, presenting with seizures.

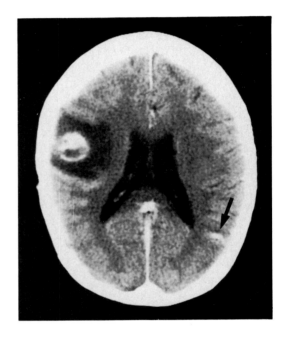

The deep, mass-like lesion with surrounding edema in this case is one of many potential appearances for cerebral toxoplasmosis in AIDS patients. Lesions are most commonly located in the basal ganglia (as seen here) or near the gray/white matter junction (as in Case 290).

Toxoplasmosis most frequently presents as multiple lesions of variable size and depth. Individual abscesses may demonstrate peripheral enhancement with central necrosis on CT studies (and a target-like morphology with a rim of relatively short T2 on MR scans).

The broad spectrum of morphologies seen in cerebral toxoplasmosis is overlapped by other pathologies. The mass seen here could equally well represent primary CNS lymphoma (see Cases 244 to 250) or another opportunistic pathogen (e.g., fungi). Because of the high incidence of toxoplasmosis in AIDS patients, appropriate therapy is often begun empirically, with biopsy reserved for nonresponding lesions.

In this case the right frontal mass was one of several lesions that had been noted to wax and wane over several months in response to courses of antimicrobial therapy. Treatment (currently with sulfadiazine and pyrimethamine) usually causes regression of toxoplasmosis within weeks, but does not eradicate the pathogen. When treatment is discontinued (in this case due to toxicity), recurrence is to be expected. A smaller focus of disease is present in the left lateral occipital region (arrow).

Intracranial mass lesions are reported in over 20% of AIDS patients. Toxoplasmosis usually ranks as the most common pathology among these cases, followed by primary CNS lymphoma. As discussed in Case 247, primary CNS lymphoma in AIDS patients may be multifocal and centrally necrotic, mimicking toxoplasmosis.

Progressive multifocal leukoencephalopathy (PML) can also cause numerous cerebral lesions in an immunocompromised host (see Cases 321 to 323). However, the lesions of PML often have a characteristic angular or scalloped morphology and rarely demonstrate contrast enhancement.

Case 291

26-year-old man.
(axial, noncontrast scan; SE 2500/90)

HIV Encephalitis.

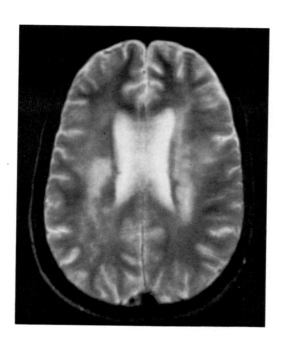

Case 292

49-year-old man (same patient as Case 267).
(axial, postcontrast scan; SE 800/20)

CMV Ventriculitis.

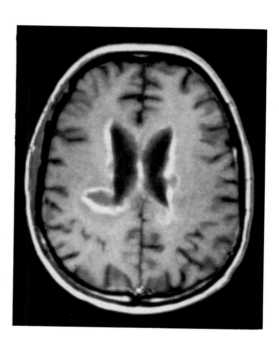

Most of the cerebral complications of AIDS are well demonstrated by CT scans. MR is occasionally helpful in characterizing lesions or in detecting small masses that are more amenable to biopsy than those apparent on a CT scan.

The more important imaging advantages of MR in AIDS relate to the detection of subtle white matter disease. Infection of glial cells by the human immunodeficiency virus (HIV) or by an opportunistic pathogen (e.g., CMV) can cause extensive leukoencephalopathy with little or no CT abnormality.

In this case a CT scan was negative. The MR study documents large areas of signal abnormality throughout the midhemisphere white matter. This "soft," symmetrical appearance of bihemispheral white matter pathology is a common finding in HIV encephalitis, but can also be caused by CMV.

Cranial CT and MR scans in AIDS patients often demonstrate sinusitis, multicystic enlargement of the parotid glands, and cervical adenopathy. These associated findings may support the diagnosis in the appropriate clinical context.

Meningeal and ependymal involvement by inflammatory processes is well demonstrated by MR (see also Case 263). Here an extensive ventriculitis due to cytomegalovirus is documented by circumferential periventricular enhancement. A similar appearance could be caused by other organisms (e.g., cryptococcus) or by primary CNS lymphoma.

A thick rind of reactive subependymal edema is inapparent on this T1-weighted scan but becomes obvious on long TR images (see Case 267). The ability of MR to demonstrate disease along CSF surfaces, highlight subtle involvement of white matter and characterize mass lesions often provides a better understanding of AIDS cases than is possible by CT.

SUBDURAL INFLAMMATORY PROCESSES

Case 293

5-month-old boy with meningitis due to *Hemophilus influenzae.*

Subdural Effusion.

Case 294

13-year-old boy.

Subdural Empyema.

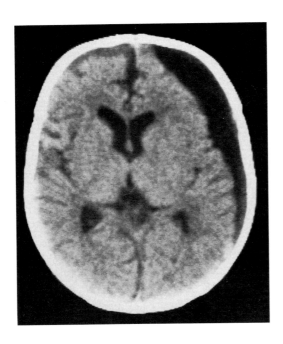

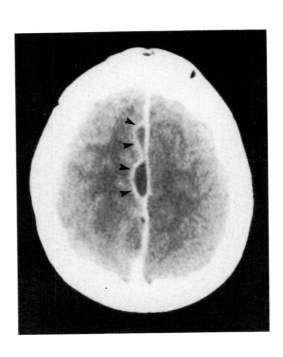

Subdural effusions are commonly associated with infection by *H. influenzae,* the leading cause of meningitis in the United States. (Meningitis due to other organisms, notably pneumococcus, may also be accompanied by subdural effusion; see Case 260.) The effusions typically contain large amounts of protein but few cells. Their appearance is nonspecific and resembles other subdural fluid collections.

The distinction between subdural effusion and subdural empyema is best made by the clinical condition of the patient. Patients with even large subdural effusions are often remarkably well, while patients with even small subdural empyemas are often remarkably ill. The relative amount of contrast enhancement within the membranes of a subdural collection is an inexact index of the degree of infection (see Case 295). In general, the membranes surrounding subdural empyemas tend to enhance more than those bordering subdural effusion.

Subdural effusions may persist beyond successful treatment of meningitis. They may increase in size like chronic subdural hematomas. Infection of the effusion produces a subdural empyema in occasional cases.

The narrow, partially loculated subdural collection adjacent to the falx in this case is typical of subdural empyemas. These abscesses are usually very thin and easily overlooked as symptoms begin. A high index of suspicion and careful examination of the scan are necessary to avoid missing such lesions.

Thin subdural empyemas are often surprisingly extensive. Multiple loculations may be present at scattered sites (see Case 296 for other sites involved in this patient). Involvement of the interhemispheric fissure, as in this case, and the tentorial surface (see Cases 295 and 296) is common. Convexity subdural empyemas are more easily detected by MR than by CT, due to the absence of artifact from adjacent bone and the availability of the coronal scan plane.

Subdural empyemas are often considered to be a surgical emergency. The course in nonoperated cases can lead to rapid morbidity and mortality.

One or more re-explorations may be necessary to remove persistent or recurrent loculations of subdural infection. The boy in this case underwent several craniotomies for recurring empyemas (see also Case 296); he is now asymptomatic 1 year after admission.

SUBDURAL EMPYEMAS ADJACENT TO THE TENTORIUM

Case 295

20-year-old man.

Subdural Empyema due to Mastoiditis.

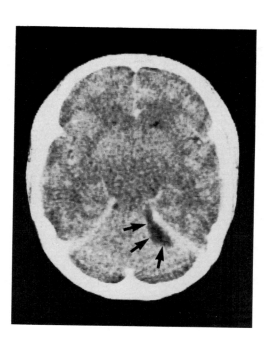

Case 296

13-year-old boy (same patient as Case 294).

Multiple Subdural Empyemas (and Cerebral Abscess).

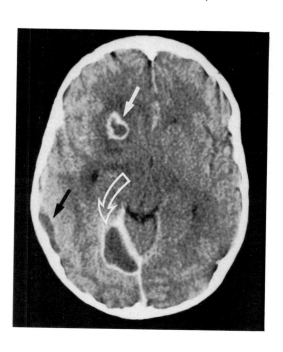

Intracranial infection may arise from sinusitis or mastoiditis of the skull base (see also Cases 277, 303, and 304). This spread of infection often involves retrograde thrombophlebitis, which can lead to subdural empyema and/or cerebritis.

In this case, infection has extended from the petrous bone to form a pocket of subdural empyema along the inferior surface of the tentorium *(arrows)*. Marginal contrast enhancement is much less prominent than in Cases 294 and 296.

In this case a subdural empyema is localized along the superior surface of the tentorium *(open arrow)*. The smaller abscess along the convexity in the right posterior temporal region *(black arrow)* is a good example of the relatively subtle appearance of many subdural empyemas. A small, peripherally enhancing right frontal abscess is also demonstrated *(solid white arrow)*.

DIFFERENTIAL DIAGNOSIS:
THICKENING AND DENSE ENHANCEMENT OF THE TENTORIUM

Case 297

42-year-old man with a history of pulmonary tuberculosis, now presenting with multiple left-sided cranial nerve palsies.
(coronal scan)

Case 298

59-year-old man.

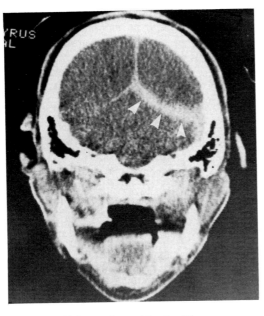

Tuberculous Meningitis.

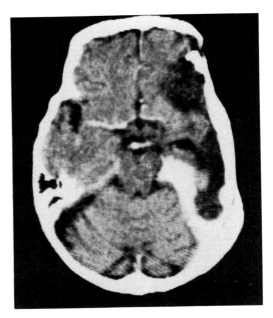

Recurrent Meningioma.

The dural surfaces of the falx and tentorium can be involved by meningitis as well as by subdural empyemas. In Case 297, a coronal scan demonstrates enhancement of the grossly thickened tentorium *(arrowheads)*, proved surgically to represent tuberculous pachymeningitis. (Compare to the example of tuberculous involvement of the subarachnoid spaces in Case 263.)

The appearance of inflammatory tentorial thickening may mimic an "en plaque" meningioma of the tentorium, as seen in Case 298. This patient had undergone several craniotomies for resection of an aggressively recurrent meningioma involving much of the left hemicranium (see discussion of Cases 43 to 45). Old encephalomalacia is present, with enlargement of the left temporal horn and depression of the craniotomy flap.

When thick meningeal enhancement is found in the basal cisterns or along dural surfaces, the differential diagnosis includes tuberculosis, fungal disease (e.g., coccidiomycosis), pyogenic meningitis, cysticercosis, sarcoidosis, and meningeal tumor (e.g., carcinomatosis, seeding from a primary CNS malignancy, lymphoma, and leukemia).

Case 299

66-year-old man.

Case 300

68-year-old woman presenting with seizures.

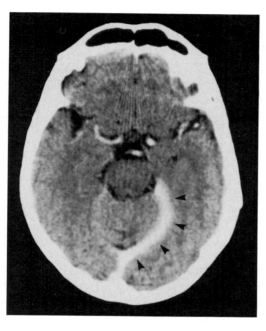

Pyogenic Pachymeningitis due to Mastoiditis.

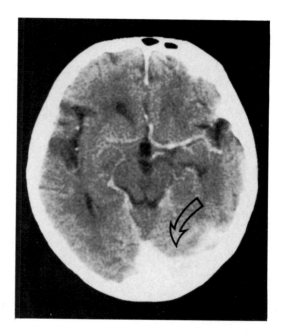

Superior Sagittal Sinus Thrombosis with Tentorial Hyperemia.

In Case 299, the tentorium has become thickened in reaction to long-standing low-grade mastoiditis involving the adjacent petrous bone (see Cases 295 and 304). This is a more chronic dural response to pyogenic infection than the formation of subdural empyemas, as seen in Cases 294 to 296. The appearance is quite similar to that of a subdural hematoma along the tentorial surface (compare to Case 348).

An additional cause of thickening and prominent enhancement of the tentorium is thrombosis of the superior sagittal sinus, as in Case 300 (see discussion Cases 468 to 471). Dural veins within the tentorium are dilated as routes of collateral circulation, and the overall impairment in venous drainage causes congestion of the dural surfaces.

EPIDURAL ABSCESSES

Case 301

15-year-old boy.

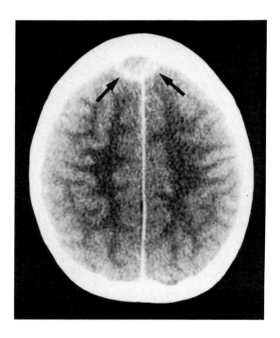

Case 302

32-year-old man with a history of head trauma
and skull fractures.

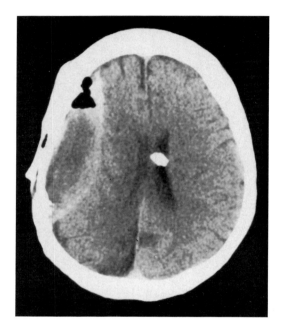

Abscesses within the epidural space may arise primarily or from secondary infection of other epidural lesions. In this case, the bifrontal epidural abscess was due to frontal sinusitis. Sinusitis may cause intracranial infection by direct extension across the skull base or by propagation through septic thrombophlebitis traversing otherwise intact bone.

The extracerebral collection in this case is established as epidural by the fact that it crosses the falx. A subdural process would be limited by the dural attachment of the falx to the convexity dura.

In this case the large epidural abscess is due to contamination associated with a skull fracture. The characteristic biconvex or "lens" shape localizes the collection to the epidural space. The morphology resembles an epidural hematoma (see Cases 366 to 368), and it is possible that the collection in fact represents an infected hematoma.

Gas is rarely seen within intracranial abscesses; the air in the anterior part of this collection is postsurgical. Mass effect compresses the right lateral ventricle. Low attenuation at the right occipital pole suggests ischemia in the distribution of the posterior cerebral artery from prior herniation (see Cases 450 and 451). The high-attenuation structure within the left lateral ventricle is the tip of a shunt catheter.

Patients with infections confined to the epidural space are usually less acutely ill than patients with comparably sized subdural empyemas (see Cases 294 to 296).

Case 303

27-year-old woman with headache and fever.
(wide window)

Acute Sinusitis.

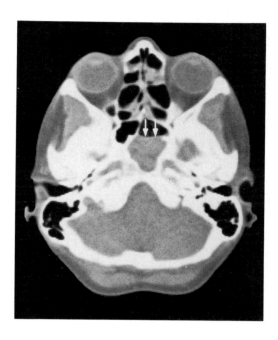

Case 304

20-year-old man (same patient as Case 295).
(wide window)

Chronic Mastoiditis.

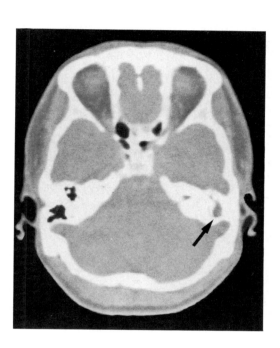

The skull base and sinuses should be evaluated with wide window on all scans. Many patients referred for possible cerebral abscesses are instead suffering from sinusitis. CT findings include mucosal thickening (seen here in the ethmoid sinuses) and air-fluid levels (seen here in the sphenoid sinus; *arrows*).

An air-fluid level is the standard radiographic hallmark of acute sinusitis in the appropriate clinical context. In the setting of trauma, the same finding (due to blood or CSF) suggests a basal skull fracture (see Case 390).

Infections spreading from the sphenoid sinus may mimic other parasellar lesions. For example, aspergillosis may cause sclerosis of bone and encasement of vessels resembling a meningioma. An expanding mucocele of the sphenoid sinus is also in the differential diagnosis of a parasellar mass.

Mastoiditis causes opacification of petrous air cells, often with associated involvement of the middle ear. Chronic infection leads to generalized sclerosis surrounding focal areas of bone erosion. Cholesteatomas often accompany chronic mastoiditis, with eventual destruction of middle ear structures.

Here the normally pneumatized right petrous bone contrasts with the opacification seen on the left. No ossicles were visible in the left tympanic cavity.

Case 295 illustrates the infratentorial subdural empyema that arose from the left petrous bone in this case. Mastoiditis infrequently leads to thrombosis of the adjacent sigmoid sinus (as in Case 474B), which may in turn cause increased intracranial pressure or hydrocephalus ("otitic hydrocephalus").

MULTIPLE SCLEROSIS: MULTIPLE LESIONS, SOME ENHANCING

Case 305

38-year-old woman presenting with seizures.

Case 306

29-year-old woman presenting with optic neuritis.

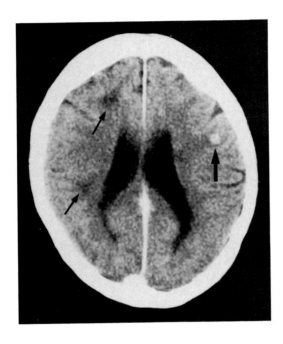

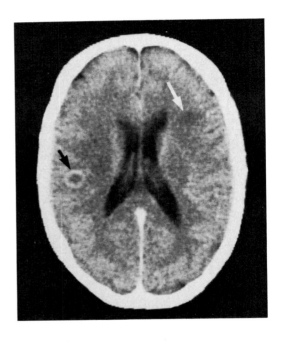

The CT appearance of multiple sclerosis is widely variable. Scans are normal in many cases of clinically definite disease. Alternatively, CT examinations may be dramatically abnormal in patients with minimal symptoms.

Nonenhancing plaques are often seen as small areas of decreased attenuation within cerebral white matter *(thin black arrows)*. These are particularly common in periventricular regions and can be confused with small infarctions in the corona radiata (see Cases 432 to 434).

Active demyelinating plaques may present as foci of contrast enhancement, usually solid as in this case *(thick black arrow)*. Although most such lesions are small, occasional enhancing plaques are large enough to resemble neoplasms (see Cases 311 and 312). Serial scans may demonstrate evolution of a plaque from an active enhancing phase to a quiescent, low-attenuation lesion.

Clinical presentation with seizures is an uncommon but recognized occurrence in multiple sclerosis.

A combination of nonenhancing and enhancing plaques is seen in this case, as in Case 305. The "target" morphology of the peripherally enhancing plaque *(black arrow)* is an unusual CT appearance, although a similar pattern has been noted on MR scans (see Case 314). MR is much superior to CT for detecting and quantitating demyelinating disease (see Cases 313 to 316).

Optic neuritis is a common manifestation of multiple sclerosis. Its occurrence with or years prior to cerebral symptoms helps to establish the diagnosis in ambiguous cases.

DIFFERENTIAL DIAGNOSIS:
MULTIPLE ENHANCING CEREBRAL NODULES

Case 307

45-year-old woman.

Case 308

29-year-old woman.

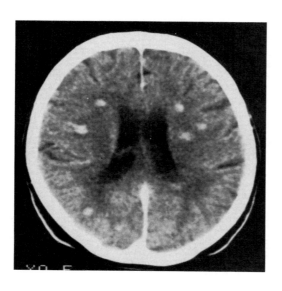

Multiple Sclerosis.

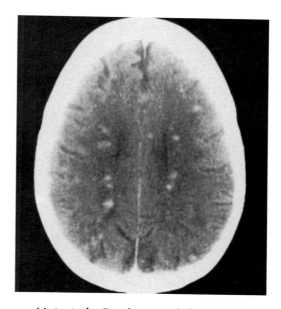

Metastatic Carcinoma of the Breast.

The enhancing plaques of multiple sclerosis may be numerous and uniform in size, as in Case 307. The pattern of the lesions then resembles the appearance of multiple metastases, as in Case 308.

Plaques usually occupy a midhemisphere location. This distribution is more central than the peripheral position of most metastases near the gray/white matter junction (see Cases 1 and 4). However, overlapping patterns are encountered, as seen here. The clinical setting usually distinguishes these two processes.

Additional pathologies in the differential diagnosis of multiple, enhancing nodules include disseminated infection (e.g., cysticercosis as in Case 288, tuberculosis, histoplasmosis, toxoplasmosis), primary CNS lymphoma (as in Case 250), subacute, multifocal infarction (arterial or venous; see Case 416), and multiple cavernous angiomas (see Case 510).

MULTIPLE SCLEROSIS: SMALL, SOLITARY LESIONS

Case 309

26-year-old man.

Case 310

38-year-old woman.

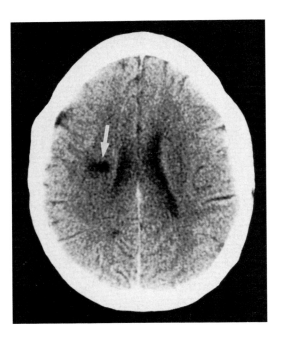

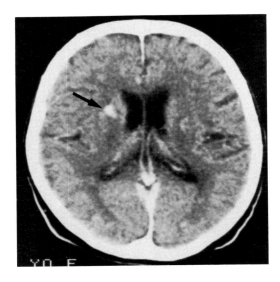

Occasionally a solitary lesion is seen on CT (or even on MR) scans of patients with multiple sclerosis. A nonenhancing plaque is detected as a focal area of low attenuation, as in this case *(arrow)*. While this appearance is nonspecific (compare to Case 436) and not diagnostic of multiple sclerosis, it does fall within the spectrum of demyelinating disease. Multiple sclerosis should be considered when such lesions are encountered, so that patients are not unnecessarily subjected to work-ups or therapies based presumptively on other diagnoses (e.g., angiography or anticoagulation for presumed cerebral infarction).

A small plaque discovered on a CT study may demonstrate contrast enhancement. Solid enhancement of a focal lesion in the periventricular white matter is the most common pattern, seen with acute or subacute lesions. As in Case 309, this appearance is not specific for demyelinating disease, but multiple sclerosis should be included in the differential diagnosis. Among other possibilities in this case would be a small vascular malformation or cavernous angioma, a subacute "lacunar" infarct, inflammatory disease such as cysticercosis, and a focal deep hemisphere metastasis.

The intensity and multiplicity of enhancing lesions in multiple sclerosis may be increased on delayed scans after large amounts of contrast material have been administered. Alternatively, the MR appearance of a case with this nonspecific CT pattern may be highly characteristic for demyelinating disease (or for another pathology such as multiple cavernous angiomas; see Cases 516 and 517).

MULTIPLE SCLEROSIS: LARGE MASS LESIONS

Case 311

29-year-old woman.

Case 312

65-year-old man presenting with rapid onset of hemiparesis.

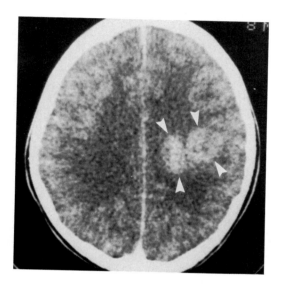

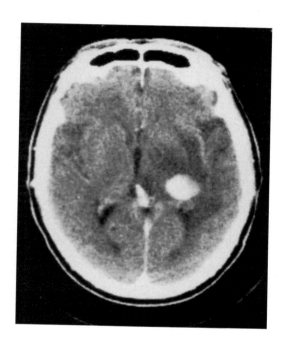

Large regions of active demyelination may cause atypical patterns of contrast enhancement. Enhancement may be solid (as in this case) or peripheral and may measure several centimeters in diameter. The resulting appearance resembles a malignant neoplasm. Such lesions are usually located in the centrum semiovale, but may also occur in the corpus callosum.

Giant MS plaques are frequently "perched" or based along the margins of the lateral ventricles. They often cause remarkably little ventricular deformity for their size. These features can combine with a very round shape to suggest the correct diagnosis on CT or MR scans.

In this case a large nodule of intense enhancement deep within the cerebral hemisphere is accompanied by extensive edema, which spreads into the internal and external capsules. A diagnosis of neoplasm was presumed, and biopsy was performed at another hospital. The pathological diagnosis of multiple sclerosis was confirmed upon review. The lesion disappeared after a month and has not recurred in over 2 years of follow-up.

The age and sex of this patient make the correct diagnosis difficult. However, a giant focus of demyelinating disease should be considered whenever a deep hemisphere mass is encountered in a young adult.

MR EVALUATION OF MULTIPLE SCLEROSIS: ACUTE DISEASE

Case 313

56-year-old woman presenting with rapidly
worsening right hemiparesis.
(axial, noncontrast scan; SE 2500/90)

Case 314

29-year-old woman.
(axial, noncontrast scan; SE 2500/90)

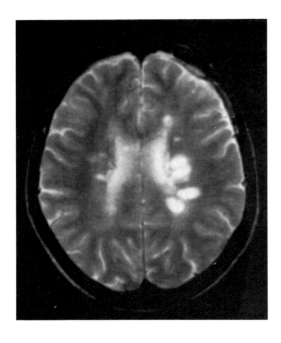

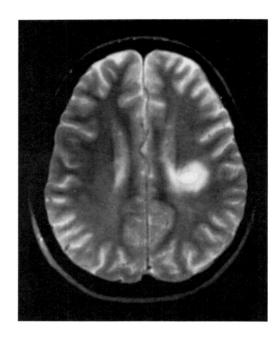

The detection of plaques in multiple sclerosis was one of the first and most dramatic demonstrations of the contrast sensitivity of magnetic resonance imaging. Although CT scans may disclose many abnormalities in patients with demyelinating disease, MR is the procedure of choice for evaluating these cases. Negative MR scans are rare in the setting of clinically documented disease. (Spinal cord involvement should be considered in such instances.)

The scan in this case demonstrates two commonly encountered types of lesions. The small, uniform, sharply defined foci of high signal intensity in the right corona radiata are typical of plaques seen in periventricular rows during quiescent clinical periods. The larger lesions with less distinct margins in the left corona radiata suggest active demyelination with associated edema. Such lesions often demonstrate contrast enhancement and may correlate with new symptoms, as in this case. The relatively elliptical shape of some periventricular lesions (with long axis directed toward the ventricular margin) has been attributed to the perivenular pathophysiology of demyelination.

As can be surmised from this case, the MR pattern of multiple sclerosis can vary from strikingly symmetrical to markedly asymmetrical, depending on the number and activity of individual lesions.

As illustrated in Cases 309 to 312, multiple sclerosis may present as a single focus of acute demyelination. Here such a lesion is seen in the posterior left corona radiata. The large size and indistinct margins of the lesion resemble the left hemisphere plaques in Case 313 and argue for active inflammation. Within the edematous zone, a thin, uniform "ring" or "rim" of shorter T2 is apparent. Such "ring lesions" are sometimes encountered on MR scans of multiple sclerosis, possibly correlating with the peripheral enhancement seen in some CT examinations (see Case 306).

A similar thin rim of relatively short T2 can be seen on MR studies of cerebral abscesses (see Cases 284 and 285). "Target" morphologies have also been noted within masses due to toxoplasmosis and primary CNS lymphoma in AIDS patients.

Case 315

30-year-old woman.
(axial, noncontrast scan; SE 3000/75)

Case 316

39-year-old woman.
(sagittal, noncontrast scan; SE 600/16)

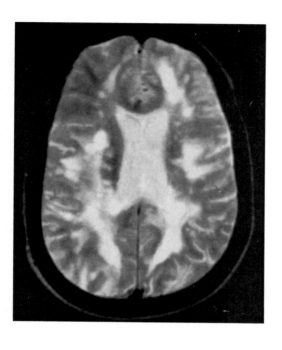

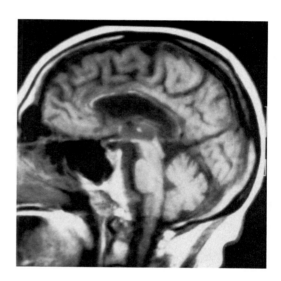

Long-standing multiple sclerosis is often associated with ventricular and sulcal enlargement, as seen here. These findings in a young patient may suggest the CT diagnosis even if individual plaques are not defined. (See Cases 336 to 337 for other causes of prominent CSF spaces in young patients.)

In this case an MR study demonstrates large areas of abnormal intensity throughout the white matter, reflecting longstanding multiple sclerosis. Although bilateral and extensive, the pattern is not as symmetrical as is usually seen in leukoencephalopathy due to vascular insufficiency or radiation (see Cases 327 and 329). The appearance is nevertheless nonspecific; a similar scan could be obtained in an AIDS patient with progressive multifocal leukoencephalopathy (see Cases 321 to 323).

The sagittal MR plane is often useful in the evaluation of multiple sclerosis. Periventricular plaques are frequently well demonstrated in the subependymal regions on parasagittal scans. More importantly, involvement of the corpus callosum is best assessed by midsagittal views.

Here the sagittal plane documents extensive atrophy, both of the hemispheres and of the corpus callosum. The sulci on the medial surface of the frontal lobe are much too large for the patient's age. The corpus callosum is markedly thinned, with abnormal signal intensity and irregular margins indicating direct involvement by severe demyelinating disease.

ACUTE DISSEMINATED ENCEPHALOMYELITIS

Case 317

11-year-old boy who developed somnolence and hemiparesis over a 4-day period, 2 weeks after a viral illness.
(postcontrast scan)

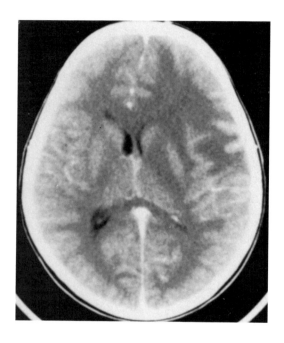

Case 318

24-year-old woman with acute deterioration in mental status 2 weeks following a viral illness.
(axial, noncontrast scan; SE 2500/90)

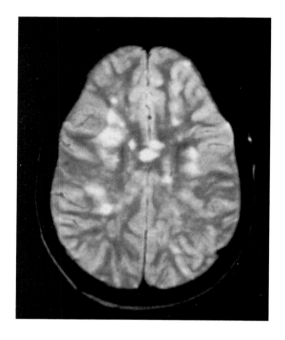

Acute disseminated encephalomyelitis (ADEM) is alternatively called "immune-mediated encephalitis" because the pathophysiology is believed to involve autoimmune demyelination. Patients typically give a history of antigenic challenge (e.g., virus or vaccination) days or weeks prior to the onset of symptoms.

Cerebral involvement primarily affects white matter, but the pattern is variable. Large, geographic regions of edema and mass effect may develop, as seen in this case. Contrast enhancement is usually absent or minimal, similar to progressive multifocal leukoencephalopathy.

Here the left frontal lesion extends into the genu of the corpus callosum. Edema thickens the internal and external capsules on the left (compare to the more normal capsular dimensions on the right). Subfalcial herniation is present.

In some cases of ADEM, multiple small lesions are scattered throughout the hemispheres, often involving the corpus callosum as seen here. The size of such lesions is typically a little larger than quiescent plaques of multiple sclerosis, and the distribution is usually more random.

Unlike multiple sclerosis, ADEM is typically monophasic. Relapse is occasionally noted.

Some cases of immune-mediated encephalitis are associated with microscopic hemorrhage. This entity, previously called "acute hemorrhagic leukoencephalitis," progresses rapidly and carries a poor prognosis.

Nonhemorrhagic cases of ADEM often respond well to steroids. Both this patient and the boy in Case 317 were clinically normal within a month after presentation.

Case 319

13-year-old boy with poor school performance
and hyperkinesia.
(postcontrast scan)

Adrenoleukodystrophy.

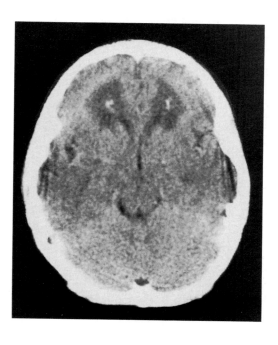

Case 320

7-year-old boy, four years after radiation and
chemotherapy for medulloblastoma.

Disseminated Necrotizing
Leukoencephalopathy.

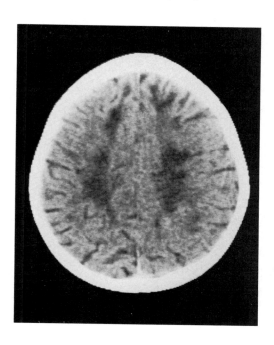

Both multiple sclerosis and ADEM can present in children (as evidenced by Case 317). Among other disorders of white matter in the pediatric population is adrenoleukodystrophy, a rare demyelinating process affecting boys. The disorder seems to be a sex-linked recessive abnormality of lipid metabolism, usually associated with adrenal hypofunction.

The typical CT pattern consists of symmetrical areas of demyelination beginning in the parieto-occipital regions and spreading anteriorly. A zone of peripheral contrast enhancement is often present at the advancing margin of demyelination.

Many atypical appearances have been reported. In this case, the frontal lobe predominance and the central contrast enhancement are unusual.

White matter damage has been noted pathologically and on CT scans following chemotherapy and/or cerebral radiation, particularly in children. The combination of radiation and chemotherapy may carry a higher risk of leukoencephalopathy than either treatment alone.

Methotrexate leukoencephalopathy has been identified in leukemia patients receiving radiotherapy, but the toxicity of other chemotherapeutic agents is less well established. The phrase "disseminated necrotizing leukoencephalopathy" is used for methotrexate-associated disease, but may apply to other combinations of chemotherapy and/or radiation. Evidence of radiation-induced demyelination may be seen on CT scans in the absence of associated chemotherapy. Such changes are more apparent and more diffuse on MR studies (see Case 329).

PROGRESSIVE MULTIFOCAL LEUKOENCEPHALOPATHY

Case 321A

29-year-old man with AIDS.
(postcontrast scan)

Case 321B

Same patient.
(postcontrast scan)

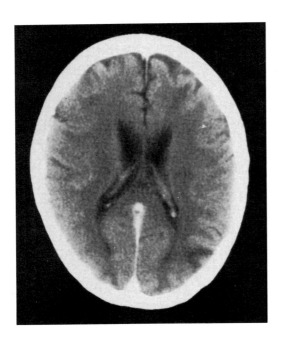

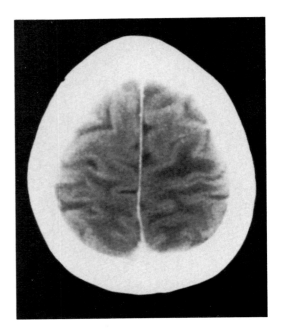

Progressive multifocal leukoencephalopathy (PML) is a demyelinating disorder representing infection by a papovavirus. The disease is usually seen in immunosuppressed hosts. Lymphoma and leukemia have been common predisposing conditions, but a rapidly increasing proportion of PML cases now occurs in AIDS patients. Iatrogenic immunosuppression may also be implicated (see Case 323 and compare with the discussion of primary CNS lymphoma, Cases 247 and 250).

The multifocal demyelination often involves subcortical white matter, as seen here. Mass effect and contrast enhancement are rare. An equivocal enhancing nodule at the tip of the right occipital horn may represent concurrent pathology of a different type.

The CT appearance of PML may resemble early cerebritis, venous infarction (see Case 471), or tumor-related edema. Diagnosis is aided by the limitation of findings to white matter and the lack of contrast enhancement. A progressive clinical course and characteristic follow-up scans are confirmatory.

Multifocal involvement in PML is rarely as symmetrical as "age-related" or "ischemic" leukoencephalopathy (see Case 327).

A prominent finding on many CT and MR scans in PML is the "heart of the gyrus" involvement demonstrated here. Individual gyri are thickened by edema of central white matter, with conspicuous sparing and margination of the overlying cortical ribbon. Involvement is prominently bilateral and multifocal, and contrast enhancement is notably absent.

MR CORRELATION: PROGRESSIVE MULTIFOCAL LEUKOENCEPHALOPATHY

Case 322A

57-year-old man.
(coronal, noncontrast scan; SE 700/17)

Case 322B

Same patient.
(axial, noncontrast scan; SE 2500/90)

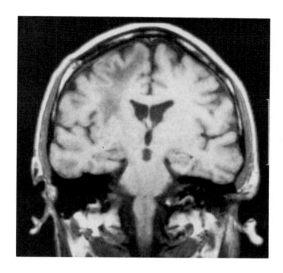

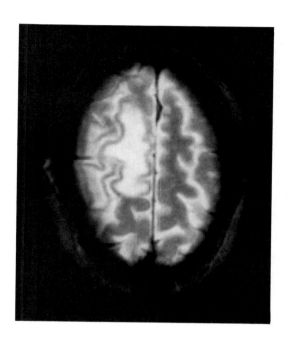

The relatively large, geographic white matter lesions of PML are well defined on MR scans. T1-weighted images demonstrate edema as zones of low signal intensity in involved regions. Here a large area of PML at the right hemisphere vertex extends into subcortical white matter, outlining the overlying cortical ribbon.

Foci of PML are most apparent and best defined on T2-weighted MR images. Here the "heart" of the right superior frontal gyrus is expanded by high-intensity edema, sharply defining the adjacent cortex. (Compare this appearance to the T1-weighted image in Case 322A and to the CT scan in Case 321B.)

Case 323

43-year-old man with a renal transplant.

Case 324

68-year-old man presenting with confusion.

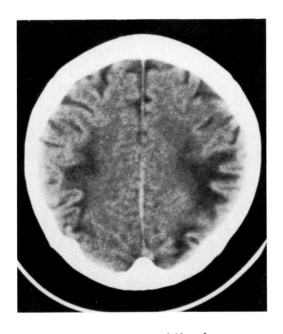

Progressive Multifocal Leukoencephalopathy.

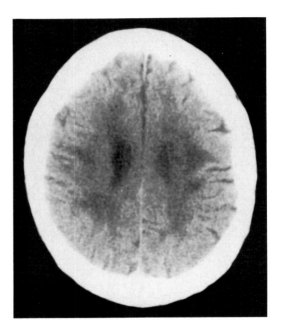

"Aging" White Matter.

Age-related changes in cerebral white mater (see Case 327) may present a pattern of multifocal low attenuation suggesting leukoencephalopathy, as in Case 324. Clues to the correct diagnosis include the general symmetry of cerebral involvement and the predominant location in midhemisphere and deep hemisphere regions.

By contrast, PML frequently affects subcortical white matter (as in Case 323) and often demonstrates less symmetry than is seen here (see Cases 321 and 322).

Both PML and white matter "aging" are usually not associated with abnormal contrast enhancement. Superior sagittal sinus thrombosis (see Cases 468 to 472) can also cause multifocal, nonenhancing cerebral edema resembling PML.

On noncontrast scans, reactive edema surrounding metastatic or inflammatory foci may mimic primary leukoencephalopathy. Contrast enhancement and the clinical context will usually clarify such cases.

IMMATURE WHITE MATTER

Case 325

Newborn boy delivered at 26 weeks' gestation.

Case 326

2-day-old boy delivered at 31 weeks' gestation.

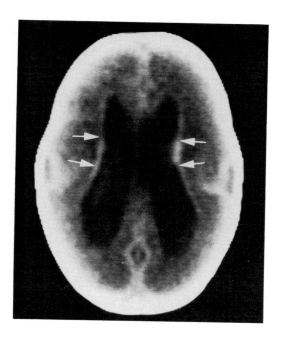

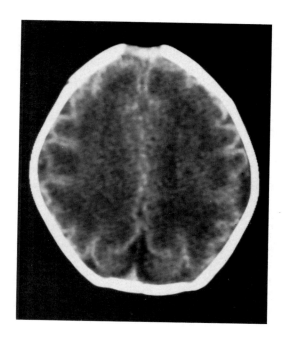

CT scans of premature infants demonstrate diffuse low attenuation throughout cerebral white matter. This normal low density is associated with immature myelination and high water content. It does not imply (or exclude) anoxic or ischemic damage. Even full-term neonates may demonstrate prominent low density in white matter for several months.

In this case, the smooth cortical ribbon is best seen in the medial occipital and sylvian regions. The dense subependymal layer of germinal matrix *(arrows)* is often prominent in premature infants and should not be mistaken for periventricular hemorrhage (see Cases 577 and 578).

The dural sinuses often appear unusually dense in neonates, probably due to hemoconcentration seen against a background of parenchymal low density. This diffuse vascular prominence should not be confused with the focal density of superior sagittal sinus thrombosis (see Case 468).

This is another example of normally immature white matter. The thin ribbon of cortex is sharply outlined by subcortical low attenuation. Both the thinness of the cortex and the watery attenuation of the centrum semiovale are within developmental expectations for the baby's gestational age. Good definition of the cortex argues against diffuse ischemia or encephalitis as the cause of white matter "edema" (but see Case 480).

AGING WHITE MATTER: "ISCHEMIC LEUKOENCEPHALOPATHY"

Case 327A

79-year-old woman presenting with a transient ischemic attack.

Case 327B

Same patient.

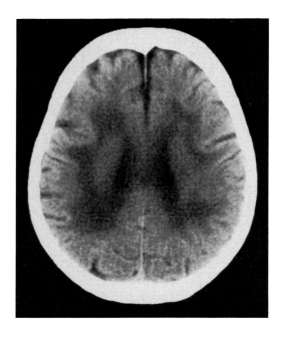

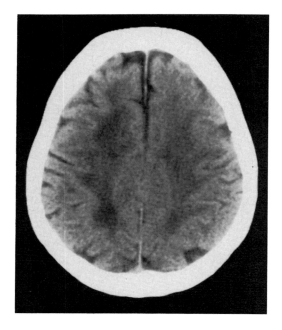

Striking low attenuation is commonly seen in the deep white matter of elderly patients. The symmetry of this low-density change distinguishes it from focal edema or infarction. Involvement may be limited to periventricular regions near the frontal horns and trigones or may extend diffusely throughout the centrum semiovale.

This white matter pattern has been considered to represent Binswanger's disease (subcortical arteriosclerotic encephalopathy). However, most cases lack a characteristic history, and the involvement is predominantly periventricular rather than subcortical. Together with the very common occurrence of this finding in elderly patients, these factors suggest that the pattern may alternatively represent a more generalized "ischemic leukoencephalopathy" associated with aging.

The diffuse nature and relative symmetry of "ischemic leukoencephalopathy" are again apparent at this level. (Contrast Case 327 with the pattern in Cases 321 and 323.) There is no associated mass effect, and no enhancement is seen on postcontrast scans.

The pattern above is also different from the multiple focal infarcts seen within the basal ganglia and deep white matter of patients with "lacunar states" due to hypertension or other small vessel disease (see Cases 434 and 435).

Radiation therapy can be followed by generalized low attenuation throughout cerebral white matter suggesting premature "aging." Such changes are particularly apparent on MR scans (see Case 329).

DIFFUSE WHITE MATTER DAMAGE

Case 328

23-year-old woman, 2 months after carbon monoxide poisoning.

Case 329

65-year-old man, 2 years after cerebral radiation for small cell carcinoma of the lung.
(axial, noncontrast scan; SE 2500/90)

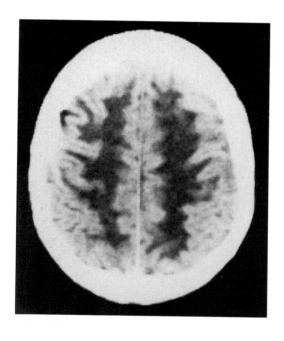

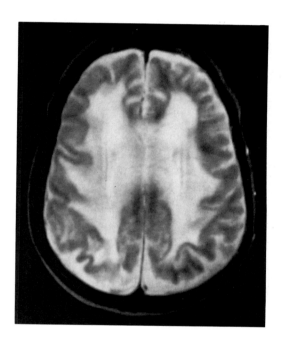

Severe leukoencephalopathy from any cause leads to extensive, confluent alteration in the CT attenuation values and MR signal intensity of white matter. Widespread injury to cerebral white matter is best demonstrated by MR scans but may also be apparent on CT studies, as in this case.

Although cerebral gray matter is particularly susceptible to anoxia (see Cases 464 to 467), anoxic damage to white matter may also be extensive (see Case 469). In some cases initial clinical recovery from an anoxic insult is followed by rapid deterioration after several weeks or months due to delayed postanoxic leukoencephalopathy.

Radiation therapy can cause diffuse changes in cerebral white matter that are more apparent on MR scans than on CT examinations. Such alterations can be seen at any age (see Case 320). In adults the extent of radiation damage as depicted by MR and its clinical significance appear to increase with patient age at the time of treatment.

Radiation may accelerate or potentiate the ongoing aging of white matter as illustrated in Case 327. In any event, the extensive, symmetrical abnormality of signal intensity seen throughout the centrum semiovale in this case favors a diffuse toxic or metabolic insult. (Contrast this appearance with the multifocal pattern of inflammatory and neoplastic diseases such as Case 321.)

MR EVALUATION OF BRAIN STEM DEMYELINATION

Case 330

39-year-old woman.
(axial, noncontrast scan; SE 3000/90)

Multiple Sclerosis.

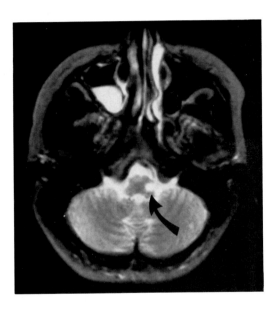

CT is of little value in evaluating patients with suspected demyelination of the brain stem. As discussed with respect to brain stem gliomas (see Cases 106 to 113), MR offers a much better view of pathology in this location.

Multiple sclerosis frequently involves the posterior fossa. The region of the brachium pontis is a particularly common site for demyelinating plaques, but they may be found at all levels of the brain stem. In this case a very well defined lesion is seen within the left medulla (arrow). Similar focal plaques may be discovered in the spinal cord (see Cases 791 and 792).

The rounded area of high signal intensity within the right maxillary sinus represents a retention cyst.

Case 331

48-year-old woman.
(axial, noncontrast scan; SE 2500/90)

Central Pontine Myelinolysis.

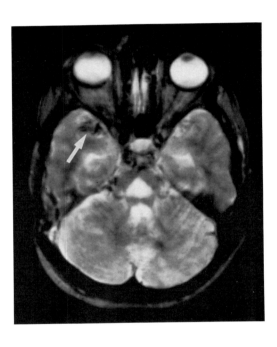

Central pontine myelinolysis is an acute demyelinating process affecting the brain stem. It is incompletely understood but may correlate with the rapid correction (or overcorrection) of severe electrolyte abnormalities. Other factors (e.g., nutritional) may contribute.

CT scans may demonstrate brain stem abnormality in cases of central pontine myelinolysis (see Case 446), but definition of the lesion is often vague. MR offers unequivocal documentation of this pathology, as seen here. In many cases involvement of the central pons with sparing of peripheral tracts results in a distinctive triangular shape as illustrated above.

A similar demyelinating pathology ("extrapontine myelinolysis") can occur within the basal ganglia and cerebral hemispheres, together with or independent of pontine involvement. Conversely, other white matter disorders (e.g., PML) may involve the pons.

A prominent tangle of vessels in the anterior portion of the right middle cranial fossa (arrow) represents proximal branches of the middle cerebral artery. This normal finding should not be mistaken for an arteriovenous malformation (compare to Case 115).

DEGENERATIVE DISORDERS

Case 332

10-year-old girl presenting with ataxia.

Friedreich's Ataxia.

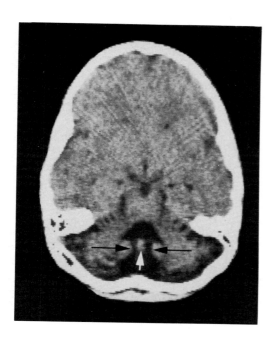

Case 333

60-year-old woman presenting with dementia and movement disorder.

Huntington's Chorea.

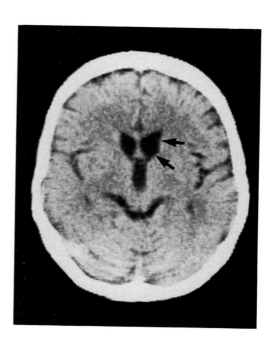

Atrophy is well defined on CT scans, with the loss of parenchymal volume clearly outlined by expanded subarachnoid spaces. In this case, the greatly enlarged posterior fossa cisterns, cerebellar sulci, and fourth ventricle contrast with the normally inconspicuous CSF spaces above the tentorium.

A number of familial syndromes (e.g., olivopontocerebellar degeneration, Marie's ataxia) may cause cerebellar degeneration with or without brain stem atrophy. Friedreich's ataxia usually presents with spinal cord involvement and less impressive cerebellar findings. Examples of acquired cerebellar atrophy include alcohol abuse, paraneoplastic syndromes, and the phenytoin/seizure combination.

Enlarged subarachnoid spaces highlight surface anatomy. Here the inferior vermis is clearly seen (white arrow) as a small nodule of tissue forming the posterior wall of the fourth ventricle and residing between the cerebellar tonsils (black arrows).

The normal caudate head bulges into the lateral aspect of the frontal horns to cause a medially convex margin. Atrophy of the caudate nucleus in advanced Huntington's disease causes this curvature to flatten and reverse, leaving a concave surface as seen here (arrows). Associated ventricular and sulcal enlargement is often present.

This characteristic CT finding is a late development in the disease and is not seen in presymptomatic carriers. Positron emission tomography can identify abnormal caudate metabolism before atrophy appears on CT scans.

CEREBRAL ATROPHY

Case 334

82-year-old man.

Case 335

74-year-old man.

Pick's Disease.

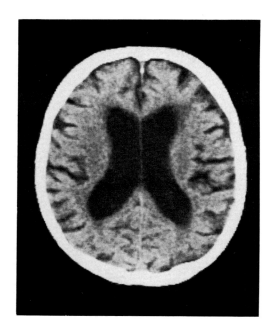

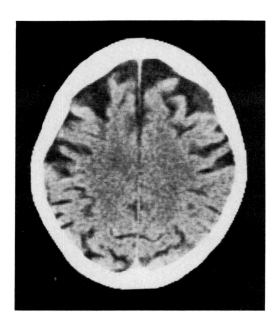

Cerebral atrophy is demonstrated on CT scans by diffuse enlargement of ventricles and subarachnoid spaces. The relative degree of ventricular and sulcal enlargement is usually similar. Prominence of the ventricular component raises the question of hydrocephalus (see Cases 604 and 605).

The correlation between enlarged CSF spaces and reduced intellectual capacity has been difficult to establish in group studies and cannot be applied to an individual case.

In some cases, the loss of cerebral volume predominantly involves the frontal lobes. The diagnosis of Pick's disease may be suggested when localized frontal atrophy is associated with prominent atrophy of the temporal lobes (inferior and middle temporal gyri).

Classic Pick's disease demonstrates strikingly thin gyri separated by gaping sulci in the frontal and temporal lobes. However, these "knife-like" gyri are not seen in all cases.

Alzheimer's disease may also be associated with focal frontal and temporal lobe atrophy.

DIFFERENTIAL DIAGNOSIS: PSEUDOATROPHY

Case 336

32-year-old man weighing 87 lb.

Case 337

30-year-old man.

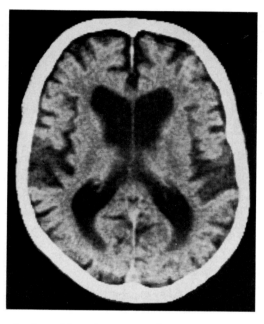

Malnutrition due to Psychiatric Disorder.

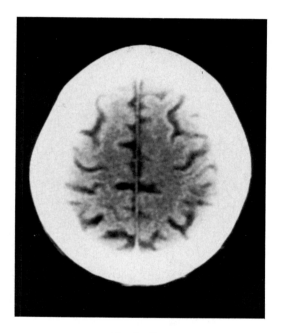

Alcoholism.

A number of conditions may cause enlargement of cerebral sulci resembling atrophy. Alcoholic "atrophy" is common, possibly due to nutritional or hydration factors as well as to direct effects of ethanol. In some patients the enlarged sulci return to more normal size after successful treatment.

Other circumstances have also been associated with abnormal enlargement of cerebral sulci. These include malnutrition (anorexia nervosa or other psychiatric causes, as in Case 336), high doses of exogenous or endogenous steroids, multiple sclerosis, lupus cerebritis, AIDS, and chronic renal disease (possibly related to dialysis and hydration or nutrition states).

When a young patient presents with enlarged sulci, these possibilities should be considered (along with presenile dementing disorders and toxic-anoxic insults).

CEREBRAL HEMIATROPHY WITH HEMICRANIAL HYPERTROPHY

Case 338

6-year-old girl with seizures.

Case 339

69-year-old woman with a history of a "stroke" as an infant.

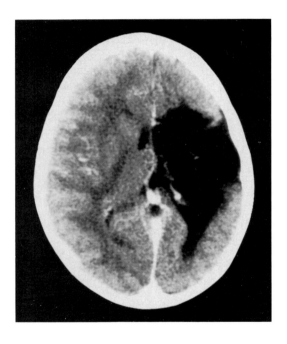

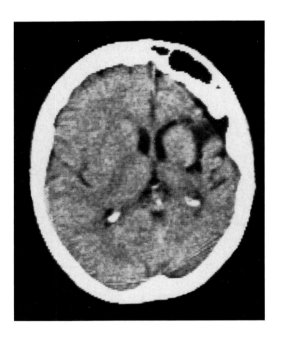

The interrelationship of brain growth and skull contour is demonstrated when a cerebrovascular accident in infancy or childhood damages one cerebral hemisphere. The reduced cerebral volume leads to ipsilateral changes in calvarial morphology.

Here, cerebral parenchyma is missing throughout much of the distribution of the left middle cerebral artery. The involved hemicranium is small, with eccentric falx position. The skull is mildly thickened on the side of cerebral atrophy.

Secondary expansion of the ipsilateral ventricle as seen here may be associated with large infarcts in patients of all ages.

In this case the occurrence of left hemisphere damage in infancy is reflected by a small hemicranium with eccentric position of the falx and mild calvarial thickening. An additional finding is asymmetric enlargement of sinuses and air cells on the affected side.

STURGE-WEBER SYNDROME

Case 340A

24-year-old man with seizures.

Case 340B

Same patient.
(wide window)

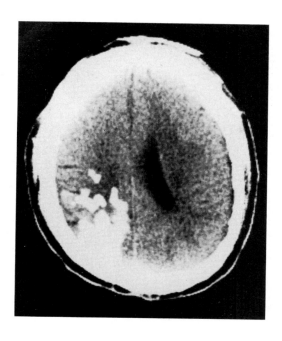

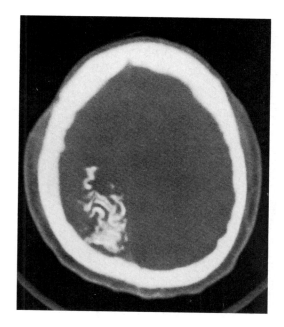

Sturge-Weber syndrome is one of the neurophacomatoses combining cutaneous and intracranial abnormalities. The external manifestation of the syndrome is a facial hemangioma or "port-wine stain" in the distribution of a division of the trigeminal nerve.

This hallmark is associated with an ipsilateral venous angioma of the meninges, most common in the parieto-occipital region. (An alternative name for the syndrome is "encephalo-trigeminal angiomatosis.")

Postcontrast CT scans may suggest vague, superficial enhancement in the region of calcification, representing the meningeal angioma. Contrast-enhanced MR scans can clearly demonstrate meningeal angiomas in Sturge-Weber syndrome that are not detectable on either postcontrast CT studies or noncontrast MR scans. On MR scans the enhancing angioma may fill sulci, resembling meningitis or meningeal carcinomatosis.

Large superficial and deep veins are often seen in the involved region on CT or MR scans, reflecting an associated abnormality of cortical venous drainage with collateral flow away from the superior sagittal sinus.

Cerebral cortex underlying the meningeal angioma of Sturge-Weber syndrome exhibits a characteristic "tram-track" pattern of dystrophic calcification. Wide window settings demonstrate this typical "gyriform" deposition of calcium. The calcification may be observed to develop in an infant or toddler over a period of weeks or months.

Gyriform calcification is probably a nonspecific response to cortical damage and can be seen in other circumstances (e.g., in children following encephalitis or meningitis, after treatment for CNS leukemia, and in association with disorders of neuronal migration).

Associated cerebral atrophy is common and may be focal or hemispheric. In this case, atrophy of the hemisphere has resulted in a small hemicranium. The falx position is eccentric and the ipsilateral calvarium is thickened. The appearance is comparable with other examples of the Dyke-Davidoff-Masson syndrome, as seen in Case 339.

VERTEX ANATOMY

Case 341

80-year-old woman.

Case 342

74-year-old woman.

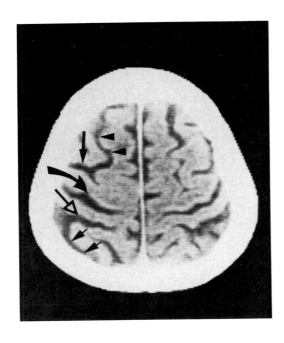

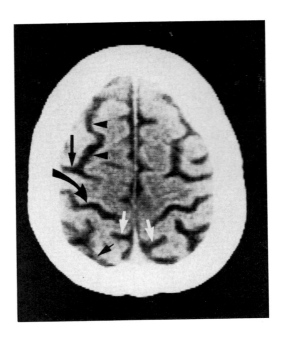

Atrophic enlargement of cerebral sulci demonstrates gyral landmarks on vertex scans.

The superior frontal sulcus *(black arrowheads)* follows a parasagittal course before intersecting posteriorly (at a right angle) with the precentral sulcus *(straight black arrow)*.

The intraparietal sulcus *(short black arrows)* angles obliquely across the posterior parietal vertex before merging anteriorly with the postcentral sulcus *(open black arrow)*.

The central sulcus *(curved black arrow)* lies between the precentral sulcus and the postcentral sulcus as the middle member of the three major laterally directed sulci.

The landmarks discussed in Case 341 are labeled with the same key in this patient.

Another vertex landmark is the marginal ramus of the cingulate sulcus, seen here as a short, paired sulcus on the medial surface of the hemisphere *(white arrows)*. The central sulcus is usually the next most anterior sulcus on the lateral surface of the convexity.

Usually one or more of these landmarks is apparent on vertex scans (compare to Case 337 for example). Their recognition localizes lesions with respect to the motor and sensory gyri, regardless of head flexion or extension.

REFERENCES: CT

1. Artmann H., Gall M.V., Hacker H., et al.: Reversible enlargement of cerebral spinal fluid spaces in chronic alcoholics. *A.J.N.R.* 2:23–27, 1981.
2. Aubourg P., Diebler C.: Adrenoleukodystrophy—Its diverse CT appearances and an evolutive of phenotypic variant: The leukodystrophy without adrenal insufficiency. *Neuroradiology* 24:33–42, 1982.
3. Benator R.M., Magill H.L., Gerald B., et al.: Herpes simplex encephalitis: CT findings in the neonate and young infant. *A.J.N.R.* 6:539–544, 1985.
4. Bursztyn E.M., Lee B.C.P., Bauman J.: CT of acquired immunodeficiency syndrome. *A.J.N.R.* 5:711–714, 1984.
5. Carroll B.A., Lane B., Norman D., et al.: Diagnosis of progressive multifocal leukoencephalopathy by computed tomography. *Radiology* 122:137–141, 1977.
6. Centeno R.S., Bentson J.R., Mancuso A.A.: CT scanning in rhinocerebral mucormycosis and aspergillosis. *Radiology* 140:383–389, 1981.
7. Chong K.H., Kim W.S., Cho S.Y., et al.: Comparative evaluation of brain CT and ELISA in the diagnosis of neurocysticercosis. *A.J.N.R.* 9:125–130, 1988.
8. Clark W.C., Acker J.D., Dohan F.C. Jr., Robertson J.H.: Presentation of central nervous system sarcoidosis as intracranial tumors. *J. Neurosurg.* 63:851–856, 1985.
9. Collins A.T., Cromwell L.D.: Computed tomography in the evaluation of congenital cerebral toxoplasmosis. *J. Comput. Assist. Tomogr.* 4:326–329, 1980.
10. Danziger A., Price H.I.: CT findings with cerebral hemiatrophy. *Neuroradiology* 19:269–271, 1980.
11. Danziger A., Price H., Schechter M.M.: An analysis of 113 intracranial infections. *Neuroradiology* 19:31–34, 1980.
12. Davis, P.C., Hoffman J.C. Jr., Pearl G.S., Braun I.F.: CT Evaluation of effects of cranial radiation therapy in children. *A.J.N.R.* 7:639–644, 1986.
13. Enzmann D.R., Britt R.H., Placone R.C. Jr.: Staging of human brain abscess by computed tomography. *Radiology* 146:703–708, 1983.
14. George A.E., de Leon M.J., Gentes C.I., et al.: Leukoencephalopathy in normal and pathologic aging. 1. CT of brain lucencies. *A.J.N.R.* 7:561–566, 1986.
15. George A.E., de Leon M.J., Stylopoulos L.A., et al.: CT diagnostic features of Alzheimer's disease: Importance of the choroidal/hippocampal fissure complex. *A.J.N.R.* 11:101–108, 1990.
16. Haughton V.M., Ho K.C., Williams A.L., et al.: CT detection of demyelinated plaques in multiple sclerosis. *A.J.R.* 132:213–215, 1979.
17. Heinz E.R., Drayer B.P., Haenggeli C.A., et al.: Computed tomography in white-matter disease. *Radiology* 130:371–378, 1979.
18. Herman T.E., Cleveland R.H., Kushner D.C., Taveras J.M.: CT of neonatal herpes encephalitis. *A.J.N.R.* 6:773–776, 1985.
19. Hong-Magno E.T., Muraki A.S., Huttenlocher P.R.: Atypical CT scans in adrenoleukodystrophy. *J. Comput. Assist. Tomogr.* 11:333–336, 1987.
20. Huckman M.S.: Computed tomography in the diagnosis of degenerative brain disease. *Radiol. Clin. North Am.* 20:169–183, 1982.
21. Inoue Y., Fukuda T., Takashima S., et al.: Adrenoleukodystrophy: New CT findings. *A.J.N.R.* 4:951–954, 1983.
22. Kido D.K., Caine E.D., LeMay M., et al.: Temporal lobe atrophy in patients with Alzheimer's disease: A CT study. *A.J.N.R.* 10:551–556, 1989.
23. Kingsley D.P., Kendall B.E.: CT of the adverse effects of therapeutic radiation of the central nervous system. *A.J.N.R.* 2:453–460, 1981.
24. Kramer L.D., Locke G.E., Byrd S.E., Daryabogi J.: Cerebral cysticercosis: Documentation of natural history with CT. *Radiology* 171:459–462, 1989.
25. Kumpe, D.A., Rao C.V., Garcia J., et al.: Intracranial neurosarcoidosis. *J. Comput. Assist. Tomogr.* 3:324–330, 1979.
26. LeMay M.: CT changes in dementing diseases: A review. *A.J.N.R.* 7:841–854, 1986.
27. LeMay M.: Radiologic changes of the aging brain and skull. *A.J.N.R.* 5:269–275, 1984.
28. Levy R.M., Rosenbloom S., Perrett L.V.: Neuroradiologic findings in AIDS: A review of 200 cases. *A.J.N.R.* 7:833–840, 1986.
29. Lotz P.R., Ballinger W.E. Jr., Quisling R.G.: Subcortical arteriosclerotic encephalopathy: CT spectrum and pathologic correlation. *A.J.N.R.* 7:817–822, 1986.
30. McCormick G.F., Zee C.S., Heiden J.: Cysticercosis cerebri: Review of 127 cases. *Arch. Neurol.* 39:534–539, 1982.
31. Noorbehesht B., Enzmann D.R., Sullender W., et al.: Neonatal herpes encephalitis: Correlation of clinical and CT findings. *Radiology* 162:813–820, 1987.
32. Otsuka S.-I., Nakatsu S., Matsumoto S., et al.: Multiple sclerosis simulating brain tumor on computed tomography. *J. Comput. Assist. Tomogr.* 13:674–678, 1989.
33. Packer R.J., Bilaniuk L.T., Zimmerman R.A.: CT parenchymal abnormalities in bacterial meningitis: Clinical significance. *J. Comput. Assist. Tomogr.* 6:1064–1068, 1982.
34. Palacios E., Rodriquez-Carbajal J., Taveras J.M. (eds.): *Cysticercosis of the Central Nervous System.* Springfield, Ill., Charles C Thomas, Publisher, 1983.
35. Popovich M.J., Arthur R.J., Helmer E.: CT of intracranial cryptococcosis. *A.J.N.R.* 11:139–142, 1990.
36. Post M.J.D., Hensley G.T., Moskowitz L.B., Fischl M.: Cytomegalic inclusion virus encephalitis in patients with AIDS: CT, clinical, and pathologic correlation. *A.J.N.R.* 7:275–280, 1986.
37. Post M.J.D., Kursunoglu S.J., Hensley G.T., et al.: Cranial CT in acquired immunodeficiency syndrome: Spectrum of diseases and optimal contrast enhancement technique. *A.J.N.R.* 6:743–754, 1985.
38. Ramos A., Quintana F., Diez C., et al.: CT findings in spinocerebellar degeneration. *A.J.N.R.* 8:635–640, 1987.
39. Rodacki M.A., Detoni X.A., Teixeira W.R.: CT features of cellulosae and racemosus neurocysticercosis. *J. Comput. Assist. Tomogr.* 13:1013–16, 1989.
40. Rosenbloom S., Buchholz D., Kumar A.J., et al.: Evolution of central pontine myelinolysis on CT. *A.J.N.R.* 5:110–112, 1984.
41. Rovira M., Romero F., Torrent D.: Study of tuberculous meningitis by CT. *Neuroradiology* 19:137–141, 1980.
42. Sadhu B.K., Handel S.F., Pinto R.S., et al.: Neuroradiologic diagnosis of subdural empyema and CT limitations. *A.J.N.R.* 1:39–44, 1980.
43. Spiegel S.M., Vinuela F., Fox A.J., Pelz D.M.: CT of multiple sclerosis: Reassessment of delayed scanning with high doses of contrast material. *A.J.N.R.* 6:533–536, 1985.
44. Suss R.A., Resta S., Diehl J.T.: Persistent cortical enhancement in tuberculous meningitis. *A.J.N.R.* 8:716–720, 1987.

45. Vinuela F.V., Fox A.J., Debrun G.M., et al.: New perspectives in computed tomography of multiple sclerosis. *A.J.N.R.* 3:277–281, 1982.
46. Wang A.M., Morris J.H., Hickey W.F., et al.: Unusual CT patterns of multiple sclerosis. *A.J.N.R.* 4:47–50, 1983.
47. Wang A.M., Skias D.D., Rumbaugh C.L., et al.: Central nervous system changes after radiation therapy and/or chemotherapy: Correlation of CT and autopsy findings. *A.J.N.R.* 4:466–471, 1983.
48. Whelan M.A., Hilal S.K.: Computed tomography as a guide in the diagnosis and follow-up of brain abscesses. *Radiology* 135:663–671, 1980.
49. Whelan M.A., Kricheff I.I., Handler M., et al.: Acquired immunodeficiency syndrome: Cerebral computed tomographic manifestations. *Radiology* 149:477–484, 1983.
50. Whelan M.A., Stern J., deNapoli R.A.: The computed tomographic spectrum of intracranial mycosis: Correlation with histopathology. *Radiology* 141:703–707, 1981.
51. Zee C.-S., Segall H.D., Apuzzo M.L.J., et al.: Intraventricular cysticercal cysts: Further neuroradiologic observations and neurosurgical implications. *A.J.N.R.* 5:727–730, 1984.
52. Zimmerman R.D., Leeds N.E., Danziger A.: Subdural empyema: CT findings. *Radiology* 150:417–422, 1984.
53. Zimmerman R.D., Russell E.J., Leeds N.E.: CT in the early diagnosis of herpes encephalitis. *A.J.R.* 134:61–66, 1980.

REFERENCES: MR

1. Aisen A.M., Gabrielson T.O., McCune W.J.: MR imaging of systemic lupus erythematosus involving the brain. *A.J.N.R.* 6:197–202, 1985.
2. Atlas S.W., Grossman R.I., Goldberg H.I., et al.: MR diagnosis of acute disseminated encephalomyelitis. *J. Comput. Assist. Tomogr.* 10:798–801, 1986.
3. Atlas S.W., Grossman R.I., Packer R.J., et al.: Magnetic resonance imaging diagnosis of disseminated necrotizing leukoencephalopathy. *C.T.* 11:39, 1987.
4. Balakrishnan J., Becker P.S., Kumar A.J., et al.: Acquired immunodeficiency syndrome: Correlation of radiologic and pathologic findings in the brain. *Radiographics* 10:201–216, 1990.
5. Barloon T.J., Yuh W.T.C., Knepper L.E., et al.: Cerebral ventriculitis: MR findings. *J. Comput. Assist. Tomogr.* 14:272–275, 1990.
6. Chang K.H., Han M.H., Roh J.K., et al.: Gd-DTPA-enhanced MR imaging of the brain in patients with meningitis: Comparison with CT. *A.J.N.R.* 11:69–76, 1990.
7. Chrysikopoulos H.S., Press G.A., Grafe M.R., et al.: Encephalitis caused by human immunodeficiency virus: CT and MR imaging manifestations with clinical and pathologic correlation. *Radiology* 175:185–192, 1990.
8. Curnes J.T., Laster D.W., Ball M.R., et al.: Magnetic resonance imaging of radiation injury to the brain. *A.J.N.R.* 7:389–394, 1986.
9. Dooms G.C., Hecht S., Brant-Zawadzki M., et al.: Brain radiation lesions: MR imaging. *Radiology* 158:149–156, 1986.
10. Drayer B.P.: Imaging of the aging brain. Part I. Normal findings. *Radiology* 166:785–796, 1988.
11. Drayer B.P.: Imaging of the aging brain. Part II. Pathologic conditions. *Radiology* 166:797–806, 1988.
12. Edwards M.K., Farlow M.R., Stevens J.C.: Multiple sclerosis: MRI and clinical correlation. *A.J.N.R.* 7:595–598, 1986.
13. Ekholm S., Simon J.H.: Magnetic resonance imaging and the acquired immunodeficiency syndrome dementia complex. *Acta Radiol.* 29:227, 1988.
14. George A.E., de Leon M.V., Kalnin A., et al.: Leukoencephalopathy in normal and pathologic aging. 2. MRI of brain lucencies. *A.J.N.R.* 7:567–570, 1986.
15. Greco A., Steiner R.E.: Magnetic resonance imaging in neurosarcoidosis. *Magn. Reson. Imaging* 5:15, 1987.
16. Grossman R.I., Braffman B.H., Bronson J.R., et al.: Multiple sclerosis: Serial studies of gadolinium-enhanced MR imaging. *Radiology* 169:117–122, 1988.
17. Guilleux M.H., Steiner R.E., Young I.R.: MR imaging of progressive multifocal leukoencephalopathy. *A.J.N.R.* 7:1033–1035, 1986.
18. Gupta R.K., Jena A., Sharma A.: MR imaging of intracranial tuberculomas. *J. Comput. Assist. Tomogr.* 12:280–285, 1988.
19. Haimes A.B., Zimmerman R.D., Morgello S., et al.: MR imaging of brain abscesses. *A.J.N.R.* 10:279–292, 1989.
20. Hayes W.S., Sherman J.L., Stern B.J., et al.: MR and CT evaluation of intracranial sarcoidosis. *A.J.N.R.* 8:841–848, 1987.
21. Horowitz A.L., Kaplan R.D., Grewe G., et al.: The ovoid lesion: A new MR observation in patients with multiple sclerosis. *A.J.N.R.* 10:303–306, 1989.
22. Jensen M.E., Sawyer R.W., Braun I.F., Rizzo W.B.: MR imaging appearance of childhood adrenoleukodystrophy with auditory, visual, and motor pathway involvement. *Radiographics* 10:53–66, 1990.
23. Kumar A.J., Rosenbaum A.E., Naidu S., et al.: Adrenoleukodystrophy: Correlating MR imaging with CT. *Radiology* 165:497–504, 1987.
24. Lester J.W. Jr., Carter M.P., Reynolds T.L.: Herpes encephalitis: MR monitoring of response to acyclovir therapy. *J. Comput. Assist. Tomogr.* 12:941–943, 1988.
25. Mark A.S., Atlas S.W.: Progressive multifocal leukoencephalopathy in patients with AIDS: Appearance on MR images. *Radiology* 173:517–520, 1989.
26. Martinez H.R., Rangel-Guerra R., Elizondo G., et al.: MR imaging in neurocysticerosis: A study of 56 cases. *A.J.N.R.* 10:1011–1020, 1989.
27. Miller G.M., Baker H.L. Jr., Okazaki H., Whisnant J.P.: Central pontine myelinolysis and its imitators: MR findings. *Radiology* 168:795–802, 1988.
28. Moriwaka F., Tashiro K., Maruo Y., et al.: MR imaging of pontine and extrapontine myelinolysis. *J. Comput. Assist. Tomogr.* 12:446–449, 1988.
29. Neils E.W., Lukin R., Tomsick T.A., Tew J.M.: Magnetic resonance imaging and computerized tomography scanning of herpes simplex encephalitis. *J. Neurosurg.* 67:592–594, 1987.
30. Nowell M.A., Grossman R.I., Hackney D.B., et al.: MR imaging of white matter diseases in children. *A.J.N.R.* 9:503–509, 1988.
31. Olsen W.L., Longo F.M., Mills C.M., Norman D.: White matter disease in AIDS: Findings at MR imaging. *Radiology* 169:445–448, 1988.
32. Post M.J.D., Sheldon J.J., Hensley G.T., et al.: Central nervous system disease in acquired immunodeficiency syndrome: Prospective correlation using CT, MR imaging, and pathologic studies. *Radiology* 158:141–148, 1986.
33. Post M.J.D., Tate L.G., Quencer R.M., et al.: CT, MR, and pathology in HIV encephalitis and meningitis. *A.J.N.R.* 9:469–476, 1988.
34. Press G.A., Weindling S.M., Hesselink J.R., et al.: Rhinocerebral mucormycosis: MR manifestations. *J. Comput. Assist. Tomogr.* 12:744–749, 1988.
35. Ragland R.L., Duffis A.W., Gendelman S., et al.: Central pontine myelinolysis with clinical recovery: MR documentation. *J. Comput. Assist. Tomogr.* 13:316–318, 1989.
36. Rippe D.J., Edwards M.K., D'Amour P.G., et al.: MR imaging of central pontine myelinolysis. *J. Comput. Assist. Tomogr.* 11:724–726, 1987.
37. Runge V.M., Price A.C., Kirshner H.S., et al.: The evaluation of multiple sclerosis by magnetic resonance imaging. *Radiographics* 6:203–212, 1986.
38. Savoiardo M., Strada L., Girotti F., et al.: Olivopontocerebellar atrophy: MR diagnosis and relationship to multisystem atrophy. *Radiology* 174:693–696, 1990.
39. Schroth G., Kretzschmar K., Gawehn J., et al.: Advantage of magnetic resonance imaging in the diagnosis of cerebral infections. *Neuroradiology* 29:120, 1987.
40. Sheldon J.J., Siddharthan R., Tobias J., et al.: MR imaging of multiple sclerosis: Comparison with clinical and CT examinations in 74 patients. *A.J.N.R.* 6:683–690, 1985.
41. Simon J.H., Holtas S.L., Schiffer R.B., et al.: Corpus callosum and subcallosal-periventricular lesions in multiple sclerosis: Detection with MR. *Radiology* 160:363–368, 1986.
42. Simon J.H., Schiffer R.B., Rudick R.A., Herndon R.M.: Quantitative determination of MS-induced corpus callosum atrophy in vivo using MR imaging. *A.J.N.R.* 8:599–604, 1987.
43. Suss R.A., Maravilla K.R., Thompson J.: MR imaging of

intracranial cysticercosis: Comparison with CT and anatomopathologic features. *A.J.N.R.* 7:235–242, 1986.

44. Sze G., Zimmerman R.D.: Magnetic resonance imaging of infectious and inflammatory disease. *Radiol. Clin. North Am.* 26:839–860, 1988.

45. Teitelbaum G.P., Otto R.J., Lin M., et al.: MR imaging of neurocysticerosis. *A.J.N.R.* 10:709–718, 1989.

46. Thompson A.J., Brown M.M., Swash M., et al.: Autopsy validation of MRI in central pontine myelinolysis. *Neuroradiology* 30:175, 1988.

47. Tsuruda J.S., Kortman K.E., Bradley W.G., et al.: Radiation effects in cerebral white matter: MR evaluation. *A.J.N.R.* 8:431–438, 1987.

48. Uhlenbrock D., Seidel D., Genlen W., et al.: MR imaging in multiple sclerosis: Comparison with clinical, CSF, and visual evoked potential findings. *A.J.N.R.* 9:59–68, 1988.

49. Wasenko J.J., Rosenbloom S.A., Duchesneau P.M., et al: The Sturge-Weber syndrome: Comparison of MR and CT characteristics. *A.J.N.R.* 11:131–134, 1990.

50. Wehn S.M., Heinz E.R., Burger P.C., Boyko O.B.: Dilated Virchow-Robin spaces in cryptococcal meningitis associated with AIDS: CT and MR findings. *J. Comput. Assist. Tomogr.* 13:756–762, 1989.

51. Weingarten K., Zimmerman R.D., Becker R.D., et al.: Subdural and epidural empyemas: MR imaging. *A.J.N.R.* 10:81–88, 1989.

52. Zee C.-S., Segall H.D., Boswell W., et al.: MR imaging of neurocysticercosis. *J. Comput. Assist. Tomogr.* 12:927–934, 1988.

53. Zeiss J., Brinker R.A.: MR imaging of cerebral hemiatrophy. *J. Comput. Assist. Tomogr.* 12:640–643, 1988.

CHAPTER 8

Traumatic Lesions

ACUTE SUBDURAL HEMATOMAS

Case 343

71-year-old man who struck his head in a fall.
(noncontrast scan)

Case 344

69-year-old man who fell 1 day prior to
admission, now hemiparetic.
(noncontrast scan)

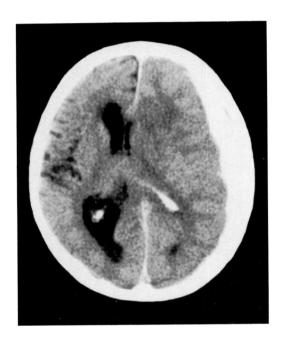

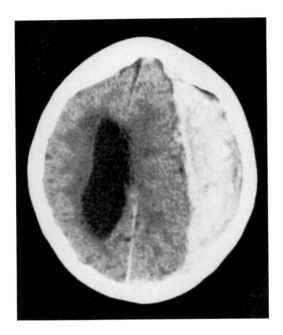

Acute subdural hemorrhages form a layer of high attenuation closely applied to the calvarium or dura. The subdural space is easily dissected by hematomas, which spread over a wide area while remaining relatively thin. This crescentic shape contrasts with the thick, biconvex morphology of epidural hematomas, as seen in Cases 366 to 368.

Subdural hematomas may appear thin on single sections while surrounding large portions of a hemisphere. Such extensive hematomas can cause more significant cerebral compression and herniations than might be expected from their narrow diameter. Mass effect is often compounded by associated cerebral contusion and edema. In this case, marked subfalcial herniation is apparent.

Small subdural hematomas may blend with the skull and can be overlooked if scans are viewed only at narrow window widths. As the display window is widened, the high attenuation of the subdural hematoma is more easily distinguished from the overlying calvarium. MR is more sensitive than CT for detecting very small subdural collections adjacent to the inner table (see Cases 356 and 357).

Acute subdural hematomas may become very large, particularly in elderly patients. The presence of pre-existing atrophy delays the onset of cerebral compression by the expanding collection. When the buffering capacity of enlarged CSF spaces has been exceeded, the development of a neurological deficit may lead to the discovery of a surprisingly thick hematoma.

The clinical presentation of patients with acute subdural hematomas can range from vague headache to generalized disorientation and confusion (see Cases 347 and 348), to focal deficits mimicking an acute cerebrovascular accident, as in this case. Elderly patients have a generally poorer prognosis than younger adults.

Many acute subdural hematomas are caused by injured cortical arteries rather than by torn bridging veins, as has been traditionally taught.

MR CORRELATION: ACUTE SUBDURAL HEMATOMAS

Case 345A

30-year-old woman scanned several days after a shunt for obstructive hydrocephalus (previous cardiopulmonary arrest). (coronal, noncontrast scan; SE 800/17)

Case 345B

Same patient, 7 days later. (coronal, noncontrast scan; SE 1000/17)

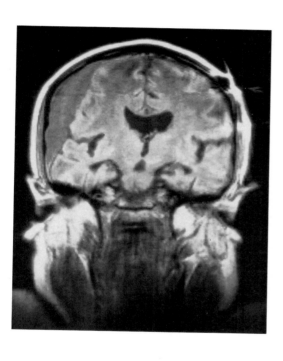

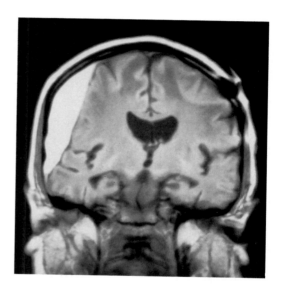

The MR appearance of hemorrhage is a complex function of many variables. In general, acute intracerebral or extracerebral hematomas are isointense or slightly lower in signal intensity than cerebral parenchyma on T1-weighted images (see Case 560A).

Here a T1-weighted coronal scan clearly documents a subdural collection overlying the right hemisphere. The signal intensity of the acute hematoma is intermediate between that of CSF and brain tissue. Metallic artifact from the shunt valve is seen adjacent to the left hemicranium. Abnormally low signal intensity throughout cerebral white matter reflects the history of severe anoxia and ischemia.

Coronal MR examinations are particularly useful for detecting small subdural hematomas over the vertex or along the falx or tentorium.

The signal intensity of the right-sided subdural hematoma has changed dramatically in the week since the previous scan. This evolution is believed to reflect the oxidation of blood pigments to methemoglobin, with consequent T1-shortening (see Case 561).

The increasing signal intensity commonly seen on T1-weighted images of intracranial hemorrhages during the first week after bleeding contrasts with the CT pattern of immediate maximal attenuation. Subsequent aging of hematomas leads to further changes in signal intensity on MR scans (see Cases 561 to 563).

INTERHEMISPHERIC SUBDURAL HEMATOMAS

Case 346

33-year-old man.

Case 347

68-year-old man, confused after head trauma.

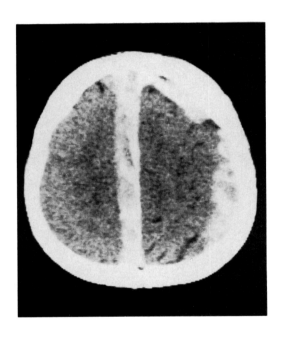

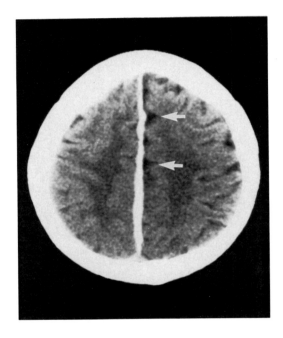

Interhemispheric subdural hematomas may accompany convexity collections or occur as isolated lesions. In this case, a large interhemispheric hematoma is associated with a contralateral convexity collection. Although both hematomas are acute, they are inhomogeneous and contain areas of relative isodensity (see discussion of Case 350).

Interhemispheric clot demonstrates a flat medial margin along the falx and a variably thick lateral extension. (Compare the location of this hematoma to the subdural empyema in Case 294.)

The acute interhemispheric subdural hematoma in this case is much thinner than in Case 346 (but still too thick and irregular to simply represent dural density). The hematoma is unilateral along the right side of the falx. Medial subarachnoid spaces at the vertex are compressed on the right and undisturbed on the left (arrows).

Posterior interhemispheric subdural hematomas (near the tentorium) are commonly seen in children subjected to shaking injuries. Such hematomas are an important hallmark of the "battered child syndrome." They may be very thin, and careful examination of the scan is often necessary for diagnosis. (Confirmation can be provided by MR; see Case 356).

SUBDURAL HEMATOMAS ALONG THE TENTORIUM

Case 348

68-year-old man, confused after head trauma (same patient as Case 347).

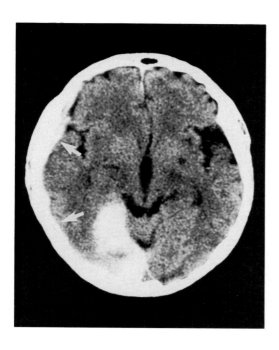

Case 349

74-year-old woman with new brain stem symptoms 1 day after surgery to remove a large acoustic schwannoma.

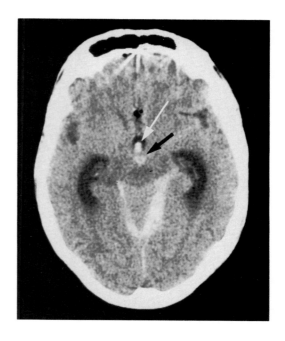

Although most subdural hematomas are found adjacent to the calvarium or falx, they may also occur along the tentorium. In this case a thick layer of subdural hemorrhage lies on the superior tentorial surface (compare to the subdural empyema in Case 296). This suboccipital subdural hematoma was continuous with thinner collections over the convexity (arrows) and in the interhemispheric fissure (shown as Case 347).

As seen here, the medial margins of the tentorium form a "chalice" or "Y" configuration enclosing the midline cerebellar vermis. A coronal scan of this case would resemble the thickened tentorium in Cases 297 to 300.

Here the "chalice" or "Y" configuration of the tentorial margin is defined by a thick layer of subdural hemorrhage along its left medial aspect.

Localization medial to the leaves of the tentorium places a lesion in the posterior fossa (see Case 132). The subdural hematoma in this case is layered along the inferior tentorial surface, like the subdural empyema in Case 295. Mass effect is evident by effacement of the quadrigeminal and superior cerebellar cisterns (compare to Case 348). Enlargement of the temporal horns and third ventricle indicates obstructive hydrocephalus.

A small amount of subarachnoid hemorrhage is present in the interpeduncular cistern (black arrow), and hemorrhage is also seen in the third ventricle (white arrow).

Case 459 presents a follow-up scan of this patient.

Case 350

83-year-old man.

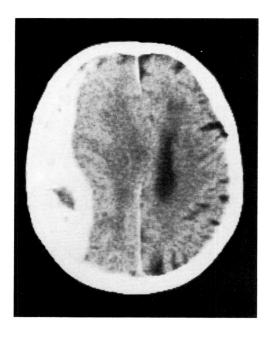

Case 351

74-year-old man presenting with headache.
(postcontrast scan)

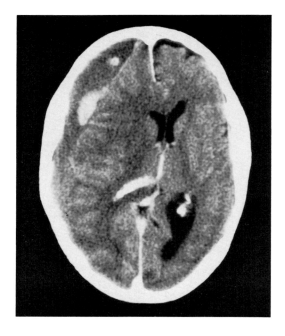

Low-attenuation pockets are occasionally found within acute subdural (and epidural) hematomas, as seen here. These areas may represent older clot surrounded by fresh blood, loculated plasma that has separated from red cells, or encysted spinal fluid from an associated arachnoid tear.

Some subdural hematomas demonstrate layers of varying attenuation. Such compartmentalization occurs when an acute hematoma is superimposed on preceding subacute or chronic collections.

Medial convexity (as seen posteriorly in this case) is an unusual feature of acute subdural hematomas. A component of epidural hemorrhage should be considered with this appearance (compare to Case 371).

Rebleeding is common in subdural hematomas, contributing to their progressive enlargement. Recurrent hemorrhages may cause a layered or laminated appearance. A gradient of attenuation values due to dependent settling of high-density components is seen in other patients (see Case 353). Nodular "islands" of recent clot may also be found within the lower attenuation of older hemorrhage, as in this case.

There is very little contrast enhancement at the margins of this subacute subdural hematoma. In other cases, prominent enhancement of subdural membranes is seen along the compressed cerebral surface. The fragile vascularity of membranes surrounding subdural hematomas is probably a major source of secondary hemorrhages.

This case is a good example of hemisphere compression by an extra-axial mass. Sulci are effaced, the cortical contour is flattened, and white matter within the hemisphere is distorted or "buckled."

ISODENSE SUBDURAL HEMATOMAS

Case 352

80-year-old woman referred for evaluation
of a "CVA."
(noncontrast scan)

Case 353

74-year-old man presenting with headaches.
(postcontrast scan)

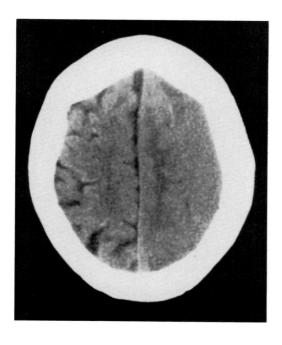

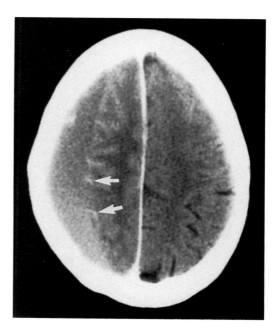

The attenuation values of subdural hematomas decrease over time, passing through an isodense period in a matter of weeks. The hematoma may be poorly defined on noncontrast scans performed at this time.

Here the effacement of sulci and the interhemispheric fissure at the left hemisphere vertex indicates mass effect. Recognition of a large, subacute subdural hematoma as the cause of this compression requires close examination. Although the hematoma is very nearly isodense to brain, the distorted internal architecture of the compressed hemisphere (with displacement of the gray/white junction) can be recognized medially and distinguished from the homogeneous subdural collection laterally. Contrast-enhanced CT (see Cases 353 and 355) or MR scans will confirm the diagnosis in ambiguous cases.

Acute subdural hematomas may be isodense in anemic patients. Alternatively, isodense subacute or chronic subdural hematomas may present acutely in elderly patients when the growth of the collection finally exceeds the "buffering" reserve of pre-existing atrophy and cerebral compliance (see Case 359).

The subacute subdural hematoma in this case is quite comparable in size and attenuation to the isodense collection in Case 352. The diagnosis is more easily made here because of the clues provided by contrast enhancement.

Enhancement of the cerebral cortex helps to define its location and morphology, increasing its attenuation values further above those of the overlying hematoma and underlying white matter. In addition, opacification of large cortical veins (arrows) confirms the displaced location of the cerebral surface (see also Case 355).

The same finding of displaced veins helps to distinguish low-attenuation subdural collections (hygroma or chronic hematoma) from widened subarachnoid spaces (see Cases 362 and 363).

BILATERAL SUBDURAL HEMATOMAS

Case 354

40-year-old man.
(noncontrast scan)

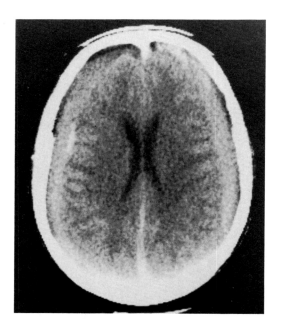

Case 355

65-year-old woman.
(postcontrast scan)

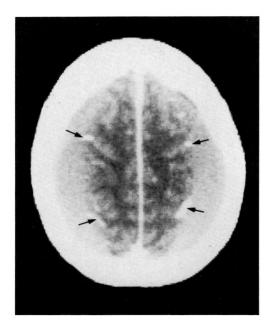

Approximately 25% of subacute and chronic subdural hematomas are bilateral. Bilateral hematomas of equal size may cause symmetrical distortions of anatomy. If the hematomas themselves are nearly isodense, the presence of balancing mass effect may be overlooked.

An important clue to the presence of bilateral mass effect from subdural hematomas is the typical deformity of the lateral ventricles. Compression and medial displacement of the ventricular bodies change their shape to elongated slits. The narrowed and straightened ventricles are abnormally close to the midline and parallel to the sagittal plane.

Such "parasagittal parentheses" are characteristic of bilateral subdural hematomas. They should suggest the diagnosis even when the hematomas are obscured by artifact or isodensity.

Extension of the patient's head will cause normal ventricles to appear elongated on axial scans. However, the ventricular bodies in such images are not straightened and flattened as illustrated in this case.

In this case a noncontrast scan had demonstrated symmetrical absence of vertex sulci. (Head tilt is a common cause of unilateral "absence" of vertex sulci.) A follow-up scan with contrast infusion clearly shows the slightly dense, bilateral subdural hematomas. The interface between the hematomas and compressed cortex is further defined by several large cortical veins *(arrows)*.

MR DETECTION OF SMALL OR SYMMETRICAL SUBDURAL HEMATOMAS

Case 356

17-year-old boy.
(sagittal, noncontrast scan; SE 700/17)

Subacute Subdural Hematoma in the Posterior Fossa.

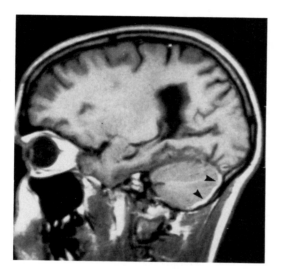

Case 357

5-year-old boy.
(axial, noncontrast scan; SE 3000/25)

Bifrontal Chronic Subdural Hematomas.

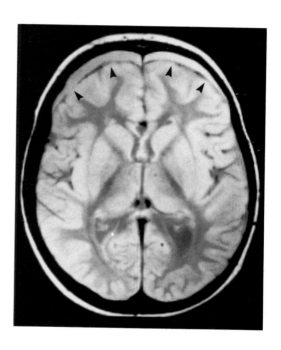

The increased attenuation of small acute or subacute subdural hematomas can be difficult to distinguish from the inner table on CT studies. MR offers two major advantages for detecting such lesions: (1) multiplanar display, and (2) high contrast between subacute hematomas and adjacent bone.

As discussed in Case 345, the T1-shortening typically seen within subacute subdural hematomas makes these lesions conspicuous on T1-weighted images. Here a sagittal scan clearly defines a very thin hematoma along the posterior wall of the posterior fossa (arrowheads). The demonstration of equally thin subdural hemorrhages along the posterior falx or tentorium can be an important clue to the diagnosis of child abuse (see discussion of Case 347).

Thin, low-attenuation subdural collections may resemble subarachnoid spaces on CT scans. MR examinations can make this distinction by demonstrating altered signal intensity in the questioned region.

In this case a CT study had demonstrated symmetrically prominent extracerebral spaces anterior to the frontal lobes. The MR scan shows that the CT appearance was due to bilateral small, chronic subdural hematomas, with higher signal intensity than CSF in the underlying subarachnoid space or ventricular system.

Case 358

79-year-old man with a history of multiple falls.
(postcontrast scan)

Case 359

83-year-old man, believed to have suffered a
"stroke" at a nursing home.
(noncontrast scan)

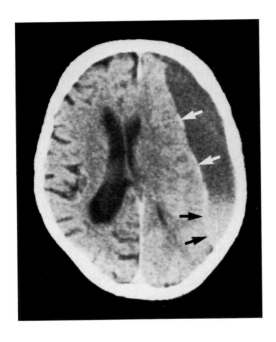

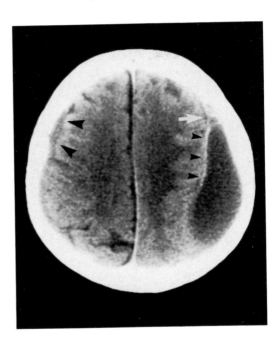

The density and morphology of subdural hematomas are time dependent. Attenuation values decrease as the hematoma ages, so that chronic collections are well defined as low-density regions. The initially thin and crescentic shape of a subdural hematoma usually widens over time, with the medial margin becoming straight or even convex (see Case 359).

As mentioned in Case 351, the mechanism of enlargement often includes recurrent hemorrhage. Reflecting this process (and the liquefaction that usually occurs by 2 to 3 weeks of age), chronic subdural hematomas may contain high-attenuation sediment *(black arrows)*. If the sedimenting component is isodense, the size of the hematoma may be underestimated as representing only the low-attenuation region.

A well-organized subdural membrane usually develops by 3 to 4 weeks. The membrane typically demonstrates linear enhancement adjacent to the cortical surface *(white arrows)*. Enhancement of lateral subdural membranes adjacent to the inner table is obscured by bone density on CT scans but can be demonstrated on MR examinations. Loculation of enhancing membranes may present a confusing appearance (see Case 397). Prominent calcification of old subdural membranes can be seen in children and adults.

Chronic subdural hematomas may become very large as they gradually displace spinal fluid from the subarachnoid spaces of an atrophic hemisphere. As the collection widens, the medial margin may become convex.

Symptoms can develop acutely when the expanding mass reaches a critical size. For this reason, chronic subdural hematomas are occasionally discovered in elderly patients being evaluated for "strokes." (Compare with the presentation in Cases 10 and 72.)

Hemiparesis may be contralateral or ipsilateral to the hematoma. The latter occurrence reflects brain stem displacement causing pressure on the contralateral cerebral peduncle.

The medial subdural membrane is visible as a thin layer of high attenuation on this noncontrast scan *(small black arrowheads)*, likely reflecting vascularity and hemorrhage. Loculation of a small portion of the subdural hematoma is seen anteriorly *(white arrow;* compare to Case 397).

A small, chronic subdural hematoma is present over the right hemisphere convexity *(large black arrowheads)*. Attenuation values within this collection are slightly but definitely higher than CSF in the interhemispheric fissure. MR may be useful in distinguishing true CSF collections (e.g., widened subarachnoid spaces or subdural hygromas) from old subdural hematomas with low attenuation values (see Case 357).

Case 360

69-year-old woman.
(coronal, noncontrast scan; SE 700/16)

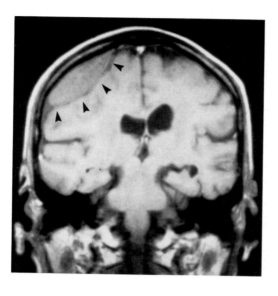

Case 361

30-year-old woman (same patient as Case 345).
(axial, noncontrast scan; SE 3000/80)

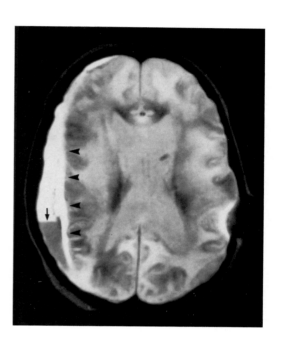

The chronic subdural hematoma over the superior right hemisphere in this case *(arrowheads)* demonstrates a biconvex morphology similar to Case 359. Mass effect is indicated by depression of the underlying cortex and displacement of the right lateral ventricle.

The signal intensity of this chronic hematoma has returned to a level intermediate between the acute and subacute stages illustrated in Case 345. Chronic subdural hematomas are often relatively isointense to cortex on T1-weighted scans (see Case 365 for another example). However, the interface between the extra-axial collection and underlying brain is usually clearly defined by a combination of compressed subarachnoid space, displaced cortical veins, and/or subdural membranes (compare to the margination of meningiomas on T1-weighted scans, as in Case 31).

The persistence of T1-shortening within a chronic subdural hematoma is evidence for rebleeding.

Two layers of subdural hemorrhage are seen over the right hemisphere in this case. The thinner, medial component *(arrowheads)* demonstrates uniformly high signal intensity, as is commonly seen in chronic subdural hematomas on T2-weighted scans.

The larger lateral collection contains a sedimentation level with a dependent zone of T2-shortening. This combination of long and short T2 components suggests a subacute or chronic collection with sedimentation of cellular material. (Compare to the CT appearance of Case 358 as well as to the MR scan of a hemorrhagic pituitary adenoma in Case 179.)

The cerebral hemispheres in this case are diffusely abnormal, with edema throughout the white matter reflecting the history of anoxia (see Cases 464 to 467).

DIFFERENTIAL DIAGNOSIS:
WIDE EXTRACEREBRAL FLUID SPACES IN AN ELDERLY PATIENT

Case 362

77-year-old man with a history of recent head trauma.

Case 363

70-year-old man.

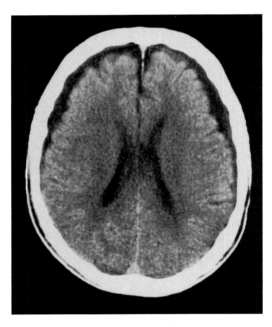

Bifrontal Subdural Hygromas.

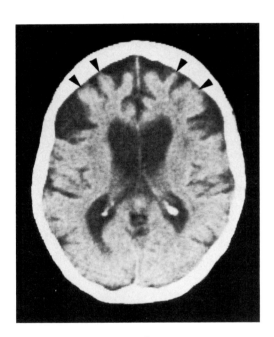

Atrophy.

Some patients develop acute low-density subdural collections following head trauma. These accumulations have been termed "subdural hygromas" because they usually contain clear spinal fluid. The fluid apparently gains access to the subdural space through an arachnoid tear. Subdural hygromas are most often seen in elderly persons and young children. Most of these collections remain small and resolve spontaneously.

Low-attenuation subdural collections (hygromas or chronic hematomas) are sometimes confused with widened subarachnoid spaces due to cerebral atrophy. These two processes are usually distinguishable on the basis of cortical contour and gyral position.

The margin of compressed cortex beneath a subdural collection is abnormally smooth, while the outline of atrophic cortex is irregular due to widened sulci. The tips of cortical gyri seldom retract significantly from the inner table even in the presence of marked atrophy (*arrows,* Case 363). In contrast, the gyral fronds are unequivocally displaced from the calvarium by subdural collections. Similarly, displacement of cortical veins from the inner table indicates subdural accumulation of fluid.

The distinction between chronic subdural hematoma and subdural hygroma may be difficult on a single scan. In Case 362, the low-density collections had been observed to triple in size over a 1-week period, implying predominant hygroma fluid. MR scans may be used to demonstrate or exclude the presence of blood products within subdural collections (see Cases 364 and 365).

Case 364

5-year-old boy.
(sagittal, noncontrast scan; SE 900/17)

Subdural Hygroma.

Case 365

79-year-old man.
(sagittal, noncontrast scan; SE 700/17)

Chronic Subdural Hematoma.

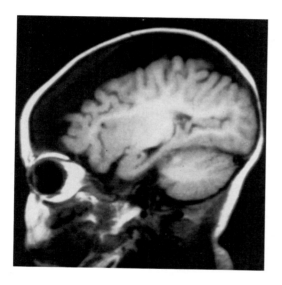

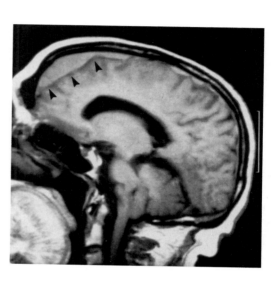

The large subdural collection in this case contains signal intensity that is very close to that of spinal fluid (compare to the temporal horn or vitreous humor of the globe; contrast to the collections in Cases 360 and 365). This appearance identifies the lesion as a subdural hygroma rather than a chronic subdural hematoma.

Some subdural hygromas are found to contain traces of hemorrhage or increased levels of protein at surgery. Such collections demonstrate signal intensities that are slightly higher than CSF on all pulse sequences (most prominent on "balanced" images with long TR and short TE). Even these "complicated" hygromas are rarely as different from CSF signal intensity as the usual chronic subdural hematomas.

The signal intensity of the subdural collection in this case is clearly different from that of ventricular CSF, contrasting with Case 364. The homogeneous isointensity with brain on T1-weighted images is typical for chronic subdural hematomas (see Case 360). The contrast between the signal intensity of the subdural collection and that of normal CSF would be much less on T2-weighted images, where both would appear "bright."

EPIDURAL HEMATOMAS

Case 366

28-year-old man found unresponsive.

Case 367

43-year-old man with the onset of intense headache, nausea, and vomiting while being treated for a scalp laceration following a bicycle accident.

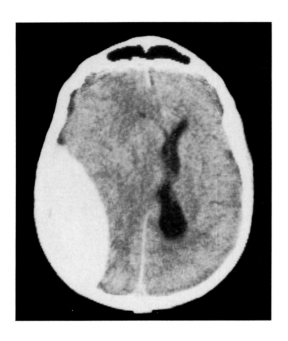

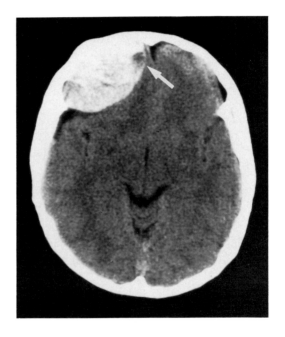

The dura functions as periosteum for the inner table and is tightly adherent to the skull. For this reason, hemorrhage accumulating between the calvarium and the dura remains relatively confined. An epidural hematoma acquires a thick "waist" with a medially convex margin before sufficient pressure has developed to strip the dura for further expansion. This biconvex or lentiform shape contrasts with the thin crescent of acute subdural hematomas (see Case 343).

Supratentorial epidural hematomas may enlarge rapidly and are considered a surgical emergency. Most are due to lacerations of branches from the middle meningeal artery at the point of skull fracture, as in this case.

This large epidural hematoma has stripped the frontal dura as far posteriorly as the pterion. Within the dense hematoma is a zone of lower attenuation (arrow), which indicates continued active bleeding. This "swirl sign" of "hyperacute" epidural hemorrhage probably represents unclotted blood.

A "lucid interval" of several hours between trauma and the rapid onset of symptoms is a characteristic clinical feature of expanding epidural hematomas.

DIFFERENTIAL DIAGNOSIS:
DENSE EPIDURAL LESIONS

Case 368

12-year-old girl with an occipital skull fracture
after being struck by a car.
(noncontrast scan)

Case 369

76-year-old woman.
(postcontrast scan)

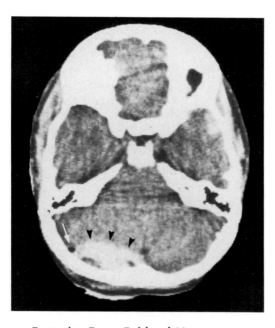

Posterior Fossa Epidural Hematoma.

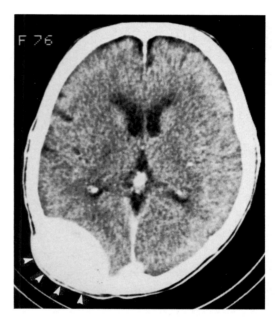

Multiple Myeloma.

Posterior fossa epidural hematomas are usually caused by venous bleeding from torn dural sinuses. They present less acutely and may have less characteristic morphology than supratentorial epidural hemorrhages. Regardless of shape, an extracerebral hematoma is established as epidural if it crosses the plane of the tentorium (or falx; compare to Case 301).

In Case 368 the posterior fossa appears "tight," with poor visualization of the fourth ventricle. The biconvex hematoma continued superiorly across the plane of the tentorium. Other findings include an air bubble *(white arrow)* of pneumocephalus adjacent to the hematoma and contusion of the contralateral temporal lobe.

The familiar biconvex configuration of epidural hematomas may also be seen with epidural masses. Epidural tumors usually represent extension of calvarial metastases, as in Case 369. An identical appearance may be seen in children with metastatic neuroblastoma (and rarely, leukemia). Occasionally primary bone tumors (e.g., calvarial epidermoid, eosinophilic granuloma) expand to involve the epidural space (see Cases 156 and 812).

CT offers an excellent cross-sectional display of skull lesions. The extent of table involvement is well demonstrated, along with any adjacent soft-tissue masses and other diagnostic features (e.g., calcification or "button sequestra").

Clues to the correct diagnosis in Case 369 include contrast enhancement, destruction of the calvarium (which would be more apparent at wider window settings), and the extracranial extent of the mass *(arrowheads)*.

ATYPICAL EPIDURAL HEMATOMAS

Case 370

36-year-old achondroplastic dwarf noted to be somnolent after a beating.

Case 371

27-year-old man, 1 day after head trauma and negative admission CT scan.

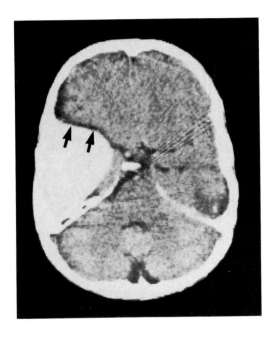

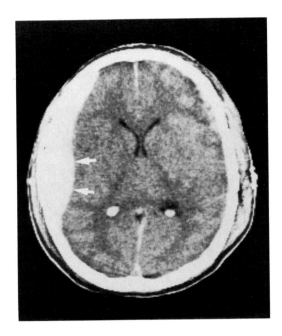

The dura in achondroplasia is abnormally adherent to the skull. As a result, the very thick morphology of this epidural hematoma represents an exaggeration of the normal restraining mechanism discussed in Case 366.

The anterior margin of this hematoma (arrows) is shaped like the sphenoid wing, suggesting confinement by dura tethered along the sphenoid ridge. These findings were confirmed at surgery. (The patient recovered completely.)

Delayed post-traumatic epidural hematomas are much less common than delayed intracerebral hemorrhages (see Case 380).

A second unusual feature of this case is the relatively thin and elongated shape of the hemorrhage. The configuration resembles an acute subdural hematoma. The biconvex posterior component (arrows) suggests the correct diagnosis, but subdural hematomas may have a similar morphology (see Case 350).

ISODENSE COMPONENTS IN EPIDURAL HEMATOMAS

Case 372

26-year-old man.

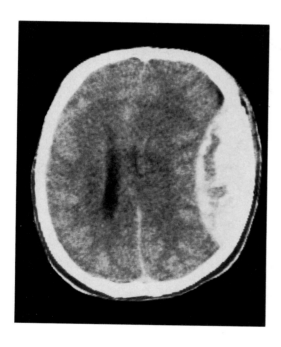

Case 373

29-year-old man, 10 days after ventriculostomy and craniotomy for a colloid cyst.

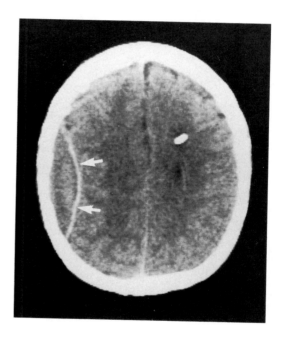

Occasional epidural hematomas contain isodense regions, as seen here. Possible explanations are those discussed in Case 350. Continued active bleeding may also cause low-attenuation zones within epidural hemorrhages (see Case 367). The overall appearance of the lesion remains diagnostic.

Few patients tolerate epidural hematomas long enough to allow the development of subacute attenuation changes. This epidural collection had been denser initially, appearing to contain a mixture of blood and spinal fluid. The dense line along the medial margin of the hematoma represents the displaced dura. (Compare with the membranes of chronic subdural hematomas as seen in Cases 358 and 359.)

CEREBRAL CONTUSION

Case 374

61-year-old man who fell, striking the back of his head.

Case 375

79-year-old man who fell backward and sustained an occipital skull fracture.

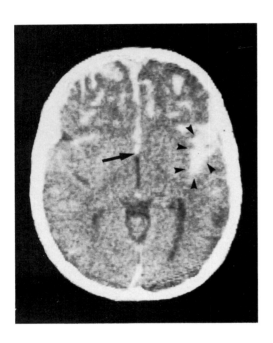

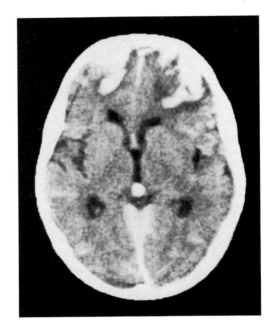

Post-traumatic intracerebral hematomas vary widely in size and number. In some cases, a region of injured brain is filled with many small hemorrhages, as seen here in the frontal lobes. This contusion pattern is soon accompanied by adjacent edema and corresponds to the surgical findings of "pulped brain."

Subarachnoid blood has accumulated in the anterior interhemispheric fissure, outlining its interface with the third ventricle at the lamina terminalis (large arrow). Sufficient subarachnoid blood to fill the left sylvian cistern (small arrowheads) is unusual following trauma. Primary subarachnoid hemorrhage might be considered if the pattern of frontal contusion were less characteristic.

Cerebral injury may be located directly across from the site of head trauma. These "contrecoup" contusions are probably caused when the brain recoils within the calvarium, moving away from the impact region and striking the opposite side of the skull.

The pattern of bifrontal hematomas in patients with occipital skull fractures (as in this case) is a common illustration of this phenomenon. Another common site of cerebral contusion is the anterior temporal lobe, which is easily bruised against the bony margins of the middle cranial fossa.

Case 375 also demonstrates interhemispheric subdural hematomas and scattered subarachnoid blood. A simple fall from the standing position can cause extensive intracranial hemorrhage in elderly patients, as seen here.

CHARACTERISTIC LOCATIONS FOR POST-TRAUMATIC HEMORRHAGES

Case 376

29-year-old man.

Case 377

34-year-old man admitted after 3 days in a detoxification center when his unintelligible speech failed to improve.

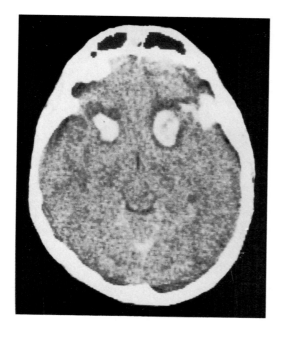

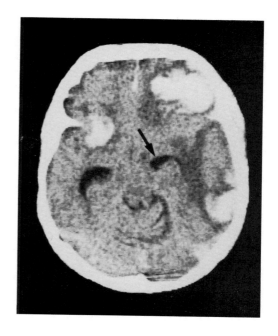

An unusual but characteristic location for post-traumatic intracerebral hemorrhage is the inferior frontotemporal region. Contusion of the brain in this area may occur against the underlying sphenoid ridge, with hemorrhages sometimes resembling imprints of the anterior clinoid processes (as in this case).

Such characteristic hematomas may establish the cause of intracerebral hemorrhage in an otherwise ambiguous context.

Clues to the traumatic origin of intracerebral hemorrhages include multiplicity and characteristic location. This case demonstrates three common sites of cerebral injury: the inferior frontal lobe (see also Cases 374 and 375), the frontotemporal surface adjacent to the sphenoid wing (as in Case 376), and the inferior temporal lobe just above the petrous ridge. In each of these locations cerebral parenchyma is easily bruised against neighboring bone.

Post-traumatic hemorrhages occurring in atypical locations must be carefully evaluated. Such hematomas may represent an initial cerebral event leading to trauma, or post-traumatic hemorrhage into a pre-existing structural lesion (see Case 95).

Marked edema may exacerbate the mass effect of post-traumatic hemorrhage. Here, the left temporal horn *(arrow)* is displaced medially, with uncal herniation obliterating the suprasellar cistern and compressing the brain stem.

LOCALIZED CEREBRAL INJURY

Case 378

78-year-old woman presenting with confusion.

Case 379

59-year-old man with a depressed fracture of the superior left frontal bone.

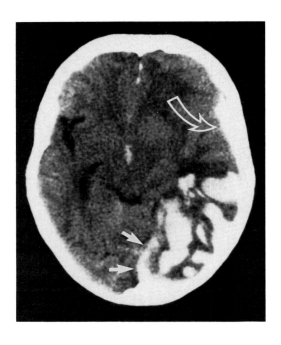

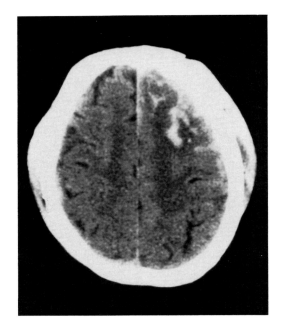

Occasionally cerebral contusion is concentrated in one area. This appearance may represent either "contrecoup" injury from an oblique force or direct trauma to the site underlying a blow (as in Case 379).

In this case the left posterior temporal and occipital lobes demonstrate severe contusion. Multiple large, coalescing hematomas are surrounded by edema. Overlying acute subdural hematomas are seen along the falx and tentorium *(small arrows)* and the convexity *(large arrow)*. A small amount of hemorrhage is also present within the third ventricle.

Here the left frontal lobe has been directly injured in association with a depressed skull fracture. Displacement of fractured bone edges may cause focal laceration of the underlying cortex in addition to generalized contusion.

Much of the hemorrhage on this scan seems to be subarachnoid, outlining sulci between edematous gyri. Localized subarachnoid hemorrhage and cortical contusion often coexist in regions of superficial injury.

DELAYED POST-TRAUMATIC INTRACEREBRAL HEMORRHAGE

Case 380A

2-year-old girl struck by a car (scan on day 1).

Case 380B

Same patient (scan on day 2).

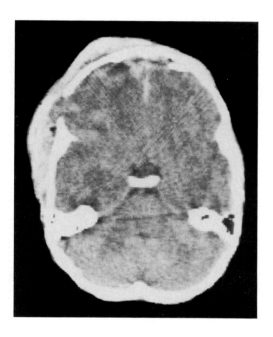

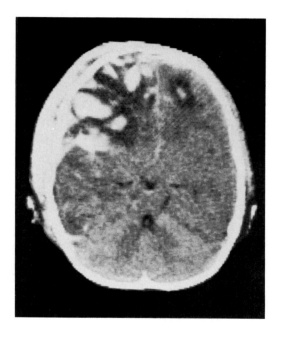

CT scans often demonstrate the development or marked enlargement of post-traumatic intracerebral hemorrhages occurring hours or days after injury. Delayed post-traumatic extracerebral hematomas have also been noted (see Case 371).

This phenomenon should be suspected in any trauma patient whose condition deteriorates or fails to improve as expected. The appearance of widespread contusion, as seen in the right frontal lobe in this case, is often the precursor of significant delayed hemorrhage.

Within 20 hours, the contused right frontal lobe has developed multinodular hematomas and marked edema. The pattern of injury now resembles Case 378. A small hematoma is seen on the contralateral side.

In some cases, the development of delayed post-traumatic intracerebral hemorrhages may be facilitated by evacuation of tamponading subdural or epidural hematomas. In other instances (including this case), delayed hemorrhage occurs without surgical intervention.

DIFFERENTIAL DIAGNOSIS:
MULTIPLE, SUPERFICIAL HEMORRHAGIC LESIONS

Case 381

71-year-old man following head trauma and evacuation of acute subdural hematoma. (noncontrast scan)

Case 382

61-year-old woman presenting with nausea and vomiting. (noncontrast scan)

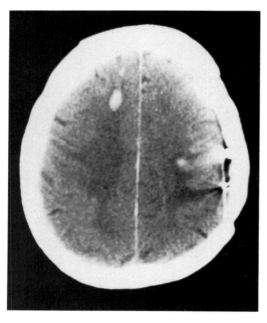

Shearing Injuries (Diffuse Axonal Injury).

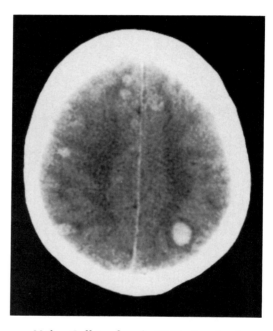

Hairy-Cell Leukemia With Cerebral Chloromas.

Small, post-traumatic cerebral hemorrhages often represent contusion, as illustrated in the previous cases. Another cause of scattered cerebral hemorrhage following head trauma is "diffuse axonal injury." (A third cause, superior sagittal sinus thrombosis, is discussed in Cases 468 to 472.)

Focal post-traumatic disruption of white matter may occur at interfaces between tissues of different rigidity. Rotational/acceleration injuries cause "shear strain" in these locations. "Shearing" injuries commonly occur near the gray/white matter junction and are frequently hemorrhagic. The hemorrhages in Case 381 are within white matter, deep to the cortical mantle.

Case 382 is a reminder that hemorrhagic lesions are not necessarily traumatic, even when multiple. The cerebral nests of leukemic cells in this case are dense on a noncontrast study, probably due to the presence of associated hemorrhage. (The alternative explanation of high attenuation due to cellularity is less likely when density is this high.) Metastatic melanoma would be a more common primary tumor to present in this manner.

The differential diagnosis of multifocal cerebral hemorrhage also includes amyloid angiopathy or other arteritis, moya moya disease (see Case 564), and coagulopathy.

MR DEMONSTRATION OF AXONAL INJURIES

Case 383

10-year-old boy.
(axial, noncontrast scan; SE 3000/80)

Case 384

30-year-old man.
(axial, noncontrast scan; SE 2500/90)

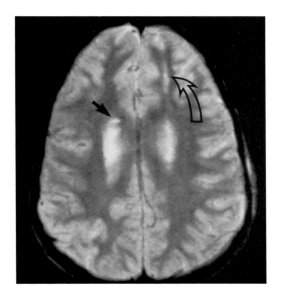

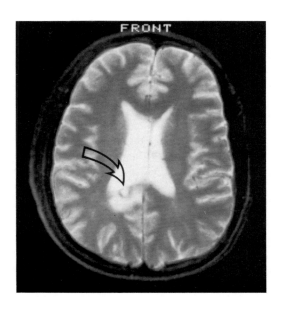

The superiority of MR over CT for disclosing white matter pathology as illustrated in Chapter 7 extends to the demonstration of shearing injuries. These foci of axonal disruption are usually invisible on CT examinations; occasionally associated hemorrhages are apparent as in Case 381. MR scans are much more sensitive to small sites of injury within white matter of the cerebral hemispheres and posterior fossa.

Shearing injuries occur in approximately 40% of patients with severe head trauma, most commonly in the frontal and temporal lobes. They may range from millimeters to centimeters in size. The majority are bland, but up to 25% are hemorrhagic. Focal hemorrhage within these lesions can be demonstrated by MR scans using gradient echo sequences to highlight the magnetic susceptibility effects of blood products.

In this case a parasagittal band of signal abnormality reflects injury within white matter of the left frontal lobe (open arrow; compare to the location of right frontal hemorrhage in Case 381). A smaller focus of abnormal signal in the right minor forceps (solid arrow) represents a second site of axonal injury.

The corpus callosum is a common site of shearing injury. (Direct callosal contusion may also occur if the commissure is bruised against the falx.) The splenium is most frequently involved, as seen in this case (arrow). A small amount of hemorrhage is present at the margins of the lesion, seen as a low-intensity zone of shortened T2.

Callosal lesions correlate strongly with the presence of diffuse axonal injury and primary brain stem injury (see also Case 383). Injuries to the corpus callosum are often associated with intraventricular hemorrhage, which can be a CT clue to the diagnosis.

Although MR is more sensitive than CT for demonstrating hemorrhagic or nonhemorrhagic shearing injuries, microscopically documented axonal damage is often undetected by either modality.

235

POST-TRAUMATIC CEREBRAL SWELLING

Case 385

6-year-old boy (same patient as Case 450).
(noncontrast scan)

Case 386

16-year-old boy presenting with diplopia after
head trauma.
(noncontrast scan)

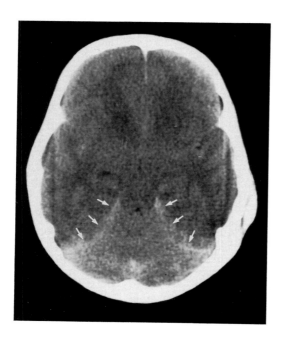

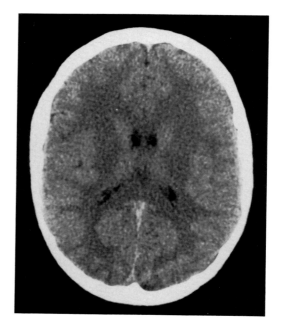

Nonhemorrhagic cerebral swelling is a dangerous consequence of head trauma. Swelling often includes a component of increased cerebral blood volume due to loss of vasomotor tone. Cerebral attenuation values may be little changed or prominently decreased, and involvement may be local or generalized.

In this case the cerebral hemispheres are diffusely swollen, demonstrating vague low attenuation and reduced gray/white matter discrimination. Widespread mass effect has completely effaced the subarachnoid spaces, including cisterns at the tentorial hiatus (compare to a later scan of this patient in Case 450). Elevated intracranial pressure and brain stem compression may be assumed when this appearance is encountered.

The relative density of the falx and tentorium in such cases probably represents a combination of margination by adjacent low-density tissue and vascular stasis due to high intracranial pressure. Here the tentorium appears bowed medially and inferiorly (arrows) by the swollen cerebral hemispheres.

The attenuation values of the cerebral hemispheres are nearly normal in this case. However, symmetrical posttraumatic swelling is suggested by the small size and indistinct margins of the lateral ventricles. This impression was confirmed by return of the ventricles to normal size and definition on follow-up scans.

Post-traumatic cerebral edema may be focal rather than diffuse. Localized areas of edema can act as mass lesions even in the absence of hemorrhage, causing secondary herniations and compression of adjacent parenchyma.

This patient's diplopia was due to a sixth nerve palsy, which is a frequent nonlocalizing sign of increased intracranial pressure.

Compare Cases 385 and 386 to the examples of cerebral swelling from other causes in Cases 252 to 255.

Case 387

20-year-old woman.

Case 388

24-year-old man.

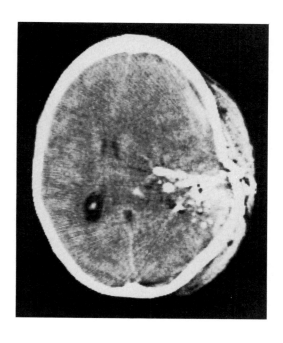

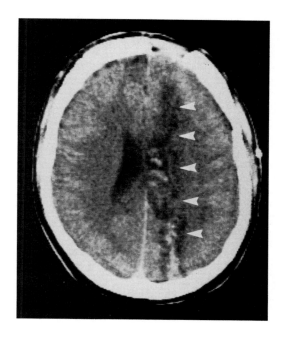

Scans may disclose multiple intracerebral densities in patients with cranial gunshot wounds. These foreign bodies include metal fragments and pieces of imbedded calvarium. Bullet fragments may be relatively inert and are often left in place, while bone fragments are a common source of infection and are usually removed if possible. The distinction between metal and bone may be difficult at normal display settings, but is usually apparent at wide windows.

In this case, a comminuted skull fracture is present. Instead of being depressed (as in Case 389), the fracture region has been elevated by the blast injury and underlying subdural and intracerebral hemorrhage.

A projectile passing through the brain may leave a trail of small hemorrhages or a track of hypodensity. This path indicates the extent and nature of cerebral injury more accurately than the final location of the bullet. In this case, the parasagittal track of the bullet (arrowheads) correlated with an excellent clinical recovery.

237

SKULL FRACTURES

Case 389

28-year-old woman who was severely beaten.

Depressed Skull Fracture.

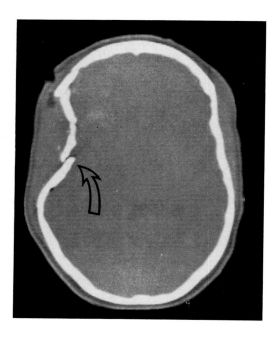

Case 390

22-year-old man injured in an automobile accident.

Basal Skull Fracture.

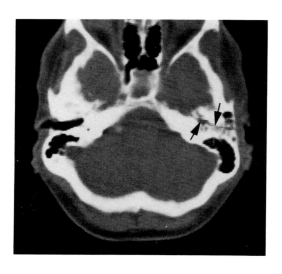

Depressed skull fractures are well evaluated in the axial plane of CT scans. These fractures are usually comminuted and are often compound. Scans demonstrate the degree of depression and localize fragments of bone for surgical debridement.

Basal skull fractures are difficult to define by standard radiographic techniques. The axial display of the skull base on CT scans aids in this evaluation.

Here a longitudinal fracture of the petrous bone is clearly seen *(arrows)*, with opacification of adjacent mastoid air cells. Opacification of the sphenoid sinus suggests blood or spinal fluid within the sinus and is a secondary sign of basal fracture. (However, trauma patients who have been supine and/or intubated for long periods may have pooled secretions in the sphenoid sinus with no adjacent fracture.)

POST-TRAUMATIC CSF RHINORRHEA

Case 391

56-year-old man who suffered head trauma one month earlier, now presenting with meningitis and watery nasal discharge.
(coronal scan, wide window)

Case 392

45-year-old man presenting with a third episode of meningitis within 5 years.
(prone coronal scan with intrathecal contrast, wide window)

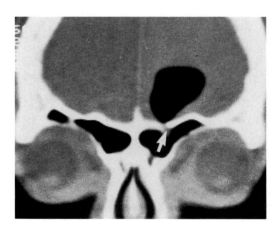

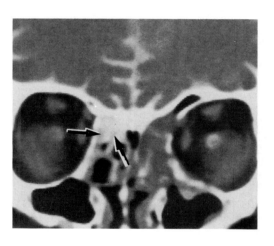

Fractures of the cribriform plate and ethmoid sinus are a common source of posttraumatic meningitis and CSF rhinorrhea. Other causes include frontal sinus fracture, parasellar fractures into the sphenoid sinus, and petrous bone fractures communicating with the middle ear and eustachian tube.

In this case, the coronal scan clearly demonstrates a fracture in the roof of the frontoethmoid sinus *(arrow)*. An unusual pocket of intracranial air ("pneumatocele") arises from this site. Surgery demonstrated communication of the sinus with a cavitated hematoma in the frontal lobe. (No abscess was found.)

The location of a fracture causing recurrent meningitis and CSF rhinorrhea is rarely as apparent as in Case 391. Most patients require special studies to demonstrate the site of a CSF leak.

One useful technique combines CT with the injection of subarachnoid contrast material. Scans are performed in coronal and/or axial planes in an effort to detect the presence of contrast within a sinus, thereby identifying the site of CSF communication.

In this case, a posterior ethmoid air cell is filled with contrast material *(arrows)*, directing the surgeon to this site. A fracture was found in the roof of the sinus, and the dural laceration was repaired.

DIFFERENTIAL DIAGNOSIS:
MULTILOCULAR, SUPERFICIAL ENHANCING MASS

Case 397

93-year-old man.

Case 398

13-year-old girl.

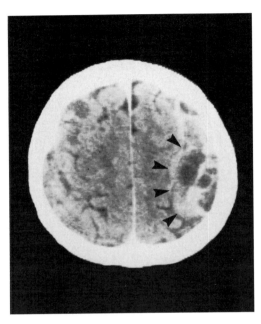

Chronic Subdural Hematoma.

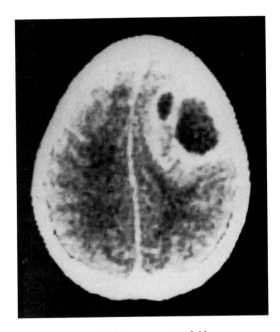

Cystic Glioblastoma Multiforme.

Some chronic subdural hematomas present an unusual appearance due to the combination of loculation and thick, enhancing membranes. The lesion in Case 397 resembles a neoplasm (or a thick-walled abscess). The differential diagnosis would include unusual metastasis or atypical meningioma (see Case 43) in addition to malignant glioma (also compare to Case 574).

Case 398 is unusual because of the patient's age. However, the thick-walled, multicystic morphology strongly suggests the correct diagnosis.

REFERENCES: CT

1. Bergstrom M., Ericson K., Levander B., et al.: Computed tomography of cranial subdural and epidural hematomas: Variation of attenuation related to time and clinic events such as rebleeding. *J. Comput. Assist. Tomogr.* 1:449–455, 1977.
2. Braun J., Borovich B., Guilbura J.N., et al.: Acute subdural hematoma mimicking epidural hematoma on CT. *A.J.N.R.* 8:171–174, 1987.
3. Bruce D.A., Alavi A., Bilaniuk L.T., et al.: Diffuse cerebral swelling following head injuries in children: The syndrome of "malignant brain edema." *J. Neurosurg.* 54:170–178, 1981.
4. Clifton G.L., Grossman R.G., Makela M.E., et al.: Neurological course and correlated computerized tomography findings after severe closed head injury. *J. Neurosurg.* 52:611–624, 1980.
5. Cohen R.A., Kaufman R.A., Myers P.A., Towbin R.B.: Cranial computed tomography in the abused child with head injury. *A.J.N.R.* 6:883–888, 1985.
6. Cornell S.H., Chiu L.C., Christie J.H.: Diagnosis of extracerebral fluid collections by computed tomography. *A.J.R.* 131:107–110, 1978.
7. Diaz F.G., Yock D.H. Jr., Larson D., et al.: Early diagnosis of delayed post-traumatic intracerebral hematomas. *J. Neurosurg.* 50:217–223, 1979.
8. Forbes G.S., Sheedy P.F., Piepgras D.G., et al.: Computed tomography in the evaluation of subdural hematomas. *Radiology* 126:143–148, 1978.
9. Ishiwata Y., Fujitsu K., Sekino T., et al.: Subdural tension pneumocephalus following surgery for chronic subdural hematoma. *J. Neurosurg.* 68:58–61, 1988.
10. Johnson D.W., Hasso A.N., Stewart C.E., et al.: Temporal bone trauma: high resolution computed tomographic evaluation. *Radiology* 151:411–415, 1984.
11. Kim K.S., Hemmati M., Weinberg P.E.: Computed tomography in isodense subdural hematoma. *Radiology* 128:71–74, 1978.
12. Lipper M.H., Kishore P.R.S., Enas G.G., et al.: Computed tomography in the prediction of outcome in head injury. *A.J.N.R.* 6:7–10, 1985.
13. Lipper M.H., Kishore P.R., Girevendulis A.K., et al.: Delayed intracranial hematoma in patients with severe head injury. *Radiology* 133:645–649, 1979.
14. Lobato R.D., Sarabia R., Cordobes F., et al.: Post-traumatic cerebral hemisphere swelling: Analysis of 55 cases studied with computerized tomography. *J. Neurosurg.* 68:417–423, 1988.
15. Manelfe C., Cellerier P., Sobel D., et al.: Cerebrospinal fluid rhinorrhea: Evaluation with metrizamide cisternography. *A.J.N.R.* 3:25–30, 1982.
16. Markwalder T.M.: Chronic subdural hematomas: A review. *J. Neurosurg.* 54:637–645, 1981.
17. Mirvis S.E., Wolf A.L., Numaguchi Y., et al.: Post-traumatic cerebral infarction diagnosed by CT: Prevalance, origin, and outcome. *A.J.N.R.* 11:355–360, 1990.
18. Monajati A., Cotanch W.W.: Subdural tension pneumocephalus following surgery. *J. Comput. Assist. Tomogr.* 6:902–906, 1982.
19. Naidich T.P., Leeds N.E., Kricheff I.I., et al.: The tentorium in axial section. II. Lesion localization. *Radiology* 123:639–648, 1977.
20. Nelson A.T., Kishore P.R., Lee S.H.: Development of delayed epidural hematoma. *A.J.N.R.* 3:583–585, 1982.
21. Pop P.M., Thompson J.R., Zinke D.E., et al.: Tension pneumocephalus. *J. Comput. Assist. Tomogr.* 6:894–901, 1982.
22. Reed D., Robertson W.D., Graeb D.A., et al.: Acute subdural hematomas: Atypical CT findings. *A.J.N.R.* 7:416–422, 1986.
23. Reith K.G., Davis D.O.: Subdural hematomas: An unusual appearance on CT. *J. Comput. Assist. Tomogr.* 3:331–334, 1979.
24. Shalen P.R., Handel S.F.: Diagnostic challenges in closed head trauma. *Radiol. Clin. North Am.* 19:53–58, 1981.
25. Smith W.P., Batnitzky S., Rengachary S.S.: Acute isodense subdural hematomas. *A.J.N.R.* 2:37–40, 1981.
26. Stein S.C., Ross S.E.: The value of computed tomographic scans in patients with low risk head injuries. *Neurosurgery* 26:638–640, 1990.
27. Stone J.L., Schaffer L., Ramsey R.G.: Epidural hematomas of the posterior fossa. *Surg. Neurol.* 11:419–424, 1979.
28. Toutant S.M., Klauber M.R., Marshall L.F., et al.: Absent or compressed basal cisterns on first CT scan: Ominous predictors of outcome in severe head injury. *J. Neurosurg.* 61:691–694, 1984.
29. Tsai F.Y., Huprich J.E., Segall H.D., et al.: The contrast-enhanced CT scan in the diagnosis of isodense subdural hematoma. *J. Neurosurg.* 50:64–69, 1979.
30. Tsai F.Y., Teal J.S., Itabashi H.H., et al.: Computed tomography of posterior fossa trauma. *J. Comput. Assist. Tomogr.* 4:291–305, 1980.
31. Tsai F.Y., Teal J.S., Quinn M.F., et al.: CT of brain stem injury. *A.J.N.R.* 1:23–29, 1980.
32. Yeakley J.W., Mayer J.S., Patchell L.L., et al.: The pseudodelta sign in acute head trauma. *J. Neurosurg.* 69:867–868, 1988.
33. Zimmerman R.A., Bilaniuk L.T.: Computed tomographic staging of traumatic epidural bleeding. *Radiology* 144:809–812, 1982.
34. Zimmerman R.A., Bilaniuk L.T., Bruce D., et al.: Computed tomography of craniocerebral injury in the abused child. *Radiology* 130:687–690, 1979.
35. Zimmerman R.A., Bilaniuk L.T., Bruce D., et al.: Computed tomography of pediatric head trauma: Acute general cerebral swelling. *Radiology* 126:403–408, 1978.
36. Zimmerman R.A., Bilaniuk L.T., Gennarelli T., et al.: Cranial computed tomography in diagnosis and management of acute head trauma. *A.J.R.* 131:27–34, 1978.
37. Zimmerman R.D., Danziger A.: Extracerebral trauma. *Radiol. Clin. North Am.* 20:105–121, 1982.
38. Zimmerman R.D., Russell E.J., Yurberg E., et al.: Falx and interhemispheric fissure on axial CT. II. Recognition and differentiation of interhemispheric subarachnoid and subdural hemorrhage. *A.J.N.R.* 3:635–642, 1981.

REFERENCES: MR

1. Ebisu T., Naruse S., Horikawa Y., et al.: Nonacute subdural hematoma: Fundamental interpretation of MR images based on biochemical and in vitro MR analysis. *Radiology* 171:449–454, 1989.
2. Fobben E.S., Grossman R.I., Atlas S.W., et al.: MR characteristics of subdural hematomas and hygromas at 1.5T. *A.J.N.R.* 10:687–694, 1989.
3. Gentry L.R., Godersky J.C., Thompson B.H.: Traumatic brain stem injury: MR imaging. *Radiology* 171:177–188, 1989.
4. Gentry L.R., Godersky J.C., Thompson B.: MR imaging of head trauma: review of the distribution and radiopathologic features of traumatic lesions. *A.J.N.R.* 9:101–110, 1988.
5. Gentry L.R., Godersky J.C., Thompson B., Dunn V.D.: Prospective comparative study of intermediate-field MR and CT in the evaluation of closed head trauma. *A.J.N.R.* 9:91–100, 1988.
6. Gentry L.R., Thompson B., Godersky J.C.: Trauma to the corpus callosum: MR features. *A.J.N.R.* 9:1129–1138, 1988.
7. Hesselink J.R., Dowd C.F., Healy M.E., et al.: MR imaging of brain contusion: A comparative study with CT. *A.J.N.R.* 9:269–278, 1988.
8. Hosoda K., Tamaki N., Masumura M., et al.: Magnetic resonance images of chronic subdural hematomas. *J. Neurosurg.* 67:677–683, 1987.
9. Kelly A.B., Zimmerman R.D., Snow R.B., et al.: Head trauma: Comparison of MR and CT—Experience in 100 patients. *A.J.N.R.* 9:699–708, 1988.
10. Levin H.S., Amparo E.G., Eisenberg H.M., et al.: Magnetic resonance imaging after closed head injury in children. *Neurosurgery* 24:223–227, 1989.
11. Levin H.S., Amparo E.G., Eisenberg H.M., et al.: Magnetic resonance imaging and computerized tomography in relation to the neurobehavioral sequelae of mild and moderate head injuries. *J. Neurosurg.* 66:706–713, 1987.
12. Moon K.L. Jr., Brant-Zawadzki M., Pitts L.H., Mills C.M.: Nuclear magnetic resonance imaging of CT-isodense subdural hematomas. *A.J.N.R.* 5:319–322, 1984.
13. Sato Y., Yuh W.T., Smith W.L., et al.: Head injury in child abuse: Evaluation with MR imaging. *Radiology* 173:653–658, 1989.
14. Snow R.B., Zimmerman R.D., Gandy S.E., Deck M.D.F.: Comparison of magnetic resonance imaging and computed tomography in the evaluation of head injury. *Neurosurgery* 18:45–52, 1986.
15. Wilberger, J.E. Jr., Deeb Z., Rothfus W.: Magnetic resonance imaging in cases of severe head injury. *Neurosurgery* 20:571–576, 1987.
16. Zimmerman R.A., Bilaniuk L.T., Hackney D.B., et al.: Head injury: Early results of comparing CT and high-field MR. *A.J.N.R.* 7:757–764, 1986.

CHAPTER 9

Infarction and Anoxia

EVOLUTION OF CT FINDINGS IN CEREBRAL INFARCTION

Case 399A

65-year-old man, 6 hours after the onset of aphasia.

Case 399B

Same patient, two days later.

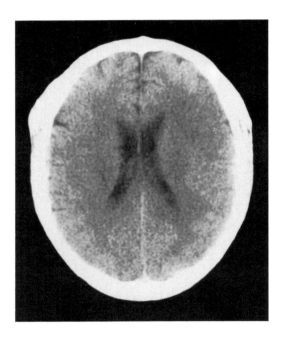

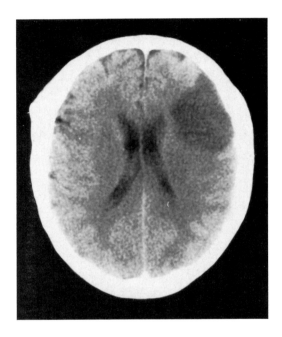

The CT appearance of cerebral infarction is highly time dependent. The rate and nature of these changes are characteristic and may be used to identify an initially ambiguous lesion.

Scans are usually normal within the first few hours of infarction. The earliest CT findings include mildly decreased attenuation values, loss of gray/white matter discrimination, and subtle mass effect.

In patients who have suffered occlusion of the middle cerebral artery (or internal carotid artery), these early changes may be first apparent at the level of the basal ganglia. Loss of the normal gray/white matter interfaces outlining the lenticular nucleus and the insula is an early sign of major hemispheric infarction.

In this case, the definition of cortical gray matter has become indistinct in the left frontal lobe, and early mass effect blurs sulcal margins (compare with the contralateral side). A wedge of low attenuation is faintly seen extending to the cerebral surface.

Low attenuation within an area of infarction is well defined by the second or third day. As in this case, the low density is usually homogeneous and often approximately wedge shaped, with widening margins reaching a broad base against the inner table. No cortical sparing is seen, in contrast to the low-density pattern of edema.

Mass effect develops concurrently, usually reaching a maximum by the second to fourth day (see Cases 404 and 405). Here the midline shift is minimal, but mass effect is indicated by effacement of ipsilateral sulci.

The region involved by this infarction is perfused by the anterior division of the middle cerebral artery.

MR CHARACTERIZATION OF EARLY INFARCTS

Case 400

43-year-old man, 36 hours after the onset of
hemiparesis.
(axial, noncontrast scan; SE 3000/75)

Case 401

28-year-old woman, 1 day after a
cerebrovascular accident.
(axial, noncontrast scan; SE 2500/30)

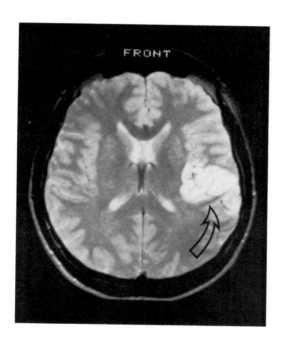

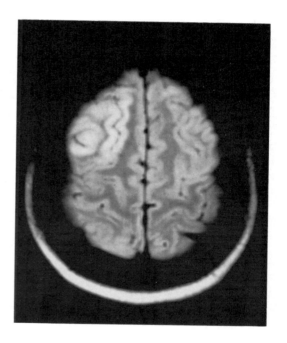

High signal intensity is seen throughout swollen cortex in the posterior left sylvian area on this T2-weighted image. The "gyriform" morphology characterizes the lesion as a regional cortical insult, most frequently caused by infarction. (Cortical reaction to overlying meningeal disease should be considered in the differential diagnosis.)

The MR demonstration of gyral edema may clarify the etiology of ambiguous zones of low attenuation on CT studies (as in Cases 399 and 405). A gyriform pattern of signal abnormality is rarely noted in cerebral gliomas.

T1-weighted MR scans of early cerebral infarctions demonstrate comparable thickening of the cortical ribbon. Gray/white matter margins are indistinct, and reduced signal intensity is seen due to prolongation of T1. Petechial hemorrhage may be apparent (see Cases 408 and 409).

MR clearly demonstrates cortical edema along sulcal margins in this case. "Gyriform" swelling of gray matter with relative sparing of subcortical white matter is a characteristic feature of recent infarction, better defined on MR examinations than CT studies.

Compare this appearance to the reverse pattern of subcortical edema with cortical sparing in Cases 321 and 322.

DIFFERENTIAL DIAGNOSIS:
VAGUE, LOW ATTENUATION IN THE SYLVIAN REGION

Case 402

82-year-old man.

Case 403

68-year-old man.

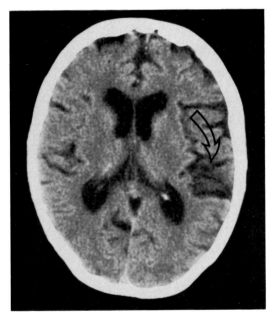

Normal (Partial Volume of Sylvian Cistern).

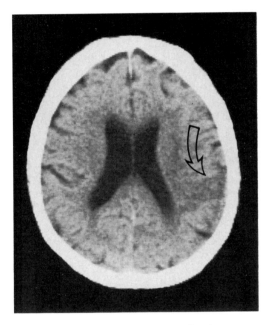

Early Infarction (Middle Cerebral Artery Distribution).

Large subarachnoid spaces are commonly found in elderly patients. When the plane of a scan passes parallel to the sulcus or cistern, a vague area of low attenuation is seen.

The posterior portion of the sylvian cistern commonly causes this appearance, as seen in Case 402 (*arrow;* see also Case 336). This poorly defined low-density region may be mistaken for early ischemic change in the middle cerebral artery distribution, as represented by Case 403.

A pseudoinfarction lacks mass effect and is usually seen at only one level. On the other hand, a true infarction involves several sections and is usually associated with loss of gray/white matter discrimination and early cerebral edema.

Other locations at which partial imaging of sulci and cisterns may mimic focal infarction include the circular sulcus/external capsule area, the lateral suprasellar cistern/hypothalamic region, the calcarine sulcus/medial occipital lobe, and the horizontal fissure/posterior cerebellar hemisphere.

The poorly defined infarction in Case 403 could also be mistaken for a low-grade glioma (see Case 62).

CEREBRAL INFARCTION: MASS EFFECT

Case 404

72-year-old man found unresponsive 1 day prior to admission.

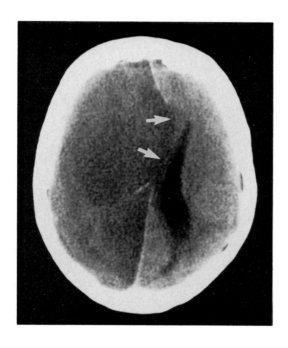

Case 405

53-year-old man, 4 days after a cerebrovascular accident.

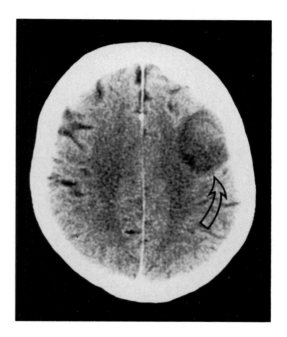

Mass effect develops during the first week of cerebral infarction, most commonly after a few days have elapsed.

This lesion is only a day old, but substantial ischemic edema is already apparent. Subfalcial herniation is present, and the right lateral ventricle is effaced.

The involved region includes the territories of the anterior, middle, and posterior cerebral arteries. This combination of vascular distributions suggests occlusion of the internal carotid artery with carotid origin of the posterior cerebral artery.

Small infarcts can also develop prominent mass effect, sometimes causing diagnostic confusion. Here a subacute left frontal lesion demonstrates rounded margins with compression of adjacent tissue. If the patient is first scanned at this stage and the clinical context is ambiguous, the possibility of a low-grade glioma such as Case 65 is raised. MR scans can resolve the issue by demonstrating the characteristic gyriform edema (see Cases 400 and 401) or petechial hemorrhage (see Cases 408 and 409) of subacute infarction.

Like Case 399, this infarct falls within the territory of the anterior division of the middle cerebral artery.

CEREBRAL INFARCTION: HETEROGENEOUS ATTENUATION

Case 406

77-year-old man, 8 days after the onset of
aphasia and hemiparesis.
(noncontrast scan)

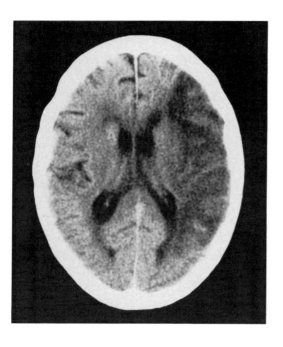

Case 407

72-year-old woman, 11 days after the acute
onset of hemiparesis.
(noncontrast scan)

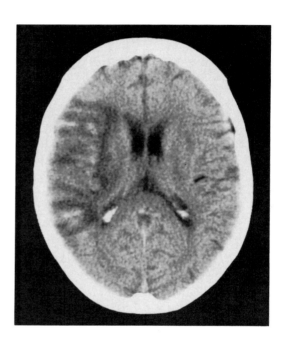

Mass effect begins to decrease by the end of the first week after infarction. In this case ventricular compression and midline shift were substantially reduced from the appearance of earlier scans.

The low attenuation of an infarct becomes less homogeneous in the second week. Islands of isodensity may appear, as seen here. (Compare the heterogeneous appearance of this lesion to the homogeneous low attenuation of the acute infarction in Case 404.) Occasionally, the entire infarct will increase in attenuation, becoming isodense and transiently invisible on a noncontrast scan ("fogging phenomenon").

Contrast scans often show intense enhancement in the isodense regions at this stage of evolution (see Cases 414 to 416). This finding suggests that the precontrast isodensity may at least partially represent the averaging of underlying low attenuation with developing hyperemia and/or blood-brain barrier breakdown.

The mixed-density pattern illustrated at this stage superficially resembles the frond-like interdigitations of cerebral edema and could be mistaken for a neoplasm.

Another cause of heterogeneous attenuation values within subacute cerebral infarcts is hemorrhage. Although frank hematomas can occur (see Case 410 to 412), hemorrhage within recent infarctions is more commonly low grade and dispersed.

This case demonstrates the "soft" and diffuse appearance of such "petechial" hemorrhage. Mildly increased attenuation values are seen in a gyriform distribution throughout the zone of infarction. MR scans have demonstrated that small amounts of hemorrhage are regularly present within the cortical ribbon of infarcted areas (see Cases 408 and 409); only occasionally is the hemorrhage sufficiently prominent to be recognized by CT.

The trapezoidal shape of the lesions in Cases 406 and 407 is typical for occlusions involving the main trunk of the middle cerebral artery. If the occlusion is at or proximal to the origins of the lenticulostriate arteries, the basal ganglia will also be involved (see Case 432). The location of the anterior and posterior limits of a middle cerebral artery infarct is determined by the variable anatomical and physiological extent of collateral flow from the neighboring distributions of the anterior and posterior cerebral arteries.

MR DEMONSTRATION OF HEMORRHAGE IN SUBACUTE INFARCTION

Case 408

69-year-old woman.
(sagittal, noncontrast scan; SE 800/20)

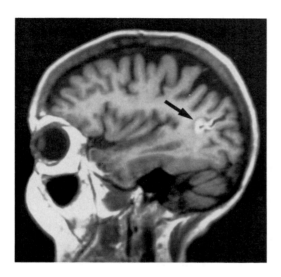

Case 409

53-year-old man.
(coronal, noncontrast scan; SE 600/20)

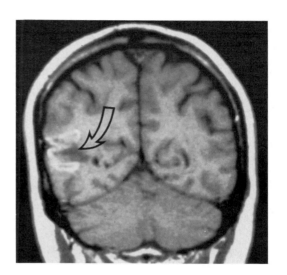

T1-weighted MR scans may demonstrate a ribbon of high signal intensity involving the cortical mantle in regions of recent infarction. This finding localizes and characterizes even small lesions, as in this case *(arrow)*. The T1-shortening is probably due to petechial hemorrhage within the infarcted gray matter, which is much more frequently noted on MR scans than on CT studies.

Gyriform high signal intensity follows the course of the cortical ribbon in this infarction, involving a branch of the posterior division of the middle cerebral artery *(arrow)*. The small amount of petechial hemorrhage causing this T1-shortening is usually below the threshold of CT detection.

A similar appearance can be seen within bland infarctions on MR scans after contrast infusion. The MR pattern of contrast enhancement is often gyriform, comparable to CT (see Cases 414 and 415).

HEMORRHAGE INTO ISCHEMIC INFARCTIONS

Case 410

80-year-old man receiving hemodialysis.

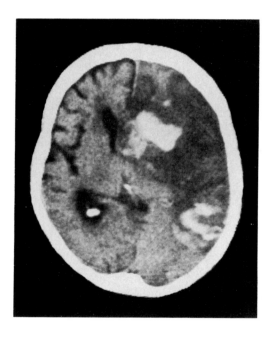

Case 411

22-year-old woman who suffered a stroke shortly after severe head trauma.

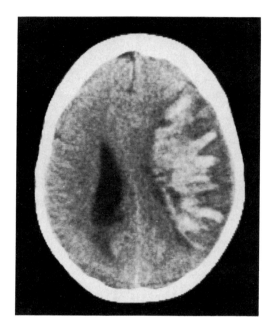

A small number of ischemic infarctions become frankly hemorrhagic, either spontaneously or following anticoagulation therapy.

Here, large areas of hemorrhage have developed at several locations within an infarction of the anterior and middle cerebral artery distributions. The patient had received anticoagulants during dialysis and probably also suffered from uremic platelet dysfunction.

A cerebrovascular accident in a young patient should suggest the possibility of an embolic source (see also Case 465). Leading causes include spontaneous dissection of the carotid or vertebral arteries or post-traumatic lesions of these vessels.

In this case, infarction was due to embolization from a traumatic dissection of the common carotid artery. Originally bland infarction became diffusely hemorrhagic 2 days after the patient began to receive anticoagulant therapy.

Dissolution of a cerebral embolus may predispose to hemorrhagic infarction by allowing reperfusion of damaged vessels.

252

Case 412

81-year-old woman presenting with confusion and hemiparesis.

Case 413

79-year-old woman referred for evaluation of a "CVA."

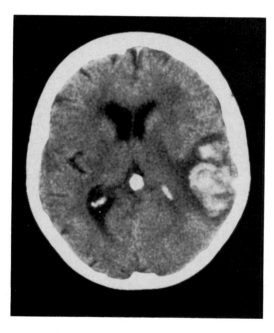

Hemorrhage Into a Middle Cerebral Artery Infarction.

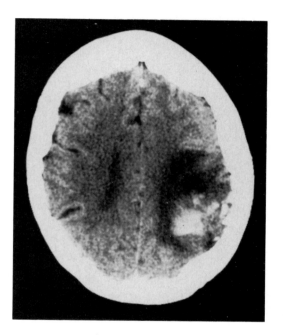

Hemorrhage Into a Low-Grade Astrocytoma.

Hemorrhage within areas of cerebral infarction can mimic other sources of "atypical" hematomas (see Cases 565 to 568).

Conversely, the presence of a low-attenuation zone surrounding an intracerebral hematoma should not be assumed to indicate hemorrhagic infarction. The small calcifications lateral to the hemorrhage in Case 413 imply a pre-existing structural lesion, in this case a glial neoplasm.

Both hemorrhage and calcification could also be seen at the site of an arteriovenous malformation (see Cases 496 to 500). Arteriovenous malformations are rarely associated with edema or ischemia as extensive as the low-attenuation regions seen here.

CONTRAST ENHANCEMENT IN INFARCTION: GENERALIZED

Case 414

72-year-old woman, 11 days after the acute onset of hemiparesis (same patient as Case 407).

Case 415

70-year-old woman, 10 days after infarction.

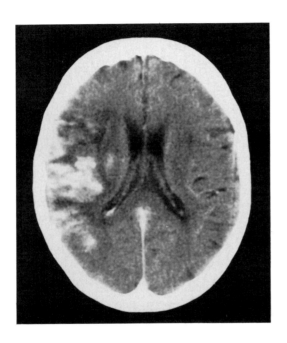

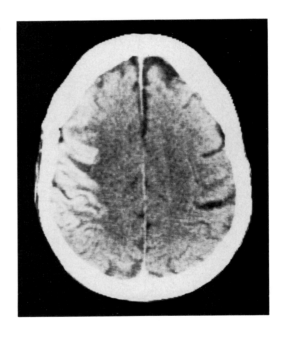

Contrast enhancement may be seen on CT scans of cerebral infarctions from the end of week 1 through week 3 or 4. Reactive "luxury perfusion" (hyperperfusion with loss of autoregulation) and breakdown of the blood-brain barrier both contribute to this phenomenon.

Enhancement is usually confined to gray matter but may demonstrate variable morphology. The most characteristic pattern is band-like, tubular, or gyriform enhancement as in Case 415. More amorphous or "smudgy" patterns can be encountered, as in this case. Solid enhancement sometimes fills the region of infarction (see Case 453), particularly when deep nuclei are involved. Ring-enhancing appearances may also occur (see Case 419).

In most cases, the enhancing lesion retains the peripherally based shape typical of large infarctions (see also Case 455). The significance of CT contrast enhancement as an indicator of adverse prognosis in cerebral infarction is controversial.

Gyriform enhancement within a subacute cerebral infarct is seen here as a thin ribbon following the cortical convolutions.

Contrast enhancement in infarction is most prominent after the period of maximal mass effect, reducing the potential resemblance to neoplasm (but see Cases 418 and 419). In the absence of mass effect, the serpentine enhancement pattern of subacute infarction can mimic a vascular malformation (see Cases 490 and 491).

MR scans may demonstrate contrast enhancement within the first few days of cerebral infarction. The initial pattern of enhancement is often superficial or "pial," suggesting meningeal inflammation or cerebritis. Within days a more characteristic "gyriform" enhancement of gray matter is seen, resembling the CT stereotype.

CONTRAST ENHANCEMENT IN INFARCTION: LOCALIZED

Case 416

66-year-old man with the abrupt onset of multiple neurological deficits 10 days earlier.

Multifocal Infarction at Watershed Sites.

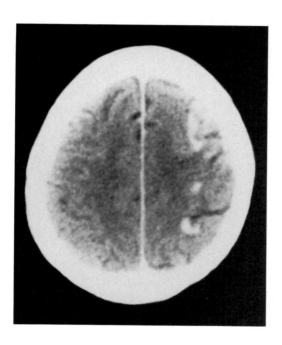

Case 417

35-year-old woman found to have the syndrome of multiple progressive intracranial arterial occlusions ("moya moya").

1-Week-Old Infarct.

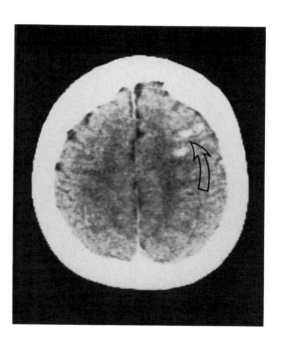

Small areas of infarction often demonstrate focal enhancement, as seen in this case. The appearance is nonspecific and could suggest inflammatory or metastatic disease. Here the clinical context and distribution along a vascular watershed (see Cases 428 and 429) aid in the diagnosis.

Multifocal infarction may be caused by hypoperfusion, multiple emboli, cerebral vasculitis (e.g., systemic lupus erythematosus), meningitis, or cortical venous thrombosis.

The focal enhancement of small cortical infarcts is best demonstrated by MR scans, where the cerebral surface is not obscured by artifact from the adjacent calvarium.

A small area of patchy enhancement is seen in the left frontal cortex. A similar appearance could be caused by a small arteriovenous malformation, focal cerebritis, a seizure focus, or an area of cortical venous infarction.

CT scans in patients with "moya moya" may demonstrate infarction, hemorrhage from rupture of telangiectatic vessels (see Case 564), or strikingly abnormal enhancement (usually in the basal ganglia) representing hypertrophied collateral channels. The caliber of the proximal anterior and middle cerebral arteries is often noticeably reduced on CT or MR scans through the circle of Willis.

DIFFERENTIAL DIAGNOSIS:
CEREBRAL LESION WITH COMPLEX BANDS AND RIMS OF CONTRAST ENHANCEMENT

Case 418

60-year-old man.

Case 419

72-year-old man.

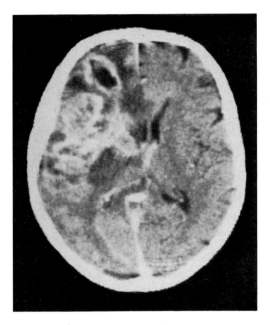

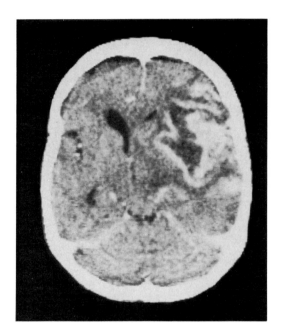

Glioblastoma Multiforme.

Infarction (19 Days After CVA).

The disorganized contrast enhancement of Case 418 is within the spectrum seen in high-grade gliomas. Case 419 illustrates the wide-ranging appearance of cerebral infarction. Rim-enhancing components are occasionally found in subacute infarcts, causing the lesions to resemble malignant neoplasms.

Clues to the diagnosis in Case 419 include the gyriform pattern of superficial enhancement and the location of the lesion within the middle cerebral artery distribution. However, a characteristic history, serial scans, or biopsy are necessary for definitive diagnosis in a lesion of this type.

OLD INFARCTION

Case 420

71-year-old woman.

Old Infarction in the Distribution of the Middle Cerebral Artery.

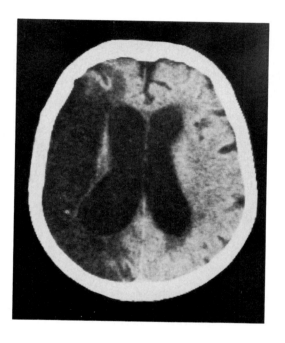

Case 421

51-year-old woman.
(axial, noncontrast scan; SE 3000/30)

Old Infarction Involving the Posterior Division of the Middle Cerebral Artery.

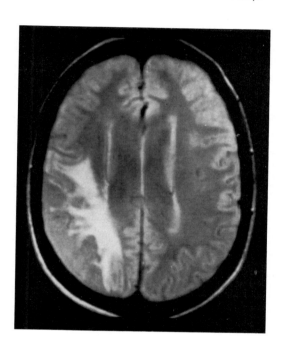

Old infarctions are seen on CT scans as sharply marginated regions of low attenuation associated with parenchymal loss. The attenuation values may be as low as spinal fluid or somewhat less "black," depending on the mixture of spared and destroyed tissue. Expansion of adjacent ventricles is characteristic, as in this case, and may lead to frank porencephaly (see Cases 629 to 632).

MR scans often demonstrate two zones of signal abnormality within an old infarction that appears homogeneous on CT examinations. The more superficial zone is usually comparable to CSF in signal intensity, reflecting the presence of spinal fluid in areas of destroyed parenchyma. (The slightly higher signal intensity of the cystic region on this scan is largely artifactual.)

The deep margin of an old infarct is seen as a zone of high signal intensity on long TR, short TE images, indicating the presence of damaged tissue. This appearance is nonspecific; a similar margin surrounds areas of encephalomalacia from other causes (e.g., after surgery).

Case 429 presents another example of the "two-tone" appearance of old infarction on MR scans.

INFARCTION IN THE DISTRIBUTION OF THE ANTERIOR CEREBRAL ARTERY

Case 422A

73-year-old woman.

Case 422B

Same patient.

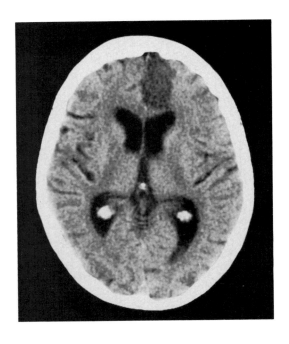

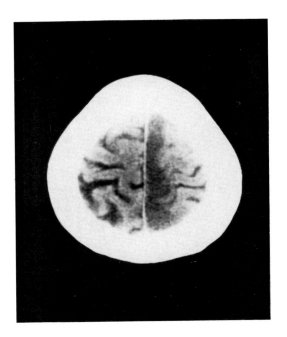

The anterior cerebral artery (ACA) supplies a parasagittal band of tissue extending from the medial frontal lobe to the parietal vertex. Uniform low attenuation in this distribution indicates obstruction of the vessel. Causes include embolization, spasm, compression by a subfrontal mass or infection (see Case 277), and marked subfalcial herniation (see Case 246).

The infarcted region in this case outlines the proximal distribution of the ACA and corresponds to the spared territory in Cases 406 and 407.

This scan illustrates infarction of the distal ACA distribution. The well-defined, homogeneous, low-attenuation region uniformly obliterates cortical morphology. A diagnosis of recent infarction is highly reliable when these features correspond to a vascular territory.

The lateral margin of infarcted tissue in this case localizes the cortical watershed between the anterior and middle cerebral arteries (see Cases 428 and 429).

INFARCTION IN THE DISTRIBUTION OF THE POSTERIOR CEREBRAL ARTERY

Case 423A

56-year-old man.

Case 423B

Same patient.

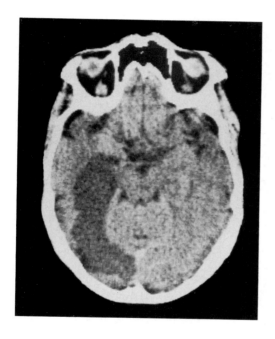

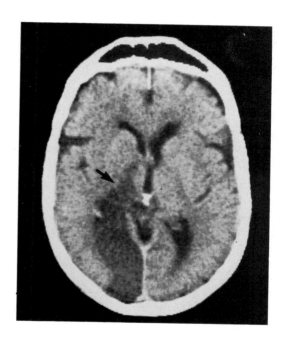

The posterior cerebral artery (PCA) supplies the medial temporal lobe, the tentorial surface of the temporal and occipital lobes, the occipital pole, and a variably extensive band of parasagittal parieto-occipital lobes.

Acute infarction in this case outlines the inferior portion of this distribution, bounded medially by the tentorial margin and laterally by the watershed with the middle cerebral artery. (Extended head position causes this scan to be parallel to the axis of the temporal lobe.)

The supply of the PCA to the medial portion of the occipital lobe is illustrated here. The superior and lateral extent of this distribution is variable and reflects reciprocal variations in the size of the anterior and middle cerebral arteries.

Thalamoperforating branches arise from the proximal posterior cerebral artery (as well as from the posterior communicating artery). For this reason, thalamic infarction (arrow) is often associated with infarctions of the medial temporal and occipital lobes.

See Cases 424 and 451 for other examples of infarction involving the PCA distribution.

LOCATION OF THE POSTERIOR CORTICAL WATERSHED

Case 424

68-year-old woman.

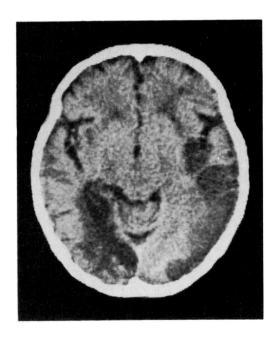

Case 425

74-year-old woman who was studied shortly after subclavian angiography at a referring hospital.

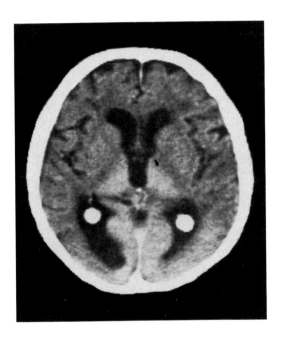

This case demonstrates an old right-sided infarction in the distribution of the posterior cerebral artery. On the left is a recent infarction involving the posterior division of the middle cerebral artery. The margin between involved and spared regions in each hemisphere represents the watershed between the middle and posterior cerebral arteries.

Uniformly increased attenuation is seen throughout the distribution of the posterior cerebral arteries, including the thalami. The margin of density indicates the watershed with supply from the middle cerebral arteries.

High attenuation values were also seen throughout the posterior fossa in this case, suggesting parenchymal penetrance of angiographic contrast material in the territory of the basilar artery. The subclavian angiogram had demonstrated embolic occlusion a short distance beyond the vertebral artery, which therefore received the bulk of the injected contrast. It is important to consider the subclavian origin of the vertebral artery when patients are evaluated for upper-extremity symptoms.

DIFFERENTIAL DIAGNOSIS:
LOW- OR MIXED-ATTENUATION MEDIAL OCCIPITAL LESION

Case 426

24-year-old man presenting with seizures.
(postcontrast scan)

Case 427

41-year-old woman with migraine headaches
presenting with a visual field cut.
(postcontrast scan)

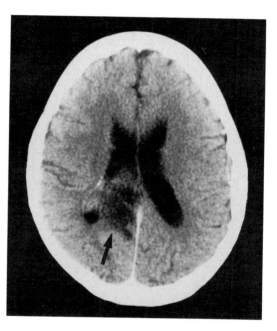

Grade 3 Astrocytoma.

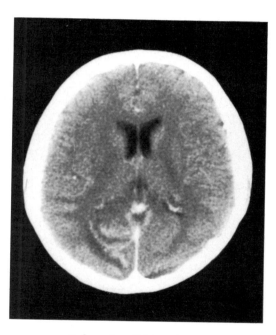

Enhancing PCA Infarct.

Case 426 illustrates that the area involved by a glioma may fall within a vascular distribution. Several CT features aid in differential diagnosis. Tumors rarely occupy the entire territory of a potentially occluded vessel. Vague or lobulated margins and cortical sparing (seen medially in Case 426) argue against infarction. Associated calcification (as in Case 413) suggests a low-grade neoplasm.

Branch occlusion may cause infarction involving only a portion of the distribution of a major cerebral artery. When such lesions are scanned in a subacute stage demonstrating mass effect and/or contrast enhancement, the appearance can resemble a tumor as in Case 427. Since this location in the major forceps is a common site for neoplasms (glioma, lymphoma, or metastasis), the correct diagnosis depends on a reliable history, characteristic evolution of CT findings, or MR demonstration of features favoring infarction.

Migraine patients sometimes develop symptoms of focal ischemia during the headaches ("hemiplegic migraine"), presumably representing vasospasm. Actual structural damage leading to CT evidence of major infarction as in Case 427 is uncommon.

CORTICAL WATERSHED INFARCTION

Case 428

70-year-old woman.

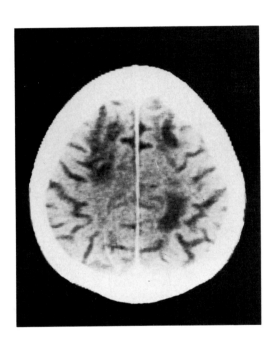

Case 429

61-year-old man.
(axial, noncontrast scan; SE 2500/28)

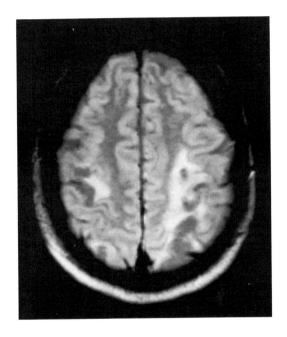

Infarction occurs along the margins of cerebrovascular territories when flow is impaired on both sides of the boundary. The cause may be generalized hypoperfusion, isolated vascular compromise, or a combination of both factors. For example, stenosis of an internal carotid artery may lead to infarction along the anterior-middle cerebral artery watershed during systemic hypotension.

The location of the cortical watersheds has been illustrated in Cases 406, 407, 422, 424, and 425. Watershed infarctions are typically small, patchy lesions, aligned along these same parasagittal boundaries.

This case illustrates typical infarctions along the cortical watershed between the anterior and middle cerebral arteries (see Case 525 for another example). Differential diagnosis of this parasagittal pattern includes venous infarction due to thrombosis of the superior sagittal sinus (see Cases 468 to 471).

Old infarctions are identified along the cortical watersheds of both cerebral hemispheres in this case. As discussed in Case 421, the MR appearance of old infarcts on long TR spin-echo images is characterized by margins of high intensity bordering zones of CSF-like signal values.

MR scans in the coronal plane clearly display the superficial, parasagittal location of ischemic lesions involving the cortical watershed. Coronal MR scans are also useful in assessing the deep hemisphere damage of "periventricular leukomalacia" in infants and children (see Cases 488 and 489).

DIFFERENTIAL DIAGNOSIS:
MULTIPLE SUPERFICIAL INFARCTS

Case 430

72-year-old man.

Case 431

70-year-old woman.

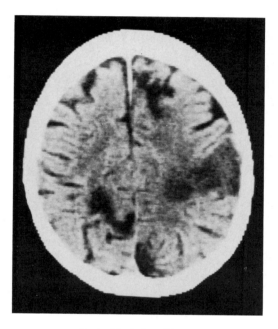

Embolic Infarctions.

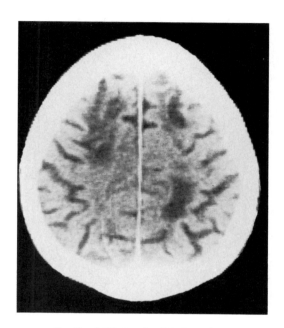

Cortical Watershed Infarctions.

The distribution of multiple cerebral infarctions may help characterize the underlying pathophysiology. In Case 430, multiple infarctions are present at scattered cortical locations, largely independent of watershed territories. The pattern suggests multifocal occlusions of distal cerebral arteries, raising the possibility of embolization, cerebral vasculitis, or coagulopathy.

By contrast, the multiple infarctions in Case 431 are aligned along watershed distributions. This pattern favors generalized hypoperfusion rather than involvement of individual cortical arteries.

Cases 440 and 441 discuss the typical location of watershed infarctions within a single hypoperfused hemisphere.

DEEP HEMISPHERE INFARCTION

Case 432

76-year-old woman, 4 days after a
cerebrovascular accident.

Case 433

84-year-old woman.

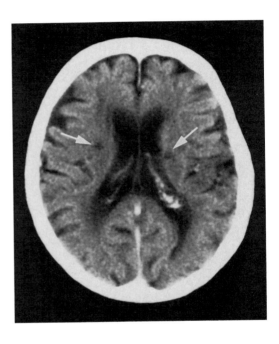

Deep hemisphere infarction may accompany large cortical infarctions or occur as an isolated event. Infarctions may involve large segments of the basal ganglia, as seen in this case, or be limited to very focal areas, as in Case 433.

The basal ganglia and internal capsule are largely supplied by lenticulostriate branches arising from the horizontal portion of the middle cerebral artery. (Other contributions include medial lenticulostriate branches from the anterior cerebral artery, the anterior choroidal artery, and thalamoperforating branches of the posterior cerebral artery.)

Infarction in this region is often due to local disease of the lenticulostriate arteries. Pathologic conditions involving the proximal portion of the middle cerebral artery (e.g., plaque, embolus, arteritis, or dissection) may also cause deep hemisphere infarction by compromising the origins of these penetrating branches. Finally, isolated deep hemisphere infarction may be seen in cases of internal carotid artery occlusion when collateral flow spares cortical tissue.

This 4-day-old infarction demonstrates typical well-defined low attenuation, with mass effect compressing the adjacent frontal horn.

Focal infarctions in periventricular white matter are a common manifestation of small artery disease. They are most frequently seen in diabetic and/or hypertensive patients (see Case 435).

Like hydrocephalus, deep hemisphere infarction is a common pathology that could be considered a form of white matter disease. The small lesions in this case might be viewed as one end of a spectrum leading toward "Binswanger's disease" or "ischemic leukoencephalopathy" (see Case 327) at the opposite extreme.

Scattered infarcts in and near the corona radiata may mimic the appearance of demyelinating plaques in multiple sclerosis, as seen here and in Case 434 (compare to Cases 305 and 306).

MULTIPLE "LACUNAR" INFARCTIONS

Case 434

80-year-old man with dementia.

Case 435

50-year-old woman with a history of diabetes mellitus and hypertension.
(axial, noncontrast scan; SE 3000/75)

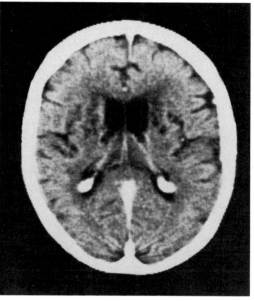

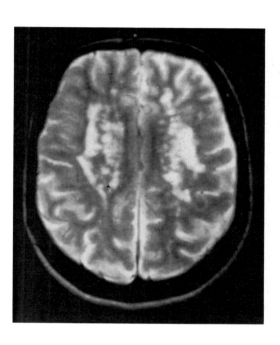

Small deep hemisphere infarctions are often called "lacunar infarcts," using the name that pathologists have given to tiny lesions found in the basal ganglia at autopsy. Large numbers of such infarcts have previously been suggested to be the cause of clinical "lacunar states," with components of dementia or pseudobulbar palsy. These clinical correlations are controversial; the symptoms of patients with multiple deep hemisphere infarcts may range from minimal to profound.

MR frequently demonstrates more "lacunar" infarcts than are visible on CT studies. In some cases these lesions are so numerous that they coalesce to form zones of ischemic leukoencephalopathy, as seen here.

The bilaterality and symmetry of the lesions favor small arterial disease as the etiology. The pattern is distinct from intrahemispheric watershed infarction due to large vessel compromise (see Cases 440 and 441).

Although periventricular "lacunes" are present, other lesions involve more peripheral portions of the centrum semiovale and subcortical white matter. This distribution may help to distinguish widespread lacunar infarcts from most cases of multiple sclerosis (compare to Case 313).

Associated parenchymal loss in this case is indicated by enlargement of sulci.

DIFFERENTIAL DIAGNOSIS:
LOW-ATTENUATION LESIONS IN THE BASAL GANGLIA

Case 436

44-year-old man.

Case 437

83-year-old man.

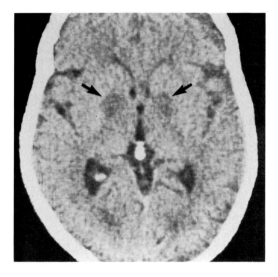

Carbon Monoxide Poisoning.

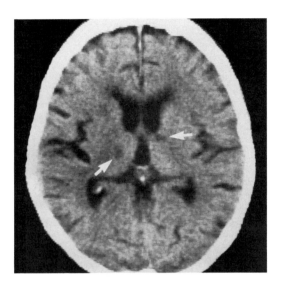

"Lacunar" Infarction.

Carbon monoxide poisoning leads to necrosis of the globus pallidus. Pallidal necrosis may be seen on CT scans as symmetrical areas of abnormal low attenuation, illustrated in Case 436 *(arrows)*. This finding is associated with a poor prognosis for recovery.

Other processes that may cause pallidal necrosis include barbiturate intoxication, cyanide poisoning, hydrogen sulfide poisoning, hypoglycemia, hypoxia (e.g., drug overdose), and hypotension. Leigh's disease (subacute necrotizing encephalomyelopathy) may cause symmetrical foci of low attenuation in the basal ganglia (usually in children and commonly associated with brain stem involvement). Myelinolysis related to electrolyte disorders (see "central pontine myelinolysis," Cases 331 and 446) may affect the basal ganglia symmetrically or asymmetrically. Wilson's disease can be associated with pallidal lucency despite the deposition of metals. The scan findings of methanol intoxication are usually seen more laterally, with hemorrhagic necrosis of the putamen.

The symmetry of involvement in Case 436 suggests a toxic or systemic cause. See Case 328 for an example of severe leukoencephalopathy following carbon monoxide exposure.

FOCAL DEEP HEMISPHERE LESIONS ALONG THE CORTICOSPINAL TRACTS

Case 438

79-year-old woman scanned 1 year after a cerebrovascular accident.

Wallerian Degeneration.

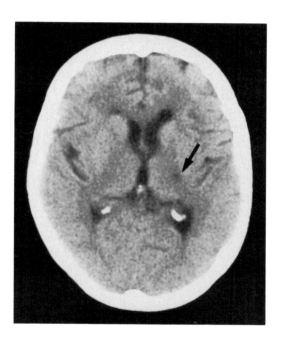

Case 439

26-year-old man presenting with paraparesis. (axial, noncontrast scan; SE 2500/45)

Amyotrophic Lateral Sclerosis.

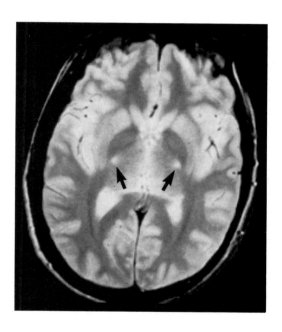

Another cause of focal low attenuation within the internal capsule or brain stem is "Wallerian degeneration." This process of axonal degeneration follows the death of neurons. When tissue damage involves a group of nerve cells that serve as the source of a major fiber tract, the aggregate degeneration of axons may become apparent on CT and MR studies.

In this case, an infarction involving the frontoparietal cortex was seen at higher levels. The focal zone of low attenuation within the internal capsule (arrow) could be followed from the centrum semiovale to the pons. On any one scan the appearance resembles a focal infarct, as seen here. The continuity across several levels of anatomy establishes the diagnosis of Wallerian degeneration parallelling the corticospinal tract.

MR studies have shown biphasic intensity changes during Wallerian degeneration. An initial period of T2-shortening within the fiber tract (possibly related to hydrophobic products of myelin breakdown) is followed by permanent prolongation of T2.

Amyotrophic lateral sclerosis (ALS) is a degenerative disorder involving the corticospinal tracts as well as lower motor neurons. Symmetrical abnormality of the pyramidal tracts can often be followed from the motor cortex through the brain stem on cranial MR studies. Zones of vague abnormal signal intensity in the centrum semiovale become increasingly concentrated and better defined as the corticospinal tracts converge on lower sections.

Small, symmetrical lesions are often seen within the posterior limb of the internal capsule, as in this case (arrows). These paired abnormalities can be followed caudally into the cerebral peduncles, pons, and medulla. A similar appearance has been noted in some cases of progressive multifocal leukoencephalopathy (PML).

Small areas of slightly high signal intensity can be seen as a normal variant on MR scans through the posterior limb of the internal capsule. These symmetrical foci, thought to represent poorly myelinated parietopontine tracts, can be mistaken for lacunar infarcts or other capsular pathologies. Clues to correct interpretation include symmetrical occurrence at a single anatomical level (unlike this case), and relative isointensity on "balanced" or "intermediate" images (long TR, short TE).

Case 440

76-year-old woman.

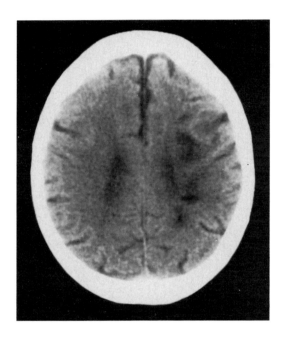

Case 441

58-year-old woman.

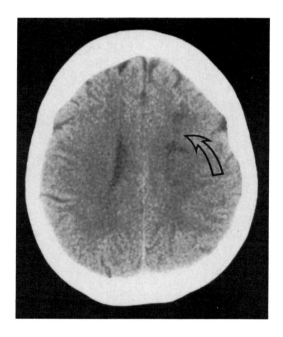

Small infarcts within cerebral white matter may reflect hypoperfusion of the hemisphere rather than small vessel disease. An intrahemispheric watershed zone occurs between the arterial supply of perforating vessels ascending from the base of the brain (e.g., lenticulostriate arteries) and the penetrating branches of arteries on the cerebral convexity. This parasagittal zone of white matter (lateral and superior to the body of the lateral ventricle) is susceptible to scattered infarction under conditions of hypoperfusion.

The CT discovery of several small infarcts clustered along the midhemispheric watershed should suggest ipsilateral carotid disease. In this case, high grade stenosis of the left internal carotid artery was found.

The short parasagittal row of intrahemispheric infarctions in this case (arrow) is less extensive than in Case 440, but the significance is the same. Occlusion of the ipsilateral internal carotid artery was found at angiography. Carotid stenosis or occlusion should be suspected when a CT (or MR) appearance resembling "unilateral multiple sclerosis" is encountered.

Cases 428 and 429 illustrate the location of cortical watershed infarctions. These superficial lesions often reflect cardiovascular impairment (causing global hyperperfusion) rather than isolated carotid disease.

Case 442

33-year-old woman with multiple neurological
deficits 1 day following cardiac surgery.
(axial, noncontrast scan; SE 2500/28)

Cortical Watershed Infarctions.

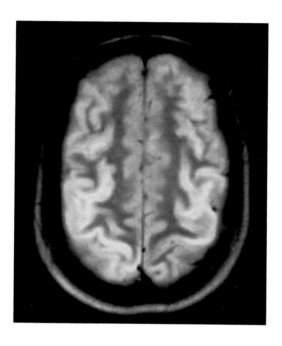

Case 443

58-year-old woman (same patient as Case 441).
(axial, noncontrast scan; SE 2500/45)

**Intrahemispheric Watershed Infarctions
due to Occlusion of the Internal Carotid
Artery.**

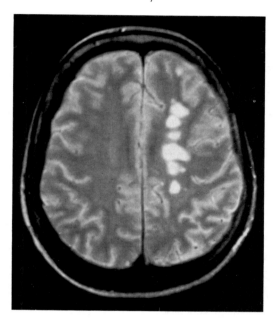

Symmetrical high signal intensity is present within gyri throughout the parasagittal zones of the cortical arterial watershed. (Compare the location of the gyral edema in this case to Cases 422, 428, and 429.) Petechial hemorrhage was apparent in the same distribution on T1-weighted images.

Small lesions within cerebral white matter are better defined by MR than by CT, whether they are demyelinating plaques or foci of ischemia. In this case, the parasagittal row of white matter infarcts is strikingly unilateral (compare to the less impressive CT appearance in Case 441). Compromise of the ipsilateral internal carotid artery should be suspected when this pattern is encountered.

BRAIN STEM INFARCTION

Case 444

63-year-old woman.
(postcontrast scan)

Case 445

74-year-old man.
(postcontrast scan)

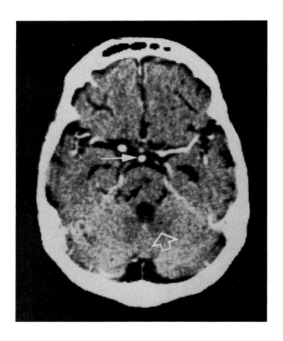

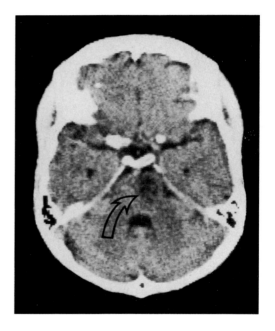

Brain stem infarctions may present as focal low-attenuation areas *(black arrow)*, most common in the midbrain or pons. These lesions are usually caused by small artery disease involving the pontine perforating vessels. MR has demonstrated a strong association between brain stem infarcts and deep hemisphere "lacunes" reflecting analogous pathology of the lenticulostriate arteries.

The precontrast and postcontrast appearance of the basilar artery is of interest in cases of brain stem ischemia. Calcification, reduced lumen size, and even intraluminal thrombus (see Case 464) may be noted. Here, the basilar artery enhances normally *(white arrow)*.

Occasionally, Wallerian degeneration (see Case 438) can cause a focal area of low attenuation resembling brain stem infarction. Associated encephalomalacia within the ipsilateral cerebral hemisphere is apparent in such cases.

The normal low attenuation of cerebellar white matter is seen posterolateral to the fourth ventricle *(open arrow)* and should not be mistaken for ischemia.

This patient was densely hemiparetic. A large hemispheric infarction was suspected, but the lesion was instead found to involve the left cerebral peduncle.

High-resolution CT scanners routinely demonstrate a midline region of low attenuation near the center of the midbrain (see Case 621 for an example). This area represents the normal decussation of the superior cerebellar peduncles. The central, symmetrical appearance high in the brain stem usually distinguishes this finding from infarction. Brain stem infarctions tend to occur at more caudal levels and are often eccentric, as seen here.

DIFFERENTIAL DIAGNOSIS:
LOW-ATTENUATION BRAIN STEM LESION

Case 446

70-year-old man.

Case 447

44-year-old man.

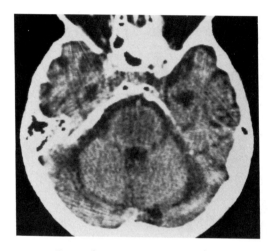

Central Pontine Myelinolysis.

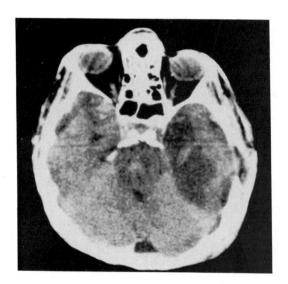

Post-traumatic Brain Stem Injury.

A number of pathologies other than infarction may cause low attenuation within the brain stem (also see discussion of Cases 108 and 109).

Central pontine myelinolysis is discussed in Case 331. The characteristic CT appearance is illustrated in Case 446, with abnormal low attenuation involving most of the pons. This patient had been admitted with a serum sodium concentration of 117 mEq/L, which had been rapidly overcorrected.

Case 447 demonstrates extensive low attenuation throughout the brain stem following trauma. (Anterior right temporal contusion and medial left temporal edema or infarction are also present.) Primary brain stem injury most often involves the posterolateral portions of the midbrain and pons. Such lesions are well demonstrated by MR scans and are frequently associated with shearing injuries of the corpus callosum and cerebral hemispheres (see Cases 381, 383, and 384).

Secondary brain stem injury after head trauma is often the result of transtentorial herniation with caudal displacement of the brain stem. This distortion stretches the penetrating branches of the basilar artery, leading to infarction and/or hemorrhage in the pons and midbrain. CT scans in such cases demonstrate diffuse low attenuation with scattered components of hemorrhage, as seen centrally in Case 447.

Extensive brain stem infarction due to occlusion of the basilar artery may resemble Cases 446 and 447. Bilateral infarcts within the cerebellum and posterior cerebral artery distributions usually accompany brain stem lesions in this setting.

Case 448

68-year-old man, after resection of a large retrosellar meningioma.

Case 449

68-year-old woman, one day after clipping of a ruptured aneurysm at the tip of the basilar artery.

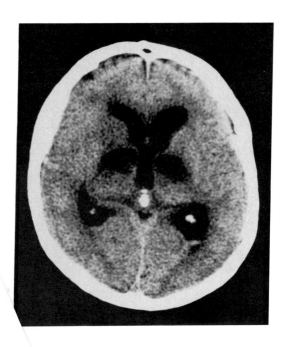

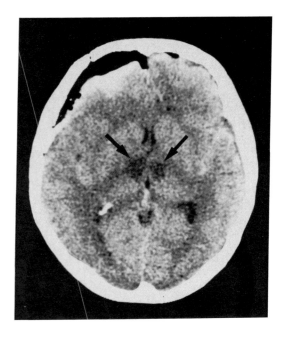

'orating branches arise near the tip of the basilar
om the posterior communicating and proximal
ral arteries) to supply the diencephalon. Addi-
the ventral thalamus and internal capsule
oidal vessels, which may be predominantly
nterior choroidal artery or the posterolateral
of the posterior cerebral artery.

these vessels at the level of the supra-
ular cistern may cause a characteristic
thalamic infarction. In this case, the
ar tumor distorted and encased the
arteries. Despite careful dissection,
followed by symmetrical capsular/

hage is present in the posterior
nes.

Bilateral infarction involving the ventral thalamus *(arrows)* is seen in this case. Small perforating arteries may have been mechanically distorted or occluded by placement of the aneurysm clip, or the vessels may have been constricted by vasospasm secondary to subarachnoid hemorrhage in the interpeduncular region.

In any event, the resultant pattern of bithalamic infarction is characteristic of small arterial compromise near the tip of the basilar artery.

Subdural pneumocephalus is present in the right frontal region from the recent craniotomy.

POSTERIOR CEREBRAL ARTERY DISTRIBUTION ISCHEMIA DUE TO UNCAL/PARAHIPPOCAMPAL HERNIATION

Case 450

6-year-old boy (same patient as Case 385).

Case 451

13-year-old girl.

PCA Ischemia due to Cerebral Swelling After Head Trauma.

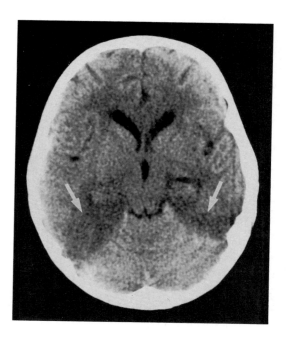

Old PCA Infarcts due to Increased Intracranial Pressure From Hydrocephalus.

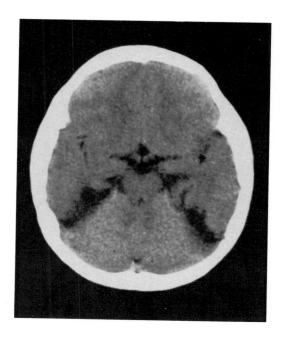

Cerebral mass effect can displace the uncus and parahippocampal gyrus of the temporal lobe medially and inferiorly, distorting the brain stem and crowding the tentorial hiatus. Such herniation may compress or kink the posterior cerebral artery as it passes from the ambient cistern to cross the tentorial margin. Secondary ischemia or infarction involving the occipital lobes can be seen as a consequence of these events, compounding the initial pathology.

Case 385 demonstrates a scan of this patient performed 9 days earlier. At that time, cerebral swelling was seen to cause bilateral uncal/parahippocampal herniation. The current scan shows reduction in mass effect with reappearance of sulci and cisterns. However, poorly defined zones of low attenuation along the tentorial surface of the occipital lobes indicate ischemia or edema in the PCA distributions due to the prior herniation.

Clinical examination failed to disclose cortical blindness or other evidence of occipital lobe dysfunction. The CT appearance returned to normal within several days, indicating that the low-attenuation pattern seen here may in some cases represent reversible edema or ischemia.

In this case the zones of abnormal low attenuation along the tentorial surface of the cerebral hemispheres are much better defined than in Case 450. This appearance indicates frank infarction within the distribution of the posterior cerebral arteries. The bilateral symmetry is evidence for a previous episode of diffusely increased intracranial pressure with bihemispheral herniation.

Cases 450 and 451 demonstrate the location of the lateral tentorial margin, which continues the 45-degree angle of the petrous ridge (see Cases 348 and 349 for localization of the medial tentorial margin).

INFARCTION IN THE DISTRIBUTION OF THE POSTERIOR INFERIOR CEREBELLAR ARTERY (PICA)

Case 452

75-year-old woman.
(postcontrast scan)

Case 453

35-year-old man.
(postcontrast scan)

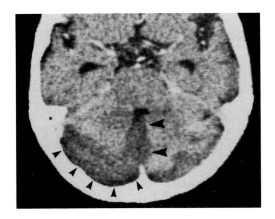

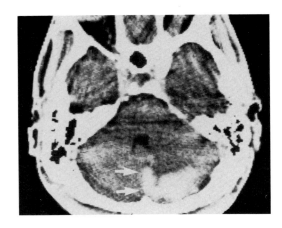

Infarction of the cerebellum may cause confusing low-attenuation changes in the posterior fossa. In many cases the diagnosis can be made by recognizing the distribution of a major cerebellar artery.

The PICA usually supplies (1) a broad rim of peripheral cerebellar hemisphere along the occipital inner table *(small arrowheads)*, and (2) a parasagittal strip of medial hemisphere and inferior vermis extending posteriorly from the fourth ventricle *(large arrowheads)*. An infarction of the PICA should be the first diagnostic consideration when a low-attenuation cerebellar lesion with this scythe-like configuration is encountered.

Incomplete infarction in the PICA distribution may cause low attenuation in either the peripheral or parasagittal region (as seen in the posterior portion of the contralateral hemisphere). Infarctions of cerebellar watershed regions or multifocal infarctions present less characteristic appearances (see Case 458).

This enhancing posterior fossa lesion in a young patient could be misinterpreted as a tumor or a vascular malformation. The clue to the correct diagnosis is the scythe-like morphology of PICA infarction. A curving, peripheral crescent of involved hemisphere is linked to a straight, parasagittal band that borders the midline. This sharp, medial margin *(arrows)* is particularly suggestive of a vascular distribution respecting an anatomical boundary.

Magnetic resonance imaging is more successful than CT in demonstrating the brain stem consequences of PICA occlusion. The lateral aspect of the medulla is typically infarcted in such cases, correlating with the clinical picture of "Wallenberg's syndrome."

Infarction in the PICA distribution is the most likely cause of acute cerebellar signs in a young adult.

INFARCTION IN THE DISTRIBUTION OF THE SUPERIOR CEREBELLAR ARTERY (SCA)

Case 454

54-year-old man.
(noncontrast scan)

Case 455

78-year-old woman.
(postcontrast scan)

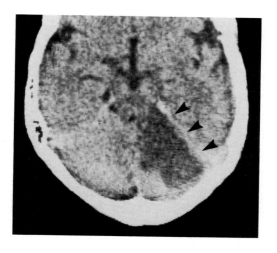

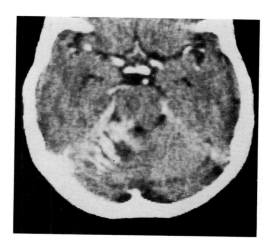

The SCA supplies the superior portion of the cerebellar hemisphere and vermis. Infarction in the distribution of this vessel involves the hemisphere but may spare the vermis due to collateral circulation from the inferior vermian arteries.

As in supratentorial infarctions, the lesion demonstrates homogeneous low attenuation with a broad peripheral base. A straight, diagonal, lateral margin *(arrowheads)* is a hallmark of infarction in the SCA distribution, which is bounded laterally by the tentorium. The medial margin is variable and less distinct, depending on collateral flow patterns.

Associated mass effect compresses the ipsilateral quadrigeminal cistern.

In this case, the hemispheric distribution of the SCA is outlined by gyriform contrast enhancement. The shape and location of the lesion are more specific than its internal appearance, which could be confused with a vascular malformation.

Compare the parallel pattern of enhancing cerebellar folia in this case to the enhancement of leptomeningeal tumor within cerebellar sulci in Case 121.

DIFFERENTIAL DIAGNOSIS:
LOW-ATTENUATION CEREBELLAR MASS

Case 456

80-year-old man.

Case 457

70-year-old woman.

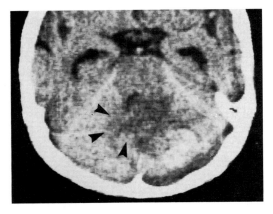

**Metastatic Bronchogenic Carcinoma, Left
Cerebellar Hemisphere.**

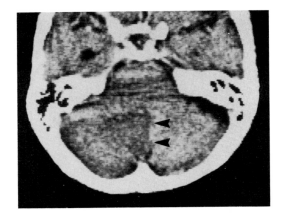

**Cerebellar Infarction, Right Cerebellar
Hemisphere.**

Metastases are the most common cause of cerebellar masses in adults. The lesion in Case 456 is unusually poorly defined. Adjacent edema compresses the fourth ventricle and crosses the midline through the vermis *(arrowheads)*.

Acute cerebellar infarction may also produce extensive low attenuation and mass effect, as seen in Case 457. Swelling may compress the brain stem and require acute decompression, similar to a cerebellar hematoma (see Case 569).

A clue to the diagnosis in Case 457 is the very straight medial margin of the lesion *(arrowheads)*, which suggests a vascular boundary. This appearance contrasts with the vague medial margin of edema in Case 456.

CEREBELLAR INFARCTION: PITFALLS

Case 458

74-year-old woman.
(noncontrast scan)

Multifocal Cerebellar Infarction.

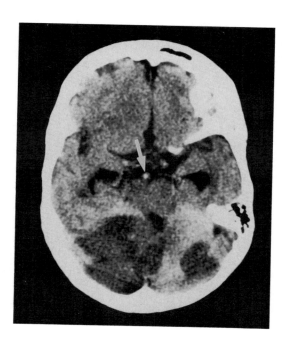

Case 459

74-year-old woman 1 month after resection of a large acoustic schwannoma (same patient as Case 349).

Chronic Subdural Hematoma along the Inferior Surface of the Tentorium.

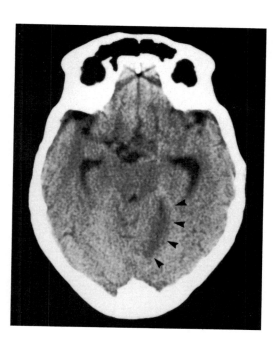

The linear margins emphasized in Cases 452 to 457 can be an important clue to the diagnosis of cerebellar infarction. However, subacute cerebellar infarcts may demonstrate convex borders mimicking mass lesions (and comparable to some cerebral infarcts, as noted in Case 405).

In this case, substantial mass effect is associated with the subacute cerebellar lesions. The rostral fourth ventricle is displaced and deformed, and the right side of the brain stem is flattened.

It is important to remember that vertebrobasilar disease often causes bilateral cerebellar and/or occipital infarctions. Ischemia should be considered (along with metastases or inflammatory foci) when multiple lesions are encountered in the basilar artery distribution.

Density within the basilar artery in this case (arrow) may represent calcification and/or fresh thrombus (see Case 479).

Although infarctions involving the superior cerebellar artery are characteristically marginated by the tentorium (see Cases 454 and 455), other pathologies can mimic this appearance.

In Case 459 a chronic subdural hematoma is seen as a low-attenuation zone adjacent to the tentorial surface. Mass effect compresses the superior vermis and ipsilateral quadrigeminal cistern. Enlarged temporal horns reflect mild obstructive hydrocephalus.

MR CORRELATION: BRAIN STEM INFARCTION

Case 460

82-year-old woman.
(axial, noncontrast scan; SE 3000/90)

Case 461

75-year-old man presenting with the sudden
onset of hemiparesis.
(axial, noncontrast scan; SE 2500/90)

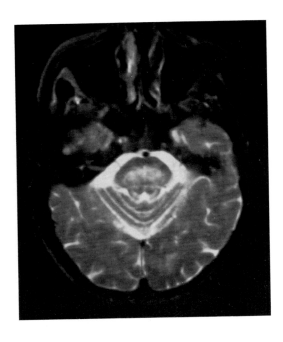

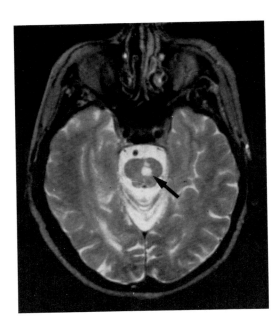

Small arterial disease affecting the brain stem is usually most apparent at the pontine level. This case is a typical example, with multiple foci of increased signal intensity clustered centrally. Patients with this MR appearance may have surprisingly minimal symptoms.

Cerebral scans in patients with multiple pontine infarcts usually demonstrate associated "lacunar" lesions in the basal ganglia and periventricular white matter (see Cases 433 to 435).

CT scans may fail to define recent brain stem infarcts. These lesions are often small, and their subtle attenuation changes are obscured by interpetrous artifact. MR is valuable for confirming and localizing the clinical diagnosis of brain stem ischemia.

In this case, a focal lesion is seen just to the left of midline in the caudal midbrain (compare to the larger CT lesion in Case 445). Small brain stem infarcts may resemble involvement by multiple sclerosis (see Case 330), but the clinical setting usually distinguishes between these pathologies. Brain stem metastases can present a similar appearance and should be considered in the appropriate context.

MR CORRELATION: CEREBELLAR INFARCTION

Case 462

73-year-old woman.
(axial, noncontrast scan; SE 2500/90)

PICA Distribution Infarction.

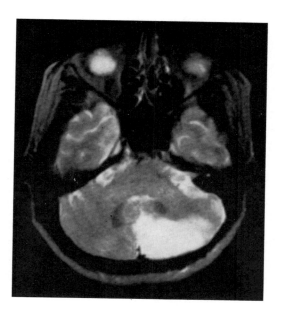

Case 463

60-year-old woman.
(axial, noncontrast scan; SE 2500/90)

SCA Distribution Infarction.

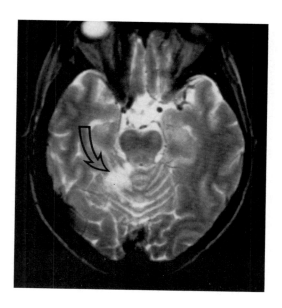

The margins of cerebellar infarctions are clearly defined on MR studies. As a result, the typical morphology of specific vascular distributions is usually apparent.

In this case, the wedge-shaped region of high signal intensity involving the medial and posterior portions of the cerebellar hemisphere indicates recent infarction in the PICA distribution (compare to Cases 452 and 453). The greater contrast sensitivity of MR often "fills in" the center of the scythe-like shape of PICA infarction as seen by CT.

The small area of high signal intensity involving the superior right cerebellar hemisphere in this case (arrow) represents infarction within the distribution of the superior cerebellar artery. The location adjacent to the tentorial surface and the mildly serrated morphology paralleling cerebellar folia are characteristic on MR scans as in CT studies (compare to Cases 454 and 455).

Case 464

27-year-old man recently treated for subacute bacterial endocarditis, now presenting with acute diplopia.
(noncontrast scan)

Saddle Embolus in the Basilar Artery.

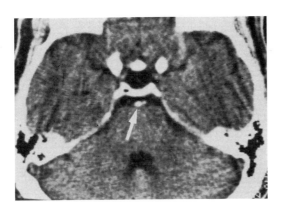

Case 465

15-year-old boy involved in a fight 10 hours before the acute onset of hemiparesis.
(noncontrast scan)

"Supernormal" Occluded Middle Cerebral Artery.

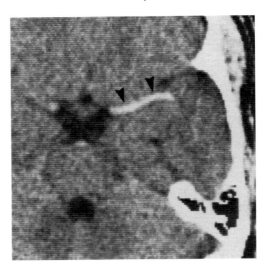

Thromboemboli can occasionally be seen as small densities within cerebral arteries. The density of an embolus may be due to calcification (e.g., a fragment of atheroma) or to the dense fibrin network within a thrombus.

Common locations for lodged emboli include the horizontal segment of the middle cerebral artery and the anterior cerebral artery bifurcation near the genu of the corpus callosum. Small densities near vessels in the subarachnoid cisterns may also be caused by calcified atherosclerotic plaque, falx calcification, and intracranial iophendylate (Pantopaque) droplets.

In this patient, an abnormal density occupies the tip of the basilar artery on the noncontrast scan *(arrow)*. The density was angiographically proved to represent a "saddle embolus" lodged at the basilar bifurcation. The patient later suffered subarachnoid hemorrhage, and autopsy confirmed a noncalcified, septic thromboembolus associated with erosion of the basilar artery tip.

Occlusion of the middle cerebral artery may be associated with abnormal prominence of the proximal segment on CT scans *(arrowheads)*. This "supernormal" or "hyperdense" horizontal segment may represent intraluminal stasis and/or thrombus. Angiograms in such cases have shown occlusion both distal and proximal to the dense arterial segment.

The "supernormal" artery may be seen before infarction is apparent and can provide the earliest CT clue to the diagnosis. MR scans demonstrate a corresponding lack of normal "flow void" in such occluded arterial segments (see Case 466).

Angiography in this case showed dissection of the internal carotid artery with embolic occlusion of the MCA origin (compare to the history in Case 411).

Case 466

59-year-old woman.
(axial, noncontrast scan; SE 2500/90)

Absence of "Flow Void" due to Arterial Occlusion.

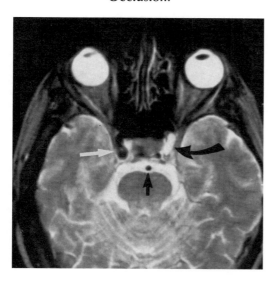

Case 467

56-year-old man with a 2-day history of neck pain, now presenting with transient ischemic attacks.
(axial, noncontrast scan; SE 2500/45)

Dissecting Intramural Hematoma.

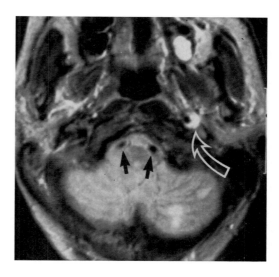

The characteristic appearance of rapidly flowing blood on routine spin-echo MR scans is an absence of signal intensity or "flow void." When this expected lack of signal is replaced by measurable intraluminal intensity, slow flow or thrombus should be suspected.

Here high signal from the left supraclinoid internal carotid artery (curved arrow) contrasts with the normal "flow void" of the right paraclinoid carotid artery (white arrow) and rostral basilar artery (short black arrow). The left parasellar internal carotid artery was found to be completely occluded at angiography.

The signal intensity of intraluminal thrombus is variable. Arterial ("white") thrombi are often isointense to cerebral parenchyma. Venous ("red") thrombi containing more erythrocytes may demonstrate T1- and T2-shortening (see discussion of Cases 560 and 561).

Reduced caliber of patent arteries at the skull base is another MR and CT sign of vascular compromise. This finding may be associated with extracranial or intracranial stenoses (see discussion of "moya moya" syndrome in Case 564).

MR can diagnose arterial dissection by direct demonstration of the intramural hematoma. Scans perpendicular to the long axis of an artery define crescentic thickening of the vessel wall, eccentrically narrowing the lumen at the level of dissection.

In this case the intramural hematoma involving the left internal carotid artery at the skull base (curved white arrow) is seen as a high-intensity crescent along the lateral wall of the vessel. (Compare this appearance to the normal wall thickness of the distal vertebral arteries; black arrows.) The right internal carotid artery was severely narrowed due to an old dissection. Small cerebellar infarcts are present on the left, and a retention cyst is seen in the left maxillary sinus.

Spontaneous or post-traumatic dissections of the internal carotid artery commonly extend to the petrous segment. The dissection itself is usually associated with headache and a Horner's syndrome; neurological deficits often reflect secondary cerebral embolization.

SUPERIOR SAGITTAL SINUS THROMBOSIS

Case 468

10-month-old boy who suffered a midline parietal skull fracture 2 days earlier, now lethargic and vomiting.
(noncontrast scan)

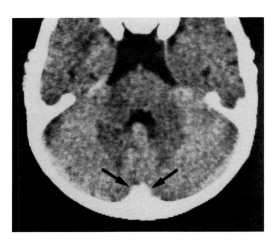

Case 469

21-year-old man injured in an automobile accident 6 days earlier, now presenting with impaired level of consciousness.
(postcontrast scan)

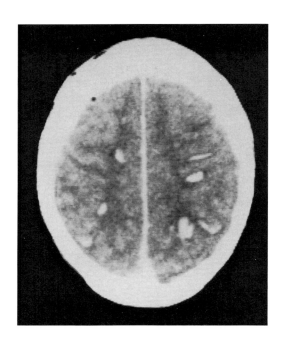

The CT findings of superior sagittal sinus thrombosis (SSST) depend on the age of the process and the presence or absence of contrast material. Acute SSST may present as an abnormally dense sinus on noncontrast scans (*arrows;* see Cases 325 and 640 for discussion of normally dense sinuses in neonates). The density of acute thrombosis may be masked by contrast enhancement of the sinus and adjacent dura.

Other potential clues to the diagnosis of SSST on noncontrast scans include parasagittal hemorrhages or edema (see Cases 469 and 471) and cerebral swelling.

Magnetic resonance imaging (and/or MR angiography) is a noninvasive means of assessing sinus patency in equivocal cases (see Case 474).

Parasagittal hemorrhages due to cortical venous infarction are a highly suggestive secondary finding in SSST. The parasagittal densities in this case were present on noncontrast scans, with no additional enhancement on this postcontrast study.

Patchy parasagittal edema without hemorrhage is also suggestive of SSST, although the appearance may be similar to that of arterial watershed infarction (see Cases 428 and 429) or white matter pathology such as progressive multifocal leukoencephalopathy (see Cases 321 and 322). Occasional gyriform enhancement may be seen in the same parasagittal areas.

Postcontrast scans in SSST may also show abnormally intense enhancement of the tentorium, probably due to a combination of collateral venous flow and stasis (see Case 300).

SUPERIOR SAGITTAL SINUS THROMBOSIS: SUBTLE PRESENTATIONS

Case 470

68-year-old woman presenting with seizures
(same patient as Case 300).
(noncontrast scan)

Case 471

64-year-old woman with progressive
bihemispheral symptoms, thought to have
suffered bilateral cerebral infarctions.
(noncontrast scan)

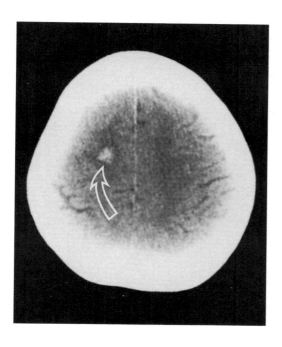

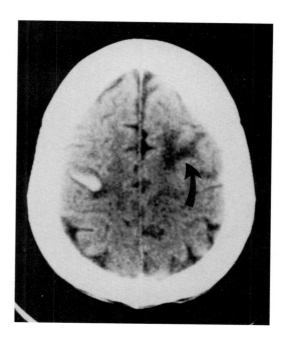

Scans early in the course of superior sagittal sinus thrombosis may demonstrate no parenchymal abnormality or only subtle parasagittal lesions. In this case, one tiny hemorrhage *(arrow)* is seen in a characteristic location near the vertex.

Since head trauma may predispose to SSST (as in Cases 468 and 469), small areas of parasagittal hemorrhage and edema should not be casually attributed to "contusion" or "shearing injury."

Here an area of focal, parasagittal edema at the left hemisphere vertex accompanies a small hemorrhage in the corresponding zone of the right hemisphere. Either of these lesions should raise the possibility of superior sagittal sinus thrombosis (with associated cortical venous thrombosis). The combination of two such foci is highly diagnostic.

Scattered areas of cerebral edema due to SSST may resemble the appearance of primary white matter lesions such as progressive multifocal leukoencephalopathy (see Cases 321 to 323).

DIFFERENTIAL DIAGNOSIS:
THE "EMPTY TRIANGLE" SIGN

Case 472

21-year-old man (same patient as Case 469).
(postcontrast scan, high window level, narrow
window width)

Case 473

25-year-old man suffering head trauma.
(noncontrast scan)

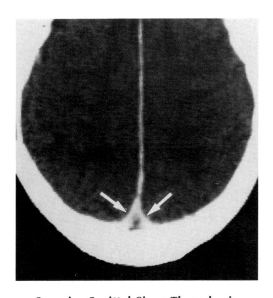

Superior Sagittal Sinus Thrombosis.

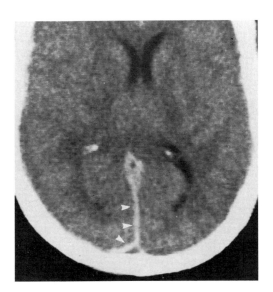

**Interhemispheric Hemorrhage Outlining a
Patent Sagittal Sinus.**

Clot within a dural sinus may be seen as a filling defect when surrounded by contrast material in the residual lumen or outlined by the enhancing margins of the sinus. On axial scans, the superior sagittal sinus is viewed in cross section as a triangular structure near the occipital inner table. Thrombus filling this portion of the sinus creates the "empty triangle" sign of SSST on postcontrast images, as seen in Case 472 *(arrows)*. Optimal demonstration of the sign may require adjustment of display settings, with high window levels and narrow window widths.

The appearance of an "empty triangle" on noncontrast scans is usually due to subdural or subarachnoid blood outlining the sinus margins and does not imply thrombosis (Case 473). As discussed in Case 468, the diagnosis of SSST on a noncontrast scan should be based on a *dense* sinus or on the characteristic secondary findings.

Another false "empty triangle" appearance may be caused by artifact crossing the posterior portion of the superior sagittal sinus on postcontrast scans. Prominent ridges of bone at the edges of the sinus groove favor this low-density band, analogous to the interpetrous ("Hounsfield") artifact in the posterior fossa.

Finally, the normal sinus may separate slightly from the occipital inner table as it nears the torcular. This variation causes a nonenhancing zone along the posterior wall of the sinus that may be misinterpreted as thrombus.

MR CORRELATION: DURAL SINUS THROMBOSIS

Case 474A

32-year-old woman presenting with headache
and papilledema.
(sagittal, noncontrast scan; SE 750/20.)

Superior Sagittal Sinus Thrombosis.

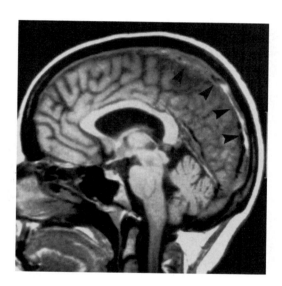

Case 474B

Same patient.
(axial, noncontrast scan; SE 3000/45)

Transverse Sinus Thrombosis.

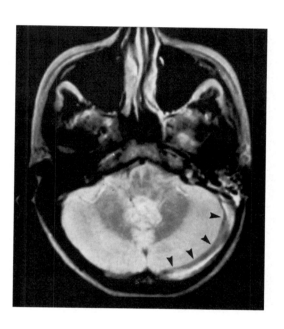

The sagittal and coronal planes of MR are useful for assessing patency of the superior sagittal sinus. On normal spin-echo noncontrast scans (away from the margins of the imaging volume), the sinus should contain little signal. Thrombosis and stasis replace this normal "flow void" with variable intraluminal intensity.

Here the superior sagittal sinus is filled with a mixture of isointense and high-intensity components. Other thrombosed dural sinuses may be completely isointense or strikingly hyperintense on T1-weighted images. Gradient-echo pulse sequences (maximizing flow-related enhancement) may be used to distinguish between slow flow and thrombus within a vascular structure.

The differential diagnosis of this MR appearance on midsagittal scans includes subdural or epidural hematoma or neoplasm (e.g., neuroblastoma, leukemia, lymphoma, or metastasis). Coronal scans are useful to exclude these possibilities.

The straight sinus is also thrombosed in this case.

The etiology of dural sinus thrombosis in this case was found to be left mastoiditis, with associated septic thrombophlebitis of the sigmoid and transverse sinuses. (Compare the bright signal intensity from mucosal thickening within the left petrous bone to the normal lack of signal in the mastoid region as seen on the right side.) The left transverse sinus *(arrowheads)* demonstrates uniformly high intensity due to thrombus replacing the expected "flow-void."

The clinical course of patients with SSST reflects the extent to which thrombus propagates into cortical veins. In this case there was no clinical or MR evidence of venous infarction. Anticoagulation therapy was begun, and the patient recovered completely.

CEREBRAL ANOXIA: DIFFUSE INVOLVEMENT

Case 475

5-month-old boy following cardiopulmonary arrest with prolonged hypotension and seizures.

Case 476

65-year-old woman suffering seizures 1 day after cardiopulmonary arrest.
(noncontrast scan)

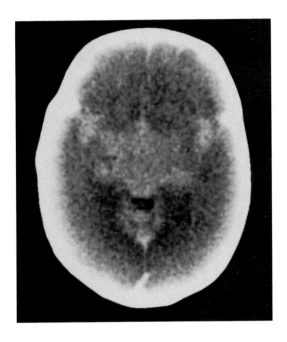

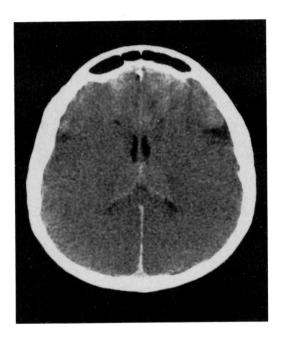

Anoxia may cause diffuse ischemic and cytotoxic edema leading to low attenuation and cerebral swelling. Gray matter is severely affected and may become lower in density than the underlying white matter. Reversal of the normal density relationship of gray and white matter can be seen along the horizontal segment of the sylvian cisterns in this case, and is more clearly demonstrated in Cases 478 and 482.

Deep-seated structures may be relatively spared, as seen here in the diencephalon and quadrigeminal plate. Diffuse cerebral swelling has completely effaced ventricles, cisterns, and sulci.

Case 483 illustrates the appearance of a similar insult in the subacute stage, and Case 485 illustrates the result of severe anoxia as displayed on later scans.

Symmetrical cerebral swelling causes ventricular compression in this case. Most sulci and cisterns are also effaced. Diffuse low attenuation obliterates gray/white matter discrimination and accentuates the normal density of the posterior falx and superior sagittal sinus.

CEREBRAL ANOXIA: BASAL GANGLIA INVOLVEMENT

Case 477

14-year-old boy who fell from a dock during a seizure.

Near Drowning.

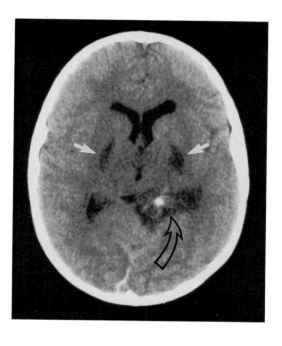

Case 478

3-month-old boy.

Sudden Infant Death Syndrome.

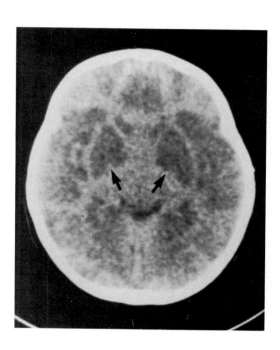

Some cases of anoxia show selective damage in the deep cerebral nuclei. Since the basal ganglia are perfused by "end arteries," they are particularly vulnerable to an anoxic insult.

Here the main abnormality is well-defined low attenuation involving the globus pallidus bilaterally *(white arrows)*. (Compare this scan to the appearance of carbon monoxide poisoning in an adult in Case 436.)

The cause of the patient's seizure was the calcified, low-grade glioma involving the medial posterior left temporal lobe *(open arrow)*.

The lenticular nucleus *(arrows)* may be strikingly involved along with cortical gray matter in some cases of cerebral anoxia. Here the cortical gyri and basal ganglia demonstrate equivalent and symmetrical low attenuation, while the density of white matter is relatively preserved.

Involvement of the deep hemisphere nuclei with or without cortical changes is usually a sign of severe anoxia; milder hypoxia or hypoperfusion may manifest only gyral abnormalities.

DIFFERENTIAL DIAGNOSIS:
LOW ATTENUATION THROUGHOUT CEREBRAL WHITE MATTER IN AN INFANT

Case 479

2-day-old boy.

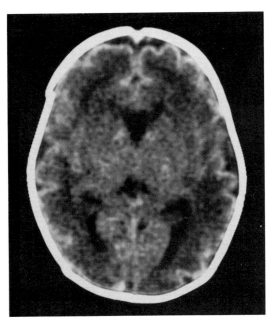

Normal (31 Weeks Gestation).

Case 480

10-day-old boy.

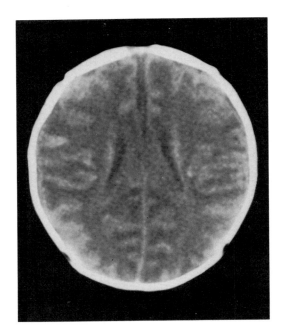

Anoxia due to Sudden Infant Death Syndrome.

As discussed in Cases 325 and 326, the white matter of premature infants is poorly myelinated and contains a large amount of water. The resultant low attenuation is accentuated by the normal thinness of the cortical mantle, mimicking diffuse edema as in Case 479.

The infant in Case 480 is full term (compare the degree of gyral folding and invagination to Case 479). The low attenuation throughout white matter in this case represents abnormal edema due to an anoxic insult.

Anoxic encephalopathy can affect the white matter acutely or chronically in both children and adults. (See Case 328 for an example of predominant white matter change following adult anoxia.) The factors causing white matter edema as opposed to the more common cortical low density in anoxia are poorly understood. Diffuse hemispheric low attenuation as seen in some cases of anoxia (e.g., Cases 475 and 476) probably represents a combination of gray and white matter injury.

DIFFERENTIAL DIAGNOSIS:
DIFFUSE CEREBRAL LOW ATTENUATION AND SWELLING IN AN INFANT

Case 481

10-week-old boy.

Case 482

15-month-old girl.

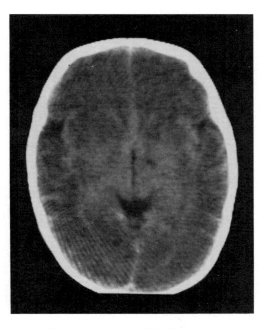

Herpes Encephalitis (Type 2).

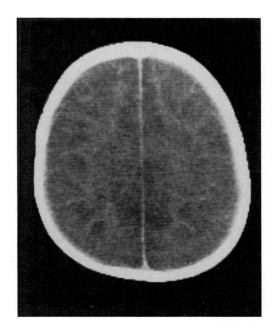

Anoxia (Cardiopulmonary Arrest Following Aspiration of Food).

Scans in the acute phases of infantile encephalitis and anoxia may be similar. Both processes demonstrate widespread swelling and low attenuation change.

The edema of encephalitis in Case 481 involves white matter regions and shows relative sparing of basal ganglia and some cortical areas. In contrast, the anoxia in Case 482 causes low attenuation throughout the cortex with relatively less abnormality of white matter ("gray/white reversal"; see also Cases 475 and 478).

Cases 268C and 269 illustrate the atrophy and calcification that commonly follow neonatal encephalitis such as Case 481.

Case 483A

3-month-old girl, 8 days after an anoxic insult.

Case 483B

Same patient.

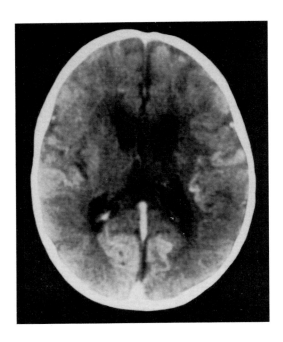

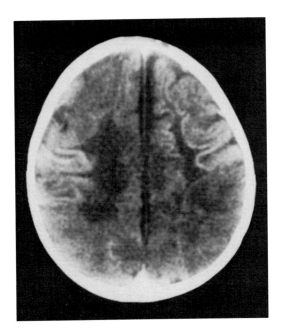

Widespread contrast enhancement involving portions of the cortical ribbon is seen in this case. The pattern resembles the "gyriform" enhancement seen in subacute cerebral infarction, but multiple arterial distributions are involved.

A scan 5 days earlier had demonstrated swollen, featureless cerebral hemispheres comparable to Cases 475 and 476. The enlarging ventricles on this study indicate rapidly developing parenchymal loss, which will result in a final appearance similar to Case 485.

The gyral enhancement seen in subacute anoxia may persist for hours or days after contrast injection. This "stain" indicates severe cortical injury and resembles the appearance in some cases of infantile encephalitis (compare to Case 268B).

DIFFERENTIAL DIAGNOSIS:
LARGE VENTRICLES WITH PERIPHERAL ZONES OF LOW ATTENUATION IN AN INFANT

Case 484

1-month-old boy.

Case 485

8-month-old girl, 3 months after smoke inhalation.

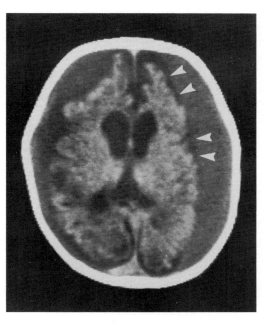

Viral Meningoencephalitis; Subdural Fluid Collections.

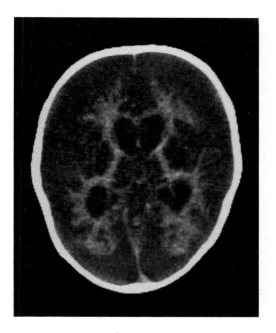

Cerebral Anoxia.

Perinatal viral meningitis and/or encephalitis often causes rapid and extensive damage to the immature brain (see Cases 268 and 269). The result is a diffuse loss of parenchymal volume, which presents the appearance of atrophy.

In Case 484 the cerebral cortex has collapsed away from the inner table and large subdural fluid collections have developed. The subdural fluid is slightly higher in attenuation than the thin ribbon of CSF surrounding the collapsed hemispheres *(arrowheads)*. Despite severe infectious parenchymal damage, the morphology of cortical gray matter is relatively preserved, in contrast to Case 485.

Primary subdural hematomas may cause communicating hydrocephalus with secondary ventricular enlargement. The atrophic cortical surface and large sulci in Case 484 argue against this interpretation.

Acute anoxia causes swelling (see Cases 475 and 476), which is rapidly replaced by parenchymal loss. In Case 485 the enlarged ventricles are surrounded by a halo of relatively preserved white matter. Cortical regions are seen as a featureless zone of low attenuation.

Case 486

14-year-old boy (same patient as Case 477).
(axial, noncontrast scan; SE 2500/90)

Near Drowning.

Case 487

14-year-old boy (different patient).
(axial, noncontrast scan; SE 3000/75)

Near Hanging.

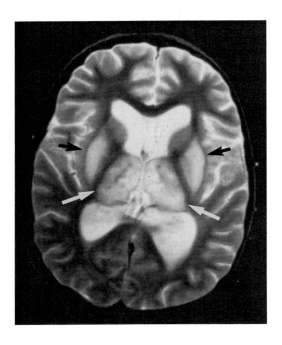

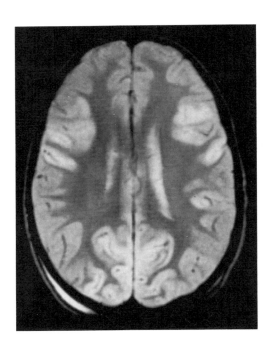

MR sensitively demonstrates anoxic injury to cerebral gray matter. In this case, uniformly increased signal intensity throughout the lenticular nuclei *(black arrows)* and thalami *(white arrows)* indicates cytotoxic edema. T1-weighted scans showed symmetrical petechial hemorrhages in the same regions.

In this case symmetrical injury to cortical gray matter is apparent. Zones of gyral edema are seen bilaterally, predominantly affecting the frontal lobes. Signal intensity was also diffusely increased throughout the basal ganglia on lower sections of the scan.

MR DEMONSTRATION OF PERIVENTRICULAR LEUKOMALACIA

Case 488

8-year-old boy with spastic diplegia.
(axial, noncontrast scan; SE 3000/90)

Case 489

2-year-old girl with developmental delay.
(coronal, noncontrast scan; SE 2500/90)

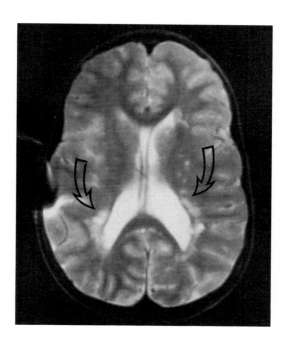

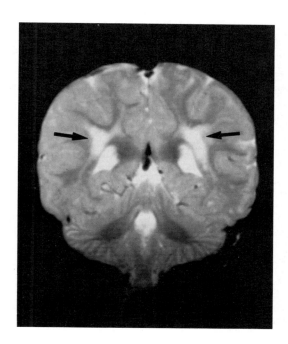

Periventricular leukomalacia (PVL) is a syndrome of multifocal damage within deep hemisphere white matter in premature infants. The etiology of PVL has traditionally been assumed to be a hypoxic/ischemic insult to the watershed zones in the developing brain. Other contributing factors (toxic, metabolic, and immune-mediated) have been suggested recently.

White matter near the posterior bodies and trigones of the lateral ventricles is most frequently and most severely affected in such cases. Infants who incur PVL characteristically develop spastic diplegia or quadriplegia and often carry the diagnosis of "cerebral palsy."

MR scans offer direct evidence of periventricular injury. In this case, multiple posterior periventricular foci of signal abnormality indicate sites of white matter necrosis. The posterior bodies of the lateral ventricles are expanded due to the loss of adjacent parenchyma. (Superficial artifact in the right sylvian region is due to a shunt valve.)

The perinatal diagnosis of PVL is based on ultrasound studies, which demonstrate abnormal echogenicity and subsequent cyst formation in the periventricular regions. CT scans later in childhood often show reduced bulk of the periventricular white matter. Cortical sulci may penetrate far into the hemisphere, nearly reaching the ventricular margin. The ventricular borders themselves may be irregular due to loss and cavitation of subependymal white matter.

MR scans can document periventricular injury even when associated volume loss is minimal. In this case, symmetrical zones of signal abnormality involve peritrigonal white matter (arrows). The ventricles are mildly dilated.

These zones of signal abnormality from PVL are larger and nearer to the ventricular margins than the normal areas of slow myelination in parietal white matter (which occur posterior and superior to the ventricular trigones).

REFERENCES: CT

1. Becker H., Desch H., Hacker H.: CT fogging effect with ischemic cerebral infarcts. *Neuroradiology* 18:185–192, 1979.
2. Bird C.R., Drayer B.P., Gilles F.H.: Patholophysiology of "reverse" edema in global cerebral ischemia. *A.J.N.R.* 10:95–98, 1989.
3. Cobb S.R., Mehringer C.M., Itabashi H.H., Pribram H.: CT of subinsular infarction and ischemia. *A.J.N.R.* 8:221–228, 1987.
4. Fieback B.J., Dabir K., Hermie P., et al.: Cerebral CT in fatal courses of resuscitated sudden infant death. *A.J.N.R.* 4:689–691, 1983.
5. Flodmark O., Roland E.H., Hill A., Whitfield M.F: Periventricular leukomalacia: Radiologic diagnosis. *Radiology* 162:119–124, 1987.
6. Ford K., Sarwar M.: Computed tomography of dural sinus thrombosis. *A.J.N.R.* 2:539–543, 1981.
7. Goldberg A.L., Rosenbaum A.E., Wang H., et al.: Computed tomography of dural sinus thrombosis. *J. Comput. Assist. Tomogr.* 10:16–20, 1986.
8. Han B.K., Towbin R.B., De Courten-Myers, et al.: Reverse sign on CT: Effect of anoxic/ischemic cerebral injury in children. *A.J.N.R.* 10:1191–1198, 1989.
9. Henrickson G.C., Patel D.V.: Enhancing cerebral infarction simulating arteriovenous malformation on computed tomography. *J. Comput. Assist. Tomogr.* 9:502–506, 1985.
10. Houser O.W., Campbell J.K., Baker H.L., et al.: Radiologic evaluation of ischemic cerebrovascular syndromes with emphasis on computed tomography. *Radiol. Clin. North Am.* 20:123–142, 1982.
11. Inoue Y., Takemoto K., Miyamoto T., et al.: Sequential computed tomography scans in acute cerebral infarction. *Radiology* 135:655–662, 1980.
12. Kendall B.E., Pullicino P.: Intravascular contrast injection in ischaemic lesions. II. Effect on prognosis. *Neuroradiology* 19:241–243, 1980.
13. Kim K.S., Walczak T.S.: Computed tomography of deep cerebral venous thrombosis. *J. Comput. Assist. Tomogr.* 10:386–390, 1986.
14. Kricheff I.I.: Arteriosclerotic ischemic cerebrovascular disease. *Radiology* 162:101–110, 1987.
15. Liwnicz B.H., Mouradian M.D., Ball J.B. Jr.: Intense brain cortical enhancement on CT in laminar necrosis verified by biopsy. *A.J.N.R.* 8:157–160, 1987.
16. Masdeu J.C.: Infarct versus neoplasm on CT: Four helpful signs. *A.J.N.R.* 4:522–524, 1983.
17. Miura T., Mitomo M., Kawai R., Harada K.: CT of the brain in acute carbon monoxide intoxication: Characteristic features and prognosis. *A.J.N.R.* 6:739–742, 1985.
18. Nelson R.F., Pullicino P., Kendall B.E., et al.: Computed tomography in patients presenting with lacunar syndromes. *Stroke* 11:256–261, 1980.
19. Paltice H.J., O'Gorman A.M., Meagher-Villemure K., et al.: Subacute necrotizing encephalomyelopathy (Leigh disease): CT study. *Radiology* 162:115–118, 1987.
20. Paroni Sterbini G.L.P., Agatiello L.M., Stocchi A., Solivetti F.M.: CT of ischemic infarctions in the territory of the anterior choroidal artery: A review of 28 cases. *A.J.N.R.* 8:229–232, 1987.
21. Pressman B.D., Tourje E.J., Thompson J.R.: An early CT sign of ischemic infarction: Increased density in a cerebral artery. *A.J.N.R.* 8:645–648, 1987.
22. Pullicino P., Kendall B.E.: Contrast enhancement in ischemic lesions. I. Relationship to prognosis. *Neuroradiology* 19:235–239, 1980.
23. Pullicino P., Nelson R.F., Kendall B.E.: Small deep infarcts diagnosed on computed tomography. *Neurology* 30:1090–1096, 1980.
24. Rao K.C., Knipp H.C., Wagner E.J.: Computed tomographic findings in cerebral sinus and venous thrombosis. *Radiology* 140:391–398, 1981.
25. Sato M., Tanaka S., Kohama A. Fujii C.: Occipital lobe infarction caused by tentorial herniation. *Neurosurgery* 18:300–305, 1986.
26. Schellinger D., Grant E.G., Richardson J.D.: Neonatal leukoencephalopathy: A common form of cerebral ischemia. *Radiographics* 5:221–242, 1985.
27. Schellinger D., Grant E.G., Richardson J.D.: Cystic periventricular leukomalacia: Sonographic and CT findings. *A.J.N.R.* 5:439–446, 1984.
28. Takahashi S., Goto K., Fukasawa H., et al.: Computed tomography of cerebral infarction along the distribution of the basal perforating arteries. Part I. Striate arterial group. *Radiology* 155:107–118, 1985.
29. Takahashi S., Goto K., Fukasawa H., et al.: Computed tomography of cerebral infarction along the distribution of the basal perforating arteries. Part II. Thalamic arterial group. *Radiology* 155:119–130, 1985.
30. Takeuchi S., Kobayashi K., Tsuchida T., et al.: Computed tomography in moyamoya disease. *J. Comput. Assist. Tomogr.* 6:24–32, 1982.
31. Taneda M., Ozaki K., Wakayama A., et al.: Cerebellar infarction with obstructive hydrocephalus. *J. Neurosurg.* 57:83–91, 1982.
32. Taylor R., Holgate R.C.: Carbon monoxide poisoning: Asymmetric and unilateral changes on CT. *A.J.N.R.* 9:975–977, 1988.
33. Taylor S.B., Quencer R.M., Holzman B.H., Naidich T.P.: Central nervous system anoxic-ischemic insult in children due to near-drowning. *Radiology* 156:641–646, 1985.
34. Tomura N., Inugami A., Kanno I., et al.: Differentiation between cerebral embolism and thrombosis on sequential CT scans. *J. Comput. Assist. Tomogr.* 14:26–31, 1990.
35. Tomura N., Vemura K., Inugami A., et al.: Early CT findings in cerebral infarction: Obscuration of the lentiform nucleus. *Radiology* 168:463–468, 1988.
36. Tsai F.Y., Teal J.S., Heishima G.B., et al.: Computed tomography in acute posterior fossa infarcts. *A.J.N.R.* 3:149–156, 1982.
37. Virapongse C., Cazenave C., Quisling R., et al.: The empty delta sign: Frequency and significance in 76 cases of dural sinus thrombosis. *Radiology* 162:779–786, 1987.
38. Vonofakos D., Marcu H., Hacker H.: CT diagnosis of basilar artery occlusion. *A.J.N.R.* 4:525–528, 1983.
39. Wall S.D., Brant-Zawadzki M., Jeffry R.B., et al.: High frequency CT findings within 24 hours after cerebral infarction. *A.J.N.R.* 2:553–557, 1981.
40. Yagnik P., Gonzalez C.: White matter involvement in anoxic encephalopathy in adults. *J. Comput. Assist. Tomogr.* 4:788–790, 1980.
41. Yock D.H. Jr.: CT demonstration of cerebral emboli. *J. Comput. Assist. Tomogr.* 5:190–196, 1981.
42. Zimmermann R.A., Bilaniuk L.T., Packer R.J., et al.: Computed tomographic-arteriographic correlates in acute basal ganglionic infarction of childhood. *Neuroradiology* 24:241–248, 1983.

REFERENCES: MR

1. Anderson S.C., Shah C.P., Murtagh F.R.: Congested deep subcortical veins as a sign of dural venous thrombosis: MR and CT correlations. *JCAT* 11:1059–1061.
2. Baker L.L., Stevenson D.K., Enzmann D.R.: End-stage periventricular leukomalacia: MR evaluation. *Radiology* 168:809–816, 1988.
3. Barkhof F., Valk J.: "Top of the basilar" syndrome: A comparison of clinical and MR findings. *Neuroradiology* 30:293, 1988.
4. Biller J., Adams H.P. Jr., Dunn V., et al: Dichotomy between clinical findings and MR abnormalities in pontine infarction. *J. Comput. Assist. Tomogr.* 10:379–385, 1986.
5. Braffman B.H., Zimmerman R.A., Trojanowski J.Q., et al.: Brain MR: Pathologic correlation with gross and histopathology. 1. Lacunar infarction and Virchow-Robin spaces. *A.J.N.R.* 9:621–628, 1988.
6. Brant-Zawadzki M., Weinstein P., Bartkowski H., Moseley M.: MR imaging and spectroscopy in clinical and experimental cerebral ischemia: A review. *A.J.N.R.* 8:39–48, 1987.
7. Brown J.J., Hesselink J.R., Rothrock J.F.: MR and CT of lacunar infarction. *A.J.N.R.* 9:477–482, 1988.
8. Cordes M., Henkes H., Roll D., et al.: Subacute and chronic cerebral infarctions: SPECT and gadolinium-DTPA-enhanced MR imaging. *J. Comput. Assist. Tomogr.* 13:567–571, 1989.
9. Flodmark O., Lupton B., Li D., et al.: MR imaging of periventricular leukomalacia in childhood. *A.J.N.R.* 10:111–118, 1989.
10. Fox A.J., Bogousslavsky J., Carey L.S., et al.: Magnetic resonance imaging of small medullary infarctions. *A.J.N.R.* 7:229–234, 1986.
11. Fujisawa I., Asato R., Nishimura K., et al.: Moyamoya disease: MR imaging. *Radiology* 164:103–106, 1987.
12. Goldberg H.I., Grossman R.I., Gomori J.M., et al.: Cervical internal carotid artery dissecting hemorrhage: Diagnosis using MR. *Radiology* 158:157–162, 1986.
13. Hecht-Leavitt C., Gomori J.M., Grossman R.I., et al.: High field MRI of hemorrhagic cortical infarction. *A.J.N.R.* 7:581–586, 1986.
14. Heinz E.R., Yeates A.E., Djang W.T.: Significant extracranial carotid stenosis: Detection on routine cerebral MR images. *Radiology* 170:843–848, 1989.
15. Horowitz A.L., Kaplan R., Sarpel G.: Carbon monoxide toxicity: MR imaging in the brain. *Radiology* 162:787–788, 1987.
16. Hulcelle P.J., Dooms G.C., Mathurin P., et al.: MRI assessment of unsuspected dural sinus thrombosis. *Neuroradiology* 31:217, 1989.
17. Imakita S., Nishimura T., Naito H., et al.: Magnetic resonance imaging of human cerebral infarction: Enhancement with GD-DTPA. *Neuroradiology* 29:422, 1987.
18. Imakita S., Nishimura T., Yamada N., et al.: Magnetic resonance imaging of cerebral infarction: Time course of Gd-DTPA enhancement and CT comparison. *Neuroradiology* 30:372, 1988.
19. Jungreis C.A., Kanal E., Hirsch W.L., et al.: Normal perivascular spaces mimicking lacunar infarction: MR imaging. *Radiology* 169:101–104, 1988.
20. Katz B.H., Quencer R.M., Kaplan J.O., et al.: MR imaging of intracranial carotid occlusion. *A.J.N.R.* 10:345–350, 1989.
21. Knepper L., Biller J., Adams H.P. Jr., et al.: MR imaging of basilar artery occlusion. *J. Comput. Assist. Tomogr.* 14:32–35, 1990.
22. Kuhn M.J., Johnson K.A., Davis K.K.: Wallerian degeneration: evaluation with MR imaging. *Radiology* 168:199–202, 1988.
23. Kuhn M.J., Mikulis D.J., Ayoub D.M., et al.: Wallerian degeneration after cerebral infarction: Evaluation with sequential MR imaging. *Radiology* 172:179–182, 1989.
24. Macchi P.J., Grossman R.I., Gomori J.M., et al.: High field MR imaging of cerebral venous thrombosis. *J. Comput. Assist. Tomogr.* 10:10–15, 1986.
25. Marshall V.G., Bradley W.G., Marshall C.E., et al.: Deep white matter infarction: Correlation of MR imaging and histopathologic findings. *Radiology* 167:517–522, 1988.
26. McArdle C.B., Mirfakhraee M., Amparo E.G., Kulkarni M.V.: MR imaging of transverse/sigmoid dural sinus and jugular vein thrombosis. *J. Comput. Assist. Tomogr.* 11:831–838, 1987.
27. McArdle C.B., Richardson C.J., Hayden C.K., et al.: Abnormalities of the neonatal brain: MR imaging. Part II. Hypoxic-ischemic brain injury. *Radiology* 163:395–404, 1987.
28. McMurdo S.K., Brant-Zawadzki M., Bradley W.G., et al: Dural sinus thrombosis: Study using intermediate field strength MR imaging. *Radiology* 161:83–86, 1986.
29. Medina L., Chi T.L., DeVivo D.C., Hilal S.K.: MR findings in patients with subacute necrotizing encephalomyelopathy (Leigh syndrome): Correlation with biochemical defect. *A.J.N.R.* 11:379–384, 1990.
30. Miromitz S., Sartor K., Gado M., Torack R.: Focal signal intensity variations in the posterior internal capsule: Normal MR findings and distinction from pathologic findings. *Radiology* 172:535–540, 1989.
31. Rippe D.J., Boyko O.B., Spritzer C.E., et al.: Demonstration of dural sinus occlusion by the use of MR angiography. *A.J.N.R.* 11:199–201, 1990.
32. Salomon A., Yeates A.E., Burger P.C., Heinz E.R.: Subcortical arteriosclerotic encephalopathy: Brain stem findings with MR imaging. *Radiology* 165:625–630, 1987.
33. Soges L.C., Cacayorin E.D., Petro G.R., Ramachandran Y.S.: Migraine: evaluation by MR. *A.J.N.R.* 9:425–430, 1988.
34. Sze J., Simmons B., Krol G., et al.: Dural sinus thrombosis: Verification with spin-echo techniques. *A.J.N.R.* 9:679–686, 1988.
35. Uhlenbrock D., Sehlen S.: Value of T1-weighted images in the differentiation between MS, white matter lesions, and subcortical arteriosclerotic encephalopathy (SAE). *Neuroradiology* 31:203, 1989.
36. Virapongse C., Mancuso A., Quisling R.: Human brain infarcts: Gd-DTPA-enhanced MR imaging. *Radiology* 161:785–794, 1986.
37. Zimmerman R.A., Gill F., Goldberg H.I., et al.: MRI of sickle cell cerebral infarction. *Neuroradiology* 29:232, 1987.

CHAPTER 10

Vascular Lesions and Hemorrhage

ARTERIOVENOUS MALFORMATIONS

Case 490

32-year-old woman presenting with seizures.
(postcontrast scan)

Case 491

14-year-old girl presenting with right body
numbness.
(postcontrast scan)

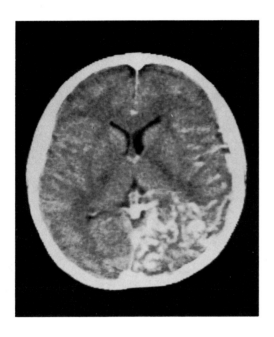

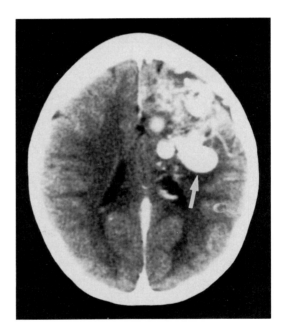

Arteriovenous malformations (AVMs) cause a variety of CT appearances. The characteristic lesion is a closely packed tangle of serpentine, enhancing vascular channels, as seen here in the left temporal and occipital lobes.

Mass effect is unusual in the absence of associated hemorrhage, although some AVMs do contain bulky vascular components (see Cases 502 and 503). Encephalomalacia may be present due to old hemorrhage or to parenchymal damage from the pulsations or "steal" of the malformation.

Patients with AVMs commonly present with seizures, as in this case. Other symptoms include headache and focal hemispheric deficits (see Case 491). Hemorrhage is the initial manifestation of a cerebral AVM in about 50% of cases (see Cases 496 and 497).

Ectatic feeding arteries or draining veins may be prominent components of high-flow AVMs. In this case, the large, tubular collection of contrast along the posterior margin of the lesion *(arrow)* was angiographically seen to represent a varix (compare to the noncontrast scan in Case 500).

Aneurysms of arteries feeding a vascular malformation may also cause large, rounded contrast collections within or adjacent to the lesion (see Case 497).

MR CORRELATION: ARTERIOVENOUS MALFORMATIONS

Case 492

36-year-old man.
(axial, noncontrast scan; SE 2500/30)

Case 493

21-year-old woman.
(axial, noncontrast scan; SE 3000/75)

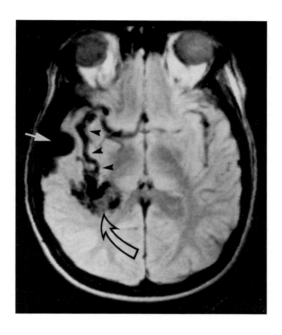

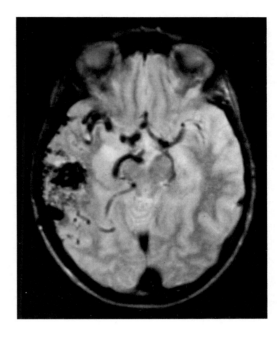

The rapid blood flow through an AVM causes a conspicuous lack of signal intensity on standard MR pulse sequences. (Gradient-echo pulse sequences that emphasize flow-related enhancement will demonstrate high signal intensity within arterial components of vascular malformations.)

In this case, the nidus of the AVM is seen as a nodular zone of mixed intensity in the deep posterior temporal region *(open arrow)*. The higher intensity components interspersed with "flow void" inside the lesion may represent zones of slow flow, hemorrhage, and/or intervening parenchyma.

Hypertrophied feeding branches of the middle cerebral artery are apparent *(black arrowheads)*, as are enlarged superficial draining veins *(white arrow)*.

The tangle of abnormal vascular channels seen here in the right temporal lobe is highly characteristic of an arteriovenous malformation. "Flow void" can be seen within large vessels associated with intracranial tumors (see Cases 33 and 76), but the pattern is rarely as tightly interwoven as in AVMs.

In this case, the proximal right middle and posterior cerebral arteries are both hypertrophied, indicating combined supply to the lesion. Venous drainage is both superficial and deep, as evidenced by enlargement of the straight sinus and superior sagittal sinus.

DIFFERENTIAL DIAGNOSIS:
LARGE LESION WITH DENSE, TUBULAR, AND SERPENTINE CONTRAST ENHANCEMENT

Case 494

58-year-old woman presenting with an apparent cerebrovascular accident.

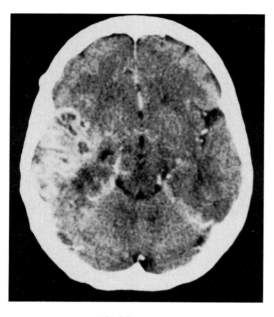

Glioblastoma.

Case 495

72-year-old woman presenting with an apparent cerebrovascular accident.

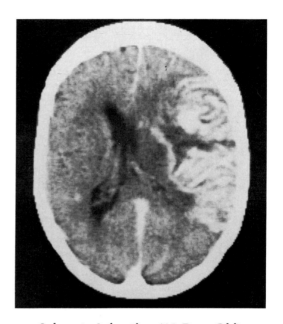

Subacute Infarction (19 Days Old).

Tubular or serpentine contrast enhancement is characteristic of AVMs. However, a similar appearance may be encountered in other lesions, particularly tumors and subacute cerebral infarctions.

The pattern of contrast enhancement within malignant gliomas is highly variable (see Cases 72 to 74). In some tumors a band-like or serpentine morphology predominates, mimicking an AVM as in Case 494.

Gyriform enhancement within areas of subacute infarction may also resemble the tortuous, curvilinear morphology of a vascular malformation. A clue to the correct diagnosis is the vascular distribution of ischemic lesions. In Case 495, the shape of the enhancing zone matches the characteristic trapezoidal territory of the middle cerebral artery (compare to Cases 406 and 407).

Clinical information often distinguishes among these lesions. However, AVMs can present with acute symptoms suggesting a "CVA" (due to "steal," hemorrhage, or seizure), matching the histories of the two patients illustrated here. As demonstrated in Cases 492 and 493, magnetic resonance imaging may be used to establish or exclude the diagnosis of AVM in ambiguous cases.

Case 496

81-year-old woman presenting with a
cerebrovascular accident.
(postcontrast scan)

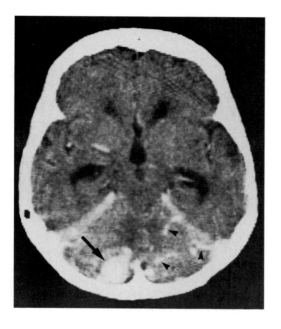

Case 497

49-year-old man presenting with seizures.
(postcontrast scan)

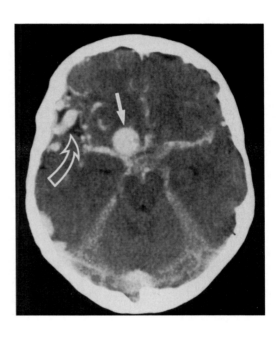

Hemorrhage is the most common presentation of AVMs, occurring in one third to two thirds of patients in most series. The majority of these hemorrhages are intracerebral rather than subarachnoid.

CT scans usually demonstrate both the hematoma and the responsible vascular malformation. Rarely a small AVM is destroyed at the time of rupture or compressed by the resulting hematoma.

In this case, a small cerebellar hematoma is seen *(large arrow)*, associated with several tortuous vascular channels *(small arrowheads)*. This particular pattern of enlarged cortical veins without a parenchymal nidus often indicates a predominantly dural AVM, as was true in this case.

Large veins are normally present near the tentorium (see Cases 506, 512, and 553B). These prominent vessels drain the inferior surface of the temporal and occipital lobes, passing through or near the tentorial dura to reach the transverse sinuses. Their location immediately adjacent to the tentorium distinguishes normal veins from the more scattered components of a true AVM, as seen here.

Case 568 presents another example of parenchymal hemorrhage from an AVM.

The high attenuation values filling the suprasellar cistern in this case represent subarachnoid hemorrhage, which was apparent on a precontrast scan. An AVM is present, involving the anterior right sylvian region *(open arrow)*.

In addition, a large, round collection of contrast is seen at the bifurcation of the right supraclinoid internal carotid artery (solid arrow). This structure was angiographically demonstrated to be an aneurysm and surgically proven to be the source of subarachnoid hemorrhage.

One or more aneurysms are frequently found along the course of arteries feeding an AVM. The occurrence of these aneurysms is likely flow related; they may thrombose spontaneously after the AVM is resected.

Among patients who present with subarachnoid hemorrhage and are found to have aneurysms associated with AVMs, the aneurysm is the more frequent source of bleeding.

CALCIFICATION IN AVMS

Case 498

49-year-old man presenting with seizures (same patient as Case 497).
(noncontrast scan)

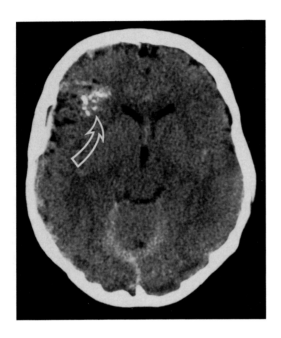

Case 499

10-year-old boy presenting with seizures.
(noncontrast scan)

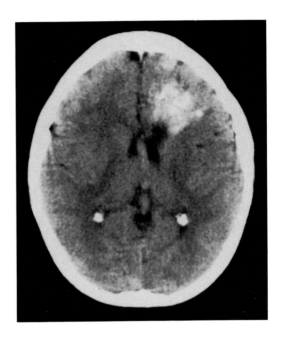

Many AVMs are associated with intracerebral calcification. The calcium may occur within the walls of vascular channels or within dystrophic cerebral parenchyma.

In this case, the cluster of right frontal calcifications is not associated with abnormal low attenuation or mass effect, as would be expected in a low-grade glioma (compare to Cases 66, 413, and 466). A contrast scan (see Case 497) demonstrated characteristic serpentine enhancement throughout the lesion.

Some AVMs are angiographically inapparent or "cryptic" due to thrombosis and/or low flow. Such lesions are usually detected on CT scans as small, high-attenuation regions. Their density may be due to calcification, blood volume, and/or contrast enhancement.

Calcification within an AVM may be very dense, suggesting a mass lesion. In this case, the presence of abnormal low attenuation deep to the lesion and associated deformity of the left frontal horn further support the possibility of a neoplasm (compare to Case 66).

Low-attenuation areas can be encountered within or adjacent to AVMs, usually reflecting encephalomalacia but occasionally representing active edema or recent infarction. Mass effect is also seen in a small number of AVMs, due to the bulk of the lesion or to associated hemorrhage and/or edema.

When the combination of these features is present, careful evaluation of the postcontrast scan and possible further evaluation by MR and/or angiography may be necessary to distinguish between AVM and tumor.

DIFFERENTIAL DIAGNOSIS:
CEREBRAL LESION WITH EXTENSIVE CALCIFICATION

Case 500

14-year-old girl presenting with right body numbness (same patient as Case 491).
(noncontrast scan)

Case 501

79-year-old woman presenting with "CVA."
(noncontrast scan)

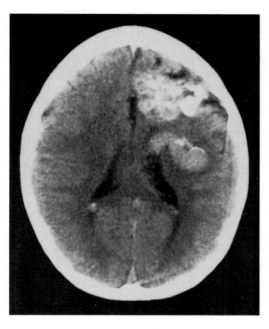

Arteriovenous Malformation.

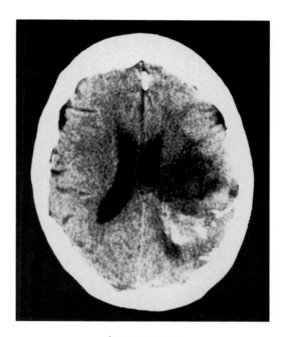

Astrocytoma.

The pattern of calcification within AVMs is highly variable. Rings or arcs of calcium may be seen in the walls of large arteries or veins, as demonstrated near the posterior margin of the lesion in Case 500. Other areas of an AVM may contain calcification that is finely granular or coarsely nodular, as seen anteriorly in Case 500.

An important clue to the correct diagnosis in Case 500 is atrophy associated with the lesion. The interhemispheric fissure and overlying cortical sulci are enlarged, arguing against a mass lesion and favoring a chronic process with long-standing parenchymal damage. Recognition of the draining varix posteriorly (compare to Case 491) clinches the diagnosis.

The calcification pattern of the glioma in Case 501 is nonspecific and could also be seen within an AVM. However, the associated mass effect and extensive abnormal low attenuation would be atypical for a vascular lesion and make neoplasm more likely.

The reason for the acute, stroke-like presentation of the mass in Case 501 is unclear (see discussion of Case 10).

VEIN OF GALEN ANEURYSMS

Case 502

2-day-old boy with congestive heart failure.
(noncontrast scan)

Case 503

2-month-old girl.
(noncontrast scan)

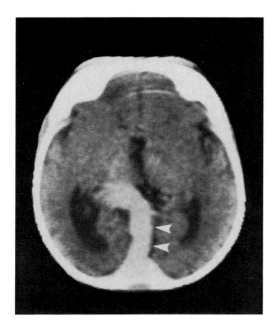

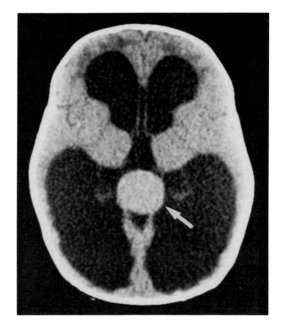

Some AVMs contain hugely dilated vascular channels. These structures may represent expansion of anatomically normal veins, as is commonly seen with malformations draining into the vein of Galen. Malformations in this region often contain direct arteriovenous shunts. The associated high flow causes marked enlargement of the receiving veins, traditionally misnamed as a "vein of Galen 'aneurysm.' "

This scan demonstrates expansion of the straight sinus (arrowheads) leading from a "vein of Galen aneurysm" to the torcular. High flow through a cerebral AVM is an important cause of neonatal heart failure, as in this patient. Case 505 presents a "vein of Galen aneurysm" in an adult.

High flow vascular malformations are often associated with distal stenosis of draining veins or dural sinuses, which contributes to their distension more proximally.

"Vein of Galen aneurysms" may cause hydrocephalus in children or adults. Venous hypertension may impair resorption of CSF, leading to communicating hydrocephalus (analogous to "otitic" hydrocephalus following dural sinus thrombosis; see Cases 304 and 474). More frequently the mass effect of the varix causes obstructive hydrocephalus by compressing the posterior third ventricle and aqueduct.

The central high attenuation of the "lesion" in this case is due to circulating blood. Intense enhancement would be seen throughout the varix after contrast injection (see Case 505). Such a uniformly dense and enhancing mass indenting the posterior third ventricle could be confused with a pineal region neoplasm (see Cases 224 to 226). Alternatively, variceal components of AVMs may mimic the precontrast density and intense contrast enhancement of a meningioma or a giant aneurysm (see Cases 504, 505, and 552).

Spin-echo MR scans of such cases demonstrate a large region of "flow void," establishing the vascular nature of the mass (see Case 509).

DIFFERENTIAL DIAGNOSIS:
INTENSELY ENHANCING MASS NEAR THE VEIN OF GALEN

Case 504

30-year-old woman with neurofibromatosis.
(postcontrast scan)

Case 505

33-year-old woman scanned because of head
trauma.
(postcontrast scan)

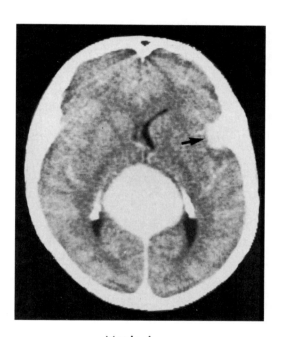

Meningioma.

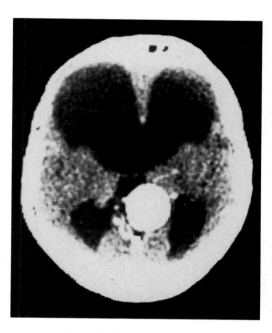

Vein of Galen Aneurysm.

The large subsplenial meningioma in Case 504 splays the posterior bodies of the lateral ventricles. A second, small meningioma is present near the pterion *(arrow)*.

Case 505 illustrates the adult presentation of a "vein of Galen aneurysm" that has caused long-standing hydrocephalus. Large, round aneurysms or varices demonstrate uniform density and intense contrast enhancement resembling the CT features of meningiomas.

Magnetic resonance imaging can easily differentiate these lesions, demonstrating lack of signal due to rapid blood flow in varices draining AVMs (see Case 509).

VENOUS ANGIOMAS

Case 506

12-year-old girl with seizures.

Case 507

65-year-old man.

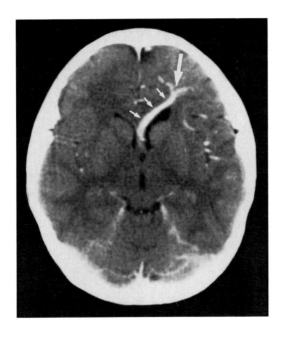

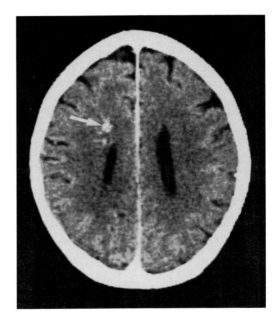

Venous angiomas have a characteristic morphology that is often recognizable on CT scans. The lesion has two components: (1) a group of radially oriented tributary veins converging like spokes of an umbrella to a central point, and (2) a single, abnormally large draining vein, formed at the confluence of the tributaries and following an aberrant route through cerebral parenchyma.

Here, the confluence of tributary channels is seen anteriorly *(large arrow),* with the draining vein *(small arrows)* coursing medially along the margin of the left frontal horn.

The prominent veins near the tentorium are a normal anatomical feature in this region (compare to Case 496).

This scan demonstrates a cross section of the enlarged draining vein as it is formed deep within the cerebral hemisphere. Radially oriented tributaries are faintly visible in the adjacent parenchyma. The aberrantly located, dilated "stem" of a venous angioma is highly characteristic even when tributary veins are inconspicuous.

Venous angiomas are most often incidental "anomalies" rather than threatening "malformations." They are infrequently associated with seizures, as in Case 506. Hemorrhage is uncommon; a possibly increased incidence in cerebellar lesions is controversial.

Venous angiomas are often found together with an adjacent cavernous angioma (see Cases 510 to 512), which may be mistaken for evidence of hemorrhage.

MR SPECTRUM OF VENOUS MALFORMATIONS

Case 508

24-year-old man.
(axial, noncontrast scan; SE 3000/80 with
gradient motion refocusing)

Venous Angioma of the Cerebellum.

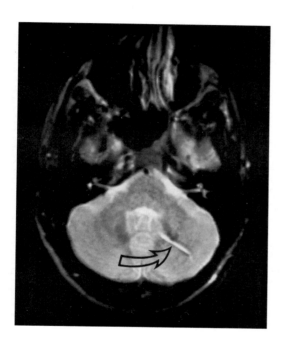

Case 509

2-month-old girl (same patient as in Case 503).
(axial, noncontrast scan; SE 2500/90 with
gradient motion refocusing)

Vein of Galen Aneurysm.

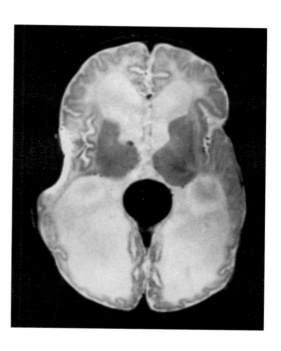

The MR appearance of a venous malformation depends on the rate of flow through the lesion and the nature of the pulse sequence.

In this case, a large, aberrant transparenchymal vascular channel within the left cerebellar hemisphere is typical for the "stem" vein of a venous angioma. These lesions are commonly found within the cerebellum, often arising near or draining to the fourth ventricle.

The high intensity within the large vein is due to rephasing of the signal from slowly flowing protons. This recovery of signal (i.e., avoidance of "flow void") is mainly due to refocusing features of current spin-echo pulse sequences. (Such sequences are designed primarily to reduce mismapping of CSF signal from pulsating cisterns.) Rephasing can also be seen on "even echoes" of non-refocused spin-echo sequences.

High signal intensity is regularly seen in slowly flowing veins (normal and pathological) after the injection of contrast material.

Rapid flow through the arterialized veins of a vascular malformation exceeds the rephasing capability of nonangiographic MR sequences. The signal void within such structures also persists after the injection of contrast material.

Here the dilated vein of Galen is strikingly defined as a midline zone of absent signal. Other sources of signal loss (e.g., dense calcification or marked T2-shortening) are rarely as uniform, severe, and sharply marginated as seen in this case.

CAVERNOUS ANGIOMAS (HEMANGIOMAS)

Case 510

43-year-old man.
(postcontrast scan)

Case 511

26-year-old woman with right arm weakness.
(noncontrast scan)

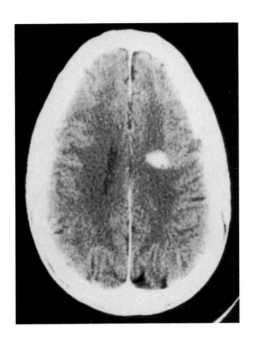

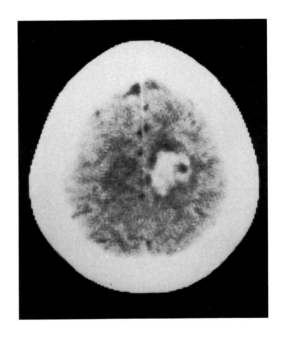

Cavernous hemangiomas or "angiomas" are collections of sinusoidal vascular spaces without intervening neuroglial tissue. Although well recognized pathologically as one of the major categories of cerebrovascular malformations, these lesions have been difficult to diagnose prior to CT scanning. Their frequent discovery by CT (and MR) requires recognition and distinction from other masses.

Noncontrast CT scans typically demonstrate a mixed- or high-attenuation lesion, which may be several millimeters to several centimeters in diameter. The high density represents blood volume, thrombosed channels, and/or associated calcification. Low attenuation may reflect adjacent encephalomalacia or old, clotted portions of the malformation.

Contrast enhancement varies from minimal to intense, as in this case. The CT appearance of small lesions may resemble an active demyelinating plaque, a focal subacute infarct, or a small metastasis (compare to Cases 11A, 310, and 417).

Large cavernous angiomas may resemble neoplasms, as seen here (and in Cases 514 and 516). Precontrast density is an important clue to the benign etiology and correct diagnosis of such lesions.

Another helpful characteristic of cavernous angiomas is frequent multiplicity, with occasional familiar incidence. Ambiguous lesions are commonly accompanied by other more typical angiomas, best demonstrated on MR scans (see Cases 516 and 517).

Cavernous angiomas are often apparent on CT studies despite their lack of angiographic visualization. (The angiogram in this case showed no abnormal vascularity or stain.) They account for a substantial number of the so-called "cryptic" vascular malformations.

The walls of the cavernous channels within hemangiomas are often thickened, with calcification or even ossification. Heavily calcified lesions have been termed "hemangioma calcificans."

DIFFERENTIAL DIAGNOSIS:
FOCAL, HIGH-ATTENUATION BRAIN STEM LESION

Case 512

59-year-old man with long-standing internuclear ophthalmoplegia.

Case 513

71-year-old man.

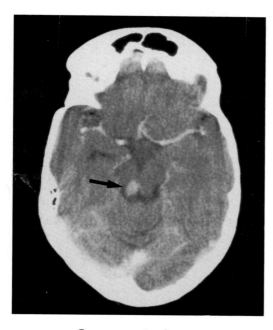

Cavernous Angioma.

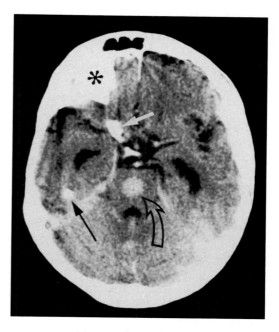

Metastatic Melanoma.

Cavernous angiomas commonly occur in the brain stem, where they may mimic primary or metastatic tumors. (The indolent or relapsing/remitting clinical course associated with these lesions may alternatively resemble multiple sclerosis.) Further characterization of such lesions is best accomplished by magnetic resonance imaging (see Cases 516 and 517).

Metastatic melanoma as in Case 513 *(open arrow)* may closely resemble a cavernous angioma by virtue of precontrast density and association with additional lesions at other sites. As discussed in Case 108, metastasis should be a strong consideration when a brain stem mass is encountered in an adult.

Normally prominent vessels are seen near the tentorium in Case 512. Case 513 demonstrates the false impression of calcified lesions caused by unilateral partial volume imaging of the orbital roof *(asterisk)*, anterior clinoid process *(white arrow)* and arcuate eminence of the petrous bone *(thin black arrow)* in the presence of head tilt.

DIFFERENTIAL DIAGNOSIS:
LARGE, ENHANCING BRAIN STEM MASS

Case 514

44-year-old man scanned because of schizophrenia.

Case 515

4-year-old boy presenting with ataxia and diplopia.

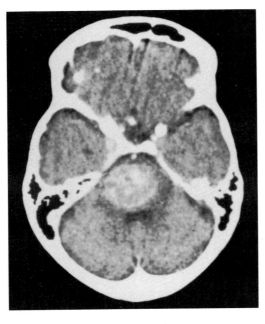

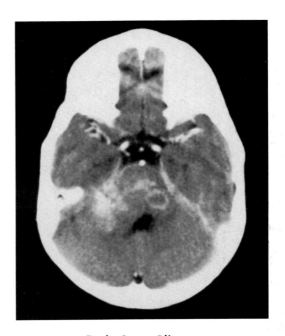

Cavernous Angioma.

Brain Stem Glioma.

Cavernous angiomas of the brain stem may be large lesions as in Case 514. The benign and chronic nature of these masses is usually reflected by minimal symptomatology and lack of progression. It is likely that many previously confusing cases of "stable" brain stem gliomas have in fact represented cavernous hemangiomas.

An appearance similar to that in Case 514 could be caused by a longstanding prepontine mass invaginating into the brain stem (e.g., chordoma, meningioma, or aneurysm; see Case 553).

Other varieties of vascular malformations may also involve the brain stem. The pathologically common capillary telangiectasia is rarely evident on CT scans, but may cause pontine hemorrhage. True AVMs of the brain stem occur, often bordering the fourth ventricle. Bulky components of an AVM may fill the ventricle, with their prominent enhancement suggesting an intraventricular tumor. In other cases, the poorly defined margin of a brain stem AVM may combine with nonspecific symptoms to mimic a glioma. The usual absence of mass effect in true AVMs favors the correct diagnosis.

Tumors of the brain stem are usually associated with early symptoms and a deteriorating course. The glioma in Case 515 is extensive, with mass effect expanding the pons and deforming the fourth ventricle (compare to Cases 106, 109, and 110).

MR CHARACTERIZATION OF CAVERNOUS ANGIOMAS

Case 516

45-year-old woman who had carried the diagnosis of "brain stem tumor" for 10 years. (sagittal, noncontrast scan; SE 700/16)

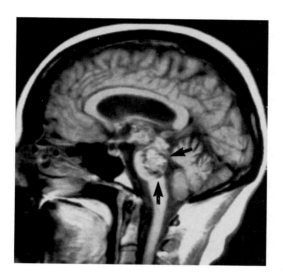

Case 517

38-year-old woman with a long history of seizures. (coronal, noncontrast scan; SE 3000/90)

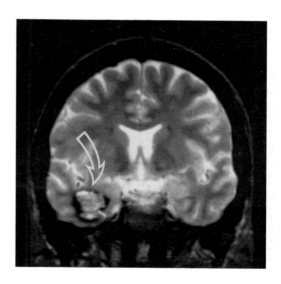

The MR appearance of cavernous angiomas is highly characteristic. An aggregate, multinodular, or "popcorn" morphology with prominent central zones of T1-shortening is surrounded by a characteristic rind of T2-shortening. Septations and focal areas of additional T2-shortening are often seen within the lesion. The brain stem "mass" seen here matches this typical pattern and almost certainly represents a cavernous angioma (compare to the CT scan in Case 514).

MR is highly sensitive to the detection of cavernous angiomas, which are often multiple. The demonstration of additional lesions may establish the diagnosis of an individual mass in equivocal cases. Gradient echo techniques exploiting susceptibility effects are more sensitive for this purpose than spin-echo sequences. (Gradient echo techniques are also more sensitive for detecting subtle hemorrhages associated with other pathologies such as shearing injuries or small vascular metastases.)

The MR study of this patient showed several other angiomas within the cerebral hemispheres. The patient's sister subsequently had an MR examination because of seizures and was found to also harbor multiple cavernous angiomas.

Cavernous angiomas are commonly found in the temporal lobes, where they represent an important cause of seizures. Mixed attenuation and frequent calcification in these lesions may resemble low-grade gliomas on CT scans.

The coronal plane and absence of bone artifact make MR superior to CT for evaluation of temporal lobe pathology (see Cases 104 and 105). Here, these imaging advantages demonstrate the familiar MR stereotype of a cavernous angioma within the right temporal lobe. The absence of edema and mass effect support the diagnosis of a low-grade, long-standing lesion.

Occasionally hemorrhage into a neoplasm (e.g., metastatic melanoma or hypernephroma) can mimic the MR characteristics of cavernous angiomas. Care should be taken to assess the clinical context and secondary scan features (e.g., surrounding edema) when "angiomas" are diagnosed.

Thrombosed or low-flow AVMs may also have a similar MR appearance and "mixed" vascular malformations containing several histological patterns are common.

Thrombosed aneurysms may present with a mixture of signal intensities resembling that of cavernous angiomas. However, the pattern or structure of such lesions is often lamellar (see Cases 543 and 545), in contrast to the nodular or "honeycomb" architecture of most cavernous angiomas.

SUBARACHNOID HEMORRHAGE

Case 518

58-year-old man with sudden headache
followed by loss of consciousness.
(noncontrast scan)

Ruptured Aneurysm of the Anterior
Communicating Artery.

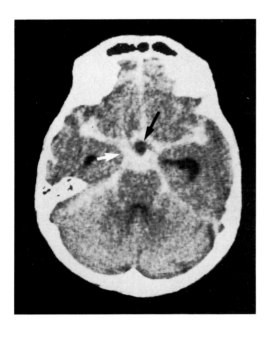

Subarachnoid hemorrhage is usually apparent on CT scans. The high attenuation of blood replaces the low density of spinal fluid, causing normally "black" CSF spaces to become "white." The hemorrhage may be symmetrical and diffuse, as in this case, or localized to a single cistern (see Case 520).

Blood within the spinal fluid serves as a subarachnoid contrast agent, outlining surface anatomy. Here the brain stem is well defined, as is the uncus *(white arrow)*. The filling defect in the suprasellar cistern *(black arrow)* is a combined image of the optic chiasm (anterior, transverse band) and the dilated anterior recesses of the third ventricle (circular posterior component).

Case 519

67-year-old woman presenting with sudden
headache and nausea.
(noncontrast scan)

Ruptured Aneurysm of the Anterior
Communicating Artery.

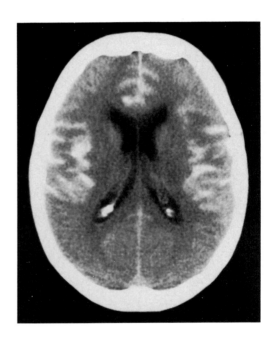

Subarachnoid blood may fill the sylvian cisterns, interhemispheric fissure, and cortical sulci. Symmetrical subarachnoid hemorrhage as in this case is often seen with ruptured aneurysms of the anterior communicating artery. The sylvian hemorrhages document the deep medial extension of the insular cisterns.

SUBTLE SUBARACHNOID HEMORRHAGE

Case 520

50-year-old woman.
(noncontrast scan)

Ruptured Aneurysm of the Middle Cerebral Artery.

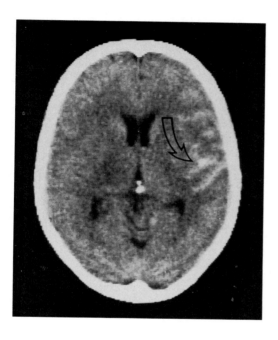

Case 521

57-year-old man scanned 6 days after rupture of an aneurysm of the anterior communicating artery.

Isodense Subarachnoid Spaces.

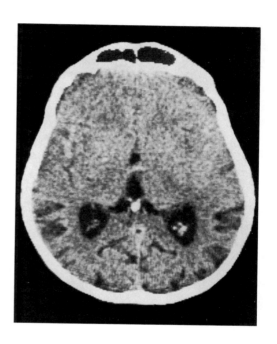

A small amount of subarachnoid hemorrhage may remain localized near the site of bleeding. Focal high attenuation within sulci or cisterns will then predict the source of hemorrhage. Angiography in this case demonstrated an aneurysm of the left middle cerebral artery.

The attenuation of blood within the subarachnoid space depends on the amount and age of the hemorrhage. Cases with small or subacute hemorrhages may demonstrate isodense cisterns and sulci, as seen here in the frontal and sylvian regions. (Compare the lack of surface topography anteriorly with the normal sulcal markings posteriorly; see also Case 536.)

Other causes for isodense subarachnoid spaces include filling of the cisterns by inflammatory exudate (*i.e.*, meningitis; see Cases 256 and 257) or tumor spread (e.g., CSF seeding from medulloblastoma, ependymoma, or germinoma; see Case 121).

MR CORRELATION: SUBARACHNOID HEMORRHAGE

Case 522

64-year-old woman, 1 week after hemorrhage
from an aneurysm at the PICA origin.
(sagittal, noncontrast scan; SE 600/17)

Case 523

74-year-old woman 2 days after subarachnoid
hemorrhage of undetermined origin.
(sagittal, noncontrast scan; SE 750/20)

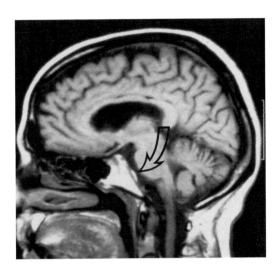

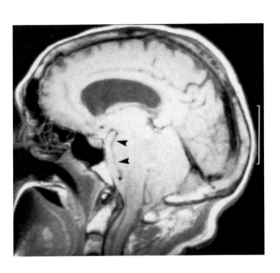

Magnetic resonance imaging is less sensitive than CT for the diagnosis of acute subarachnoid hemorrhage. A number of factors probably contribute to the inconspicuity of subarachnoid blood on MR scans. High oxygen tension within the CSF, spinal fluid pulsation, and averaging of subtle signal changes with the long T1 and T2 values of CSF have been suggested as possible causes.

On the other hand, MR can confirm the suspicion of subacute subarachnoid hemorrhage at a stage when the CT attenuation of cisterns has returned to near normal. In this case, the small area of T1-shortening along the posterior surface of the clivus (arrow) represents residual subacute thrombus. Similar remnants of clot may be found on MR scans adjacent to a ruptured aneurysm, helping to localize the site of bleeding.

MR scans in patients with massive subarachnoid hemorrhage may demonstrate replacement of CSF spaces by altered signal intensity, as seen here. The prepontine cistern is filled with nearly isointense hemorrhage, surrounding and defining the lumen of the basilar artery (arrowheads).

This appearance is not specific. A similar pattern might be seen in meningeal carcinomatosis or exudative meningitis (see Case 262).

COMPLICATIONS OF SUBARACHNOID HEMORRHAGE

Case 524

69-year-old woman.

Acute Hydrocephalus Associated With Ruptured MCA Aneurysm

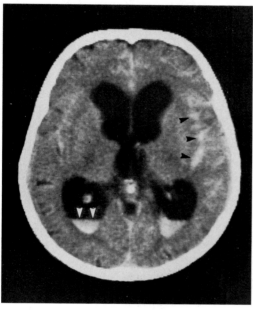

Case 525

65-year-old woman.

Widespread Infarction due to Vasospasm.

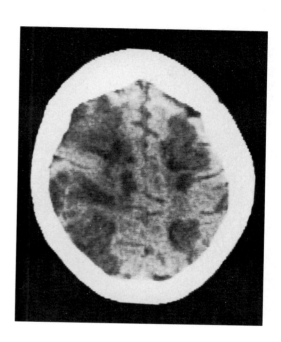

Hydrocephalus may develop at several stages following subarachnoid hemorrhage. Acute hydrocephalus as in Case 524 may be obstructive (due to clot within the ventricular system) or communicating (attributed to clogging of arachnoid granulations by erythrocytes). Delayed communicating hydrocephalus (see Cases 527 and 602) is thought to be caused by postinflammatory changes in meningeal CSF pathways, including the arachnoid granulations. Hydrocephalus may compound parenchymal damage by increasing intracranial pressure at a time when cerebral perfusion is marginal due to developing vasospasm.

Intraventricular hemorrhage, as seen here in the lateral ventricular trigones *(white arrowheads),* is commonly associated with subarachnoid blood. An aneurysm may rupture directly into the ventricular system, or a parenchymal hematoma adjacent to an aneurysm may secondarily decompress into the ventricles. In other cases, no direct communication from the aneurysm site can be demonstrated, and blood appears to have flooded retrograde through the fourth ventricle and aqueduct.

Blood/fluid levels in the trigones or occipital horns of the lateral ventricles may be the only CT clue to recent subarachnoid bleeding.

Spasm of cerebral arteries is a common and serious complication of subarachnoid hemorrhage. Spasm typically develops a few days after hemorrhage, reaching a maximum in the late first week to early second week and subsiding thereafter. The vessels most severely involved tend to be those in areas of densest subarachnoid hemorrhage.

Infarction due to spasm may present at watershed regions, as in this case (compare to Cases 428 and 429), or in major arterial distributions.

In addition to hydrocephalus and infarction, recurrent bleeding is a third cause of delayed deterioration in patients suffering subarachnoid hemorrhage. Ten percent to 20% of patients experience a second hemorrhage within 2 weeks of initial presentation.

DIFFERENTIAL DIAGNOSIS:
ENHANCING SUBARACHNOID SPACES WITH COMMUNICATING HYDROCEPHALUS

Case 526

76-year-old woman.

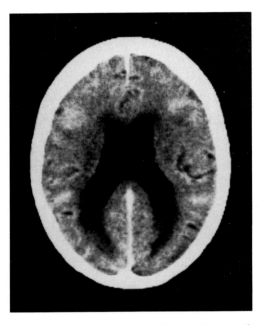

Meningeal Carcinomatosis From Metastatic Carcinoma of the Breast.

Case 527

79-year-old woman.

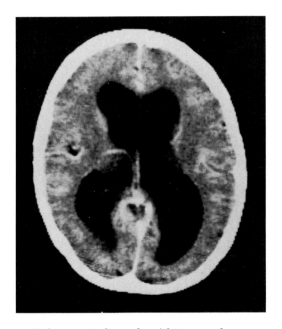

Subacute Subarachnoid Hemorrhage.

Enhancing subarachnoid spaces may reflect a variety of pathologies, including meningeal spread of CNS or systemic neoplasm as in Case 526. Enhancing sulci filled with meningeal tumor contrast with the normal low attenuation of adjacent uninvolved subarachnoid spaces.

Contrast enhancement is often seen in cisterns and sulci recently exposed to subarachnoid hemorrhage. In Case 527, the subarachnoid spaces were isodense on a precontrast scan. Diffuse enhancement of most sulci is demonstrated.

The mechanism of contrast enhancement following subarachnoid hemorrhage is unclear but may include components of contrast extravasation as well as meningeal hyperemia. Cisternal enhancement may be more apparent than the underlying subarachnoid hemorrhage, offering an important clue to the diagnosis.

The differential diagnosis of enhancing subarachnoid spaces also includes meningitis (see Cases 258 and 259). The subarachnoid spaces of children may normally appear dense on postcontrast scans when enhancing vessels almost fill the small sulci. A similar finding may be seen within compressed cisterns in the presence of hydrocephalus or increased intracranial pressure (see Cases 222 and 224). When this appearance accompanies hydrocephalus due to a tumor, the possibility of CSF "seeding" may be difficult to exclude.

As discussed in Case 524, communicating hydrocephalus may be seen both acutely and as a delayed complication in subarachnoid hemorrhage. Communicating hydrocephalus can also accompany enhancing subarachnoid spaces in meningitis (see Cases 256 to 259) or meningeal carcinomatosis, as in Case 526.

HEMORRHAGE FROM ANEURYSMS OF THE ANTERIOR COMMUNICATING ARTERY

Case 528

67-year-old woman presenting with acute nausea and headache (same patient as Case 519).

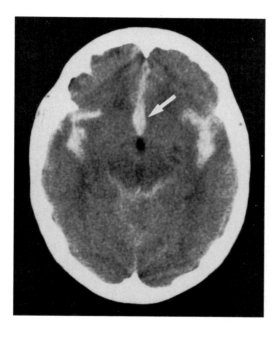

Case 529

50-year-old man.

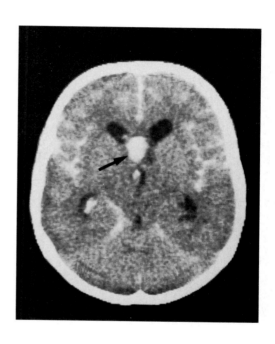

Hemorrhage from anterior communicating artery (ACoA) aneurysms may include subarachnoid and intracerebral components. The subarachnoid blood is often symmetrically distributed, as seen here and in Cases 518, 519, and 521.

The cistern of the lamina terminalis (CLT) is a characteristic location for a small amount of hemorrhage from a ruptured ACoA aneurysm. This small interhemispheric component of the subarachnoid space is located immediately anterior to the third ventricle (see Case 374). Normally, the low attenuation of CSF within the two regions is continuous. Here the CLT is filled with blood *(arrow),* sharply defining the anterior wall (lamina terminalis) of the mildly distended third ventricle.

Parenchymal hematomas from ruptured aneurysms of the anterior communicating artery often involve anterior midline structures. A hematoma within the inferior portion of the septum pellucidum *(arrow)* is highly specific but occurs in a minority of cases. Such hematomas are often continuous with clot distending the cistern of the lamina terminalis, as illustrated in Case 528.

Ruptured aneurysms of the anterior communicating artery may also cause eccentric intracerebral hematomas, often demonstrating a "tail" or track leading back to the aneurysm site (see Case 567).

Inferior frontal hematomas resembling the appearance of a ruptured ACoA aneurysm are occasionally seen as the presentation of dural AVMs involving the floor of the anterior cranial fossa. Such malformations are usually fed by ethmoidal branches of the opthalmic artery and are often associated with fragile draining varices.

HEMORRHAGE FROM ANEURYSMS OF THE MIDDLE CEREBRAL ARTERY

Case 530

69-year-old woman.

Case 531

48-year-old woman.

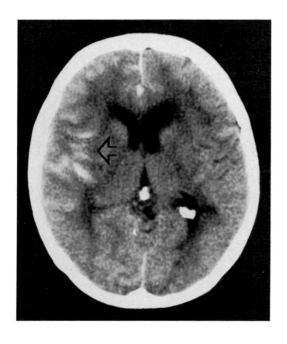

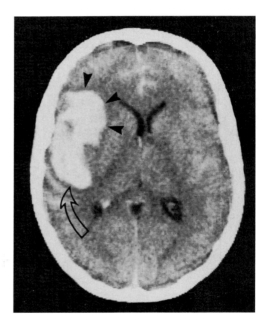

Subarachnoid hemorrhage from rupture of middle cerebral artery aneurysms often accumulates asymmetrically in the ipsilateral sylvian cistern, as seen here (and in Cases 520 and 531). The appearance of blood within sylvian sulci may mimic the morphology of hemorrhagic infarction involving the distribution of the middle cerebral artery; compare this scan to Case 407.

The distribution of subarachnoid blood is not an infallible guide to the location of a responsible aneurysm. Considerable overlap occurs in the patterns of hemorrhage from different aneurysm sites. For example, ruptured aneurysms of the anterior or posterior communicating artery could produce an image comparable to this case.

Apart from predicting aneurysm location, the amount and distribution of subarachnoid blood is important for estimating the likelihood and location of subsequent vascular spasm (see Case 525).

Intracerebral hemorrhage from aneurysms of the middle cerebral artery usually occurs in the inferior frontotemporal region *(arrowheads)*. A more common finding is a cisternal hematoma in the sylvian area *(open arrow)*.

Such a clot represents accumulation of subarachnoid blood within the confines of the expanded sylvian cistern. The resulting subarachnoid hematoma acts like an intracerebral mass, but can be removed from the cistern without a cortical incision. (Similar loculation of subarachnoid blood may occur within the spinal canal, causing focal mass effect and cord compression.)

A tiny clot at the foramen of Monro, as seen here on the right, is occasionally an isolated clue to recent intraventricular hemorrhage.

HEMORRHAGE FROM ANEURYSMS OF THE POSTERIOR CIRCULATION

Case 532

64-year-old man.

Ruptured Aneurysm of the Posterior Communicating Artery.

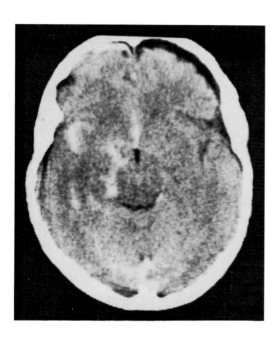

The so-called "posterior communicating artery" aneurysms arise from the supraclinoid internal carotid artery at the origin of the posterior communicating artery. Rupture of these aneurysms may produce a typical distribution of subarachnoid blood, as illustrated here.

Hemorrhage is most dense within the ipsilateral portions of the suprasellar, perimesencephalic, and proximal sylvian cisterns. A small subdural hematoma is present at the frontal pole, and a small subdural hygroma is seen on the opposite side, suggesting superimposed trauma.

Rupture of aneurysms may cause acute subdural hematomas, most commonly associated with aneurysms of the internal carotid and middle cerebral arteries. On the other hand, head trauma rarely causes dense, basal subarachnoid hemorrhage. An underlying aneurysm should be suspected whenever such hemorrhage is found, even with the history of trauma.

Case 533

52-year-old woman.

Ruptured Aneurysm at the Tip of the Basilar Artery.

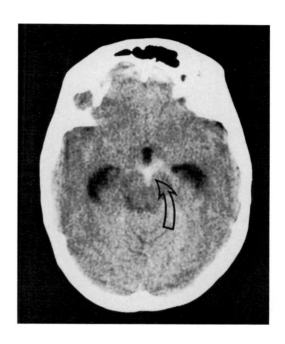

The small amount of subarachnoid hemorrhage in this case is concentrated in the interpeduncular cistern, implicating the basilar artery as the source of bleeding. Aneurysms at the tip of the basilar artery are difficult to manage and carry the risk of secondary diencephalic infarction (see Case 449).

Enlargement of the temporal horns and anterior recesses of the third ventricle is due to associated hydrocephalus, as discussed in Case 524.

Subarachnoid hemorrhage localized to the posterior fossa usually indicates a ruptured aneurysm of the vertebrobasilar system. A spinal source of subarachnoid bleeding should also be considered in such cases, particularly if cerebral angiography is initially negative.

VISUALIZATION OF UNRUPTURED ANEURYSMS

Case 534

82-year-old woman.
(noncontrast scan)

Aneurysm at the Genu of the Middle Cerebral Artery.

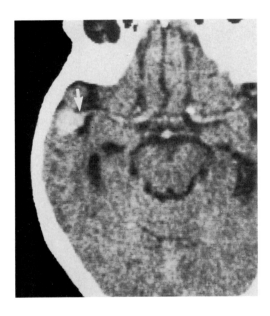

Case 535

72-year-old man.
(postcontrast scan)

Posterior Cerebral Artery Aneurysm.

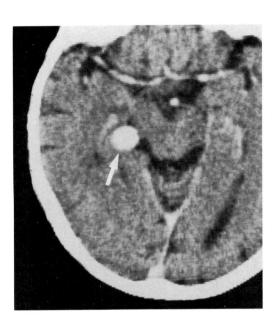

Unruptured aneurysms are sometimes discovered incidentally. They present as small, round masses with central high attenuation due to the blood they contain. A few flecks of peripheral calcification are common (see Cases 166 and 538).

The relationship of the aneurysm to a parent vessel may be clearly demonstrated, as in this case (*arrow;* see also Case 537).

Aneurysms may be found at sites distant from the circle of Willis. Peripheral aneurysms exhibit the same characteristics of extra-axial location and intense contrast enhancement seen in conventional lesions. In this case the aneurysm is well defined as an extra-axial mass displacing the adjacent cerebral peduncle and widening the perimesencephalic cistern.

When aneurysms are found in peripheral locations, the possibility of mycotic, traumatic, or neoplastic origin should be considered. This lesion was found to be an unusual congenital aneurysm arising from the perimesencephalic portion of the posterior cerebral artery.

DIFFERENTIAL DIAGNOSIS:
SMALL, MIDLINE HIGH-ATTENUATION STRUCTURE NEAR THE ANTERIOR CIRCLE OF WILLIS

Case 536

37-year-old woman.
(noncontrast scan)

Case 537

73-year-old man.
(postcontrast scan)

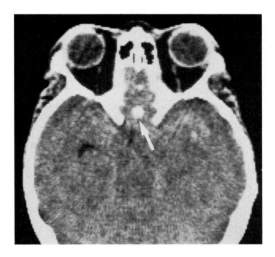

Tuberculum Sellae (with Subarachnoid Hemorrhage from a Posterior Communicating Artery Aneurysm).

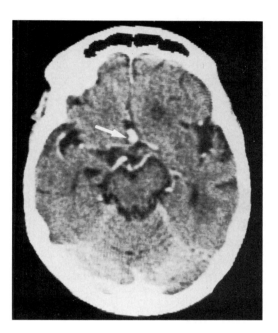

Unruptured Anterior Communicating Artery Aneurysm.

The superior surface of the tuberculum sellae is often imaged as a small area of high attenuation on scans passing through the circle of Willis (*arrow*, Case 536). This midline density may be mistaken for calcification, contrast, or clot within an aneurysm of the anterior communicating artery.

Partial imaging of an anterior clinoid process may produce a "pseudoaneurysm" near the supraclinoid internal carotid artery. These spurious islands of density are comparable to the partial visualization of the petrous bone in Cases 513 and 583A.

Pneumatization of the tuberculum sellae or anterior clinoid process may cause similar confusion on MR scans. Partial volume of such air-containing bony prominences may mimic the "flow-void" of small patent aneurysms at these locations (see Case 542).

In Case 536, hemorrhage within CSF spaces causes them to appear isodense (see Case 521, and compare to the appearance of meningitis in Case 257).

DIFFERENTIAL DIAGNOSIS:
CALCIFIED, ENHANCING MASS AT THE FORAMEN MAGNUM

Case 538

73-year-old woman.

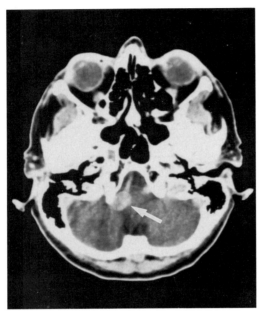

**Unruptured Aneurysm at the Origin of the
Posterior Inferior Cerebellar Artery.**

Case 539

85-year-old woman.

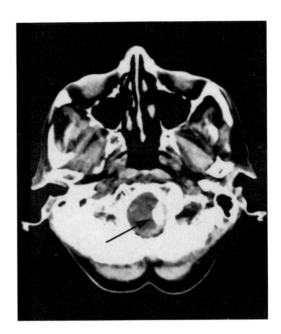

Meningioma.

The frequent calcification and intense contrast enhancement of aneurysms may resemble extra-axial tumors in several common locations. Among these is the foramen magnum, where aneurysms arising from the distal vertebral arteries are encountered as in Case 538. Such lesions can mimic the appearance of meningiomas that occur commonly at this site, particularly in elderly patients.

Clues to the correct diagnoses include continuity of the lesion with the vertebral artery in Case 538 and the solid pattern of calcification favoring a mass in Case 539. Neither feature is decisive and these lesions can be indistinguishable on CT examinations.

MR studies are useful in evaluating such cases. Coronal and sagittal scans provide an excellent view of the foramen magnum (see Cases 161 and 162), and the characteristic signal void of flowing blood localizes the vertebral arteries with respect to adjacent masses.

Occasionally the odontoid process rises into the foramen magnum and can be mistaken for a calcified lesion (see Case 809).

DIFFERENTIAL DIAGNOSIS:
UNIFORMLY ENHANCING PARASELLAR MASS

Case 540

86-year-old woman with a 2-year history of diplopia and right sided ptosis.

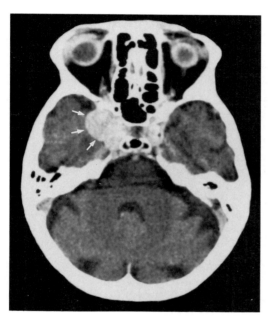

Aneurysm of the Parasellar Internal Carotid Artery.

Case 541

62-year-old woman presenting with decreased vision in the right eye (same patient as Case 215).

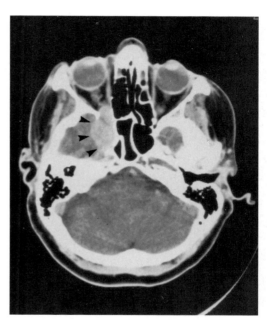

Meningioma.

Aneurysmal ectasia of the internal carotid artery is a common parasellar mass in adults. The vessel is often calcified, with little intraluminal thrombus. The resulting precontrast density and marked contrast enhancement may closely resemble a parasellar meningioma.

In Case 540, the lateral margin of the intracavernous aneurysm *(arrows)* bulges into the medial portion of the middle cranial fossa. The meningioma in Case 541 occupies a similar location, extending through the superior orbital fissure to involve the orbital apex. Both of these long-standing masses have caused erosion of the sphenoid bone.

Magnetic resonance imaging can distinguish between these lesions (see Cases 542 through 545). Patent aneurysms demonstrate "flow void" or lack of signal on standard pulse sequences. Partially thrombosed aneurysms often contain a lamellar pattern with components of short T1 and short T2. Such findings contrast with the variable but more uniform tissue intensity seen within meningiomas. Alternatively, flow-sensitive sequences may be used to demonstrate augmentation of signal intensity within a patent aneurysm, distinguishing it from a solid neoplasm.

Other enhancing parasellar masses include lateral extensions of pituitary adenomas (see Case 214), metastases (see Cases 212 and 213), chordomas and chondromas (see Cases 157 and 158), carotid-cavernous fistulas distending the cavernous sinus (see Case 665), inflammatory processes extending from the sphenoid sinus (e.g., mucocele, aspergillosis) and inflammatory disorders involving the cavernous sinus (e.g., Tolosa-Hunt syndrome, Wegener's granulomatosis).

Case 542

61-year-old woman.
(axial, noncontrast scan; SE 3000/90)

Small, Patent Aneurysms of the Supraclinoid Internal Carotid Artery and Middle Cerebral Artery.

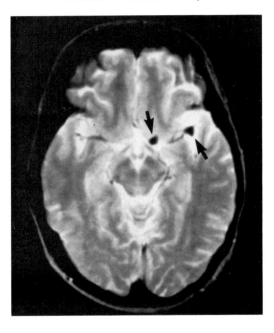

Case 543

59-year-old woman.
(sagittal, noncontrast scan; SE 600/17)

Thrombosed Aneurysm of the Rostral Basilar Artery.

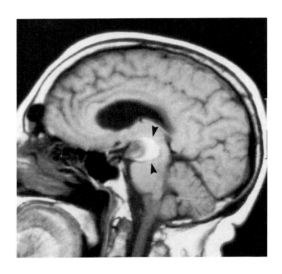

Small, patent aneurysms can be identified on spin-echo MR studies as nodular expansions of "flow void" along the course of cerebral arteries. Such lesions are particularly well outlined by the high signal intensity of CSF on T2-weighted sequences, as in this case (arrows).

Large, patent aneurysms may present a more complicated appearance. Zones of slow flow or stasis within giant aneurysms can generate regions of variable signal that may be difficult to distinguish from thrombus. Gradient echo sequences emphasizing flow-related enhancement help to separate these intraluminal components. (Both slow flow and thrombus may be associated with enhancement on post-contrast MR scans.)

As discussed in Case 536, partial volume imaging of a pneumatized anterior clinoid process may mimic the MR appearance of a small aneurysm of the paraclinoid internal carotid artery.

Partially or completely thrombosed aneurysms present a variety of MR appearances depending on the age of intraluminal clot and the parameters of the pulse sequence. On T1-weighted images, thrombosed aneurysms often demonstrate a mixture of isointensity and high signal zones, as in this case.

Here the interpeduncular cistern is occupied by a mass containing a broad, crescentic layer of T1-shortening posteriorly. This indication of subacute thrombus combines with the location adjacent to the basilar tip to establish the correct diagnosis.

Compare the morphology of this lesion to other suprasellar masses containing hemorrhage in Cases 178 and 205.

Case 544

86-year-old woman (same patient as Case 540).
(axial, noncontrast scan; SE 3000/28 without motion compensation)

Partially Thrombosed Aneurysm of the Parasellar Internal Carotid Artery.

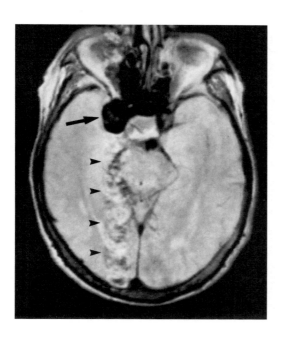

Case 545

59-year-old woman (same patient as Case 543).
(axial, noncontrast scan; SE 2500/28)

Thrombosed Aneurysm of the Rostral Basilar Artery.

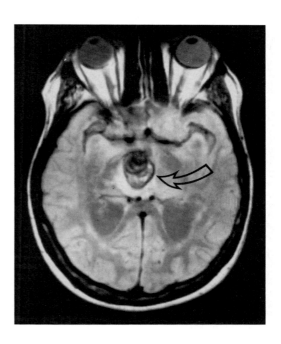

Low signal intensity may be found within cerebral aneurysms on long TR spin echo images due to marked T2-shortening within thrombus. This effect is probably due to old blood products such as hemosiderin (see Cases 562 and 563). The resultant loss of signal may blend with the "flow void" in patent portions of the aneurysm lumen.

In this case a CT scan had identified a parasellar mass, and MR was performed to distinguish between meningioma and aneurysm (see Cases 538 to 541). The MR study makes the diagnosis of aneurysm by demonstrating characteristic T2-shortening *(arrow)* and marked pulsation artifact *(arrowheads)*. This spatial mismapping of signal intensity from moving structures occurs along the phase-encoding axis and is most marked on long TR sequences without motion compensation.

A reliable hallmark of thrombosed aneurysms on CT or MR scans is lamination. Long TR MR images often highlight this feature, as seen here. Such characteristic layered morphology distinguishes thrombosed aneurysms from other suprasellar or midbrain masses.

A small amount of edema is seen surrounding the aneurysm.

Compare this MR scan to the CT study in Case 551.

Case 546

70-year-old woman.
(noncontrast scan)

Ruptured Giant Aneurysm of the Supraclinoid Internal Carotid Artery.

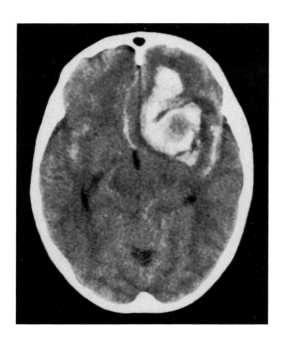

Case 547

64-year-old woman.
(postcontrast scan)

Unruptured Giant Aneurysm of the Basilar Artery.

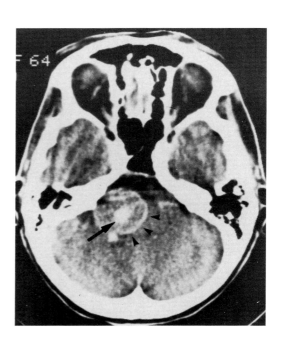

Large aneurysms have been angiographically described as "giant" when their diameter reaches 2.5 cm. Giant aneurysms most commonly arise from the supraclinoid internal carotid artery or the middle cerebral artery. They often present as mass lesions, but hemorrhage is not as rare as previously believed.

In this case, a rind of hemorrhage surrounds the largely thrombosed giant aneurysm, which is seen as a filling defect within the hematoma. Blood has dissected anteriorly into the frontal lobe, and subarachnoid hemorrhage is present.

Giant aneurysms frequently demonstrate peripheral arcs or rims of calcification. Their lumens are usually at least partially occupied by thrombus, which often has a lamellar or concentric appearance. The association of hemorrhage with a large, marble-like mass near the skull base is highly characteristic of a ruptured giant aneurysm.

When giant aneurysms occur in a suprasellar location, the combination of peripheral calcification and segmental enhancement may resemble a craniopharyngioma (see Case 189).

Contrast enhancement within giant aneurysms may take several forms. Occasionally the lumen is entirely patent. The uniform precontrast density of circulating blood and the intense enhancement following injection of contrast may then mimic a meningioma (analogous to the appearance of a variceal vein of Galen; see Cases 503 and 505). Thrombosed giant aneurysms typically demonstrate a thin rim of surrounding enhancement due to adventitia or "capsule."

Many lesions present a combination or "target" appearance, as in this case. A small, slightly eccentric lumen (arrow) is surrounded by a large zone of nonenhancing thrombus, which is in turn bordered by a rim of peripheral enhancement (small arrowheads).

GIANT ANEURYSMS AS MASS LESIONS

Case 548A

76-year-old man with progressive aphasia referred from an outside hospital for resection of a "brain tumor."
(noncontrast scan)

Case 548B

Same patient.
(coronal, noncontrast scan; SE 600/15)

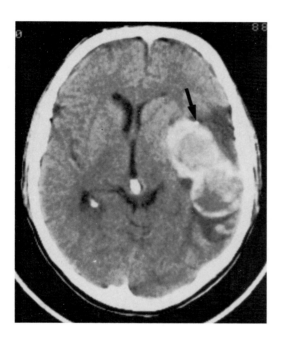

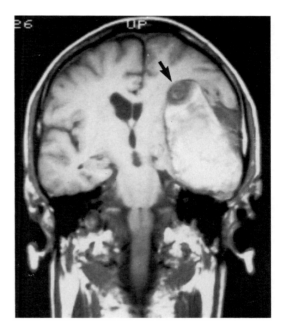

The clinical presentation of patients with giant intracranial aneurysms often reflects the mass effect of the lesion. In this case the bilobed mass in the left sylvian region has caused midline shift with compression of the ipsilateral ventricle. Low attenuation surrounding the mass could be interpreted as edema, and high attenuation values within the lesion could be considered to represent intratumoral hemorrhage.

The recognition of this mass as a thrombosed giant aneurysm is based on several points. While hemorrhage may occur in malignant tumors (see Cases 10, 94, 95, 413, and 566), the peripheral or rim-like pattern seen here would be unusual. An important second clue to the diagnosis of giant aneurysm is the small amount of calcification in the wall of the lesion (arrow). Finally, the "mass" occupies a location which is potentially extra-axial, with the surrounding "edema" representing distorted cisterns.

A coronal MR scan in this case demonstrates that the middle fossa "tumor" is an extra-axial mass, filled with subacute thrombus. The appearance suggests a giant aneurysm of the middle cerebral artery.

Giant aneurysms can reach remarkable size through slow expansion, gradually deforming the surrounding brain. (Compare to the prolonged growth of intracranial meningiomas, as in Case 33.) Here the midline shift is quite small for the size of the mass, attesting to its long-standing nature.

At angiography, the horizontal segment of the middle cerebral artery was draped over the top of the aneurysm. A small patent lumen was found, corresponding to the low-intensity zone at the dome of the lesion (arrow).

BASILAR ARTERY ANEURYSMS

Case 549	Case 550
77-year-old man.	70-year-old woman.
Saccular Aneurysm (Partially Thrombosed).	**Fusiform Aneurysm (Partially Thrombosed).**

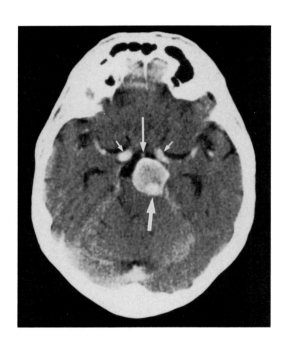

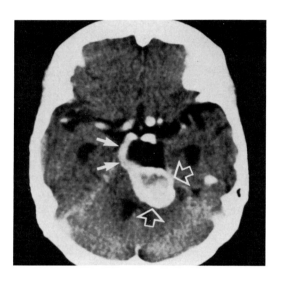

Two categories of aneurysms may involve the basilar artery. Saccular or "berry" aneurysms are usually seen as discrete vascular masses near the vertebrobasilar junction (as in Case 547) or at the basilar artery tip, as seen here.

In this case the aneurysm is largely thrombosed, with an enhancing rim and a residual enhancing lumen seen posteriorly *(thick arrow)*. A small "dot" of enhancement at the ventral margin of the aneurysm *(thin arrow)* is the pituitary infundibulum. Mild ectasia of the supraclinoid internal carotid arteries is also present *(small arrows)*.

A second type of basilar artery aneurysm is due to fusiform, atherosclerotic ectasia of the vessel, which may reach aneurysmal proportions. This dilatation is often combined with elongation (see "dolichoectasia," Cases 554 and 555).

This case demonstrates a combination of dolichoectatic and aneurysmal features. A calcified aneurysm *(open arrows)* is superimposed on an elongated basilar artery *(solid arrows)*. This long-standing extra-axial mass has become imbedded against the brain stem, deforming the fourth ventricle. Posterior displacement of the brain stem has widened the prepontine cistern.

DIFFERENTIAL DIAGNOSIS:
MASS ADJACENT TO THE ROSTRAL BASILAR ARTERY

Case 551

59-year-old woman.
(noncontrast scan)

Case 552

56-year-old man.
(postcontrast scan)

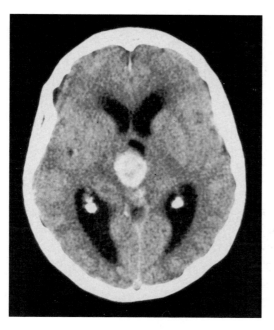

Basilar Artery Aneurysm.

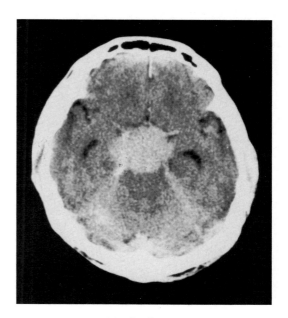

Meningioma.

Aneurysms arising from the tip of the basilar artery may ascend to deform the diencephalon and third ventricle. Such lesions may be mistaken for suprasellar or pineal region tumors.

In Case 551 a thrombosed aneurysm of the basilar artery compresses the posterior third ventricle, causing moderate hydrocephalus. The extensive invagination of this extra-axial lesion mimics an intrinsic mass such as a diencephalic glioma (compare to Cases 226 and 227). Patent aneurysms of the basilar tip can present as uniformly enhancing masses in the suprasellar region, mimicking meningioma or germinoma.

The peripheral rim of high attenuation surrounding the dense center of the lesion in Case 551 is characteristic of a thrombosed aneurysm (compare to Cases 547 and 549). The CT suspicion of a thrombosed or patent aneurysm may be confirmed by magnetic resonance imaging, as illustrated in Cases 542 to 545 and 548.

The retrosellar meningioma in Case 552 closely resembles the other uniformly enhancing suprasellar masses discussed above and illustrated in Cases 165 to 168. Compare also to Cases 504 and 505.

BASILAR ARTERY ECTASIA MIMICKING A BRAIN STEM LESION

Case 553A

60-year-old woman.

Case 553B

Same patient.

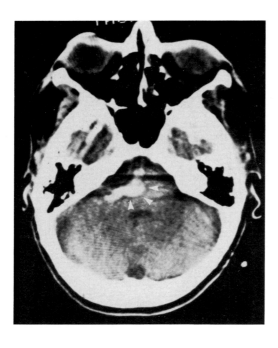

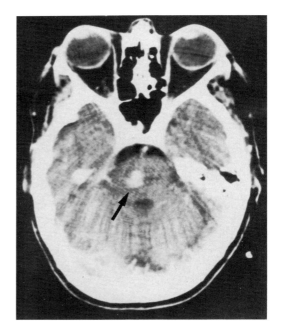

Atherosclerotic ectasia and tortuosity of the basilar artery may cause substantial deformity of the brain stem and/or cranial nerves. Associated symptoms may suggest an intra-axial process, and CT scans may be mistakenly interpreted to support the diagnosis of an intrinsic brain stem lesion.

In this case, focal dilatation *(arrowheads)* is superimposed on generalized ectasia at the vertebrobasilar junction.

Prepontine extra-axial lesions may indent the ventral surface of the brain stem. Axial scans passing through the superoposterior portion of such embedded lesions cause them to appear intra-axial. Tumors that may present in this manner include meningioma, epidermoid cyst, and chordoma.

The dome of the aneurysm in Case 553A is partially imaged on this scan, mimicking a brain stem lesion. The course of the basilar artery should be carefully followed on adjacent scans when this appearance is encountered.

Sagittal (and coronal) MR scans are valuable to define the extra-axial origin of lesions deforming the brain stem (see also Case 231).

This scan incidentally demonstrates two pseudolesions: (1) partial volume of the right petrous ridge appears as a calcification within the inferior temporal lobe, and (2) prominent veins near the tentorium could be misinterpreted as a vascular malformation.

DOLICHOECTASIA

Case 554

74-year-old man.
(noncontrast scan)

Case 555

70-year-old man.
(noncontrast scan)

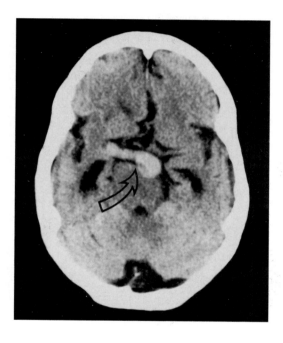

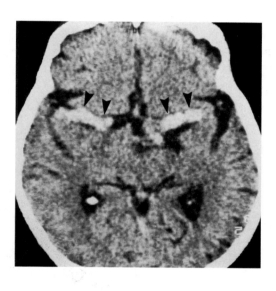

The basilar artery may undergo striking elongation and ectasia in elderly patients. This so called "dolichoectasia" may cause the tip of the artery to rise as far superiorly as the foramen of Monro. The vessel may then appear as an enhancing mass impinging on the third ventricle and causing hydrocephalus. (Hydrocephalus may alternatively be caused by increased intraventricular "pulse pressure" due to the invaginating basilar artery tip.) The "lesion" can usually be followed inferiorly through the series of scans and identified as a tubular structure originating in the prepontine area.

In this case the tortuous and ectatic rostral basilar artery is seen as a transverse tubular structure of high attenuation (arrow). An elongated basilar artery is often tortuous, and its aberrant course may distort cranial nerves with consequent neuropathies. Hemorrhages are rare in true dolichoectasia; brain stem infarction is more common. (Hemorrhage does occur from more fusiform atherosclerotic aneurysms of the basilar artery, such as Case 550.)

Dolichoectasia of the internal carotid or middle cerebral arteries may accompany or exceed involvement of the basilar artery. In this case, the horizontal segments of the middle cerebral arteries are grossly ectatic (arrowheads), appearing dense because of their blood content. (Compare this scan with the noncontrast density of dilated veins as in Case 502.)

SPONTANEOUS INTRACEREBRAL HEMATOMAS

Case 556

86-year-old woman presenting with acute right hemiparesis.

Case 557

53-year-old man presenting with malignant hypertension and a sudden visual field cut.

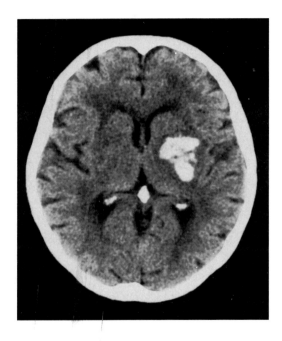

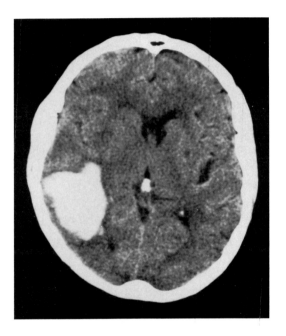

The clear demonstration of intracerebral hemorrhage was one of the earliest achievements of cerebral CT scanning. The characteristic high attenuation of hematomas is due primarily to the x-ray absorption (via Compton scatter) of the globin protein in red blood cells.

Spontaneous intraparenchymal hemorrhages tend to occur in a few specific locations, notably the basal ganglia, thalamus, pons, and cerebellum. Many patients experiencing "spontaneous" hemorrhages have a history of systemic hypertension. In these cases, angiopathic changes of small arteries (e.g., Charcot's aneurysm formation) may predispose to bleeding.

Here the deep hemisphere hematoma is of medium size. It has arisen in the putamen, the site of most ganglionic hemorrhages.

Small hematomas displace more tissue than they destroy. They often have a better long-term prognosis than cerebral infarctions causing equal initial deficits.

Spontaneous and/or hypertensive intracerebral hemorrhages may become very large, occupying much of the cerebral hemisphere and causing rapid uncal herniation. Large ganglionic hematomas frequently rupture into the ventricular system (see Cases 558 and 580).

In this case, the large hematoma has arisen superficial to the deep nuclei. Hypertensive hemorrhages can occur in lobar locations, but the differential diagnosis of atypical hematomas (see Cases 565 to 568) should be considered in such instances.

Sedimentation levels may be seen within intracerebral hematomas when clotting is impaired (i.e., coagulopathy) or liquifaction has occurred. The appearance of such lesions resembles hemorrhages into a pre-existing tumor or cyst.

DIFFERENTIAL DIAGNOSIS:
LARGE, MIDHEMISPHERIC INTRACEREBRAL HEMATOMA

Case 558

68-year-old woman.

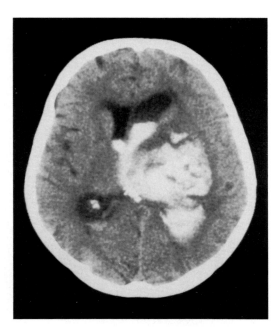

Spontaneous Hemorrhage.

Case 559

69-year-old woman.

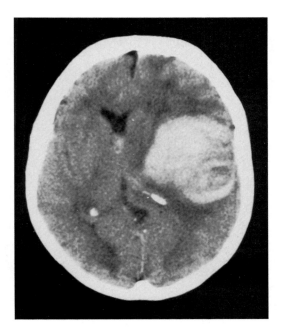

Hemorrhage into Metastatic Hypernephroma.

As demonstrated in Case 557, not all spontaneous or hypertensive hemorrhages are ganglionic. Conversely, not all midhemisphere hemorrhages are spontaneous.

The geographic center of the hematoma in Case 559 suggests that it originated lateral to the lenticular nucleus, which raises the possibility of nonspontaneous etiology. The "ghost" of a low attenuation mass within the hematoma is a second clue to the correct diagnosis. (Compare to Cases 94 and 566; see Cases 9 to 11 for discussion of hemorrhagic metastases.)

Spontaneous ganglionic hemorrhages are often multinodular, as in Case 558. The deep hematoma has ruptured into the ventricular system, "casting" the third ventricle and the trigone of the left lateral ventricle. Blood has traversed the foramina of Monro to enter the frontal horns, and a small CSF-blood layer is seen in the trigone of the right lateral ventricle.

MR CORRELATION: ACUTE INTRACEREBRAL HEMORRHAGE

Case 560A

83-year-old woman with a history of "CVA" 2
days before admission.
(sagittal, noncontrast scan; SE 600/17)

Case 560B

Same patient.
(axial, noncontrast scan; SE 3000/75)

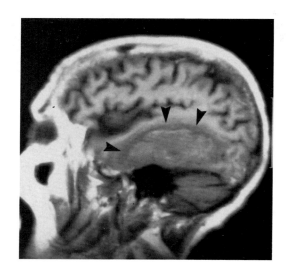

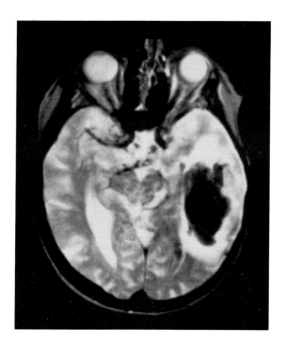

Acute intracerebral hematomas are usually seen as nearly isointense masses on T1-weighted MR scans. Mild prolongation of T1 may be present, causing slightly decreased signal intensity within the lesion.

Here a large hematoma in the middle cranial fossa is slightly lower in intensity than adjacent parenchyma.

Acute hematomas typically demonstrate very low signal intensity on T2-weighted images, as seen here. Selective T2 proton relaxation enhancement due to intracellular deoxyhemoglobin and clot retraction have been suggested as major contributions to this loss of signal. In any event, the combination of isointensity on T1-weighted scans and markedly low signal intensity on T2-weighted images is characteristic of an acute hematoma.

A zone of "bright" edema commonly surrounds the hematoma, as seen here.

Hyperacute intracerebral hematomas may present a less distinctive MR appearance. Such fresh hemorrhages represent a solution of nonparamagnetic oxyhemoglobin; and their MR behavior resembles that of proteinaceous fluid with uniform prolongation of T1 and T2. Hyperacute hematomas can therefore mimic other homogeneous cystic or solid masses.

Compare the homogeneous appearance of signal changes in this case and in Case 561 to the heterogeneity of blood products within a hemorrhagic neoplasm, as in Case 99.

MR CORRELATION: SUBACUTE INTRACEREBRAL HEMORRHAGE

Case 561A

33-year-old man who suffered a "stroke" 5 days
earlier.
(sagittal, noncontrast scan; SE 600/17)

Case 561B

Same patient.
(axial, noncontrast scan; SE 3000/80)

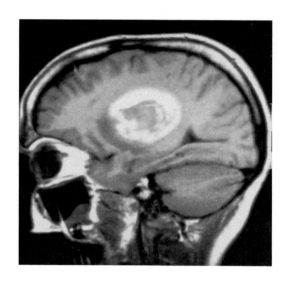

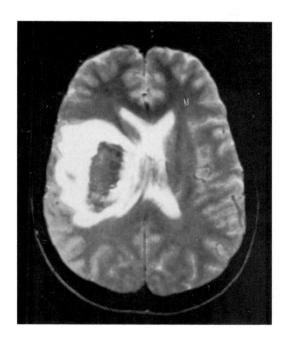

The MR appearance of intracerebral hemorrhage on T1-weighted scans changes during the first week of age. Prominent T1-shortening usually begins near the periphery of the lesion, gradually extending toward the center over a period of days to weeks. This alteration in signal intensity has been ascribed to the oxidation of deoxyhemoglobin to intracellular methemoglobin, which acts as a paramagnetic agent shortening T1.

The thick rind of high signal intensity surrounding an isointense center in this case is a typical presentation for an early subacute hematoma on a T1-weighted scan. (Contrast this appearance to Case 560A.) A follow-up scan with the same parameters after an additional week showed uniformly high signal intensity throughout the lesion.

Cell lysis and watery dilution of blood products accompanies the oxidation of intracerebral hematomas, progressing inward from the periphery of the lesion. The combination of these events converts the initially low signal intensity of acute hematomas on T2-weighted scans to high signal intensity over a period of weeks.

This case demonstrates the typical appearance of an early subacute intracerebral hematoma. Although a core of T2-shortening remains, the broadening perimeter of the lesion evidences high signal intensity (compare to Case 560B). After another week or two, the entire lesion would be expected to demonstrate high intensity on a T2-weighted sequence.

Case 562

39-year-old woman with a history of an old "stroke." (axial, noncontrast scan; SE 3000/75)

Case 563

56-year-old woman. (axial, noncontrast scan; SE 3000/75)

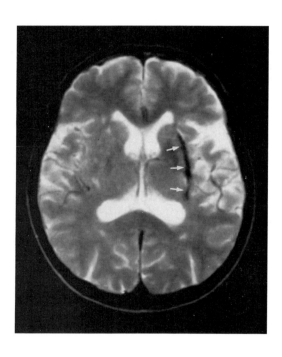

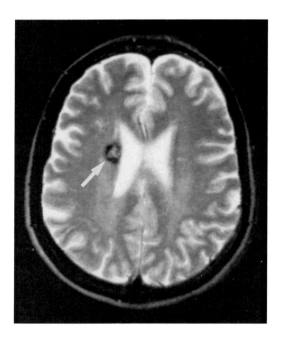

Another characteristic MR feature of cerebral hemorrhage is the "signature" of T2-shortening left at the site of such lesions. As aging hematomas are resorbed, blood products are accumulated by macrophages at the perimeter of the organized hemorrhage. This intracellular debris, mainly in the form of hemosiderin, is associated with selective T2 relaxation enhancement. The resultant T2-shortening causes a rim of low signal intensity, which is initially seen at the margin of intracerebral hematomas in the subacute phase.

This finding remains as a hallmark of prior hemorrhage even after the lesion has been completely resorbed. (This is strictly true only in areas of "normal" brain involved by hemorrhage; hemosiderin-laden macrophages within hemorrhagic neoplasms may gain abnormal vascular access and leave the region.)

In this case, T2-shortening causes prominently low signal intensity along the margins of an old hematoma in the region of the left putamen (arrows). This finding suggests an old "spontaneous" hemorrhage that has been resorbed and has collapsed, leaving a hemosiderin-lined cleft.

Hemosiderin-laden macrophages have long been noted as evidence of previous intracerebral hemorrhage by pathologists. MR allows similar characterization in vivo.

Here a focal lesion with thick margins of T2-shortening is seen in the mid-right corona radiata. The MR appearance indicates the presence of old hemorrhage at this site. The differential diagnosis would include spontaneous hematoma or cavernous hemangioma (see Cases 516 and 517).

Gradient echo images are more sensitive than spin-echo sequences to paramagnetic blood breakdown products. For this reason, gradient echo sequences may be helpful in identifying small hemorrhagic lesions (e.g., remote hemorrhages, shearing injuries, vascular metastases, or small angiomas).

DEEP HEMISPHERE HEMORRHAGE IN "MOYA MOYA" SYNDROME

Case 564A

49-year-old man presenting with a "CVA."

Case 564B

Same patient.

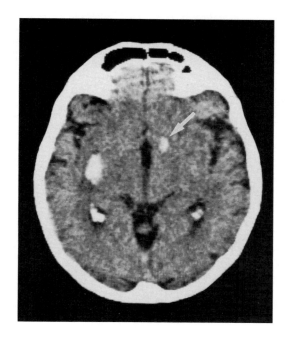

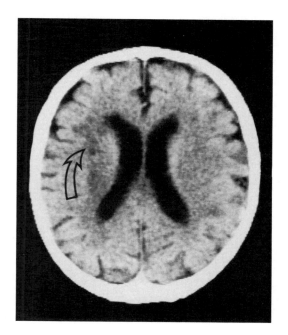

Small intracerebral hematomas are present in the region of the left hypothalamus and right putamen. Simultaneous hemorrhages at several sites raise considerations of trauma (see Cases 374 to 381), sagittal sinus thrombosis (see Case 469), hemorrhagic metastases (see Cases 9 and 382), coagulopathy, arteritis, or amyloid angiopathy (usually involving more superficial locations in older patients). The correct diagnosis in this case was provided by higher scan sections.

At this level a row of intrahemispheric infarcts is noted on the right side, with a few isolated lesions more peripherally in the left hemisphere. While these could represent "lacunar" lesions, the pattern on the right matches the typical morphology of ischemia along the intrahemispheric watershed (see Cases 440 and 441).

This suggestion of impaired hemisphere perfusion provides a new context for interpreting the small hemorrhages in the ganglionic region. The diagnosis of "moya moya" disease (progressive occlusion of cerebral arteries at the skull base) can account for the combination of ischemic changes and superimposed hemorrhages from the rupture of hypertrophied collateral channels.

Angiography confirmed high-grade stenosis of the supraclinoid internal carotid arteries and middle cerebral arteries, with a "cloud" of hypertrophied lenticulostriate vessels traversing the basal ganglia. MR scans in such cases may demonstrate both reduced caliber of basal arteries and prominent "dots" of low intensity within cerebral parenchyma representing enlarged collateral channels.

DIFFERENTIAL DIAGNOSIS:
ATYPICAL INTRACEREBRAL HEMATOMA

Case 565

20-year-old Vietnamese man presenting with seizures.

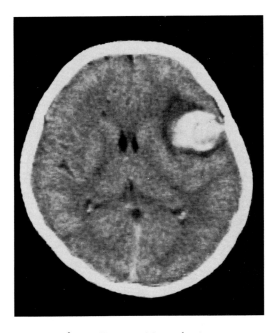

Hemorrhage From a Mycotic Aneurysm.

Case 566

30-year-old man presenting with a CVA.

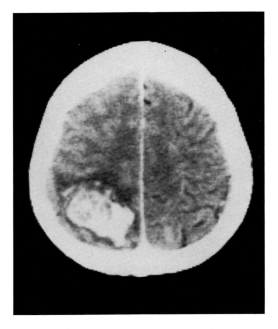

Hemorrhage Into Metastatic Melanoma.

The discovery of an intracerebral hematoma should be followed by critical assessment of its location and morphology. The diagnosis of "spontaneous hemorrhage" is reserved for hematomas occupying typical sites and demonstrating no unusual features. Superficial hematomas as seen in these cases are highly suspicious, and clues to an underlying cause should be sought.

In Case 565, the history of recent immigration and the appearance of concentric hemorrhage originating near the cortical surface suggested the correct diagnosis of mycotic aneurysm. Hemorrhage from other peripheral aneurysms (e.g., those associated with tumor emboli or meningitis) or from a small AVM could cause a similar appearance.

In Case 566, the structure of an underlying mass can be seen through the hematoma. Melanoma is one of the primary tumors known to cause vascular metastases, and intracerebral hemorrhage is a recognized presentation of this disease (compare with Cases 9 to 11, 94, 95, and 413).

Postcontrast scans performed days or weeks after intracerebral hemorrhage may demonstrate peripheral enhancement attributable to the organizing hematoma itself (see Cases 573 to 575). Such enhancement does not imply (or exclude) an underlying lesion.

DIFFERENTIAL DIAGNOSIS (CONTINUED):
ATYPICAL INTRACEREBRAL HEMATOMA

Case 567

27-year-old woman presenting with sudden
headaches.
(noncontrast scan)

Case 568

19-year-old man presenting with the acute onset
of headache, nausea, and stiff neck.
(postcontrast scan)

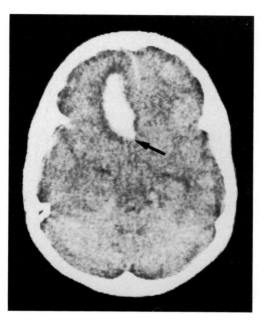

**Ruptured Aneurysm of the Anterior
Communicating Artery.**

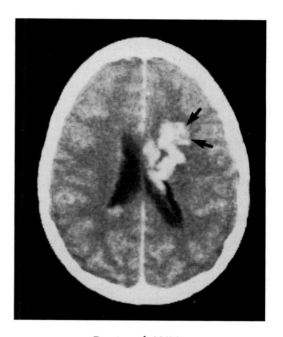

Ruptured AVM.

The frontal lobe hematoma in Case 567 is unusual in location and morphology. The posterome-
dial margin of the hemorrhage approaches the midline near the anterior circle of Willis *(arrow)*.
When a hematoma can be traced to a common aneurysm site in this manner, a clue to the origin
of the hemorrhage is obtained.

Although the hematoma in Case 568 occupies a deep hemisphere location, its occurrence in a
teenager argues strongly against a "spontaneous" etiology. The statistically best choice for an underlying lesion in these circumstances is an AVM.

Careful comparison of the precontrast and postcontrast scans in Case 568 established abnormal
contrast enhancement in a small region at the margin of the hematoma *(arrows)*. Angiography and
surgery confirmed a small AVM at this site.

When hematomas are found in an atypical location with no other clues as to cause, the possibility of underlying coagulopathy or vasculopathy (e.g., amyloid angiopathy; see Case 574) should
be considered.

Case 569

80-year-old woman with the acute onset of coma.

Cerebellar Hematoma.

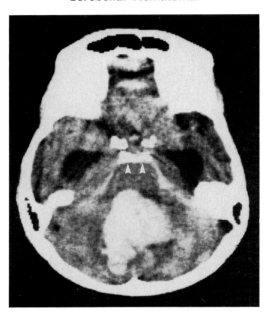

Case 570

32-year-old woman with the acute onset of headaches and facial paresis.

Brain Stem Hematoma.

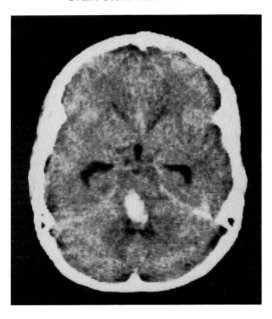

About 10% to 15% of spontaneous and/or hypertensive hematomas occur in the posterior fossa. They may involve the cerebellum or the brain stem, usually the pons. It is important to distinguish between cerebellar and brain stem hemorrhages, since the former may be evacuated with life-saving results.

Cerebellar hematomas may be midline or hemispheric (see also Case 571). Here a large vermian hematoma has effaced the fourth ventricle, causing obstructive hydrocephalus. The brain stem is displaced anteriorly, with its ventral margin compressed against the clivus and dorsum (arrowheads).

The apparent AP diameter of the brain stem varies with the angle of the scan. When the head is flexed, the usual axial scan (0-degree gantry angle) passes obliquely through the brain stem from anterosuperior to posteroinferior. For example, a typical scan may demonstrate the cerebral peduncles (midbrain) ventrally while passing through the fourth ventricle (pons) dorsally. Routine axial scans performed with head extension result in a truer cross section of the brain stem with less elongation. This apparently "small" brain stem diameter may cause confusion in localizing lesions. The cerebellar hemorrhage in this case had originally been misinterpreted as a brain stem hematoma because of its apparent anterior location (caused by head extension of the intubated patient and brain stem compression by the cerebellar mass).

Brain stem hematomas are seen anterior to the plane of the fourth ventricle, as illustrated in this case. Compression of the fourth ventricle or aqueduct usually causes superimposed hydrocephalus, indicated here by the large temporal horns.

Although spontaneous and/or hypertensive hemorrhages are seen in the brain stem, the age of this patient suggests a possible underlying vascular malformation.

Small hemorrhages from low-flow vascular malformations within the brain stem (commonly cavernous angiomas) may cause less devastating and more recurrent symptoms than spontaneous hematomas. The clinical course of such patients may suggest a slowly progressive brain-stem tumor or demyelinating disease.

DIFFERENTIAL DIAGNOSIS:
HIGH ATTENUATION NEAR THE DENTATE NUCLEI

Case 571

74-year-old hypertensive man presenting with acute nausea and disequilibrium.

Case 572

79-year-old man referred to evaluate a CVA.

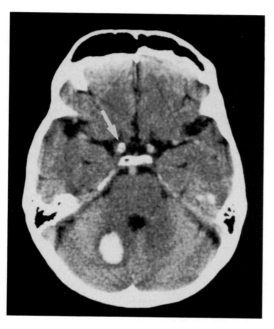

Cerebellar Hematoma.

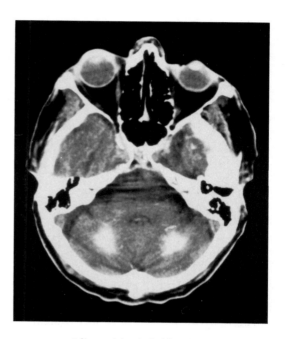

Idiopathic Calcification.

Spontaneous and/or hypertensive hemorrhage within the cerebellum often originates near the dentate nucleus, as in Case 571.

Calcification is occasionally encountered in this region as seen in Case 572. Apart from rare cases of parathyroid dysfunction or "Fahr's disease" (ferrocalcinosis), the etiology is usually undetermined.

Such calcification is typically higher in attenuation values than an acute hematoma. Infrequently foci of less dense calcification have a "softer" appearance and can initially mimic parenchymal hemorrhage. The typical bilateral symmetry establishes the correct diagnosis (in the absence of head tilt). In addition, the margins of nuclear calcification are often more irregular or "feathered" than those of a hematoma, as noted in the above cases.

The same considerations apply to distinguishing hemorrhage from calcification within the lenticular nucleus, a more common site for both processes.

Partial volume of the arcuate eminence in Case 571 simulates a calcified left temporal lesion. Calcification is present in the wall of the right supraclinoid internal carotid artery in the same case (arrow).

Case 573

73-year-old woman.
(postcontrast scan)

Case 574

53-year-old woman, 1 month after intracerebral
hemorrhage due to amyloid angiopathy.
(postcontrast scan)

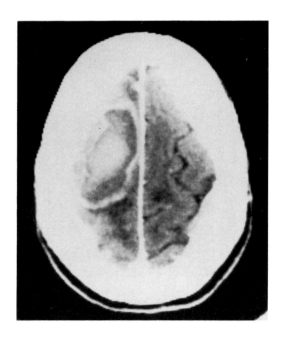

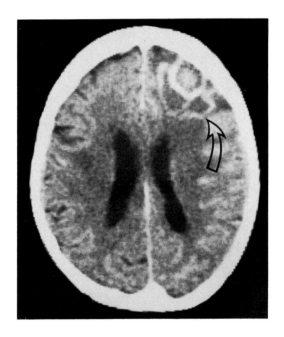

The attenuation values of an intracerebral hematoma decrease gradually over a period of weeks. Dissolution and organization of the clot simultaneously begin from the periphery (see Case 561). This process leads to a rim of contrast enhancement at the margins of a resolving hematoma.

A scan performed several weeks after hemorrhage may demonstrate the enhancing rim of the lesion, with little remaining high attenuation. The resolving hematoma may then resemble an abscess or neoplasm, as seen here. The lesion in this scan represented an unusual superior extension of a large, but otherwise typical, ganglionic hematoma.

Clues to the correct diagnosis in most cases are: (1) a history of recent CVA; (2) location at a common site of spontaneous hemorrhage; (3) a smooth, uniform rim, *not* well seen on the precontrast scan; (4) faint residual high attenuation near the center of the mass; and (5) lack of adjacent edema.

Hematomas may occur in unusual locations, have irregular contours, and cause marked edema. Such lesions may create bizarre rim-enhancement patterns as they resolve, as seen in this case. Since hemorrhage may secondarily occur into pre-existing lesions, enhancement patterns must be closely evaluated before being ascribed to evolution of a spontaneous hematoma.

"Benign" enhancement around an intracerebral hematoma has been seen within days of the original hemorrhage. The finding may persist for 1 or 2 months.

Amyloid (or "congophilic") angiopathy is a leading cause for lobar hemorrhage in elderly patients. This pathologically proven case in a younger adult is somewhat unusual.

DIFFERENTIAL DIAGNOSIS:
RIM-ENHANCING MASS WITH CENTRAL HEMORRHAGE

Case 575

58-year-old man with a history of "CVA"
3 weeks earlier.

Case 576

57-year-old woman with a history of "CVA"
2 weeks earlier.

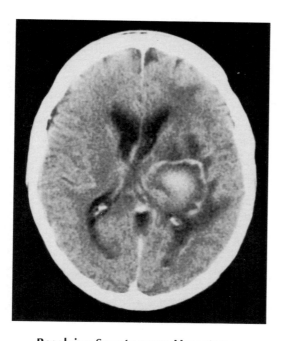

Resolving Spontaneous Hematoma.

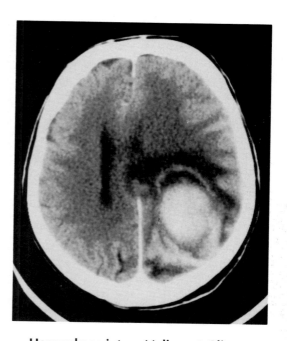

Hemorrhage into a Malignant Glioma.

The rim of contrast enhancement surrounding a "benign" resolving hematoma is usually uniformly thin and almost completely circumferential, as in Case 575.

When the enhancing rim of a hemorrhagic mass demonstrates variable thickness and discontinuity as in Case 576, an underlying neoplasm should be considered.

The appearance of the subacute central hematoma is similar in both cases, and both demonstrate surrounding edema. Since the clinical histories are also similar, the differential diagnosis is based primarily on the character of rim enhancement (supported by typical/atypical locations for spontaneous hemorrhage).

GERMINAL MATRIX HEMORRHAGE IN PREMATURE INFANTS

Case 577

2-day-old girl born at 33 weeks gestation.

Case 578

2-week-old boy born at 31 weeks gestation.

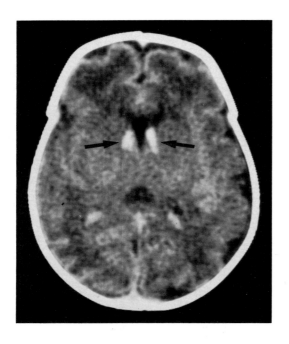

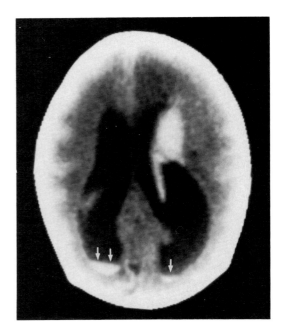

Hemorrhage commonly arises from fragile vessels in the periventricular layer of germinal matrix in premature newborns. Small hematomas may remain confined to the subependymal region, as seen here near the caudate nuclei.

Care must be taken to not misinterpret the normal, mildly increased attenuation of the germinal matrix as symmetrical hemorrhage (compare this case to Case 325). Symmetrical high attenuation within the lateral ventricular trigones represents normal choroid plexus.

Signs of prematurity in this case include the thin cortical mantle and the prominent low attenuation of cerebral white matter (see Cases 325 and 326).

Subependymal hemorrhage in premature infants commonly ruptures into the ventricular system causing secondary hydrocephalus. This case demonstrates CSF/blood levels within the dilated lateral ventricles *(arrows)*. A strand of thrombus within the left lateral ventricle is likely adherent to choroid plexus.

Cribside ultrasound (using the open fontanelles as acoustic windows) is the procedure of choice for following the course of such cases.

INTRAVENTRICULAR HEMORRHAGE

Case 579

80-year-old woman in a coma (same patient as Case 569).

Case 580

68-year-old man.

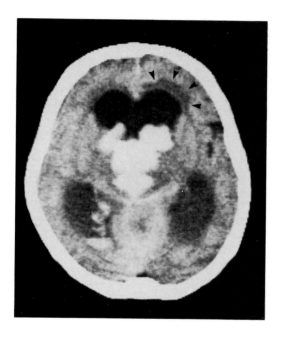

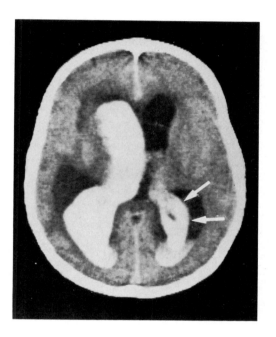

Hematomas in the posterior fossa or basal ganglia may rupture into the fourth or third ventricles. The ventricles may be grossly expanded by clot, as in this case. The intraventricular hematoma acts as a mass lesion and causes obstructive hydrocephalus.

Here the massa intermedia is faintly seen as a filling defect in the distended third ventricle. Clot extends through the foramina of Monro into the frontal horns (compare to Case 558).

Periventricular edema due to acute hydrocephalus is seen in the frontal lobes *(arrowheads)*. Ascending, transtentorial herniation has impacted the cerebellar vermis and brain stem at the tentorial hiatus.

In this case, a primary hematoma within the caudate nucleus has ruptured into the ventricular system. The right lateral ventricle has filled with blood.

Such "casting" forms a clot having the shape and size of the ventricle at the time of hemorrhage. A small cast is present within the trigone of the left ventricle *(arrows)*, which has evidently enlarged since the original hemorrhage. Superimposed on the cast is a sedimentation level.

TORTUOUS NORMAL VESSELS ASSOCIATED WITH CRANIAL NERVE SYNDROMES

Case 581

69-year-old man presenting with left-sided
tinnitus and hemifacial spasm.
(postcontrast scan)

Case 582

35-year-old woman with left hemifacial spasm.
(postcontrast scan)

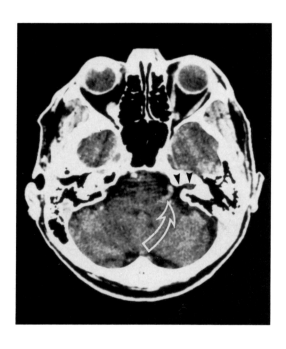

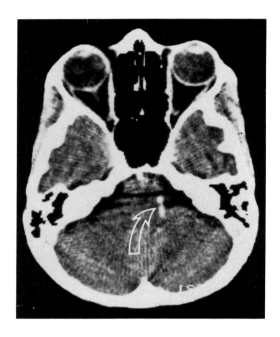

Some patients experience recurrent symptoms due to distortion of cranial nerves by adjacent vessels. Both tic douloureux (trigeminal nerve) and hemifacial spasm (facial nerve) may be caused by contact of an artery or vein with the nerve near its junction with the brain stem ("entry zone"). Although CT and MR scans rarely give an image of the microvascular anatomy responsible for most cases of nerve irritation, occasional symptomatic arterial loops can be identified.

Here a prominent cephalic loop of the left vertebral artery *(open arrow)* extends high into the cerebellopontine angle. The tortuous vessel has reached the plane of the internal auditory canal *(arrowheads)*, and may be reasonably supposed to distort the cisternal segments of the seventh and eighth cranial nerves. In any event, the location of this large arterial loop is important preoperative information for a surgeon contemplating microvascular decompression.

In this case a loop of the tortuous distal left vertebral artery lies against the brain stem near the level of the facial nerve. The vessel behaves as an extra-axial mass, deforming the brain stem and widening the cerebellopontine angle cistern (compare to Case 550).

Surgery confirmed compression and distortion of the seventh nerve by the large arterial loop. Separation of the artery from the nerve resulted in cessation of facial spasms.

REFERENCES: CT

1. Adams H.P. Jr., Kassell N.F., Torner J.C., et al.: CT and clinical correlations in recent aneurysmal subarachnoid hemorrhage: A preliminary report of the cooperative aneurysm study. *Neurology* 33:981–988, 1983.

2. Ahmadi J., Miller C.A., Segall H.D., et al.: CT patterns in histopathologically complex cavernous hemangiomas. *A.J.N.R.* 6:389–394, 1985.

3. Albright L., Fellows R.: Sequential CT scanning after neonatal intracerebral hemorrhage. *A.J.N.R.* 2:133–137, 1981.

4. Batjer H., Suss R.A., Samson D.: Intracranial arteriovenous malformations associated with aneurysms. *Neurosurgery* 18:29–35, 1986.

5. Broderick J.P., Brott T.J., Tomsick T., et al.: Ultra-early evaluation of intracerebral hemorrhage. *J. Neurosurg.* 72:195–199, 1990.

6. Byrd S.E., Bentson J.R., Winter J., et al.: Giant intracranial aneurysms simulating brain neoplasms on computed tomography. *J. Comput. Assist. Tomogr.* 2:303–307, 1978.

7. Davis K.R., Kistler J.P., Heros R.C., et al.: Neuroradiologic approach to the patient with the diagnosis of subarachnoid hemorrhage. *Radiol. Clin. North Am.* 20:87–94, 1982.

8. Diebler C., Dulac O., Renier D., et al.: Aneurysms of the vein of Galen in infants aged 2 to 15 months: Diagnosis and natural evolution. *Neuroradiology* 21:185–197, 1981.

9. Fierstien S.B., Pribham H.W., Hieshima G.: Angiography and computed tomography in the evaluation of cerebral venous malformations. *Neuroradiology* 17:137–148, 1979.

10. Golding R., Peatfield R.C., Shawdon H.H., et al.: Computer tomographic features of giant intracranial aneurysms. *Clin. Radiol.* 31:41, 1980.

11. Goldstein S.J., Sacks J.G., Lee C., et al.: Computed tomographic findings in cerebral arterial ectasia. *A.J.N.R.* 4:501–504, 1983.

12. Graeb D.A., Robertson W.D., Lapointe J.S., et al.: Computed tomographic diagnosis of intraventricular hemorrhage: Etiology and prognosis. *Radiology* 143:91–96, 1982.

13. Inoue Y., Saiwai S., Miyamoto T., et al.: Post-contrast computed tomography in subarachnoid hemorrhage from ruptured aneurysms. *J. Comput. Assist. Tomogr.* 5:341–344, 1981.

14. Kistler J.P., Crowell R.M., Davis K.R., et al.: The relation of cerebral vasospasm to the extent and location of subarachnoid blood visualized by CT scan: A prospective study. *Neurology* 33:424–436, 1983.

15. Kumar A.J., Vinuela F., Fox A.J., Rosenbaum A.E.: Unruptured intracranial arteriovenous malformations do cause mass effect. *A.J.N.R.* 6:29–32, 1985.

16. Kumar A.J., Fox A.J., Vinuela F., Rosenbaum A.E.: Revisited old and new CT findings in unruptured larger arteriovenous malformations of the brain. *J. Comput. Assist. Tomogr.* 8:648–655, 1984.

17. Laster D.W., Moody D.M., Ball M.R.: Resolving intracerebral hematoma: Alteration of the ring sign with steroids. *A.J.R.* 130:935–939, 1978.

18. Leblanc R., Ethier R., Little J.R.: Computerized tomography findings in arteriovenous malformations of the brain. *J. Neurosurg.* 51:765–772, 1979.

19. Lee Y.-Y., Moser R., Bruner J.M., Van Tassel P.: Organized intracerebral hematoma within acute hemorrhage: CT patterns and pathologic correlations. *A.J.N.R.* 7:409–416, 1986.

20. Little J.R., Tubman D.E., Ethier R.: Cerebellar hemorrhage in adults. *J. Neurosurg.* 48:575–579, 1978.

21. Loes D.J., Smoker W.R.K., Biller J., Cornell S.H.: Nontraumatic lobar intracerebral hemorrhage: CT/angiographic correlation. *A.J.N.R.* 8:1027–1030, 1987.

22. Martell A., Scotti G., Harwood-Nash D.C.: Aneurysms of the vein of Galen in children: CT and angiographic correlations. *Neuroradiology* 20:123–133, 1980.

23. McCormack J., Peyster R.G., Brodner R.A., Cooper V.R.: CT visualization of ruptured berry aneurysm within hematoma: The flip-flop sign. *J. Comput. Assist. Tomogr.* 10:28–31, 1986.

24. Mitnick J.S., Pinto R.S., Lin J.P., et al.: CT of thrombosed arteriovenous malformations in children. *Radiology* 150:385–389, 1984.

25. Mosely I.F., Holland I.M.: Ectasia of the basilar artery: The breadth of the clinical spectrum and the diagnostic value of computed tomography. *Neuroradiology* 18:83–91, 1979.

26. Newell D.W., LeRoux P.D., Dacey R.G. Jr., et al.: CT infusion scanning for the detection of cerebral aneurysms. *J. Neurosurg.* 71:175–179, 1989.

27. Norman D., Price D., Boyd D., et al.: Quantitative aspects of computed tomography of the blood and cerebrospinal fluid. *Radiology* 123:335–338, 1977.

28. Olson E., Gilmor R.L., Richmond B.: Cerebral venous angiomas. *Radiology* 151:97–104, 1984.

29. Patel D.V., Hier D.B., Thomas C.M., et al.: Intracerebral hemorrhage secondary to cerebral amyloid angiopathy. *Radiology* 151:397–400, 1984.

30. Pinto R.S., Cohen W.A., Kricheff I.I., et al.: Giant intracranial aneurysms: Rapid sequential computed tomography. *A.J.N.R.* 3:495–499, 1982.

31. Pinto R.S., Kricheff I.I., Butler A.R.: Correlation of computed tomographic, angiographic, and neuropathological changes in giant intracranial aneurysms. *Radiology* 132:85–92, 1979.

32. Rothfus W.E., Albright A.L., Casey K.F., et al.: Cerebellar venous angioma: "Benign" entity? *A.J.N.R.* 5:61–66, 1984.

33. Schellinger D., Grant E.G., Manz H.J., Patronas N.J.: Intraparenchymal hemorrhage in preterm neonates: A broadening spectrum. *A.J.N.R.* 9:327–333, 1988.

34. Schubiger O., Valavanis A., Hayek J.: Computed tomography in cerebral aneurysms with special emphasis on giant intracranial aneurysms. *J. Comput. Assist. Tomogr.* 4:24–32, 1980.

35. Scott B.A., Weinstein Z., Pulliam M.W.: Computed tomographic diagnosis of ruptured giant posterior cerebral artery aneurysm. *Neurosurgery* 22:553–557, 1988.

36. Shirkhoda A., Whaley R.A., Boone S.C., et al.: Varied CT appearance of aneurysm of the vein of Galen in infancy. *Neuroradiology* 21:265–270, 1981.

37. Silver A.J., Pederson M.E., Ganti S.M., et al.: CT of subarachnoid hemorrhage due to ruptured aneurysm. *A.J.N.R.* 2:13–22, 1981.

38. Simard J.M., Garcia-Bengochea F., Ballinger W.E. Jr., et al.: Cavernous angioma: A review of 126 collected and 12 new clinical cases. *Neurosurgery* 18:162–172, 1986.

39. Smoker W.R.K., Corbett J.J., Gentry L.R., et al.: High resolution computed tomography of the basilar artery. 2. Vertebrobasilar dolichoectasia: Clinical-pathological correlation and review. *A.J.N.R.* 7:61–72, 1986.

40. Sobel D., Li F.C., Norman D., et al.: Cisternal enhancement after subarachnoid hemorrhage. *A.J.N.R.* 2:549–552, 1981.
41. Sugita K., Kobayashi S., Takemae T., et al.: Giant aneurysms of the vertebral artery: Report of five cases. *J. Neurosurg.* 68:960–966, 1988.
42. Taneda M., Hayakawa T., Mogami H.: Primary cerebellar hemorrhage: Quadrigeminal cistern obliteration on CT scans as a predictor of outcome. *J. Neurosurg.* 67:545–552, 1987.
43. Valavanis A., Wellauer J., Yasargil M.G.: The radiological diagnosis of cerebral venous angioma: Cerebral angiography and computed tomography. *Neuroradiology* 24:193–199, 1983.
44. Wagle W.A., Smith T.W., Weiner M.: Intracerebral hemorrhage caused by cerebral amyloid angiopathy: Radiographic-pathologic correlation. *A.J.N.R.* 5:171–176, 1984.
45. Wharen R.E., Scheithauer B.W., Laws E.R.: Thrombosed arteriovenous malformations of the brain. *J. Neurosurg.* 57:520–526, 1982.
46. Yeakley J.W., Patchall L.L., Lee K.F.: Interpeduncular fossa sign: CT criterion of subarachnoid hemorrhage. *Radiology* 158:699–700, 1986.
47. Yeates A., Enzmann D.: Cryptic vascular malformations involving the brain stem. *Radiology* 146:71–75, 1983.
48. Yock D.H. Jr., Larson D.A.: Computed tomography of hemorrhage from anterior communicating artery aneurysms with angiographic correlation. *Radiology* 134:399–407, 1980.
49. Zimmerman R.D., Leeds N.E., Naidich T.P.: Ring blush associated with intracerebral hematoma. *Radiology* 122:707–711, 1977.

REFERENCES: MR

1. Atlas S.W.: Intracranial vascular malformations and aneurysms: Current imaging applications. *Radiol. Clin. North Am.* 26:821–838, 1988.
2. Atlas S.W., Grossman R.I., Goldberg H.I., et al.: Partially thrombosed giant intracranial aneurysms: Correlation of MR and pathologic findings. *Radiology* 162:111–114, 1987.
3. Atlas S.W., Mark A.S., Fram E.K., Grossman R.I.: Vascular intracranial lesions: Applications of gradient-echo MR imaging. *Radiology* 169:455–462, 1988.
4. Atlas S.W., Mark A.S., Grossman R.I., Gomori J.M.: Intracranial hemorrhage: Gradient-echo MR imaging at 1.5T. Comparisons with spin echo imaging and clinical applications. *Radiology* 168:803–808, 1988.
5. Augustyn G.T., Scott J.A., Olson E., et al.: Cerebral venous angiomas: MR imaging. *Radiology* 156:391–396, 1985.
6. Barkovich A.J., Atlas S.W.: Magnetic resonance imaging of intracranial hemorrhage. *Radiol. Clin. North Am.* 26:801–820, 1988.
7. Brooks R.A., Di Chiro G., Patronas N.: MR imaging of cerebral hematomas at different field strengths: Theory and applications. *J. Comput. Tomogr. Assist.* 13:194–206, 1989.
8. Brooks B.S., El Gammal T., Adams R.J., et al.: MR imaging of moyamoya in neurofibromatosis. *A.J.N.R.* 8:178–179, 1987.
9. De Marco J.K., Dillon W.P., Halbach V.V., Tsuruda J.S.: Dural arteriovenous fistulas: Evaluation with MR imaging. *Radiology* 175:193–200, 1990.
10. Ebeling J.O., Tranmer B.I., Davis K.A., et al.: Thrombosed arteriovenous malformations: A type of occult vascular malformation. Magnetic resonance imaging and histopathological correlations. *Neurosurgery* 23:605–610, 1988.
11. Gaen A.D., Pile-Spellman J., Heros R.C.: A pneumatized anterior clinoid mimicking an aneurysm on MR imaging: Report of two cases. *J. Neurosurg.* 71:128–132, 1989.
12. Gomori J.M., Grossman R.I.: Mechanisms responsible for the MR appearance and evolution of intracranial hemorrhage. *Radiographics* 8:427–440, 1988.
13. Gomori J.M., Grossman R.I., Bilaniuk L.T., et al.: High field MR imaging of superficial siderosis of the central nervous system. *J. Comput. Assoc. Tomogr.* 9:972–975, 1985.
14. Gomori J.M., Grossman R.I., Goldberg H.I., et al.: High-field spin-echo MR imaging of superficial and subependymal siderosis secondary to neonatal intraventricular hemorrhage. *Neuroradiology* 29:339, 1987.
15. Gomori J.M., Grossman R.I., Goldberg H.I., et al.: Occult cerebral vascular malformations: High field MR imaging. *Radiology* 158:707–714, 1986.
16. Gomori J.M., Grossman R.I., Goldberg H.I., et al.: Intracranial hematomas: Imaging by high-field MR. *Radiology* 157:87–94, 1985.

17. Gomori J.M., Grossman R.I., Hackney D.B., et al.: Variable appearances of subacute intracranial hematomas on high-field spin-echo MR. *A.J.N.R.* 8:1019–1026, 1987.
18. Hackney D.B., Lesnick J.E., Zimmerman R.A., et al.: MR identification of the bleeding site in subarachnoid hemorrhage with multiple intracranial aneurysms. *J. Comput. Assist. Tomogr.* 10:878–880, 1986.
19. Jaspan T., Wilson M., O'Donnell H., et al.: Magnetic resonance imaging with even-echo rephasing sequences in the assessment and management of giant intracranial aneurysms. *Br. J. Radiol.* 61:351, 1988.
20. Jenkins A., Hadley D., Teasdale G.M., et al.: Magnetic resonance imaging of acute subarachnoid hemorrhage. *J. Neurosurg.* 68:731–736, 1988.
21. Kashiwagi S., Van Loueren H.R., Tew J.M. Jr., et al.: Diagnosis and treatment of vascular brain stem malformations. *J. Neurosurg.* 72:27–34, 1990.
22. Kucharczyk W., Lemme-Pleghos L., Uske A., et al.: Intracranial vascular malformations: MR and CT imaging. *Radiology* 156:383–390, 1985.
23. Leblanc R., Levesque M., Comair Y., Ethier R.: Magnetic resonance imaging of cerebral arteriovenous malformation. *Neurosurgery* 21:15–20, 1987.
24. Lee B.C.P., Herzberg L., Zimmerman R.D., Deck M.D.F.: MR imaging of cerebral vascular malformations. *A.J.N.R.* 6:863–870, 1985.
25. Lemme-Plaghos L., Kucharczyk W., Brant-Zawadzki M., et al.: MR imaging of angiographically occult vascular malformations. *A.J.N.R.* 7:217–222, 1986.
26. McArdle C.B., Richardson C.J., Hayden C.K., et al.: Abnormalities of the neonatal brain: MR imaging. Part I. Intracranial hemorrhage. *Radiology* 163:387–394, 1987.
27. Naseem M., Leehey P., Russell E., et al.: MR of basilar artery dolichoectasia. *A.J.N.R.* 9:391–392, 1988.
28. New P.F.J., Ojemann R.G., Davis K.R., et al.: MR and CT of occult vascular malformations of the brain. *A.J.N.R.* 7:771–780, 1986.
29. Noorbehesht B., Fabrikant J.I., Enzmann D.R.: Size determination of supratentorial arteriovenous malformations by MR, CT, and angio. *Neuroradiology* 29:512, 1987.
30. Olsen W.L., Brant-Zawadzki M., Hodes J., et al.: Giant intracranial aneurysms: MR imaging. *Radiology* 163:431–436, 1987.
31. Rapacki T.F.X., Brantley M.J., Furlow T.W., et al.: Heterogeneity of cerebral cavernous hemangiomas diagnosed by MR imaging. *J. Comput. Assist. Tomogr.* 14:18–25, 1990.
32. Rigamonti D.E., Drayer B.P., Johnson P.C., et al.: The MRI appearance of cavernous malformations (angiomas). *J. Neurosurg.* 67:518–524, 1987.
33. Saton S., Kadoya S.: Magnetic resonance imaging of subarachnoid hemorrhage. *Neuroradiology* 30:361, 1988.
34. Seidenwurm D., Meng T.-K., Kowalski H., et al.: Intracranial hemorrhagic lesions: Evaluation with spin-echo and gradient-refocused MR imaging at 0.5 and 1.5T. *Radiology* 172:189–194, 1989.
35. Smith H.J., Strother C.M., Kikuchi Y., et al.: MR imaging in the management of supratentorial intracranial AVMs. *A.J.N.R.* 9:225–236, 1988.
36. Stone J.L., Crowell R.M., Gandhi Y., Jafar J.V.: Multiple intracranial aneurysms: Magnetic resonance imaging for determination of the site of rupture. *Neurosurgery* 23:97–100, 1988.
37. Strother C.M., Eldevik P., Kikuchi Y., et al.: Thrombus formation and structure and the evolution of mass effect in intracranial aneurysms treated by balloon embolization: Emphasis on MR findings. *A.J.N.R.* 10:787–796, 1989.
38. Sze G., Krol G., Olsen W.L., et al.: Hemorrhagic neoplasms: Mimics of occult vascular malformations. *A.J.N.R.* 8:795–802, 1987.
39. Tash R.E., Kier E.L., Chyatte D.: Hemifacial spasm caused by a tortuous vertebral artery: MR demonstration. *J. Comput. Assist. Tomogr.* 12:492–494, 1988.
40. Toro V.E., Gever C.A., Sherman J.L., et al.: Cerebral venous angiomas: MR findings. *J. Comput. Assist. Tomogr.* 12:935–940, 1988.
41. Wong B.W., Steinberg G.K., Rosen L.: Magnetic resonance imaging of vascular compression in trigeminal neuralgia: Case report. *J. Neurosurg.* 70:132–134, 1989.
42. Yoon H.C., Lufkin R.B., Vinuela F., et al.: MR of acute subarachnoid hemorrhage. *A.J.N.R.* 9:404–405, 1988.
43. Yousem D.M., Flamm E.S., Grossman R.I.: Comparison of MR imaging with clinical history in the identification of hemorrhage in patients with cerebral arteriovenous malformations. *A.J.N.R.* 10:1151–1154, 1989.
44. Zimmerman R.D., Heier L.A., Snow R.B., et al.: Acute intracranial hemorrhage: Intensity changes on sequential MR scans at 0.5T. *A.J.N.R.* 9:47–58, 1988.

CHAPTER 11

Hydrocephalus, Cysts, and Developmental Abnormalities

Case 583A

19-month-old girl.

Case 583B

Same patient.

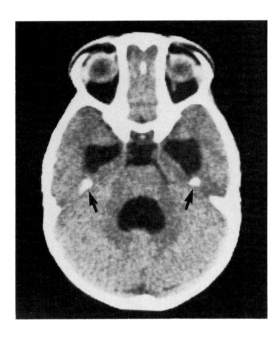

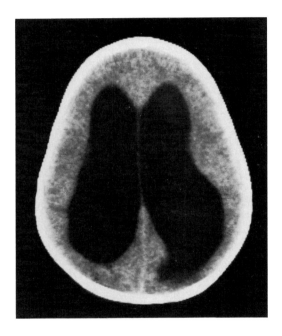

Hydrocephalus ranks among the CNS pathologies most clearly demonstrated on CT scans. Expanded components of the ventricular system are easily defined because of the contrast provided by spinal fluid.

In this case, the fourth ventricle is enlarged along with the temporal horns. The dilated anterior recesses of the third ventricle occupy the suprasellar cistern (compare with Case 590).

Hydrocephalic expansion of all four ventricles suggests impairment of cerebrospinal fluid (CSF) flow or absorption along the surface pathways from the foramen magnum through the tentorial incisura to the parasagittal arachnoid granulations. This "communicating" pathophysiology contrasts with intraventricular obstruction and is one common cause of infantile hydrocephalus. It is usually idiopathic, but may follow perinatal meningitis or intracranial hemorrhage.

Small densities in the posterior temporal region are seen where the scan passes along the superior surface of the petrous bones (arrows). The "arcuate eminence" roofing the superior semicircular canal is partially imaged on such sections.

Hydrocephalic lateral ventricles may become hugely dilated, occupying most of the supratentorial compartment. Except in extreme cases, the thinness of the residual cortical mantle is an unreliable predictor of postshunt recovery.

In severe hydrocephalus the septum pellucidum may become markedly thinned or frankly dehiscent. The resulting communication between the lateral ventricles may resemble lobar holoprosencephaly (see Case 588).

The posterior bodies, atria, and occipital horns of hydrocephalic ventricles are often larger than the frontal horns. This disparity may increase after shunting, with the greatest reduction in ventricular size occurring anteriorly.

AQUEDUCTAL STENOSIS

Case 584

19-year-old woman.
(sagittal, noncontrast scan; SE 600/20)

Case 585

32-year-old woman.
(coronal, noncontrast scan; SE 700/16)

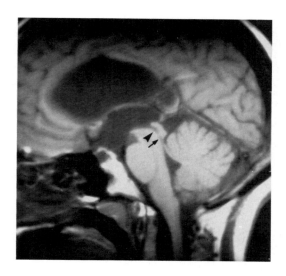

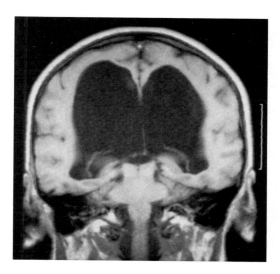

Aqueductal stenosis is a major cause of infantile hydrocephalus. Most cases are due to a congenital abnormality, usually "forking" or "gliosis." Acquired aqueductal stenosis may follow ependymitis from infection or intraventricular hemorrhage. Cases of congenital origin may present in adulthood when the borderline capacity of a narrowed lumen is further compromised or exceeded by some superimposed event.

Magnetic resonance imaging is superior to CT for evaluation of aqueductal stenosis. Multiplanar display and the absence of bone artifact contribute to an excellent view of midbrain anatomy.

In this case, the small fourth ventricle contrasts with the dilated lateral and third ventricles, localizing obstruction to the aqueductal level (compare to Case 583). The proximal aqueduct is dilated (arrowhead), while the lumen of the distal aqueduct is small (arrow), further defining the precise site of stenosis.

The midbrain tectum is normal. Contrast this case with the example of aqueductal compression by a tectal glioma in Case 111.

Adults presenting with hydrocephalus due to aqueductal stenosis often demonstrate evidence of longstanding ventricular enlargement. Here the markedly dilated lateral ventricles are associated with a relatively small posterior fossa. This finding suggests intrauterine or infantile onset of aqueductal compromise, with developmental expansion of the supratentorial compartment at the expense of the posterior fossa.

The typical CT appearance of aqueductal narrowing is seen in Case 590. The CT diagnosis of aqueductal stenosis is based on (1) enlargement of the lateral and third ventricles without fourth ventricular expansion, and (2) the absence of other lesions mimicking obstruction at the aqueductal level (see Cases 591 to 593).

DIFFERENTIAL DIAGNOSIS:
LARGE LATERAL VENTRICLES IN A CHILD

Case 586

3-year-old boy examined for large head size.

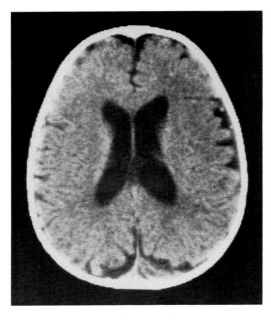

Megalencephaly.

Case 587

7-year-old boy retarded since birth.

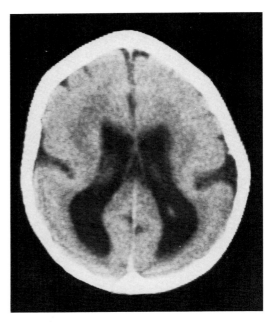

Developmental Abnormality (Pachygyria; Dysgenesis of the Corpus Callosum).

Some children have large heads as a consequence of having large brains. Several pathological syndromes (e.g., mucopolysaccharidoses, gangliosidoses) are associated with "megalencephaly," but many children with large brains are functionally normal. Clinical clues to "benign megalencephaly" include normal head shape, head growth curves parallel to standards, the absence of increased intracranial pressure, normal neurological development, and large head size of a parent. The child in Case 586 is a functionally normal boy whose father wears a cap over an unusually large head.

Children with benign megalencephaly often have large ventricles. They may also demonstrate prominent subarachnoid spaces. The latter finding provides a clue to the diagnosis, since hydrocephalic expansion of ventricles usually effaces sulcal markings. Occasionally "benign" communicating hydrocephalus causes large ventricles and sulci in a child, with a stable appearance or improvement on follow-up scans.

Poor brain growth in childhood may also result in ventricular enlargement. Distinction from hydrocephalus is usually aided by small head size and a history of developmental delay. In Case 587 the thick cortex, abnormal morphological character of the sylvian fissures ("fetal" lack of opercularization), and the paucity of normal sulcal markings also suggest a developmental problem. The terms "lissencephaly" and "pachygyria" are used to describe the surface of brains with no or few cortical gyri (see Cases 633 and 634).

DIFFERENTIAL DIAGNOSIS:
DEVELOPMENTAL ABNORMALITY WITH LARGE SUPRATENTORIAL FLUID SPACES

Case 588

3-week-old boy.

Case 589

Newborn boy.

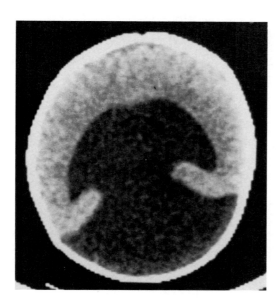

Holoprosencephaly.

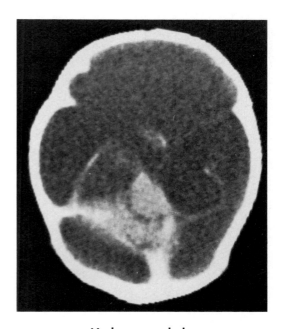

Hydranencephaly.

Several congenital abnormalities are associated with large supratentorial CSF spaces that may resemble hydrocephalic ventricles.

Holoprosencephaly is a developmental malformation (absent or incomplete cerebral hemispherization) in which a horseshoe-shaped forebrain ("holoprosencephalon") surrounds a central monoventricle. The characteristic "batwing" morphology of the single-chambered ventricle is seen anteriorly in Case 588. A midline "dorsal cyst" may be found above the brain in association with holoprosencephaly, as seen posteriorly in this case. (The posterior fossa was normal; the diencephalon was mildly malformed.)

Hydranencephaly represents loss of normal cerebral tissue due to an embryologic insult. The cerebral hemispheres are nearly or completely absent, and the supratentorial region is filled with fluid. The posterior fossa and diencephalon are characteristically preserved. This finding suggests that the hemisphere deficiency is due to agenesis, hypoplasia, and/or occlusion of the supraclinoid internal carotid arteries.

Hydranencephaly may be mistaken for severe hydrocephalus. However, the scattered remnants of cortex in hydranencephaly do not form a rim around the hemisphere, as does the compressed cortical mantle of hydrocephalus.

A diffuse anoxic or inflammatory insult may also resemble hydranencephaly due to widespread low attenuation with relative sparing of the posterior fossa and diencephalon. A "ghost" of once-normal structure is usually visible in the former circumstances (see Cases 269 and 485).

DIFFERENTIAL DIAGNOSIS:
SUPRASELLAR CYST ASSOCIATED WITH HYDROCEPHALUS

Case 590

20-year-old man.

Case 591

8-year-old boy.

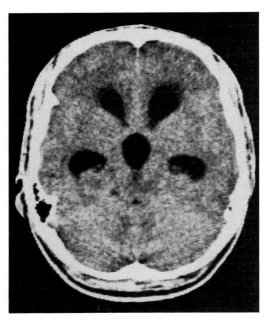

Hydrocephalic Third Ventricle (Aqueductal Obstruction due to a Midbrain Mass).

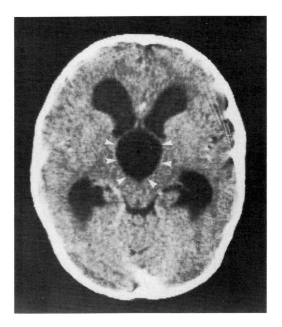

Suprasellar Arachnoid Cyst Obstructing the Third Ventricle.

The diagnosis of "benign" aqueductal stenosis requires careful exclusion of other lesions with similar appearances. Small midbrain masses can obstruct the aqueduct while causing minimal abnormalities of density or contour (see Cases 111 and 113). Alternatively, low-attenuation lesions may be overlooked as they occupy or compress the third ventricle. Such lesions can be hidden within CSF density (see Cases 592 and 593) or mistakenly interpreted as a dilated ventricle.

A hydrocephalic third ventricle is seen in Case 590. This structure may act as a suprasellar mass, causing erosion of the dorsum sella and expansion of the sella itself.

The suprasellar arachnoid cyst in Case 591 *(arrowheads)* mimics an enlarged third ventricle. The diagnosis of aqueductal stenosis could be assumed, although the very round margins of the cyst are unusual for third ventricular dilatation. Subsequent evaluation demonstrated a suprasellar cyst compressing the third ventricle and causing obstructive hydrocephalus. An ependymal cyst arising *within* the third ventricle could present an identical image.

Other midline lesions that may mimic third ventricular distention include low-density hypothalamic gliomas (see Case 592), low-attenuation craniopharyngiomas (see Case 188), and rare cysts of the septum pellucidum.

DIFFERENTIAL DIAGNOSIS:
LOW-ATTENUATION LESION WITHIN THE THIRD VENTRICLE

Case 592

9-year-old girl with neurofibromatosis.

Case 593

17-year-old girl.
(scan with intraventricular contrast)

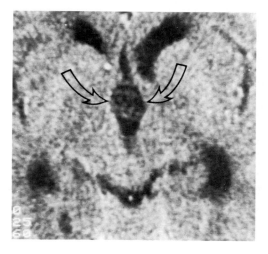

Pilocytic Astrocytoma.

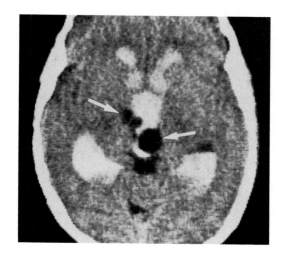

Cysticercosis.

Cysts or tumors of low attenuation (e.g., ependymal cyst, parasitic cyst, glioma, epidermoid tumor) may obstruct the third ventricle while blending with the surrounding spinal fluid. These masses can be easily overlooked, leading to the incorrect diagnosis of aqueductal stenosis.

The density of such lesions may differ slightly from CSF, allowing detection by close examination of standard scans (as in Case 592).

Other lesions may be completely hidden on CT examinations. Magnetic resonance imaging may help to define such cysts or tissues of CSF-like attenuation. In other cases, intraventricular contrast is required for diagnosis, as in Case 593.

CHIARI II ("ARNOLD-CHIARI") MALFORMATION

Case 594

4-year-old girl.

Case 595

1-year-old girl (after shunting for hydrocephalus).

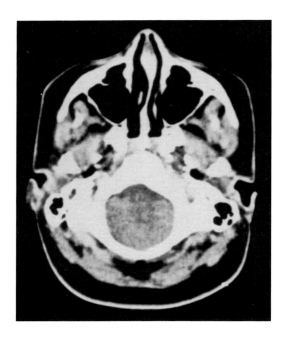

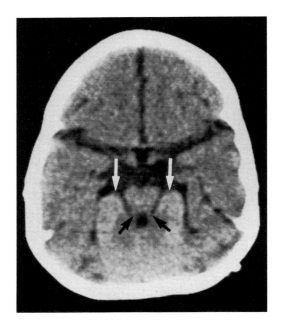

The Chiari II malformation ranks with communicating hydrocephalus and aqueductal stenosis among the major congenital causes of hydrocephalus. The malformation is a complex developmental abnormality including caudal herniation of the hindbrain through the foramen magnum into the cervical spinal canal.

In combination with associated hydrocephalus, this deformity causes a large supratentorial compartment and a small posterior fossa. Findings on CT reflect infratentorial crowding, with scalloped erosion of the petrous ridges. The foramen magnum is enlarged and filled with cerebellar tissue surrounding the brain stem, as seen here.

An additional clue to the diagnosis in infants is the associated skull dysplasia called "craniolacunae" or "lückenschädel skull." This characteristic finding is present at birth and usually disappears by age 1 year. (Mottled skull lucency due to "convolutional impressions" from increased intracranial pressure is rarely seen before age 2 years.)

In addition to the calvarial abnormalities discussed in Case 594, several parenchymal deformities are characteristic of the Chiari II malformation. The dorsal midbrain is typically "beaked," with the colliculi fused into a single peak (black arrows). The crowded cerebellum wraps around the brain stem bilaterally (white arrows). After shunting, the cerebellum towers superiorly near the midline as a pseudomass (see Case 597). Hypoplasia or fenestration of the falx and tentorium may also be noted.

The CT features described in Cases 594 and 595 are characteristic of a Chiari II malformation. The almost invariable association with myelomeningocele further supports the diagnosis.

MR CORRELATION: CHIARI II MALFORMATION

Case 596

3-year-old girl, post-shunt for hydrocephalus.
(sagittal, noncontrast scan; SE 600/17)

Case 597

11-month-old boy, post-shunt for
hydrocephalus.
(coronal, noncontrast scan; SE 700/17)

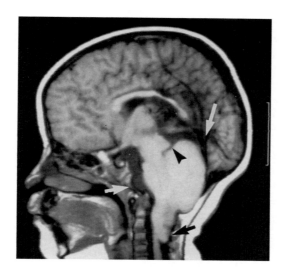

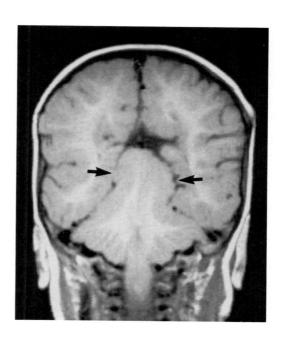

The sagittal and coronal planes of magnetic resonance imaging combine with the absence of bone artifact to provide excellent visualization of lesions involving the foramen magnum.

In this case, MR demonstrates the small, crowded posterior fossa. Prior concave erosion of the clivus *(short white arrow)* and near-vertical orientation of "flow-void" in the straight sinus *(long white arrow)* are seen. The midbrain tectum is "beaked" *(black arrowhead)*. A "cascade" of herniating tissue extends from the posterior fossa through the wide foramen magnum into the cervical spinal canal. Buckling of the caudally displaced medulla often forms a tissue layer between the herniated cerebellum and the spinal cord, as in this case *(black arrow)*.

The many CT features of the Chiari II malformation discussed in Cases 594 and 595 are well seen on axial MR scans. The coronal MR plane is useful for demonstrating the "towering" cerebellum often encountered in these patients after shunting of hydrocephalus.

The steeply sloped tentorium accentuates rostral expansion of cerebellar tissue following relief of supratentorial pressure. An axial CT scan through the superior pole of the "towering" cerebellum may be falsely interpreted as demonstrating a superior vermian mass.

DANDY-WALKER MALFORMATION

Case 598

1-year-old boy.

Case 599

3-year-old girl with a history of craniofacial surgery.

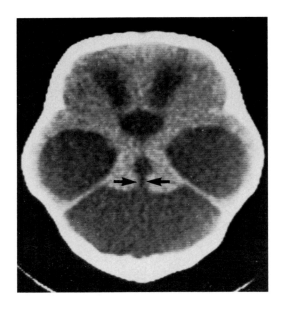

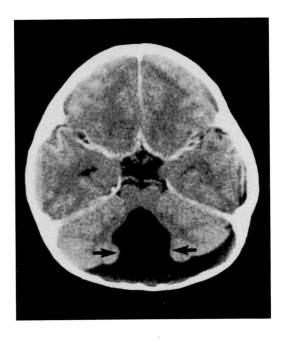

The Dandy-Walker malformation is a less common cause of congenital hydrocephalus than the previously discussed etiologies. Aplasia or hypoplasia and malrotation of the cerebellar vermis is associated with a "roofless" fourth ventricle, opening dorsally (arrows) into a large posterior fossa cyst. The cyst typically surrounds hypoplastic cerebellar hemispheres. Expansion of the posterior fossa associated with the Dandy-Walker malformation contrasts with the small posterior fossa seen in aqueductal stenosis and the Chiari II malformation.

This scan demonstrates a large infratentorial compartment at a level above the petrous ridges. The vermis defect is outlined by arrows. Chronic enlargement of the temporal horns has caused molding of the adjacent calvarium and outlines the tentorium.

The degree of vermian and hemispheric hypoplasia in the Dandy-Walker malformation is variable. In this case, a broad communication is present between the fourth ventricle and an asymmetrical posterior fossa cyst.

Posterior fossa arachnoid cysts (see Cases 622 to 626) and large cisternae magna may mimic the Dandy-Walker malformation. The integrity and position of the cerebellar vermis provide the key to differential diagnosis in such cases.

Case 600

1-year-old boy presenting with a large head.
(sagittal, noncontrast scan; SE 500/20)

Case 601

8-month-old girl.
(axial, noncontrast scan; SE 2500/90)

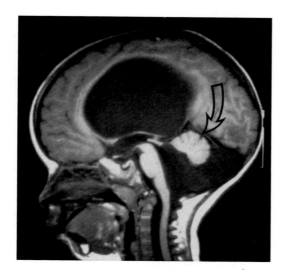

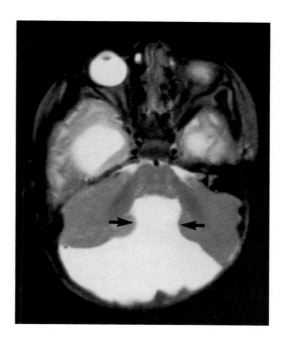

The sagittal MR plane has improved understanding of CT scans in patients with the Dandy-Walker malformation. As seen here, "absence" of the vermis on low axial scans through the posterior fossa is due more to superior rotation of this tissue than to true aplasia. The broad communication between the fourth ventricle and the posterior cyst "lifts" and rotates the vermis superiorly against the tentorial apex. Although associated vermian hypoplasia is common, the amount of residual tissue demonstrated by MR is greater than appreciated on most CT studies.

Compare this scan to the appearance of the posterior fossa arachnoid cyst in Case 624.

This scan represents the MR equivalent of Case 599. The fourth ventricle opens broadly into a posterior fossa cyst, which is slightly asymmetrical. The cerebellar hemispheres are mildly compressed and hypoplastic. Associated hydrocephalus is indicated by expansion of the temporal horns.

Case 602

57-year-old woman, 10 days after subarachnoid hemorrhage.

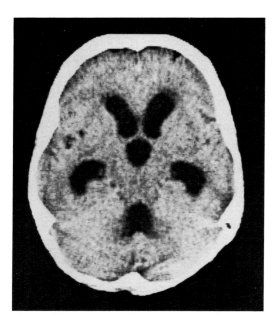

Case 603

54-year-old woman with a large acoustic schwannoma.

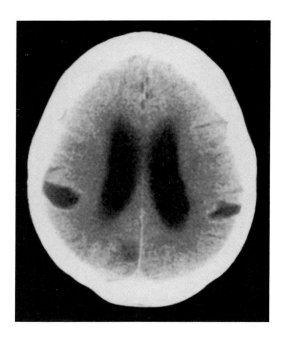

The enlargement of lateral, third, and fourth ventricles in this case places the impairment to CSF flow outside the ventricular system. (Compare this pattern of hydrocephalus to Case 590.)

Communicating hydrocephalus in adults often follows an inflammatory meningeal process, either infectious (meningitis) or hemorrhagic (trauma or aneurysm rupture). Such patients are usually good candidates for shunt procedures.

Meningitis or meningeal carcinomatosis may present as communicating hydrocephalus in adults (see Case 526). Contrast-enhanced scans (preferably MR) and CSF analysis to exclude meningeal pathology should precede a diagnosis of "normal pressure hydrocephalus" (see Case 604).

Intracranial and spinal tumors may be associated with communicating hydrocephalus due to high CSF loads of cells, hemorrhage, and/or protein. Choroid plexus papillomas, ependymomas, and acoustic schwannomas are among the masses with this tendency.

Some cases of communicating hydrocephalus demonstrate widening of subarachnoid spaces over the entire cerebral convexity. In other cases there is focal enlargement of individual cisterns and sulci, as seen here (see also Case 609).

DIFFERENTIAL DIAGNOSIS:
LARGE LATERAL VENTRICLES IN AN ELDERLY PATIENT

Case 604

77-year-old man.

Case 605

82-year-old woman.

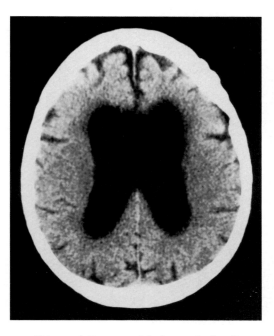

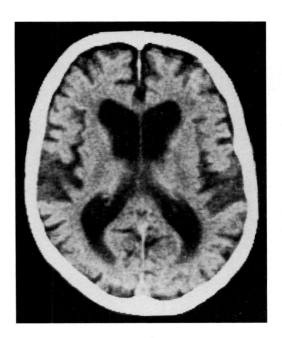

"Normal Pressure Hydrocephalus."

Atrophy.

Some adults develop low-grade, communicating hydrocephalus with no history of meningitis, subarachnoid hemorrhage, or tumor. This "normal pressure hydrocephalus" is often superimposed on a background of atrophy in an elderly patient. Associated periventricular edema may mimic the low attenuation "normally" seen in "old" white matter (see Case 327). For these reasons, the distinction between atrophic ventricular expansion and "normal pressure" hydrocephalus can be difficult.

Several clues are helpful in this situation. (1) The margins of hydrocephalic ventricles as in Case 604 appear "tight" and stretched, while the margins of atrophic ventricles as in Case 605 are less distended. (2) A halo or fringe of periventricular edema may cause the borders of hydrocephalic ventricles to become indistinct (as in Cases 606 and 607), while atrophic ventricles remain sharply defined. (3) Hydrocephalic expansion of the lateral ventricles includes prominent temporal horn enlargement, while the temporal horns are less dilated in most cases of cerebral atrophy (see Case 335 regarding temporal atrophy in Pick's and Alzheimer's diseases). (4) Enlargement of the third ventricle is definite in hydrocephalus but less impressive in patients with atrophy. (Sagittal MR scans are helpful in assessing third ventricular distention.) Enlargement of the fourth ventricle favors hydrocephalus when present, but many cases of communicating hydrocephalus do not show significant expansion of the fourth ventricle.

Tests of CSF dynamics using subarachnoid contrast material may help to document normal pressure hydrocephalus. However, the best predictor of shunt response is usually the clinical triad of gait abnormality, urinary incontinence, and dementia. A short history and a prominent degree of hydrocephalus also favor a good result.

SECONDARY FINDINGS IN HYDROCEPHALUS: PERIVENTRICULAR EDEMA

Case 606

57-year-old woman.

Hydrocephalus due to a Colloid Cyst of the Third Ventricle.

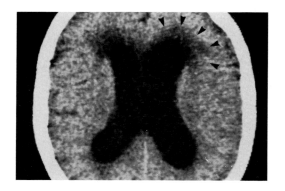

Case 607

15-month-old boy.
(narrow window)

Hydrocephalus due to an Optic Glioma.

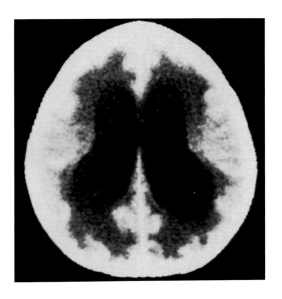

As the lateral ventricles enlarge in hydrocephalus, the tight junctions between ependymal cells are eventually disrupted. This discontinuity may allow spinal fluid under pressure to "leak" into the periventricular white matter. The normal centripetal movement of interstitial fluid from the brain through the subependymal region into the ventricles is also impaired by high intraventricular pressure.

These factors cause a localized or diffuse "fringe" of low attenuation around the ventricular margins. The low density may be appreciated as a definite zone, as in this case *(arrowheads)*, or as haziness of the normally sharp ventricular margins.

When diffuse periventricular edema occurs in an elderly patient, the appearance can mimic the aging white matter pattern illustrated in Case 327.

The zone of periventricular edema may be strikingly demonstrated in some cases of acute, severe hydrocephalus. Here the low-attenuation "halo" surrounding the ventricles has been accentuated by photographing at a narrow window width. Hydrocephalus could be considered a type of white matter disease, since distortion and edema of white matter are prominent features of the condition.

Cases 125, 192, 193, 264, and 579 illustrate other examples of periventricular edema in hydrocephalus.

Case 608

5-year-old boy with hydrocephalus due to a
cerebellar astrocytoma; recent placement of a
right frontal ventriculostomy.
(axial, noncontrast scan; SE 2500/45)

Case 609

66-year-old woman with communicating
hydrocephalus secondary to an acoustic
schwannoma.
(coronal, noncontrast scan; SE 650/15)

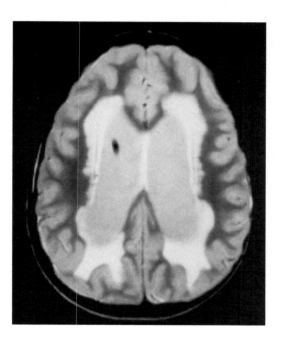

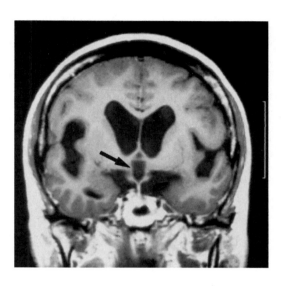

Periventricular edema due to hydrocephalus is well demonstrated by MR, like other causes of increased water content in cerebral white matter. Cases with an equivocal CT appearance may be obvious on MR studies.

Here prominent periventricular edema demonstrates a broad, irregular or "shaggy" morphology, resembling Case 607. This pattern is seen with acute and/or severe elevation of intraventricular pressure. A thinner and more uniform layer of periventricular edema is usually associated with more chronic or less severe hydrocephalus.

Multiplanar MR can support the diagnosis of communicating hydrocephalus by documenting widened superficial CSF pathways in addition to diffuse ventricular enlargement. In this case, the sylvian cisterns are prominently expanded with a "tight" contour that suggests active distention. The absence of atrophic sulci in other sites supports the interpretation of focal cisternal enlargement as a manifestation of communicating hydrocephalus (compare to Case 603).

The distended anterior recesses of the third ventricle are seen in the suprasellar region (arrow), immediately superior to the optic chiasm and pituitary infundibulum.

Case 610

15-month-old boy.

Diverticulum of the Third Ventricle.

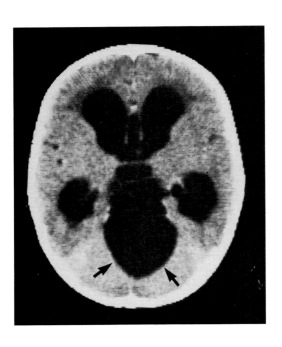

Case 611

1-year-old boy.

Diverticulum of the Lateral Ventricular Trigone.

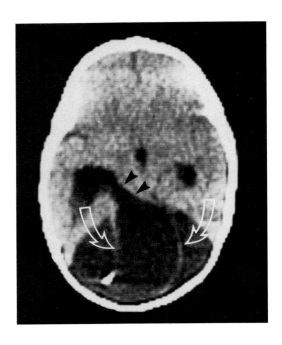

Hydrocephalic ventricles may expand into areas of relatively low resistance. For example, the posterior third ventricle may bulge into the quadrigeminal cistern. Continued enlargement of this diverticulum may extend inferiorly through the tentorial hiatus.

The diverticulum is then seen as a midline mass in the posterior fossa, as in this case. Such diverticula may be confused with primary cysts or masses and erroneously implicated as the cause of hydrocephalus (compare to Case 623).

The thinned walls of distended ventricles may also perforate, immediately relieving symptoms ("spontaneous ventriculostomy").

Another common location for the formation of ventricular diverticula is the medial wall of the trigone (lateral ventricle). A diverticulum from this site (arrowheads) often extends into the posterior fossa.

Here, shunting of a Dandy-Walker cyst has allowed infratentorial expansion of the ventricular diverticulum (arrows).

COMPLICATIONS OF VENTRICULAR SHUNTING

Case 612

8-year-old boy.

Subdural Hematomas.

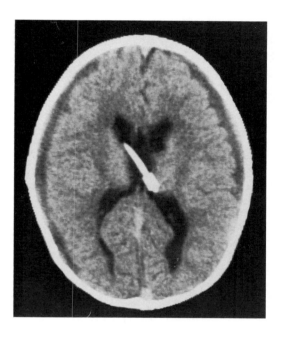

Case 613

5-year-old boy presenting 1 year after shunting with headache and vomiting.

"Slit-like" (Collapsed) Ventricles.

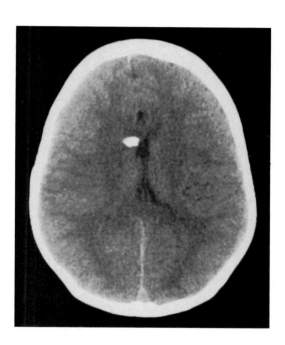

Decompression of dilated ventricles may lead to collapse of the cerebral cortex, favoring the development of secondary subdural hematomas (compare to Case 484). Large subdural collections may present acutely, while smaller lesions follow a more chronic course, as in this case. Subdural hematomas should be a primary consideration (along with shunt malfunction) when symptoms recur or head size increases in a child who has undergone shunting.

Shunted ventricles sometimes collapse to tiny residual slits, as in this case. (Compare the morphology of the lateral ventricles seen here to the ventricular distortion from bilateral subdural hematomas in Case 354.)

Chronic ventricular collapse may be associated with low compliance. Subsequent shunt malfunction can cause a rapid increase in pressure with little expansion of ventricular volume. Small ventricular size does not exclude shunt malfunction in such cases.

Infection is another complication of ventricular shunts, occurring in about 1% to 10% of cases. Shunt-related infection often involves the subependymal tissue (see Case 265). Periventricular cysts or loculations may form. These can enlarge and bulge into the ventricle, mimicking intraventricular septations.

Case 614

27-year-old man.
(postcontrast scan; wide window width)

Case 615

42-year-old woman examined because of a
"lytic lesion" on skull x-rays.

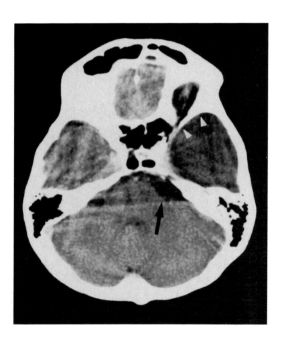

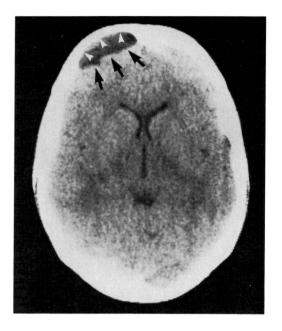

Arachnoid cysts account for about 1% of intracranial masses. They are often discovered incidentally, presenting as low-attenuation lesions in a number of characteristic locations. The middle cranial fossa is a common site, as illustrated here.

Long-term pressure from arachnoid cysts frequently causes expansion or erosion of bone. In this case, the sphenoid wing has been thinned and anteriorly displaced *(arrowheads)*.

A similar appearance is occasionally seen in children with chronic "juvenile" subdural hematomas of the middle cranial fossa. In adults, the major differential diagnosis is a middle fossa epidermoid cyst.

Extension across the petrous apex as seen here *(arrow)* is rare in arachnoid cysts (and more commonly encountered in epidermoid cysts; see Cases 236 and 241).

Arachnoid cysts are most common near the skull base but may occur over the cerebral convexities. Erosion of the adjacent inner table is often associated with such lesions *(white arrowheads)*. The medial margin or cerebral interface of the cyst is often characteristically straight and angular *(black arrows; see also Cases 617 and 619).*

MR CORRELATION: ARACHNOID CYSTS

Case 616

56-year-old woman.
(coronal, noncontrast scan; SE 800/22)

Case 617

26-year-old woman.
(axial, noncontrast scan; SE 3000/80)

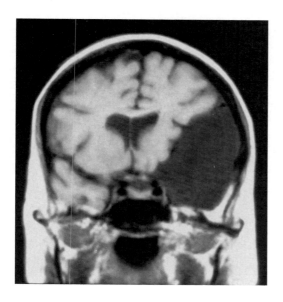

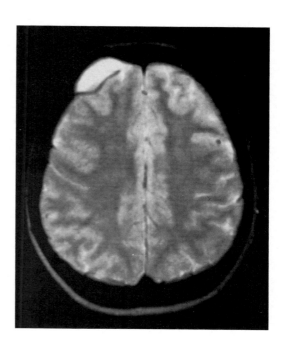

Low-attenuation CT lesions can be confirmed as CSF-containing cysts by magnetic resonance imaging. The signal intensity of such masses follows that of cisternal or ventricular fluid on all pulse sequences.

In this case a large arachnoid cyst has extended superiorly from the middle cranial fossa. The low-grade, long-standing nature of the lesion is indicated by hypoplasia of the adjacent left hemisphere with minimal midline shift (compare to Case 548B). The left middle cranial fossa has been expanded by the cyst, as in Case 614.

This scan represents the MR equivalent of Case 615. A small convexity cyst with CSF-like intensity values is associated with mild erosion of the overlying inner table. The interface of the cyst with adjacent cerebral cortex is relatively linear or "flat."

DIFFERENTIAL DIAGNOSIS:
LOW-ATTENUATION LESION EXTENDING OVER THE CEREBRAL CONVEXITY

Case 618

54-year-old woman.

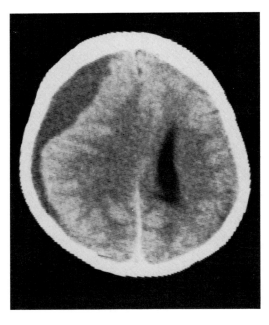

Chronic Subdural Hematoma.

Case 619

27-year-old man.

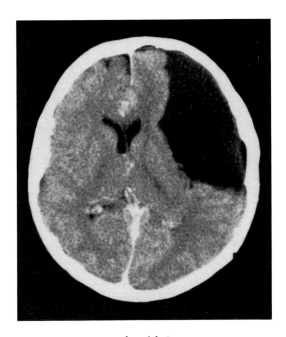

Arachnoid Cyst.

Arachnoid cysts may extend over large portions of the cerebral convexity. The appearance of such lesions can resemble a chronic subdural hematoma.

A useful diagnostic feature of arachnoid cysts is the frequently linear contour of their medial margin, as demonstrated in Case 619. This angular boundary contrasts with the smoothly compressed cerebral cortex underlying a subdural hematoma, as in Case 618.

MR scans can distinguish the intensity values of chronic hematomas from those of CSF collections in equivocal CT cases (see Cases 364 and 365).

DIFFERENTIAL DIAGNOSIS:
LOW-ATTENUATION SUPRASELLAR MASS

Case 620

25-year-old man with a 4-year history of headache.

Case 621

52-year-old man (same patient as Case 237).

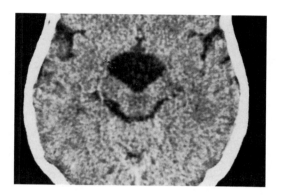

Epidermoid Cyst.

Arachnoid Cyst.

Both arachnoid cysts and epidermoid cysts may occur in the suprasellar region. Cysts or low-density tumors in this location may mimic an enlarged third ventricle (see Cases 591 to 593).

The arachnoid cyst in Case 620 causes lateral displacement of the temporal lobes and supraclinoid internal carotid arteries, and extends into the choroid fissure on the right (arrow). The epidermoid cyst in Case 621 has expanded posteriorly into the interpeduncular cistern, splaying the cerebral peduncles.

Attenuation values within an arachnoid cyst are often lower and usually more homogeneous than those of an epidermoid cyst. The distinction may also be made with subarachnoid contrast material (see Case 237) or by magnetic resonance imaging (see Case 241).

POSTERIOR FOSSA ARACHNOID CYSTS

Case 622

70-year-old man presenting with hydrocephalus.

Case 623

40-year-old man.

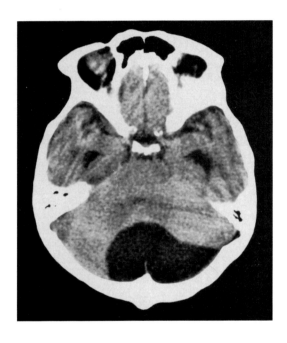

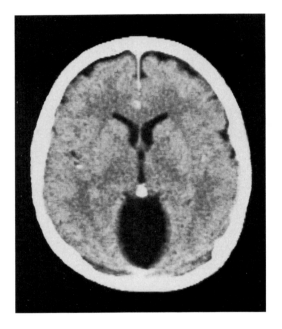

Arachnoid cysts near the occipital bone may be confused with a large and/or asymmetric cisterna magna. Evidence of mass effect favors the diagnosis of a true cyst.

In this case the bulging margin of the cyst has compressed the cerebellar vermis and fourth ventricle. The pons is ventrally displaced toward the dorsum sella. Enlargement of the temporal horns indicates obstructive hydrocephalus. Calcification of the paraclinoid internal carotid arteries is present.

Posterior fossa arachnoid cysts should not be confused with the Dandy-Walker malformation, since they are not associated with defects or malrotation of the vermis. (Compare the fourth ventricular morphology on this scan to Cases 598 and 599).

This arachnoid cyst has displaced the vermis inferiorly and occupies the apex of the posterior fossa, defined by the tentorial margins. A supracerebellar arachnoid cyst may extend through the tentorial hiatus, compressing the brain stem and posterior third ventricle. The resultant combination of transtentorial cyst and hydrocephalus may resemble the appearance of a third ventricular diverticulum, as in Case 610.

The quadrigeminal cistern is a common location for both epidermoid cysts and arachnoid cysts. As illustrated in Case 237, the CT distinction between these lesions can be made with subarachnoid contrast agents. Epidermoid cysts characteristically have a papillary surface, while arachnoid cysts demonstrate smooth margins. Arachnoid cysts may fill with subarachnoid contrast material, particularly on delayed scans.

Small lipomas are also commonly found in the quadrigeminal cistern, but their very low attenuation values should prevent confusion with cystic masses. MR scans also clearly distinguish the short T1 values of lipoma from the long T1 values usually seen in arachnoid and epidermoid cysts.

MR CORRELATION: POSTERIOR FOSSA ARACHNOID CYSTS

Case 624

25-year-old woman presenting with symptoms
of syringomyelia.
(sagittal, noncontrast scan; SE 600/20)

Case 625

87-year-old woman.
(coronal, noncontrast scan; SE 600/17)

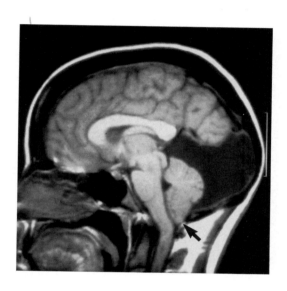

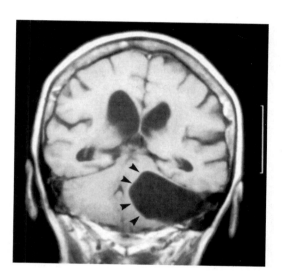

Sagittal and coronal MR scans can help to clarify the identity and morphology of arachnoid cysts in the posterior fossa. MR highlights the relationship of a cyst to the fourth ventricle and the presence of mass effect, which are important features in distinguishing these lesions from Dandy-Walker malformations or large cisternae magna.

In this case a large arachnoid cyst surrounds the cerebellum posteriorly and superiorly, representing a combination of the locations in Cases 622 and 623. The cyst is clearly not an expansion of the fourth ventricle (compare to Case 600).

Mass effect is present, with enlargement of the posterior fossa and erosion of the occipital bone. More importantly, the cerebellum has been displaced anteriorly and inferiorly into the foramen magnum. The resultant crowding of cerebellar tissue dorsal to the cervicomedullary junction resembles a Chiari I malformation, and is similarly associated with hydromyelia in this case (faintly seen at the caudal margin of the scan).

This arachnoid cyst of the cerebellopontine angle has invaginated far into the adjacent cerebellar hemisphere. Although this occurrence is common with other long-standing extra-axial lesions (e.g., meningioma or acoustic schwannoma, see Cases 33, 135, and 138), it is unusual for arachnoid cysts. As a result, the axial CT studies in this case raised the question of a cystic cerebellar neoplasm.

Coronal MR scans help to establish the correct diagnosis by demonstrating the CSF-like content of the cyst, its base against the petrous bone, and the absence of a mural nodule. The relatively small shift of the fourth ventricle also favors a long-standing lesion, similar to Case 616.

DIFFERENTIAL DIAGNOSIS:
LOW-ATTENUATION LESION IN THE CEREBELLOPONTINE ANGLE

Case 626

9-year-old girl.

Case 627

58-year-old man.

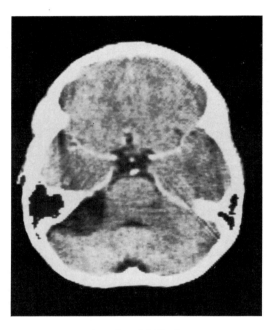

Arachnoid Cyst.

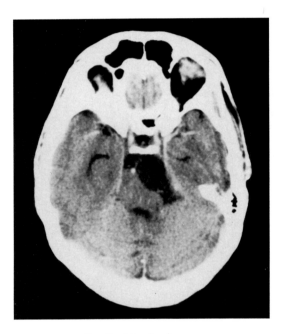

Cystic Meningioma.

The cerebellopontine angle is another common location for arachnoid cysts. They rank high in the differential diagnosis of low-attenuation, extra-axial lesions at this site, along with epidermoid cysts (see Cases 236, 239, and 241).

"Racemose cysts" of cysticercosis may involve the cerebellopontine angle (or the suprasellar, sylvian, or prepontine cisterns). Occasional schwannomas within the cerebellopontine angle are predominantly cystic or low-attenuation masses, as seen in Cases 137 and 138. Infrequently a cystic meningioma is encountered at this site, as in Case 627. Coronal and sagittal MR scans help to establish the correct diagnosis in such cases by demonstrating the solid component of complex tumors.

Magnetic resonance imaging is also useful in distinguishing between arachnoid cysts and epidermoid cysts of the cerebellopontine angle. Although the signal intensity of these lesions may be similar, their morphologies are usually characteristic. Epidermoid cysts are soft, lobulated, infiltrating masses that tend to surround vessels and cranial nerves (see Case 241). By contrast, arachnoid cysts are usually unilocular and smoothly marginated, stretching and displacing adjacent neurovascular structures. Bone erosion is commonly associated with arachnoid cysts and rarely seen with epidermoid cysts.

CYSTIC ENCEPHALOMALACIA

Case 628A

2-month-old boy studied because of large head size.

Case 628B

Same patient 1 month later, following shunt placement and injection of intraventricular contrast material.

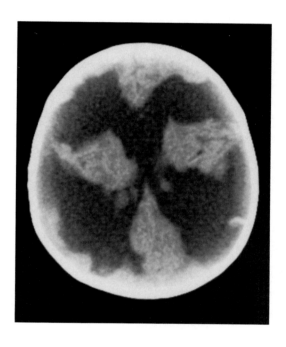

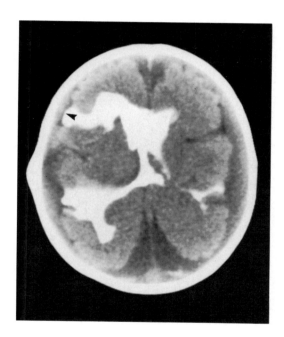

Areas of cystic encephalomalacia may occur as the result of ischemia, infection, or developmental insults. These regions may be small and numerous ("multicystic encephalomalacia") or large and unilocular as in "porencephaly" (see Cases 629 to 632). The gliotic reaction that surrounds and contains zones of cystic encephalomalacia is a more mature response to cerebral injury than the generalized dissolution of tissue often seen in other cases of perinatal damage (compare to Cases 268 and 269).

Here zones of CSF-like attenuation are seen adjacent to the anterior and posterior margins of the hydrocephalic lateral ventricles. The bilateral symmetry suggests a developmental etiology. It is not possible to comment on loculation or ventricular communication, since thin septations may be inapparent on routine CT studies.

Both the ventricular system and the adjacent areas of cystic encephalomalacia have decreased in size after shunting. Injection of contrast confirms that the parenchymal cysts are unilocular and communicate with the ventricular system.

The cystic zones appear to represent encephaloclastic clefts traversing the cerebral hemisphere from the ventricles to the cortical surface. Contrast within these cysts remains largely distinct from the overlying subarachnoid space (*arrowhead*), and the clefts do not seem to be lined by gray matter. (Contrast these features with the appearance of schizencephaly in Cases 635 and 636.)

Small extracerebral fluid spaces present on the initial scan have enlarged after shunting.

PORENCEPHALIC CYSTS

Case 629

51-year-old woman with a history of a childhood "stroke," now presenting with seizures.

Case 630

72-year-old woman with a history of an old stroke.

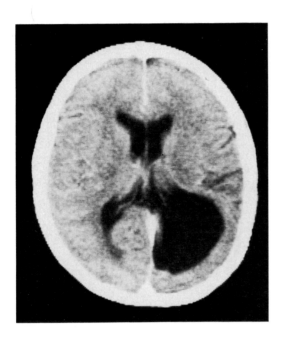

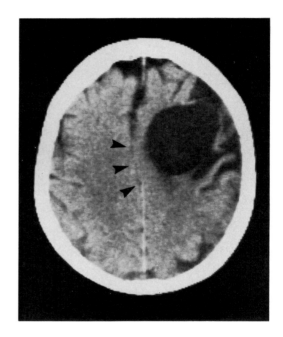

The term "porencephalic cyst" is variously applied to cystic lesions that form in regions of cerebral encephalomalacia. The strict application of the phrase refers to localized expansion of the ventricular system into an area of parenchymal damage.

In this case porencephalic expansion of the ventricular trigone probably indicates the site of the childhood cerebrovascular accident. (Compare this scan to Case 420.)

Porencephalic cysts may grow and exert pressure, probably due to incomplete communication with the parent ventricle or subarachnoid pathways. Such lesions present a paradoxical appearance of mass effect in the midst of atrophy.

The cyst in this case is surrounded by large sulci, reflecting an old parenchymal insult. The cyst itself appears "tight," with mass effect evidenced by mild subfalcial herniation (arrowheads).

Although porencephalic cysts may be superficial as seen here (and in Cases 631 and 632), they are intra-axial lesions. (Compare to the extra-axial origin of arachnoid cysts with secondary cerebral deformity or invagination as illustrated in Cases 614 through 626.)

MR CORRELATION: PORENCEPHALIC CYSTS

Case 631

22-year-old man presenting with seizures.
(coronal, noncontrast scan; SE 2500/28)

Case 632

27-year-old man presenting with seizures.
(coronal, noncontrast scan; SE 3000/80)

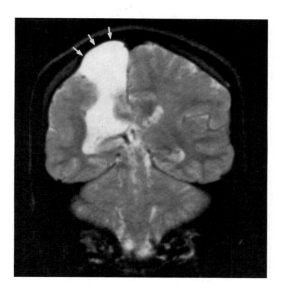

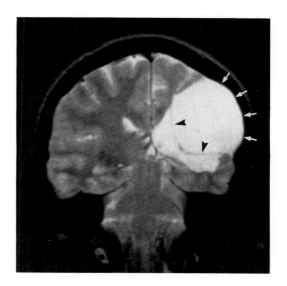

Here a superficial cyst with CSF-like intensity values is seen at the right hemisphere vertex. The location and content of the lesion might suggest an arachnoid cyst, with associated erosion of the overlying calvarium.

A clue to the correct diagnosis is the status of the underlying cerebral parenchyma. The right hemisphere is small, with expansion of the right lateral ventricle. These features imply old volume loss and suggest that the superficial cyst has arisen in a region of encephalomalacia (compare to Cases 338 and 339). Adjacent gliosis is not well seen on this scan but supports the MR diagnosis of porencephaly in many cases.

A large cyst of CSF-like intensity extends from the ventricular margin to the cortical surface of the mid-left hemisphere. The overlying inner table is mildly eroded. A thin layer of tissue (black arrowheads) separates the cyst from the ventricular chamber.

Although the cyst itself is clearly "tight" and associated with mass effect, ipsilateral ventricular enlargement suggests a porencephalic origin. The left hemicranium is slightly smaller than the right, supporting a history of parenchymal damage.

Compare the lack of tissue separating this intra-axial cyst from the adjacent ventricle to the appearance of an invaginating extra-axial arachnoid cyst in Case 625.

LISSENCEPHALY/PACHYGYRIA

Case 633

6-week-old boy.

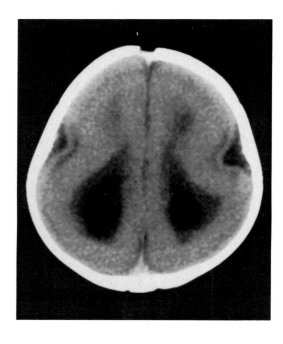

Case 634

26-year-old woman presenting with seizures.

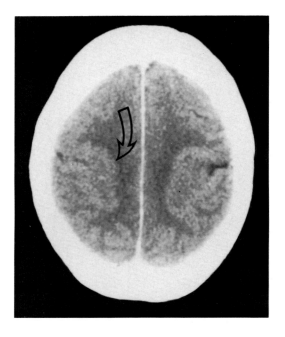

Abnormalities of neuronal migration lead to a variety of recognizable developmental malformations. Among these is lissencephaly, or "smooth brain." This disorder is characterized by thick cerebral cortex that lacks normal gyration.

Associated features include poor opercularization in the sylvian region, with the shallow sylvian grooves giving the brain a "figure of eight" appearance on axial images. Hypoplasia of white matter accompanies the abnormal cortical mantle, and ventricles are typically enlarged and dysmorphic.

Abnormally smooth, thick cortex is apparent in this case. The low-attenuation stripe within the cortex in the midhemisphere region may represent the "cell sparse zone" of presumed laminar necrosis typically found in lissencephaly.

The severe involvement seen here is usually associated with a very limited prognosis. (Case 587 presents a milder example of this syndrome.)

Evidence of abnormal neuronal migration is often less severe or more limited than true lissencephaly. Zones of abnormally thick cortex may be unilateral or may symmetrically involve localized portions of the hemispheres. The term "pachygyria" is used to describe these milder variants of the lissencephaly spectrum.

Here the cortex surrounding the rostral margin of the central sulcus is abnormally thick bilaterally. (The appearance resembles a "closed-lip schizencephaly," as seen in Case 636). Localized pachygyria, like gray matter heterotopia (see Case 639), is often correlated with seizures.

Polymicrogyria is another abnormality of cortical development, characterized by multiple tiny gyri on the cerebral surface. The small size and crowding of these microgyri causes them to blend together on CT images, often resembling the appearance of pachygyria. Involvement of the sylvian and rolandic regions is common, and pathological examination of this case could demonstrate polymicrogyria rather than true pachygyria. MR scans may define tiny interdigitations between small gyri (particularly at the interface with underlying white matter), establishing the diagnosis of polymicrogyria.

SCHIZENCEPHALY

Case 635

1-year-old boy with a history of "cerebral palsy."

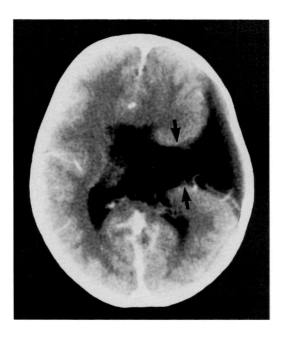

Case 636

8-year-old boy presenting with seizures and a history of "cerebral palsy."
(axial, noncontrast scan; SE 3000/75)

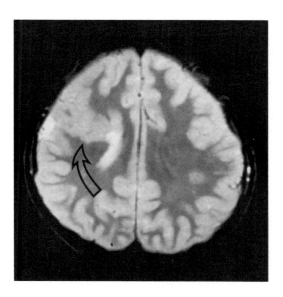

Schizencephaly is a disorder of neuronal migration characterized by a transcerebral cleft from the lateral ventricle to the cerebral surface. Unlike encephaloclastic clefts from damage to normally formed parenchyma (as in Case 628), schizencephalic clefts are lined by abnormal gray matter. The margin of transparenchymal cortex clearly seen here distinguishes this developmental malformation from acquired encephalomalacia.

The transcerebral clefts of schizencephaly may be unilateral or bilateral. They most frequently occur at the midhemisphere level, near the central sulcus. The margins of the cleft may be widely separated as in this case, or closely opposed ("fused lip schizencephaly"). In the latter instance small diverticular deformities at the ventricular and cortical terminations of the cleft provide a clue to the nature of the intervening abnormality (see Cases 636 and 638).

Patients with schizencephaly often present with seizures. Focal neurological deficits may also occur, reflecting the location and size of the cleft.

The excellent gray/white matter differentiation on MR scans helps to identify abnormalities of neuronal migration. In this case a transcerebral column of gray matter is seen in the right frontal lobe, extending from the cerebral surface to the ventricular margin. The tissue along this band demonstrates the same signal intensity as cortical gray matter in other locations.

Small, CSF-containing diverticuli at the ventricular and superficial margins of the "lesion" are remnants of a largely closed cleft ("fused-lip schizencephaly"; see Case 638).

Polymicrogyria is common along the borders of schizencephalic clefts.

Case 637

5-year-old boy.
(coronal, noncontrast scan; SE 750/20)

Pachygyria.

Case 638

8-year-old boy presenting with seizures (same patient as Case 636).
(sagittal, noncontrast scan; SE 600/17)

Schizencephaly.

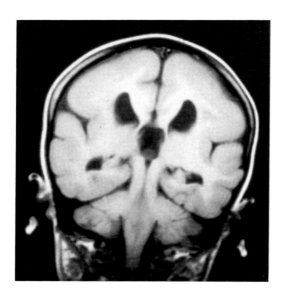

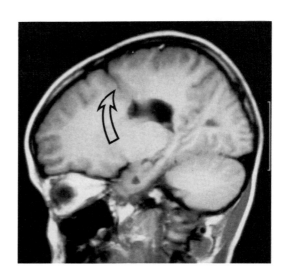

Multiplanar display and the absence of calvarial artifact enable MR to demonstrate cortical morphology better than CT.

In this case the abnormally smooth and thick cortex of the frontal lobes is well seen on a coronal scan. The temporal gyri are also abnormally wide. Hypoplasia of subcortical white matter is present, along with partial agenesis of the corpus callosum and dysmorphic ventricular enlargement.

In cases of asymmetrical pachygyria or gray matter heterotopia, the prominent density and contrast enhancement of the malformed cortex on CT scans may be mistaken for a mass. Magnetic resonance imaging is valuable for demonstrating that the region in question maintains signal intensity equal to that of normal gray matter on all pulse sequences.

A narrow schizencephalic cleft may be missed on scans that are parallel or oblique to its plane. Multiplanar MR is more effective than CT for documenting schizencephaly by means of images that are perpendicular to the cleft.

This scan is a sagittal view of the patient in Case 636. The thin residual cleft of schizencephaly is directly identified in this plane, lined by gray matter (arrow). A small deformity is seen along the ventricular margin at the inferior end of the cleft.

Case 639A	Case 639B
5-month-old boy. (sagittal, noncontrast scan; SE 700/20)	Same patient. (axial, noncontrast scan; SE 3000/90)

Heterotopic Gray Matter.

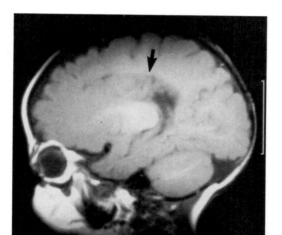

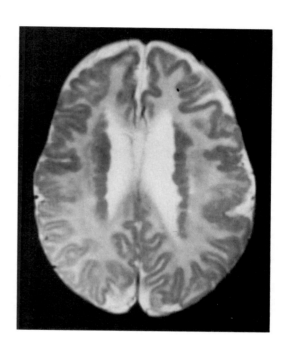

The "cobblestone" texture along the wall of the lateral ventricle in this case is due to multiple nodules of heterotopic gray matter. The subependymal rests seen here are unusually numerous and uniform. In other cases, the appearance of heterotopic gray matter may resemble tuberous sclerosis (see Case 641).

Heterotopic gray matter is well demonstrated on T2-weighted MR scans (see Case 636). Zones of incomplete neuronal migration may be seen as amorphous islands within white matter or as nodules along the ventricular surface. Cerebral involvement may be bilaterally symmetrical or strikingly unilateral.

In this case, symmetrical rows of heterotopic nodules line the walls of the lateral ventricles. The neurons within these nodules failed to migrate from the germinal matrix (see Case 325) to the cortical mantle. Abnormally high signal intensity throughout cerebral white matter sharply outlines both the nodules and the cortex.

Heterotopic gray matter may demonstrate mild contrast enhancement (comparable to normal cortex) on CT or MR studies.

AGENESIS OF THE CORPUS CALLOSUM

Case 640

Newborn boy with microcephaly.
(noncontrast scan)

Case 641

16-year-old boy presenting with headaches.

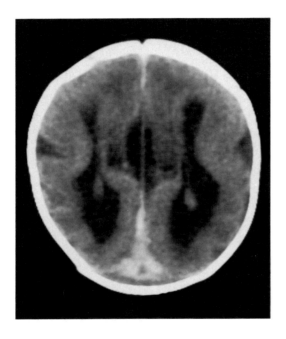

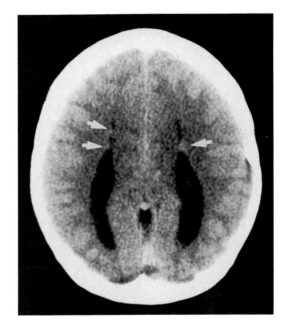

Absence of the corpus callosum allows the third ventricle to rise high in the midline as an interhemispheric cyst. (A separate and larger dorsal interhemispheric cyst may be seen in some cases of callosal agenesis, as in other congenital abnormalities such as Case 588.) This "high-riding" third ventricle is best appreciated on coronal scans, which may also demonstrate deep extension of the falx and comma-shaped frontal horns.

The density of the dural sinuses seen here near the torcular is a common feature of CT scans in newborns. The finding likely represents hemoconcentration accentuated by the relative low attenuation of adjacent parenchyma. Sinus thrombosis (or subdural or subarachnoid hemorrhage) may be mistakenly diagnosed from this appearance.

Callosal agenesis is characterized by wide separation of lateral ventricles which are abnormally parallel. This "classic" parasagittal configuration is not present in all cases, and other CT features are more reliable (see Case 645).

Agenesis of the corpus callosum may be incomplete, with absence of only the posterior portion. In such cases the CT findings are correspondingly less characteristic.

"Colpocephaly," or dilatation of the posterior portion of the lateral ventricles, accompanies many congenital malformations. This feature may be especially prominent in agenesis of the corpus callosum, since the normal bulk of the major forceps is missing from the medial occipital lobes.

Several small nodules of heterotopic gray matter are seen along the ventricular margins in this case (arrows). These foci are isodense to cortical gray matter (see discussion in Case 639).

MR CORRELATION: CALLOSAL AGENESIS

Case 642

21-year-old man.
(sagittal, noncontrast scan; SE 800/17)

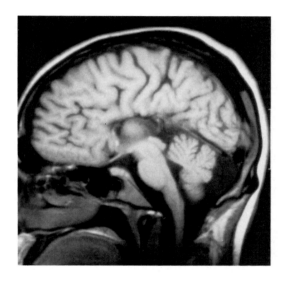

Case 643

16-year-old boy.
(coronal, noncontrast scan; SE 900/17)

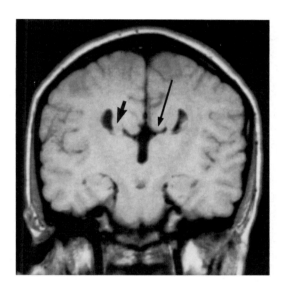

The demonstration of midline anatomy was one of the early accomplishments of cerebral MR scanning. The corpus callosum is well seen on sagittal MR studies and can be easily evaluated. (Cases 82, 83, and 316 illustrate examples of callosal pathology.)

In this case the structure of the corpus callosum is missing on a midsagittal image. The sulci on the medial surface of the hemisphere have an abnormal radial pattern, extending inferiorly to nearly reach the third ventricle and velum interpositum.

Coronal MR scans document the multiple anatomical abnormalities associated with agenesis of the corpus callosum. The high-riding third ventricle meets the interhemispheric fissure, with no separation by crossing callosal tissue. The lateral ventricles are widely separated, forming a "longhorn steer" pattern with the third ventricle.

The narrowed diameter of the lateral ventricles is due to indentation of their medial margin by the bundles of Probst (short arrow). These longitudinal fiber bands represent axons that would normally cross in the corpus callosum but have instead formed parasagittal tracts. Malrotated cingulate gyri (long arrow) are seen medial to the bundles of Probst.

DIFFERENTIAL DIAGNOSIS:
MIDLINE CYST BETWEEN THE LATERAL VENTRICLES

Case 644

40-year-old woman.

Case 645

1-year-old boy.

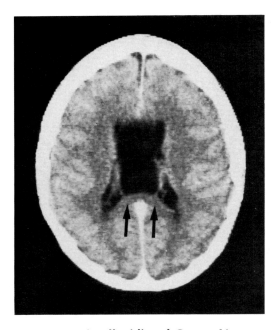

Cavum Septi Pellucidi and Cavum Vergae.

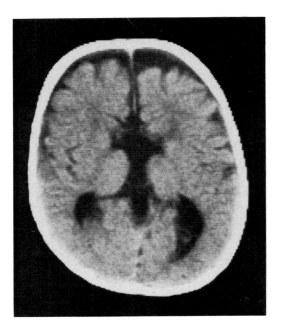

Agenesis of the Corpus Callosum.

Cysts within the septum pellucidum are a normal feature of developing brains (see Case 577) but are usually obliterated soon after birth. Persistent cysts are most commonly found at the level of the frontal horns and are termed "cavum septi pellucidi."

Larger cysts occupying most of the septum pellucidum and extending posterior to the fornix ("cavum vergae"), as in Case 644, are unusual. Case 644 has no other features to suggest agenesis of the corpus callosum; the splenium is clearly seen posteriorly (arrows).

In Case 645 the midline "cyst" represents the third ventricle and adjacent interhemispheric fissure. The absence of normal callosal tissue allows the anterior interhemispheric fissure to adjoin the elevated third ventricle. This continuity of interhemispheric fissure and superior third ventricle is a reliable sign of callosal agenesis.

Postcontrast scans in cases of agenesis of the corpus callosum may show the pericallosal arteries following an abnormally straight and posterior course as they ascend close to the anterior wall of the third ventricle. Occasionally an azygous anterior cerebral artery is seen. The high position of the third ventricle may separate and bow the internal cerebral veins.

LIPOMA OF THE CORPUS CALLOSUM

Case 646

10-month-old girl with seizures.

Case 647

1-month-old girl.
(sagittal, noncontrast scan; SE 700/16)

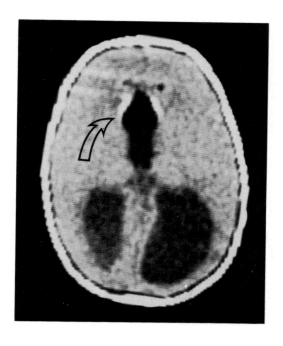

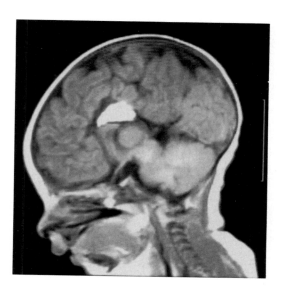

"Lipoma of the corpus callosum" is probably better considered to be an "interhemispheric lipoma with callosal dysgenesis." The lesion is believed to result from lipomatous maldifferentiation of primitive meningeal tissue in the interhemispheric fissure. The presence of the interhemispheric lipoma may secondarily impair callosal development, resulting in variable agenesis or hypoplasia.

CT scans demonstrate a characteristic morphology of midline low attenuation, often bordered by thin rims of calcification, as seen here. Attenuation values of fat within the lipoma are much lower than those of CSF within an "interhemispheric cyst" of "standard" callosal agenesis. Satellite lipomas may extend through the choroid fissure into the lateral ventricles on one or both sides.

The posterior portions of the lateral ventricles in this case are dilated and deformed, as discussed in Case 641.

Magnetic resonance imaging highlights lipid-containing lesions as areas of high signal intensity on T1-weighted images (see also Cases 420 and 815).

Here a midsagittal scan documents lipomatous tissue in the interhemispheric fissure. There is associated dysgenesis of most of the corpus callosum, with an abnormal sulcal pattern on the medial surface of the cerebral hemispheres.

Ossification within the falx may contain a marrow component with high intensity on T1-weighted scans. These thin dural plaques should not be mistaken for interhemispheric lipomas.

385

TUBEROUS SCLEROSIS

Case 648

38-year-old woman with seizures.

Case 649

49-year-old woman, scanned after head trauma.

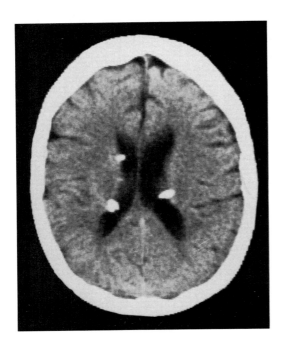

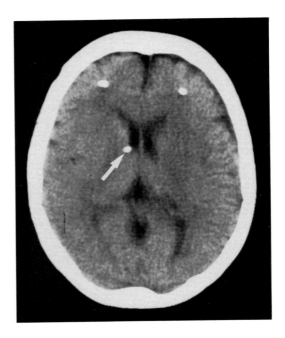

Tuberous sclerosis is one of the neurocutaneous syndromes or "neurophakomatoses," along with neurofibromatosis (see discussion of Case 136), Sturge-Weber syndrome (see Case 340), von Hippel-Lindau disease, and ataxia-telangiectasia. The disorder is inherited as an autosomal dominant trait with frequent sporadic cases. Clinical features include seizures, mental retardation, and a nodular facial rash called "adenoma sebaceum."

Subependymal calcifications as seen in this case are a CT hallmark of tuberous sclerosis. The calcification occurs within hyperplastic nodules of malformed neuroglial tissue called "tubers," which are variable in size and number.

Subependymal tubers commonly occur near the foramina of Monro, as in this case (arrow; see also Cases 219 and 221).

Tubers in this location are prone to degenerate into giant cell astrocytomas. Enlargement and contrast enhancement of a subependymal nodule are CT clues to such transformation. These low-grade gliomas demonstrate benign growth characteristics but may cause obstructive hydrocephalus because of their strategic location.

Other potential CT findings in tuberous sclerosis include calcifications within cerebral parenchyma, seen here in the frontal lobes. The white matter lesions so apparent on MR scans (see Case 654) are less prominent on CT studies. Patchy areas of calvarial sclerosis may be noted.

DIFFERENTIAL DIAGNOSIS:
PERIVENTRICULAR CALCIFICATION IN A CHILD

Case 650

13-month-old girl with microcephaly and developmental delay.

Case 651

6-year-old boy with seizures.

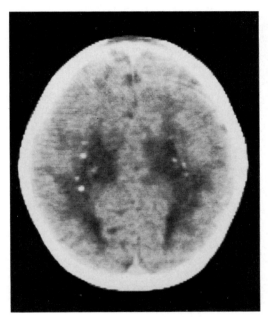

Congenital Infection With Cytomegalovirus.

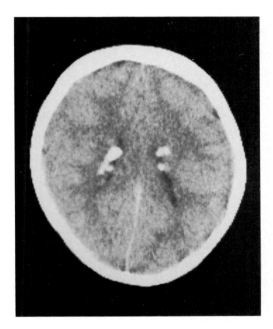

Tuberous Sclerosis.

Periventricular calcification can be an important sign of prior cerebral inflammation. Congenital infections with cytomegalovirus (CMV) typically cause this appearance, commonly in association with microcephaly as in Case 650. The ventricles are often enlarged due to cerebral damage, resembling Case 269. Congenital toxoplasmosis may also result in cerebral calcifications and ventricular enlargement. The calcifications of toxoplasmosis tend to be scattered, and the ventricular enlargement often represents true hydrocephalus. However, subependymal calcification and microcephaly may occur and be indistinguishable from CMV.

As discussed in Cases 648 and 649, subependymal calcification is characteristic of tuberous sclerosis. Calcified tubers are often larger and fewer than the periventricular calcifications of congenital inflammatory disease. In addition, subependymal tubers frequently do not calcify until the patient is several years old (see Case 652). These features and the clinical context clarify the differential diagnosis in most children.

WHITE MATTER LESIONS IN TUBEROUS SCLEROSIS

Case 652A

1-year-old boy with seizures.

Case 652B

Same patient.

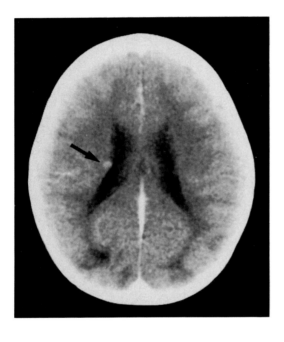

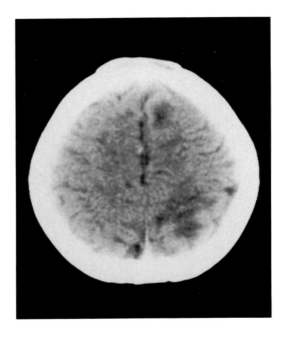

White matter abnormalities commonly accompany the subependymal and cortical hamartomas of tuberous sclerosis. These lesions may be poorly seen on CT scans and are much better defined by magnetic resonance imaging (see Case 654).

CT scans of infants with tuberous sclerosis may demonstrate only faint calcification within subependymal nodules, as seen here *(arrow)*. This appearance may resemble that of heterotopic gray matter along the ventricular margins (compare to Case 641). Recognition of associated white matter lesions may help to establish the correct diagnosis in such cases.

Here several areas of abnormal low attenuation are seen in white matter of the occipital lobes. These typical lesions range from 1 to 2 cm in diameter and have irregular, angular margins.

A scan near the vertex demonstrates additional foci of abnormality within subcortical white matter of the left hemisphere. Such lesions are due to heterotopic islands of abnormal neurons associated with localized demyelination and gliosis. Calcification is occasionally seen in these foci (see Case 649); contrast enhancement has not been observed.

When white matter lesions are prominent and subependymal nodules are inconspicuous, tuberous sclerosis may be confused with various leukoencephalopathies (compare to Cases 317 to 322).

MR CORRELATION: TUBEROUS SCLEROSIS

Case 653

6-month-old boy.
(axial, noncontrast scan; SE 1000/20)

Case 654

1-year-old boy presenting with seizures.
(axial, noncontrast scan; SE 3000/75)

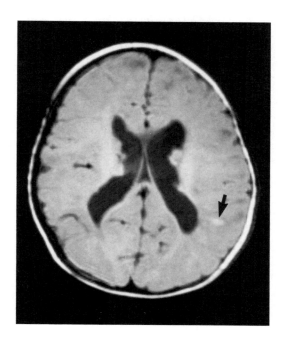

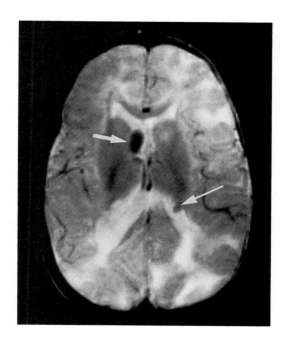

The subependymal nodules of tuberous sclerosis are well seen as irregularities along the ventricular margin on MR examinations. The characteristic calcification of these tubers so apparent on CT scans may not be appreciated on MR studies. (Compare this case to the MR appearance of heterotopic gray matter in Case 639.)

Subependymal and parenchymal tubers may demonstrate areas of T1-shortening *(arrow)*, of undetermined etiology.

MR is much more sensitive than CT for defining the white matter lesions of tuberous sclerosis. These characteristic zones of long T2 may make the diagnosis before the clinical findings or CT appearance are specific.

This case demonstrates typically large, irregular, poorly marginated, midhemispheric and subcortical white matter lesions. A densely calcified subependymal tuber is seen at the right foramen of Monro as an area of low signal intensity *(thick arrow)*. A smaller periventricular nodule is present near the trigone of the left lateral ventricle *(thin arrow)*.

DIFFERENTIAL DIAGNOSIS:
PERIVENTRICULAR MASS IN AN ADULT

Case 655

49-year-old woman (same patient as Case 649).
(noncontrast scan)

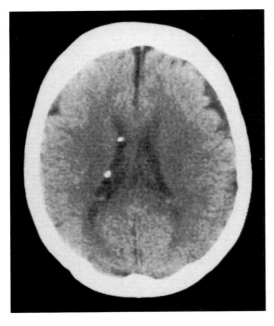

Tuberous Sclerosis.

Case 656

67-year-old man.
(postcontrast scan)

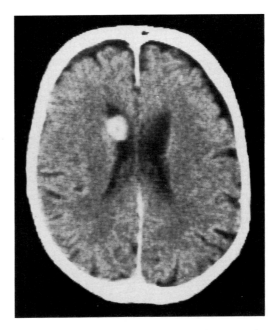

Metastatic Squamous Cell Carcinoma of the Lung.

The pattern of multiple periventricular calcifications without contrast enhancement in Case 655 is characteristic of uncomplicated tuberous sclerosis. Subependymal tubers may develop into enhancing astrocytomas, and a solitary lesion could have an appearance indistinguishable from that of Case 656.

Intraventricular metastases may arise from choroid plexus or from subependymal deposits (see Cases 22 and 23). Differential diagnosis in Case 656 would include intraventricular growth of subependymal astrocytoma or oligodendroglioma, ependymoma, subependymoma, arteriovenous malformation, and rare inflammatory granuloma. The location is unusual for intraventricular meningioma (see Case 96) or choroid plexus papilloma (see Case 222).

Heterotopic gray matter may occur along the lateral ventricular margins in adults as well as in children. These "masses" appear as slightly dense subependymal nodules without calcification or prominent contrast enhancement. Associated developmental anomalies (e.g., agenesis of the corpus callosum or absence of the septum pellucidum) may be present (see Case 641).

DIFFERENTIAL DIAGNOSIS:
SCATTERED CEREBELLAR CALCIFICATION

Case 657

35-year-old woman.
(noncontrast scan)

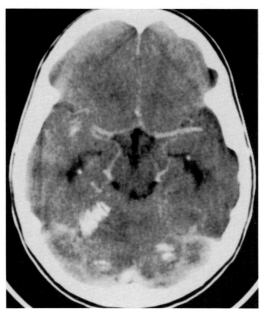

Tuberous Sclerosis.

Case 658

66-year-old woman.
(noncontrast scan)

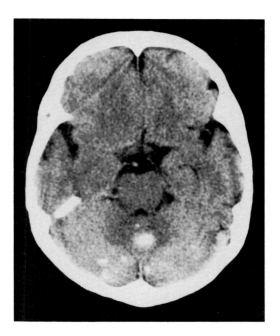

**Calcified Metastases From Breast
Carcinoma.**

Cerebellar involvement occurs in a minority of cases of tuberous sclerosis. White matter lesions and cortical hamartomas are comparable to the cerebral foci discussed in Cases 648 to 654. In Case 657, the areas of cortical calcification have an unusual gyriform morphology.

Case 658 is a reminder that metastatic disease should be considered whenever cerebellar pathology is encountered in an adult. The largest lesion in the vermis is surrounded by edema and mass effect. The smaller foci likely represent dystrophic calcification in "miliary" metastatic nodules (compare to Cases 16 and 308).

Dystrophic cerebral or cerebellar calcification is occasionally seen near the gray/white junction in patients with chronic venous hypertension (e.g., from a dural arteriovenous malformation). Similar calcifications may be noted following cranial radiation and chemotherapy.

BASAL ENCEPHALOCELES

Case 659A

62-year-old man presenting with a nasal mass.
(wide window)

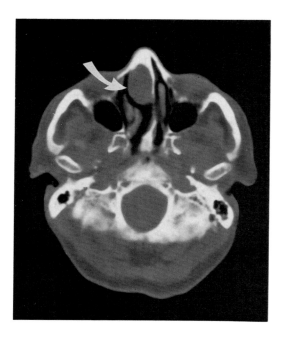

Case 659B

Same patient.
(wide window)

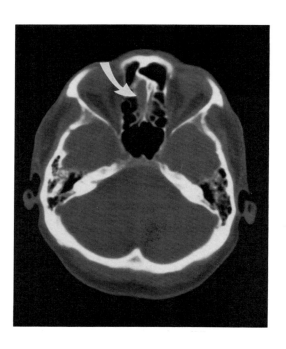

Encephaloceles are extracranial extensions of brain tissue, most commonly encountered along the skull base. Potential locations include the nose, sphenoid sinus, and petrous bones.

In this case the smoothly rounded mass within the right nasal cavity appears to be long standing. There is associated deviation of the nasal septum and deformity of the ipsilateral turbinates.

This appearance should raise the possibility of a nasal encephalocele. Biopsy or removal of such masses carries the risk of CSF leak and meningitis. Important vessels or functional neural tissue may extend into an encephalocele and be susceptible to surgical injury.

Occasionally the stalk connecting a nasal encephalocele with its origin in the anterior cranial fossa is obliterated. The resulting island of neural tissue within the nose is often called a "nasal glioma."

Dermal sinus tracts may also span the skull base with nasal and intracranial components. Like basal encephaloceles or meningoceles, congenital dermal sinuses may be associated with recurrent meningitis.

This scan passes through the level of the cribriform plate. The widened soft tissue space on the right side of the displaced crista galli represents the neck or pedicle of the encephalocele, connecting the nasal component with the anterior cranial fossa. Discovery of a soft tissue mass beneath the skull base should prompt a careful search for similar bone defects or anatomical distortions linking the lesion with the intracranial compartment.

Sagittal and coronal MR scans offer excellent demonstration of basal encephaloceles. The nature of the herniating neural tissue (i.e., content of the meningocele or encephalocele sac) is displayed in addition to the size and location of the bone defect.

DIFFERENTIAL DIAGNOSIS:
EXTRACRANIAL CYST ADJACENT TO THE OCCIPITAL BONE IN AN INFANT

Case 660

Newborn girl.

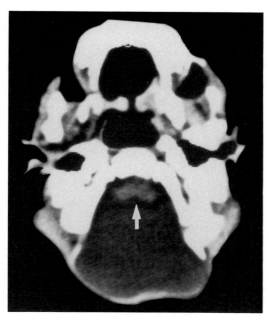

Occipital Meningocele.

Case 661

Newborn boy.

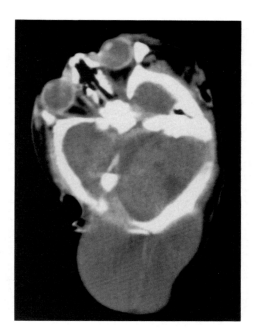

Cystic Hygroma.

Meningoceles and encephaloceles may involve the occipital region. In Case 660 a broad bone defect along the posterior margin of the foramen magnum is filled by a CSF-containing sac. The caudal brain stem is clearly seen anteriorly *(arrow),* and the sac does not contain neural tissue. The meningocele in this case represented herniation of a large Dandy-Walker cyst (see Cases 598 to 601).

Not all cystic masses at the skull base are meningoceles or encephaloceles. The lesion in Case 661 did not communicate with the intracranial compartment at any scan level. Cystic hygromas are loculated collections of serous fluid resulting from malformation and dilatation of cervical lymph channels. They usually arise in the posterior triangle of the neck but may enlarge along the skull base, as in this case.

REFERENCES: CT

1. Altman N.R., Altman D.H., Sheldon J.J., Leborgne J.: Holoprosencephaly classified by computed tomography. *A.J.N.R.* 5:433–438, 1984.
2. Archer C.R., Darwish H., Smith K.: Enlarged cisternae magnae and posterior fossa cysts simulating Dandy-Walker syndrome on computed tomography. *Radiology* 127:681–686, 1978.
3. Armstrong E.A., Harwood-Nash D.C., Hoffman H., et al.: Benign suprasellar cysts: The CT approach. *A.J.N.R.* 4:163–166, 1983.
4. Benzel E.C., Pelletier A.L., Levy P.G.: Communicating hydrocephalus in adults: Prediction of outcome after ventricular shunting procedure. *Neurosurgery* 26:655–660, 1990.
5. Bird, C.R., Gilles F.H.: Type I schizencephaly: CT and neuropathologic findings. *A.J.N.R.* 8:451–454, 1987.
6. Byrd S.E., Harwood-Nash D.C., Fitz C.R.: Absence of the corpus callosum: Computed tomographic evaluation in infants and children. *J. Can. Assoc. Radiol.* 29:108–112, 1978.
7. Crisi G., Calo M., De Santis M., et al.: Metrizamide-enhanced computed tomography of intracranial arachnoid cysts. *J. Comput. Assist. Tomogr.* 8:928–935, 1984.
8. Day R.E., Schutt W.H.: Normal children with large heads: Benign familial megalencephaly. *Arch. Dis. Child.* 54:512–517, 1979.
9. Dobyns W.B., McCluggage C.W. Computed tomographic appearance of lissencephaly syndromes. *A.J.N.R.* 6:545–550, 1985.
10. Dublin A.B., French B.N.: Diagnostic image evaluation of hydranencephaly and pictorially similar entities with emphasis on computed tomography. *Radiology* 137:81–91, 1980.
11. Fitz C.R.: Holoprosencephaly and related entities. *Neuroradiology* 25:225–238, 1983.
12. Fitz C.R.: Midline anomalies of the brain and spine. *Radiol. Clin. North Am.* 20:95–104, 1982.
13. Galassi E., Tognetti F., Frank F., et al.: Infratentorial arachnoid cysts. *J. Neurosurg.* 63:210–217, 1985.
14. Gentry L.R., Smoker W.R.K., Turski P.A., et al.: Suprasellar arachnoid cysts. 1. CT recognition. *A.J.N.R.* 7:79–86, 1986.
15. Heinz E.R., Ward A., Drayer B.P., et al.: Distinction between obstructive and atrophic dilatation of ventricles in children. *J. Comput. Assist. Tomogr.* 4:320–325, 1980.
16. Hoffman H.J., Hendrick R.B., Humphreys R.P., et al.: Investigation and management of suprasellar arachnoid cysts. *J. Neurosurg.* 57:597–602, 1982.
17. Huckman M.S.: Normal pressure hydrocephalus: Evaluation of diagnostic and prognostic tests. *A.J.N.R.* 2:385–395, 1981.
18. Kapila A., Naidich T.P.: Spontaneous lateral ventriculocisternosotomy documented by metrizamide CT ventriculography. *J. Neurosurg.* 54:101–104, 1981.
19. Kendall B., Holland I.: Benign communicating hydrocephalus in children. *Neuroradiology* 21:93–96, 1981.
20. Kendall B.E.: Dysgenesis of the corpus callosum. *Neuroradiology* 25:239–256, 1983.
21. Legge M., Saverbrei E., Macdonald A.: Intracranial tuberous sclerosis in infancy. *Radiology* 153:667–668, 1984.
22. Leo J.S., Pinto R.S., Hulvat G.F., et al.: Computed tomography of arachnoid cysts. *Radiology* 130:675–680, 1979.
23. Masdeu J.C., Dobben G.D., Akar-Kia B.: Dandy-Walker syndrome studied by computed tomography and pneumoencephalography. *Radiology* 147:109–114, 1983.
24. Maytal J., Alvarez L.A., Elkin C.M., Shinnor S.: External hydrocephalus: Radiologic spectrum and differentiation from cerebral atrophy. *A.J.N.R.* 8:271–278, 1987.
25. Ment L.R., Duncan C.C., Geehr R.: Benign enlargement of the subarachnoid spaces in the infant. *J. Neurosurg.* 54:504–508, 1981.
26. Modic M.T., Kaufman B., Bonstelle C., et al.: Megalocephaly and hypodense extracerebral fluid collections. *Radiology* 141:93–100, 1981.
27. Mori K., Handa H., Murata T., et al.: Periventricular lucency in computed tomography of hydrocephalus and cerebral atrophy. *J. Comput. Assist. Tomogr.* 4:204–209, 1980.
28. Morimoto K., Mogami H.: Sequential CT study of subependymal giant-cell astrocytoma associated with tuberous sclerosis. *J. Neurosurg.* 65:874–877, 1986.
29. Nabawi P., Dobben G.D., Mafee M., et al.: Diagnosis of lipoma of the corpus callosum by CT in five cases. *Neuroradiology* 21:159–162, 1981.
30. Naidich T.P., Chakara T.M.H.: Multicytic encephalomalacia: CT appearance and pathological correlation. *J. Comput. Assist. Tomogr.* 8:631–636, 1984.
31. Naidich T.P., McLone D.G., Fulling K.H.: The Chiari II malformation. IV. The hindbrain deformity. *Neuroradiology* 25:179–197, 1983.
32. Naidich T.P., McLone D.G., Hahn Y.S., et al.: Atrial diverticula in severe hydrocephalus. *A.J.N.R.* 3:257–266, 1982.
33. Naidich T.P., Pudlowski R.M., Naidich J.B., et al.: Computed tomographic signs of the Chiari II malformation. I. Skull and dural partitions. *Radiology* 134:65–71, 1980.
34. Naidich T.P., Pudlowski R.M., Naidich J.B.: Computed tomographic signs of Chiari II malformation. II. Midbrain and cerebellum. *Radiology* 134:391–398, 1980.
35. Naidich T.P., Pudlowski R.M., Naidich J.B.: Computed tomographic signs of the Chiari II malformation. III. Ventricles and cisterns. *Radiology* 134:657–663, 1980.
36. Naidich T.P., Schott L.H., Baron R.L.: Computed tomography in evaluation of hydrocephalus. *Radiol. Clin. North Am.* 20:143–167, 1982.
37. Ohno K., Enomoto T., Imamoto J., et al.: Lissencephaly (agyria) on computed tomography. *J. Comput. Assist. Tomogr.* 3:92–95, 1979.
38. Ramsey R.G., Huckman M.S.: Computed tomography of porencephaly and other cerebrospinal fluid-containing lesions. *Radiology* 123:73–77, 1977.
39. Raybaud C.: Destructive lesions of the brain. *Neuroradiology* 25:265–291, 1983.
40. Sarwar M., Virapongse C., Bhimani S., et al.: Interhemispheric fissure sign of dysgenesis of the corpus callosum. *J. Comput. Assist. Tomogr.* 8:637–644, 1984.
41. Servo A., Porras M., Jaaskinen J.: Diagnosis of ependymal intraventricular cysts of the third ventricle by computed tomography. *Neuroradiology* 24:155–157, 1983.
42. Wolpert S.M., Scott R.M.: The value of metrizamide CT cisternography in the management of cerebral arachnoid cysts. *A.J.N.R.* 2:29–35, 1981.

REFERENCES: MR

1. Aboulezz A.O., Sartor K., Geyer C., Gado M.H.: Position of cerebellar tonsils in the normal population and in patients with Chiari malformations: A quantitative approach with MR imaging. *J. Comput. Assist. Tomogr.* 9:1033–1036, 1985.
2. Altman N.R., Purser R.K., Post M.J.D.: Tuberous sclerosis: Characteristics at CT and MR imaging. *Radiology* 167:527–532, 1988.
3. Aoki S., Barkovich A.J., Nishimura K., et al.: Neurofibromatosis types 1 and 2: Cranial MR findings. *Radiology* 172:527–534, 1989.
4. Atlas S.W., Zimmerman R.A., Bilaniuk L.T., et al.: Corpus callosum and limbic system: Neuroanatomic MR evaluation of developmental anomalies. *Radiology* 160:355–362, 1986.
5. Barkovich A.J., Chuang S.H., Norman D.: MR of neuronal migration anomalies. *A.J.N.R.* 8:1009–1018, 1987.
6. Barkovich A.J., Kjos B.O., Norman D., Edwards M.S.: Revised classification of posterior fossa cysts and cystlike malformations based on the results of multiplanar MR imaging. *A.J.N.R.* 10:977–988, 1989.
7. Barkovich A.J., Newton T.H.: MR of aqueductal stenosis: Evidence of a broad spectrum of tectal distortion. *A.J.N.R.* 10:471–476, 1989.
8. Barkovich A.J., Norman D.: MR imaging of schizencephaly. *A.J.N.R.* 9:297–302, 1988.
9. Barkovich A.J., Norman D.: Anomalies of the corpus callosum: Correlation with further anomalies of the brain. *A.J.N.R.* 9:493–502, 1988.
10. Barkovich A.J., Wippold F.J., Sherman J.L., Citrin C.M.: Significance of cerebellar tonsillar position on MR. *A.J.N.R.* 7:795–800, 1986.
11. Berns D.H., Masaryk T.J., Weisman B., et al.: Tuberous sclerosis: Increased MR detection using gradient echo techniques. *J. Comput. Assist. Tomogr.* 13:896–898, 1989.
12. Bognanno J.R., Edwards M.K., Lee T.A., et al.: Cranial MR imaging in neurofibromatosis. *A.J.N.R.* 9:461–468, 1988.
13. Braffman B.H., Bilaniuk L.T., Zimmerman R.A.: The central nervous system manifestations of the phakomatoses on MR. *Radiol. Clin. North Am.* 25:773–800, 1988.
14. Britton J., Marsh H., Kendall B.: MRI and hydrocephalus in childhood. *Neuroradiology* 30:310, 1988.
15. Byrd S.E., Bohan T.P., Osborn R.E., Naidich T.P.: The CT and MR evaluation of lissencephaly. *A.J.N.R.* 9:925–928, 1988.
16. Byrd S.E., Naidich T.P.: Common congenital brain anomalies. *Radiol. Clin. North Am.* 26:755–772, 1988.
17. Byrd S.E., Osborn R.E., Bohan T.P., et al.: CT and MR evaluation of migrational disorders of the brain. Part I. Lissencephaly and pachygyria. *Pediat. Radiol.* 19:151, 1989.
18. Byrd S.E., Osborn R.E., Bohan T.P., et al.: CT and MR evaluation of migrational disorders of the brain. Part II. Schizencephaly, heterotopia, and polymicrogyria. *Pediat. Radiol.* 19:219, 1989.
19. Curnes J.T., Oakes W., Boyko O.B.: MR imaging of hindbrain deformity in patients with and without symptoms of brain stem compression. *A.J.N.R.* 10:293–302, 1989.
20. Dean B., Drayer B.P., Beresini D.C., Bird C.R.: MR imaging of pericallosal lipomas. *A.J.N.R.* 9:929–932, 1988.
21. El Gammal T., Allen M.B. Jr., Brooks B.S., Mark E.K.: MR evaluation of hydrocephalus. *A.J.N.R.* 8:591–598, 1987.

22. El Gammal T., Mark E.K., Brooks B.S.: MR imaging of Chiari II malformation. *A.J.N.R.* 8:1037–1044, 1987.
23. Inoue Y., Nakajima S., Fukuda T., et al.: Magnetic resonance imaging of tuberous sclerosis: Further observations and clinical correlations. *Neuroradiology* 30:379, 1988.
24. Jack C.R., Mokri B., Laws E.R. Jr., et al.: MR findings in normal pressure hydrocephalus: Significance and comparison to other forms of dementia. *J. Comput. Assist. Tomogr.* 11:923–931, 1987.
25. Jinkins J.R., Whittemore A.R., Bradley W.G.: MR imaging of collosal and corticocallosal dysgenesis. *A.J.N.R.* 10:339–344, 1989.
26. Kemp S.S., Zimmerman R.A., Bilaniuk L.T., et al.: Magnetic resonance imaging of the cerebral aqueduct. *Neuroradiology* 29:430, 1987.
27. Kjos B.O., Brant-Zawadzki M., Kucharczyk W., et al.: Cystic intracranial lesions: Magnetic resonance imaging. *Radiology* 155:363–370, 1985.
28. McMurdo S.K. Jr., Moore S.G., Brant-Zawadzki M., et al.: MR imaging of intracranial tuberous sclerosis. *A.J.N.R.* 8:77–82, 1987.
29. Mirowitz S.A., Sartor K., Gado M.: High intensity basal ganglia lesions on T1-weighted MR images in neurofibromatosis. *A.J.N.R.* 10:1159–1164, 1990.
30. Nixon J.R., Houser O.W., Gomez M.R., Okazaki H.: Cerebral tuberous sclerosis: MR imaging. *Radiology* 170:869–874, 1989.
31. Osborn R.E., Byrd S.E., Naidich T.P., et al.: MR imaging of neuronal migration disorders. *A.J.N.R.* 9:1101–1106, 1988.
32. Poe L.B., Coleman L.L., Mahmud F.: Congenital central nervous system abnormalities. *Radiographics* 9:801–826, 1989.
33. Robertson S.J., Wolpert S.M., Runge V.M.: MR imaging of middle cranial fossa arachnoid cysts: Temporal lobe agenesis syndrome revisited. *A.J.N.R.* 10:1007–1010, 1989.
34. Smith A.S., Blaser S.I., Ross J.S., Weinstein M.A.: Magnetic resonance imaging of disturbances in neuronal migration: Illustration of an embryologic process. *Radiographics* 9:509–523, 1989.
35. Titelbaum D.S., Hayward J.C., Zimmerman R.A.: Pachygyriclike changes: Topographic appearance at MR imaging and CT and correlation with neurologic status. *Radiology* 173:663–668, 1989.
36. Truwit C.L., Barkovich A.J.: Pathogenesis of intracranial lipoma. An MR study in 42 patients. *A.J.N.R.* 11:665–674, 1990.
37. Truwit C., Williams R.G., Armstrong E.A., Marlin A.E.: MR imaging of choroid plexus lipomas. *A.J.N.R.* 11:202–204, 1990.
38. Wiener S.N., Pearlstein A.E., Eiber A.: MR imaging of intracranial arachnoid cysts. *J. Comput. Assist. Tomogr.* 11:236–241, 1987.
39. Wolpert S.M., Anderson M., Scott R.M., et al.: The Chiari II malformation: MR imaging evaluation. *A.J.N.R.* 8:783–792, 1987.
40. Wolpert S.M., Scott R.M., Platenberg C., Runge V.M.: The clinical significance of hindbrain herniation and deformity as shown on MR images of patients with Chiari II malformation. *A.J.N.R.* 9:1075–1078, 1988.
41. Yasumori K., Hasuo K., Nagata S., et al.: Neuronal migration anomalies causing extensive ventricular indentation. *Neurosurgery* 26:504–506, 1990.

CHAPTER 12

Orbital Lesions

VASCULAR MASSES

Case 662

Newborn boy with proptosis.

Hemangioma.

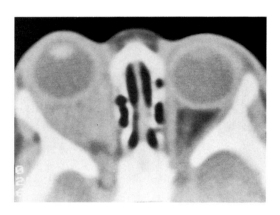

Case 663

25-year-old man with a history of proptosis when bending over.

Orbital Varix.

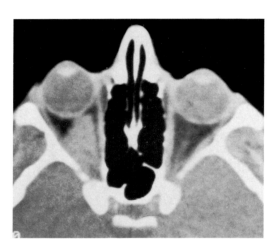

CT provides a sensitive view of orbital pathology. The normal low attenuation of retrobulbar fat contrasts with lesions of soft tissue density. In addition, the axial display of orbital anatomy allows localization of lesions with respect to the globe and muscle cone. CT also demonstrates pathologic conditions along the skull base, which may be manifested by ocular symptoms (see Case 57).

Capillary hemangiomas are the most frequent vascular masses of the infant orbit, while cavernous hemangiomas are the most common orbital masses in adults. Although benign, these tumors may have extensive intraconal and extraconal components.

Orbital hemangiomas usually present as well-defined lesions with smooth or mildly lobulated margins. They are often located superior and lateral to the globe, sparing the orbital apex. Proptosis is commonly observed, as seen here. In this case, the congenital mass is also associated with a small globe.

Hemangiomas appear dense on precontrast scan. Occasional cavernous hemangiomas contain characteristic calcified phleboliths. Uniform, intense contrast enhancement is typical.

The subcategories of vascular masses within the orbit may be indistinguishable on CT scans. This varix demonstrates well defined margins, slightly lobular contour, homogeneous density, and uniform contrast enhancement, comparable to a hemangioma or a lymphangioma.

Although the clinical history is characteristic in this case, the diagnosis was confirmed by orbital venography. Jugular vein compression or a Valsalva maneuver during CT scans may demonstrate impressive enlargement of orbital varices.

OTHER VASCULAR LESIONS

Case 664

27-year-old man.
(postcontrast scan)

Lymphangioma.

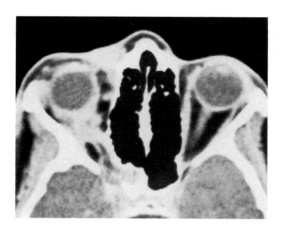

Case 665

58-year-old woman.
(postcontrast scan)

Carotid-Cavernous Fistula.

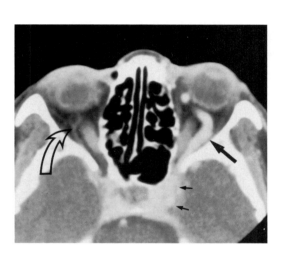

The sensitivity of orbital CT scanning exceeds the specificity of the images. The enhancing intraconal process applied to the optic nerve and globe in this case proved to be a lymphangioma. Other lymphangiomas present a more mass-like contour, identical to that of hemangiomas, while the appearance seen here resembles an inflammatory process such as orbital pseudotumor (see Case 681).

The superior ophthalmic vein is regularly seen on orbital scans as it crosses above the optic nerve on its way to the cavernous sinus (open arrow). Enlargement of the vein (solid arrow) implies increased orbital blood flow, either congenital (e.g., arteriovenous malformation) or acquired (e.g., inflammatory processes such as pseudotumor or Graves' disease, or carotid artery–cavernous sinus fistula).

Carotid-cavernous fistulae may be caused by a tear of the internal carotid artery as it passes through the venous compartment of the cavernous sinus. The resulting shunt of arterial blood floods the sinus and its tributaries, including the superior ophthalmic vein. Such high-flow fistulae are usually associated with a history of recent head trauma.

Low-flow carotid-cavernous fistulae are vascular malformations of the dura, often occurring spontaneously in middle-aged or elderly patients. Small dural branches of the internal and external carotid arteries supply a network of abnormal channels along the medial wall of the middle cranial fossa, shunting blood into the cavernous sinus.

In either case, reversal of flow in the superior ophthalmic vein is associated with evidence of orbital vascular congestion (e.g., proptosis, conjunctival injection) and is often accompanied by a bruit transmitted from the fistula. A corroborating CT finding is distention of the ipsilateral cavernous sinus, partially visualized in this case (small arrows; compare to Cases 212 to 215).

Case 666

53-year-old woman.
(postcontrast scan)

Metastatic Carcinoma of the Breast.

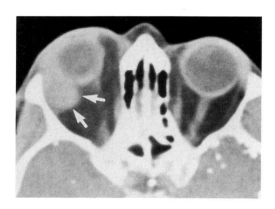

Solid tumors may arise within the globe and orbit as primary lesions or as metastases from systemic neoplasms. In children, the most frequent orbital malignancies include lymphoma, leukemia, neuroblastoma, rhabdomyosarcoma, and retinoblastoma. In adults metastases from systemic carcinomas (e.g., breast, lung, kidney, and colon) are more common.

The differential diagnosis of a mass in the superolateral quadrant of the orbit (as seen here) also includes tumors of the lacrimal gland (benign mixed tumors or adenocarcinomas), lymphoma, orbital dermoid cysts (see Case 675), sarcoidosis, and Wegener's granulomatosis. Soft tissue prominence at this site may also be seen in thyroid ophthalmopathy and in orbital pseudotumors.

Case 667

54-year-old woman.
(postcontrast scan)

Metastatic Scirrhous Carcinoma of the Breast.

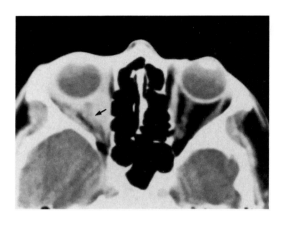

Metastatic disease within the orbit may present an infiltrating appearance resembling orbital pseudotumor (see Case 681) or a vascular mass (compare to Case 662).

In this case, enhancing tumor surrounds and outlines the nonenhancing optic nerve (arrow). The fibrotic metastasis has caused retraction of the globe rather than proptosis. Such enophthalmus is an uncommon but characteristic feature of orbital involvement by scirrhous carcinomas of the breast.

Case 668A

4-year-old girl.
(axial scan)

Histiocytosis X.

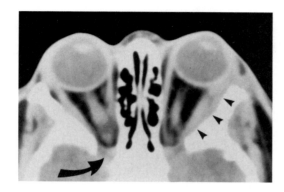

Case 668B

Same patient.
(coronal scan)

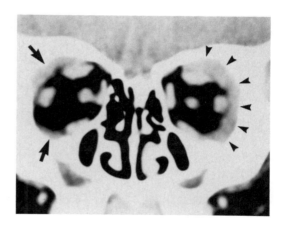

Metastatic disease is frequently detected along the orbital margins in children and adults. One common pattern is apparent thickening of a rectus muscle, as seen here on the left (arrowheads; see also Case 685). The normal fat plane between the lateral rectus muscle and the lateral wall of the orbit has been filled with soft tissue. The lateral rectus muscle itself is thickened and displaced medially.

Other childhood tumors that may cause a similar pattern of orbital involvement are neuroblastoma, leukemia, and lymphoma.

Prominent left-sided proptosis is present in this case. The scan plane passes through the superior orbital fissures (curved arrow). The optic canals are located more superiorly, at the level of the anterior clinoid processes.

Coronal CT or MR scans provide an excellent view of peripheral orbital pathology. Here the rind of neoplastic tissue along the lateral wall of the left orbit is well defined (arrowheads), medially displacing the muscle cone and retrobulbar fat. Smaller zones of histiocytosis are seen at the superolateral and inferior margins of the right orbit (arrows).

OCULAR MASSES

Case 669

49-year-old man.

Choroidal Melanoma.

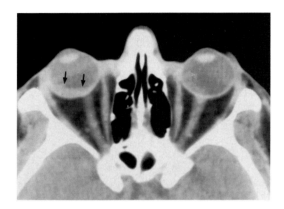

Case 670

3-year-old girl.

Retinoblastoma.

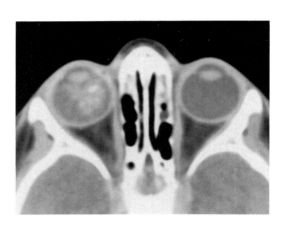

The normally low attenuation values of the ocular vitreous body outline the margins of soft tissue masses within the globe.

Here a crescentic soft tissue mass is seen along the posterior margin of the right globe *(arrows)*. The appearance is nonspecific. Focal thickening of the ocular wall could represent other tumors (e.g., metastasis or lymphoma), choroidal hemangioma, inflammatory disease (e.g., sarcoidosis), or retinal detachment with associated hematoma or subretinal fluid.

Ocular melanomas may arise in the iris, ciliary body, or choroid. Choroidal melanomas may extend within the orbit and/or give rise to hematogenous metastases.

A lobulated mass is seen within the right globe in this case. The presence of calcification is a hallmark of retinoblastoma, as discussed in Case 699. The midocular location of this lesion is somewhat unusual; most retinoblastomas are found along the posterior wall of the globe.

Retinoblastoma is the most common ocular tumor in children. Bilateral involvement occurs in about 30% of cases. An associated pineal region tumor may occasionally be seen in such patients ("trilateral retinoblastoma").

The presence of an intraocular mass is usually clinically apparent in children with retinoblastoma. CT is performed to assess extraocular invasion and to detect a possible contralateral tumor.

Case 671

60-year-old woman.
(sagittal, noncontrast scan; SE 800/20)

Choroidal Melanoma.

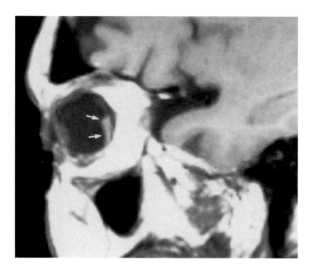

Case 672

63-year-old woman.
(coronal, noncontrast scan; SE 600/17)

Metastatic Carcinoma of the Breast.

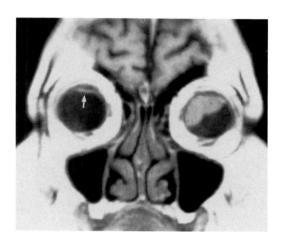

The long T1 of the vitreous body outlines many intraocular masses on T1-weighted MR scans. The advantages of multiplanar display further enhance the MR demonstration of such lesions.

In this case, a shallow choroidal melanoma is seen along the posterior wall of the globe (arrows), comparable to Case 669. The purpose of CT and MR scans in such cases is primarily to define any extraocular extension of tumor. This may be best accomplished on MR studies using pulse sequences that suppress the high signal intensity of retrobulbar fat.

Choroidal melanomas may demonstrate prominent T1-shortening and T2-shortening due to the presence of paramagnetic components (melanin and/or blood products). High signal intensity on T1-weighted images distinguishes most choroidal melanomas from most ocular metastases (in the absence of subretinal hemorrhage; see Cases 672 and 674).

Intraocular metastases in adults most commonly arise from carcinomas of the breast, lung, colon, and kidney. These lesions represent hematogenous deposits in the highly vascular uveal layer (choroid, iris, ciliary body). Choroidal metastases are commonly associated with retinal detachment, which increases the conspicuity of the lesions.

Ocular metastases may demonstrate only slightly higher signal intensity than the vitreous body on T1-weighted images. More obviously increased signal as seen in this case often reflects accompanying retinal detachment with subretinal fluid collections and hemorrhage.

Here a large metastatic retinal detachment is seen within the left globe. A smaller layer of abnormal tissue is present along the superior margin of the right globe (arrow). Ocular metastases are bilateral in approximately 25% of cases.

MR CORRELATION: ORBITAL METASTASES

Case 673

74-year-old woman.
(coronal, noncontrast scan; SE 800/17)

Metastatic Carcinoma of the Lung.

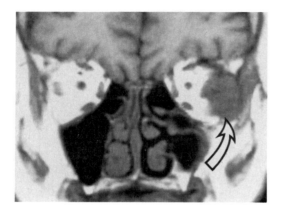

Case 674

62-year-old woman.
(axial, noncontrast scan; SE 2000/45)

Metastatic Carcinoma of the Lung With Retinal Detachment.

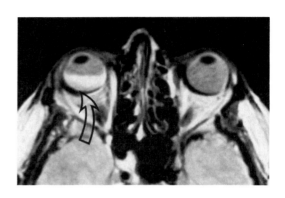

Extraocular orbital metastases are well defined on T1-weighted MR scans by the high signal intensity of surrounding fat. Here a soft tissue mass containing water protons is seen as an area of abnormally low signal occupying the lateral retrobulbar space. The lateral rectus muscle appears to be involved by the tumor (compare to Case 668). The optic nerve is medially displaced.

As discussed in Case 672, retinal detachment often accompanies ocular metastases. The typically crescentic shape of subretinal fluid collections is well seen along the posterior margin of the right globe in this case. The thin layer of metastatic tumor is faintly visible as a lower intensity mass *(arrow)* outlined by the surrounding detachment.

Most choroidal metastases are less intense than the vitreous body (and associated subretinal fluid collections) on heavily T2-weighted images. (Choroidal melanomas are moderately to markedly hypointense with respect to the vitreous on such sequences.)

DIFFERENTIAL DIAGNOSIS:
LOW-ATTENUATION MASS IN THE SUPEROLATERAL QUADRANT OF THE ORBIT

Case 675

24-year-old man.
(axial scan)

Case 676

29-year-old man with blurred vision in the left
eye for 10 years and swelling for 6 months.
(semicoronal scan)

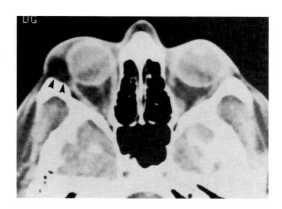

Dermoid Cyst.

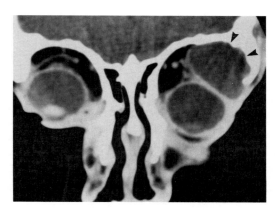

Subperiosteal Hematoma (Hematic Cyst).

Dermoid cysts often arise in the superolateral quadrant of the orbit, displacing the globe medially and inferiorly. Inferior displacement of one globe may be demonstrated on an axial scan by asymmetric visualization of the two lenses, as seen in Case 675.

The low attenuation of the lesion in Case 675 matches the density of retrobulbar fat and is characteristic of dermoid cysts (see Cases 232 to 234). Chronicity of the mass is indicated by smooth erosion of the lateral orbital rim (arrowheads).

Subperiosteal hematomas of the orbit may fail to resorb, becoming chronic fluid collections. The breakdown of blood products leads to a "hematic cyst," which can present as a long-standing mass lesion. In Case 676 the globe is displaced anteriorly and inferiorly, and the bony margins of the orbit are expanded (arrowheads; compare to the right side).

The attenuation values within a chronic subperiosteal hematoma resemble those of the vitreous but are higher than those of fat. Both dermoid cysts and subperiosteal hematomas can demonstrate short T1 and T2 values on MR scans.

Case 677

16-year-old boy with proptosis.
(noncontrast scan)

Aspergillosis of the Ethmoid and Sphenoid Sinuses.

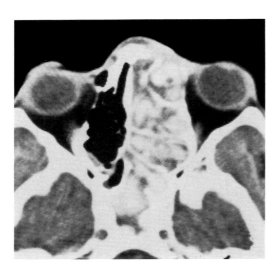

Sinus lesions are often manifested by orbital symptoms. Sinusitis may involve the orbit by direct extension as orbital cellulitis (see Cases 679 and 680) or by secondary proptosis due to expansion of the sinus (mucocele or mucopyocele).

In this case, chronic infection has caused unusual enlargement of the entire ethmoid sinus system on the left side. High attenuation within the sinus proved to be due to proteinaceous material without hemorrhage or calcification.

Dense central opacification is typical of fungal sinusitis. MR scans often demonstrate a corresponding pattern of prominent T2-shortening in the center of involved sinuses.

Case 678

38-year-old woman with proptosis.
(coronal scan)

Fibrosarcoma Arising Within the Ethmoid Sinus.

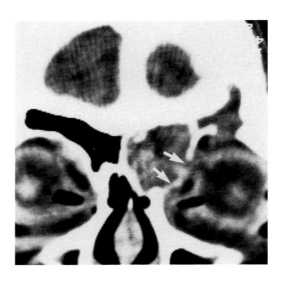

Tumors involving the paraorbital sinuses often extend into the orbit and cause secondary proptosis. Among the lesions that may present in this manner are juvenile angiofibromas, esthesioneuroblastomas, and squamous cell carcinomas.

The expansion of a sinus at the frontoethmoid junction is most commonly due to a mucocele. The irregular destruction of bone in this case (arrows) suggests a more aggressive lesion, as was confirmed at biopsy.

Case 679

13-year-old girl.

Orbital Cellulitis.

Case 680

12-year-old boy presenting with a 3-day history of orbital swelling and fever.

Subperiosteal Abscess and Preseptal Cellulitis Secondary to Sinusitis.

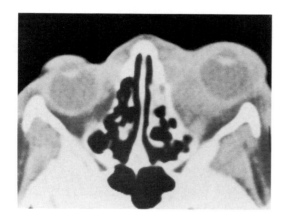

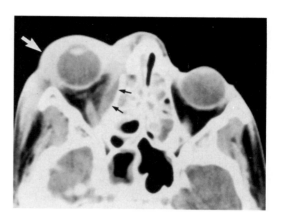

Inflammatory processes may cause edema and cellular infiltration of retrobulbar fat and/or extraocular muscles. The resulting density and swelling may mimic an orbital mass, but the clinical presentation usually clarifies the diagnosis.

Here the orbital inflammation is associated with midethmoid sinusitis and edema of preseptal tissue, favoring a diffuse cellulitis. "Orbital" cellulitis may be confined to the periorbital (preseptal) tissues, as seen anteriorly in Case 680.

In this case, the ethmoid sinuses are largely opacified, with mucosal thickening in the sphenoid sinus. Extensive swelling of preseptal tissues *(white arrow)* is comparable to Case 679 and indicates superficial cellulitis.

More importantly, an abscess pocket is present along the medial wall of the orbit *(black arrows)*. This collection occupies a subperiosteal location, displacing the medial rectus muscle and causing the patient's proptosis. (A coronal scan would demonstrate the substantial cephalocaudal extent of this "thin" abscess, analogous to Case 668.)

ORBITAL PSEUDOTUMOR

Case 681

71-year-old man presenting with painful orbital swelling.
(postcontrast scan)

Case 682

16-year-old girl presenting with painful diplopia.
(postcontrast scan)

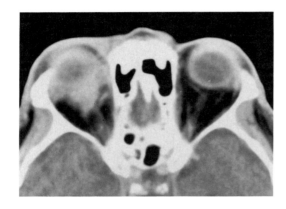

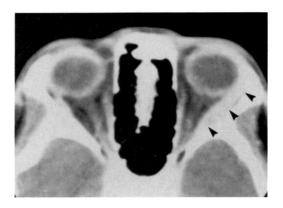

The diagnosis of "orbital pseudotumor" includes a diverse group of nonspecific lymphocytic and granulomatous inflammations. Pseudotumors may be unilateral or bilateral and may appear in many forms.

In this case a poorly defined, amorphous zone of enhancing soft tissue surrounds the right globe posteriorly and superiorly. Involvement of the retrobulbar space by this infiltrating form of pseudotumor may closely resemble orbital cellulitis, metastases, or an amorphous vascular mass (compare to Cases 664, 667, and 679). The relatively low signal intensity often seen within orbital pseudotumor on T2-weighted MR scans may help to distinguish this lesion from orbital metastases, which typically demonstrate higher intensity values.

Discrete nodules of inflammatory tissue may be seen in orbital pseudotumor, mimicking other primary or metastatic masses within the orbit or lacrimal gland. Bilaterality, associated involvement of muscles, and/or prominent scleral enhancement often narrow the diagnosis.

Clinical features (rapid onset, pain, limitation of movement, response to steroids) also help to distinguish most pseudotumors from the neoplasms or endocrinopathies that they may otherwise resemble.

This case illustrates the "myositic" form of orbital pseudotumor. The left lateral rectus muscle is markedly thickened and intensely enhancing (compare to Case 668A).

Such swelling of one or more extraocular muscles superficially mimics thyroid ophthalmopathy (see Cases 683 and 684). The clinical setting of pain and rapid onset usually supports the correct diagnosis.

Radiographic clues distinguishing myositic pseudotumor from thyroid ophthalmopathy include (1) the tendency of pseudotumor to involve the ocular insertions of the rectus muscles, which are typically spared in thyroid ophthalmopathy, and (2) the common association of myositic pseudotumor with other evidence of orbital inflammation (e.g., scleral enhancement, preseptal edema, or hazy margins of the optic nerve). Orbital myositis is also usually confined to a single muscle in adults, while thyroid ophthalmopathy is more commonly multifocal and/or bilateral.

THYROID OPHTHALMOPATHY

Case 683

69-year-old man with bilateral proptosis and diplopia.

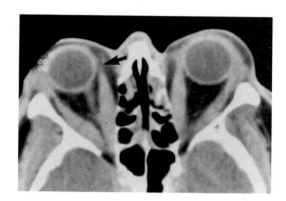

Case 684

58-year-old man with right-sided proptosis and diplopia.
(coronal scan)

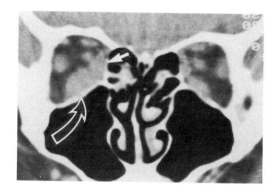

The hallmark of thyroid ophthalmopathy or "Graves' disease" is infiltration of the rectus muscles, easily detected on CT scans. The two eyes may be involved symmetrically as seen here or asymmetrically as in Case 684. Medial and inferior rectus muscles are usually affected before, and to a greater extent than, the lateral rectus or superior muscle group.

This scan demonstrates bilateral proptosis with marked thickening of the medial and lateral rectus muscles. Relative sparing of the tendinous insertions of the involved muscles *(arrow)* contrasts with the appearance of orbital myositis (see Case 682). Incidental mucosal thickening is present in the ethmoid sinuses.

Coronal CT or MR views provide a cross section of the muscle cone surrounding the optic nerve (see also Case 668). This projection is often useful for assessing the relative intracoronal and extracoronal extent of a lesion. The coronal plane also allows better visualization of the inferior rectus muscle and superior muscle bundle than is possible on axial sections. (See Case 687 for a comparable MR example.)

In this case, the right inferior rectus muscle *(open arrow)* is grossly enlarged, merging with the thickened medial rectus muscle *(small arrow)*.

DIFFERENTIAL DIAGNOSIS:
THICKENED RECTUS MUSCLES

Case 685

44-year-old man with proptosis.

Case 686

60-year-old man with proptosis.

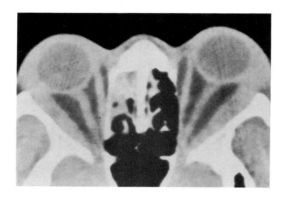

Orbital Lymphoma.

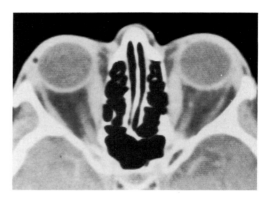

Thyroid Ophthalmopathy.

Thickening of rectus muscles may be caused by processes other than thyroid ophthalmopathy and orbital myositis. Infiltration by neoplasms such as lymphoma, leukemia, rhabdomyosarcoma, neuroblastoma, and metastasis may occur either unilaterally or symmetrically, as in Case 685. Metastatic tumor is often located *adjacent* to the muscle cone along the lateral wall of the orbit, as seen in Case 668.

Masses limited to the lateral rectus muscles, as in Case 685, would be very unusual in Graves' disease. On the other hand, bilateral thickening of the medial rectus muscles, as in Case 686, is a characteristic appearance for thyroid ophthalmopathy.

Carotid cavernous fistulae may be associated with swollen rectus muscles due to passive venous congestion. Arteriovenous malformation and orbital trauma are additional causes of extraocular muscle thickening. Occasional orbital neurofibromas may also present as thickening of a rectus muscle (or as more diffuse, nonencapsulated infiltration resembling pseudotumor or a vascular process).

MR CORRELATION: THICKENED RECTUS MUSCLES

Case 687

47-year-old woman.
(coronal, noncontrast scan; SE 700/20)

Thyroid Ophthalmopathy.

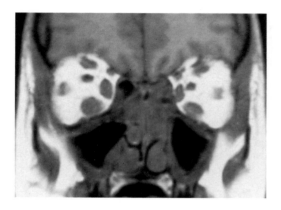

Case 688

33-year-old woman with painful restriction of
upward gaze on the right.
(coronal, noncontrast scan; SE 1000/22)

Myositic Pseudotumor.

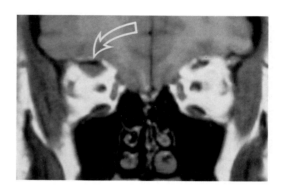

The high signal intensity of retrobulbar fat on T1-weighted MR scans clearly outlines the muscle cone. Here the inferior and medial rectus muscles are thickened bilaterally, right greater than left. This pattern of involvement is characteristic of thyroid ophthalmopathy (compare to Case 684).

The ethmoid sinuses are largely opacified, and mucosal thickening is present in the maxillary sinuses.

In this case the superior muscle group (superior rectus and levator palpebrae) on the right is swollen (arrow), while other rectus muscles are uninvolved. This pattern of involvement (and the presence of pain) would be unusual for thyroid ophthalmopathy.

The radiographic differential diagnosis instead centers on myositis versus orbital tumors such as neuromas or metastasis. The patient's age, rapid clinical onset of symptoms, and subsequent response to steroid therapy established the diagnosis of myositic pseudotumor.

OPTIC NERVE GLIOMAS

Case 689

8-year-old girl with neurofibromatosis.

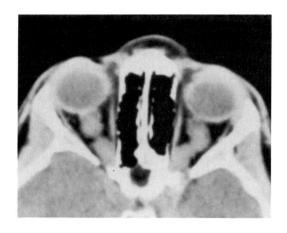

Case 690

12-year-old girl with neurofibromatosis.
(coronal scan)

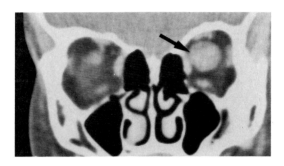

Gliomas involving the optic nerve present variable clinical patterns. Optic nerve tumors in young patients (more frequently girls) and in patients with neurofibromatosis are often low-grade lesions, behaving more like hyperplasia than neoplasm. Optic gliomas spontaneously arising in adults tend to be much more aggressive lesions (compare to the discussion of chiasmal gliomas in Cases 200 and 201).

Optic gliomas typically cause uniform thickening of the nerve, as seen here. Mild undulation or lobulation is common. The lesions are usually homogeneous, without calcification or prominent contrast enhancement.

The presence of bilateral optic gliomas is strongly suggestive of Type 1 neurofibromatosis (analogous to the presumption of Type 2 neurofibromatosis in patients with bilateral acoustic schwannomas).

Coronal CT or MR scans are valuable for defining pathology within or adjacent to the optic nerves (see also Case 695). In this case, the left optic nerve is grossly expanded by a glioma associated with neurofibromatosis.

Rotation of the head may cause coronal scans to pass through the posterior portion of one globe while demonstrating the contralateral optic nerve. This apparent asymmetry may falsely mimic an optic glioma of the posteriorly rotated side.

When an optic nerve tumor is discovered in the orbit, the optic chiasm should be closely examined to assess intracranial extension (see Case 200). Similarly, the finding of a suprasellar mass should prompt careful evaluation of the intraorbital portions of the optic nerves. Magnetic resonance imaging is now the most effective means of assessing the entire visual pathway (see Cases 695 and 696).

DIFFERENTIAL DIAGNOSIS:
THICKENING OF THE OPTIC NERVE

Case 691

7-year-old boy.
(noncontrast scan)

Case 692

24-year-old woman with decreased visual acuity
on the right.
(postcontrast scan)

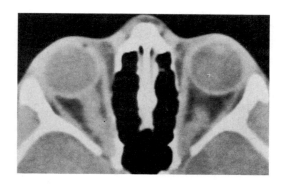

Optic Nerve Gliomas.

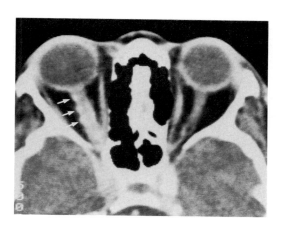

Optic Nerve Sheath Meningioma.

A wide variety of lesions may cause thickening of the optic nerve. Nonneoplastic processes such as papilledema, optic neuritis (e.g., multiple sclerosis, sarcoidosis), orbital pseudotumor, Graves' disease, and vascular malformations are included in the differential diagnosis.

Among tumors, the most important possibilities are gliomas of the nerve and meningiomas of the nerve sheath. A clinical clue to the presence of an optic nerve tumor is loss of visual acuity, which is rarely seen with other orbital masses (see Case 215).

Case 691 demonstrates the typical homogeneous, mildly lobulated thickening of optic nerve gliomas in a child with neurofibromatosis (see discussion of Cases 689 and 690).

Meningiomas of the optic nerve sheath often present as more fusiform or elliptical masses surrounding the axis of the nerve (see the calcified tumor in Case 700). Almost all optic nerve sheath meningiomas involve the orbital apex. Even relatively flat meningiomas are distinguished by the "tram-track" appearance of uninvolved nerve surrounded by calcification and/or an enhancing "collar" of tumor, as seen in Case 692 *(arrows)*.

The enhancement of optic nerve sheath meningiomas is usually more intense than that of optic nerve gliomas. Coronal CT or MR scans may convincingly demonstrate the enhancing ring of a sheath meningioma surrounding the nerve itself. MR demonstration of thin enhancement along the margins of the optic nerve often requires fat suppression techniques.

Retrobulbar metastasis can line the margins of the optic nerve, resulting in "tram-track" enhancement resembling a nerve sheath meningioma. Occasionally, optic nerve involvement by orbital pseudotumor or sarcoidosis may also produce a "tram-track" enhancement pattern.

Case 693

2-year-old girl with neurofibromatosis.
(sagittal, noncontrast scan; SE 700/17)

Case 694

3-year-old girl.
(axial, noncontrast scan; SE 3000/90)

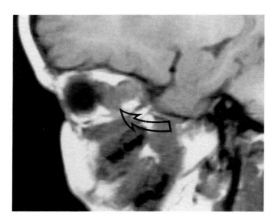

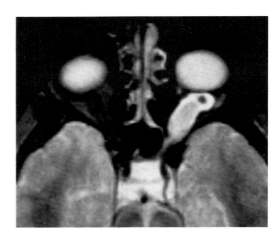

Thickening of the optic nerve is outlined by retrobulbar fat on T1-weighted MR images. In this case, the homogeneous, mildly lobulated mass extends from the globe to the orbital apex. (Compare the morphology seen here to the CT appearance of Case 689.)

Intracranial involvement of optic gliomas is also well demonstrated on axial and coronal MR scans (see Cases 695 and 696).

The glioma involving the intraorbital portion of the left optic nerve in this case demonstrates high signal intensity on a T2-weighted image. Cystic dilatation of the nerve sheath probably accounts for the very high signal at the margins of the tumor, possibly secondary to compression of the thickened nerve within the optic canal.

The absence of bone artifact on axial MR scans allows visualization of the canalicular segment of the optic nerve. This fact and multiplanar demonstration of the optic chiasm make MR more valuable than CT for assessing the potential continuity of orbital and chiasmal neoplasm.

Symmetrical dilatation of subarachnoid spaces surrounding the optic nerves may be seen as a normal variant and in cases of papilledema.

INTRACRANIAL EXTENSION OF OPTIC GLIOMAS

Case 695

10-year-old girl with neurofibromatosis.
(coronal, noncontrast scan; SE 600/17)

Case 696

7-year-old girl.
(noncontrast scan)

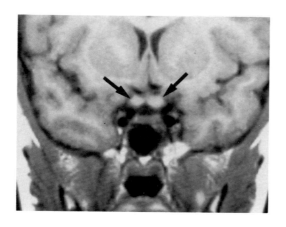

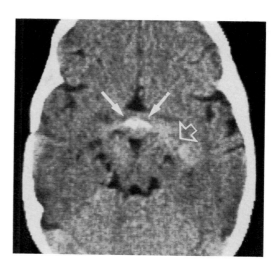

The bilobed suprasellar mass seen here *(arrows)* represents expansion of the optic nerves at the optic chiasm. Chiasmal involvement by gliomas is easily defined on coronal and sagittal MR scans (see Cases 176 to 178 and 206).

Enlargement of the chiasm may also occur in optic neuritis (e.g., multiple sclerosis), with regression following steroid therapy. Craniopharyngiomas and cavernous angiomas are occasionally intrachiasmal (see Case 206).

The chiasmal glioma in this case contains calcification *(solid arrows)*. Density along the left optic tract *(open arrow)* represents posterior extension of the tumor.

Extension of a glioma into the optic tracts and radiations is better demonstrated on MR examinations than on CT studies. Such infiltration is usually most apparent as zones of increased signal intensity on T2-weighted images. Gliomatous involvement of the optic radiations may be symmetrical or strikingly unilateral. Contrast enhancement (on either CT or MR) may be absent. When enhancement occurs, a patchy pattern is common.

Occasional craniopharyngiomas may involve the optic chiasm and follow the optic tracts. Rarely meningeal "seeding" by CNS tumors (e.g., medulloblastoma) presents a similar appearance. Sarcoidosis may also envelope the chiasm, with enhancing extension along the optic tracts.

ORBITAL CALCIFICATIONS: BENIGN

Case 697

14-year-old boy noted to have swollen optic discs.

Drusen.

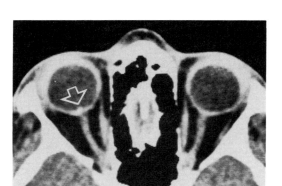

Case 698

72-year-old woman.

Senile Scleral Plaques.

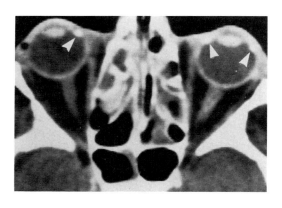

The tiny calcification near the right optic disc in this case *(arrow)* is typical of optic disc drusen. These hyaline bodies are often buried in the optic discs of children, elevating the disc and mimicking papilledema. The CT demonstration of calcification establishes the specific diagnosis, while the cerebral scan excludes increased intracranial pressure.

The differential diagnosis of globe calcification includes retinal hamartoma in tuberous sclerosis, neurofibromatosis, choroidal osteoma, melanoma, and retinoblastoma.

Small calcifications are commonly found near the junction of the horizontal rectus muscles and sclera in elderly patients. The calcium occurs within scleral plaques, possibly the result of chronic stress at the site of the rectus insertions. This benign phenomenon is usually bilaterally symmetrical.

Case 699

1-year-old boy.

Bilateral Retinoblastomas.

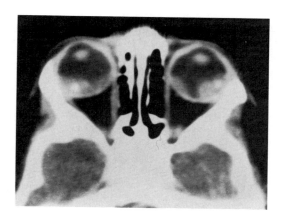

Case 700

66-year-old man.

Calcified Meningioma of the Optic Nerve Sheath.

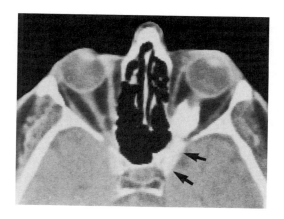

Tumors arising within the globe may be demonstrated by mass and/or calcification. In this case, the tissue density of the tumors is apparent within the globes, a finding that may also be noted with orbital melanoma or metastases to the choroid (see Cases 669 to 672).

Retinoblastomas frequently calcify and are often bilateral. CT is used mainly to assess the retrobulbar extension of a known tumor. However, a tiny focus of calcium may be a clue to involvement of the nonpresenting eye.

Calcification of the posterior globe is also seen in choroidal osteomas, benign lesions that contain cancellous bone and occur in plaques along the posterior sclera.

The tumor in this case has a fusiform shape that surrounds the axis of the optic nerve. Associated hyperostosis of the anterior clinoid process is present (arrows).

Optic nerve gliomas may be fusiform and occasionally calcify. They do not demonstrate the central core of nerve-sparing lucency characteristic of sheath meningiomas.

BLOW-OUT FRACTURES

Case 701

23-year-old man.
(coronal scan)

Case 702

46-year-old man.

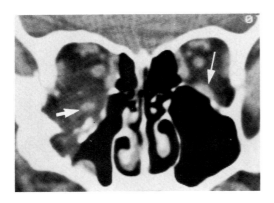

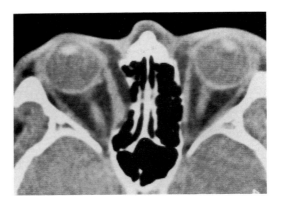

A direct blow to the eye compresses the orbital contents into the narrowing cone of the posterior orbit. The resultant increase in intraorbital pressure may cause secondary displacement of the orbital floor or medial wall.

CT scans clearly document these so-called "blow-out" fractures. Orbital fat and muscle are seen to herniate into air-containing sinuses.

The common blow-out fractures of the orbital floor are well defined on coronal CT or MR studies. In this case, the floor of the right orbit is markedly depressed. The inferior rectus muscle (short arrow) is located far below its normal location (arrow on the left).

Blow-out fractures involving the medial wall of the orbit are well seen in either coronal or axial planes. This scan demonstrates orbital fat occupying the fossa formed by displacement of the lamina papyracea. The medial rectus muscle is thickened and distorted as it is drawn toward the fracture. The position of the globes is disconjugate.

OTHER ORBITAL FRACTURES

Case 703

20-year-old man whose motorcycle left the road
and crashed into a forest.
(coronal scan)

Fractures Secondary to Wood Foreign Body.

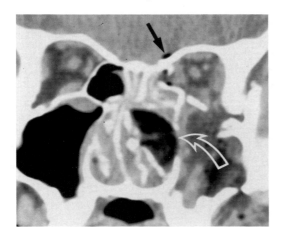

The semicircular zone of low attenuation at the junction of the nose and left maxillary sinus *(white arrow)* was found at surgery to represent a piece of a tree branch. This low-density appearance is characteristic of natural wood foreign bodies. (Manufactured and painted wood may have higher attenuation values.)

Multiple fractures involve the maxillary sinus and the medial and inferior walls of the left orbit. The small bubble of intracranial pneumocephalus *(black arrow)* indicates a fracture involving the frontal or ethmoid sinus.

Case 704

29-year-old man presenting with decreased visual acuity on the right after head trauma.
(coronal scan, bone algorithm, wide window)

Bone Fragment in the Optic Canal.

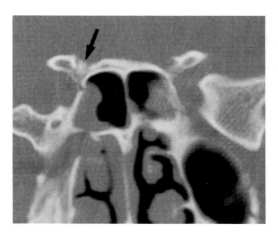

This patient sustained multiple fractures of the deep facial skeleton. A coronal CT scan demonstrates a small piece of bone *(arrow)* within the cranial end of the right optic canal. The optic nerve is located immediately medial to the anterior clinoid process, and nerve injury can be presumed from this image.

Case 705

21-year-old assault victim.

Lacerated Globe.

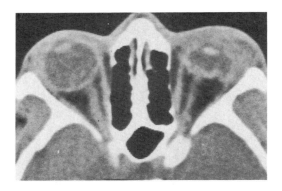

Case 706

31-year-old man following orbital laceration by
a piece of glass.

Intraocular Hemorrhage.

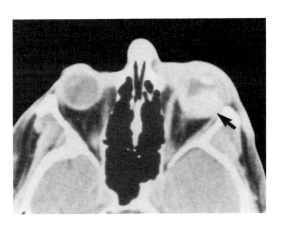

CT scans display the orbital contents in cases where facial injury may preclude ophthalmologic evaluation. In this case, a collapsed globe due to a penetrating injury is clearly demonstrated. No retrobulbar hematoma or foreign body is seen.

A small amount of head tilt may cause apparent asymmetry of normal anterior clinoid processes, as illustrated here.

Hemorrhage into the vitreous body is uncommon after blunt head trauma but may occur following penetrating injury. In this case, solid-appearing intraocular hemorrhage occupies much of the left globe. In other cases, blood-fluid levels may be recognized within the vitreous chamber after ocular laceration.

DIFFERENTIAL DIAGNOSIS:
FOCAL HIGH ATTENUATION WITHIN THE ORBIT

Case 707

24-year-old pheasant hunter.

Case 708

74-year-old woman.
(wide window)

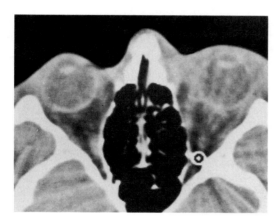

Metallic Foreign Body (Shotgun Pellet).

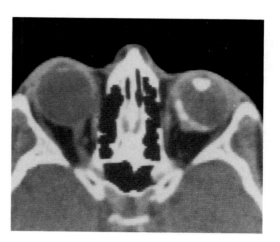

Phthisis Bulbi.

The detection and localization of dense intraorbital foreign bodies is aided by the axial display of CT scans. A pellet is seen at the apex of the left orbit in Case 707.

Foreign bodies of low attenuation (e.g., wood and plastic) can sometimes be demonstrated by CT (see Case 703). Associated ocular or retrobulbar injury is often apparent in cases of recent orbital trauma.

Ocular calcifications may be very dense, mimicking metallic foreign bodies as in Case 708. Senile scleral plaques (see Case 698) are usually paired and bilateral, assisting in their identification. Calcified drusen (see Case 697), retinal astrocytic hamartomas (seen in tuberous sclerosis or neurofibromatosis), or choroidal osteomas may be dense and solitary, resembling metallic foreign bodies at the margin of the globe.

"Phthisis bulbi" refers to decreased size and deformity of the globe due to injury or inflammation. This involution is often accompanied by calcification of the globe margin and lens, as in Case 708. A history of ocular damage clarifies any initial diagnostic confusion.

REFERENCES: CT

1. Ahmadi J., Teal J.S., Segall H.D., et al.: Computed tomography of carotid-cavernous fistula. *A.J.N.R.* 4:131–136, 1983.
2. Balchunas W.R., Quencer R.M., Byrne S.F.: Lacrimal gland and fossa masses: Evaluation by computed tomography and A-mode echography. *Radiology* 149:751–758, 1983.
3. Barrett L., Glatt H.J., Burde R.M., Gado M.H.: Optic nerve dysfunction in thyroid eye disease: CT. *Radiology* 167:503–508, 1988.
4. Berges O., Vignaud J., Aubin M.L.: Comparison of sonography and computed tomography in the study of orbital space-occupying lesions. *A.J.N.R.* 5:247–251, 1984.
5. Bryan R.N., Lewis R.A., Miller S.L.: Choroidal osteoma. *A.J.N.R.* 4:491–494, 1983.
6. Byrd W.E., Harwood-Nash D.C., Fitz C.R., et al.: Computed tomography of intraorbital optic nerve gliomas in children. *Radiology* 129:73–78, 1978.
7. Clark W.C., Theofilus C.S., Fleming J.C.: Primary optic nerve sheath meningiomas. *J. Neurosurg.* 70:37–40, 1989.
8. Curtin H.D.: Pseudotumor. *Radiol. Clin. North Am.* 25:583–600, 1987.
9. Daniels D.L., Williams A.L., Syvertsen A., et al.: CT recognition of optic nerve sheath meningioma: Abnormal sheath visualization. *A.J.N.R.* 3:181–183, 1982.
10. Danziger A., Price H.I.: CT findings in retinoblastoma. *A.J.R.* 133:695–697, 1979.
11. Davis K.R., Hesselink J.R., Dallow R., et al.: The role of CT and ultrasound in the diagnosis of cavernous hemangioma and lymphangioma of the orbit. *A.J.N.R.* 1:119, 1980.
12. Dresner S.C., Rothfus W.E., Slamovits T.L., et al.: Computed tomography of orbital myositis. *A.J.N.R.* 5:351–354, 1984.
13. Dubois P.J., Beardsley T., Klintworth G., et al.: Computed tomography of sarcoidosis of the optic nerve. *Neuroradiology* 24:179–182, 1983.
14. Enzmann D.R., Donaldson S.S., Kriss J.P.: Appearance of Graves' disease in orbital computed tomography. *J. Comput. Assist. Tomogr.* 3:815–819, 1979.
15. Flanders A.E., MaFee M.F., Rao V.M., Choi K.H.: CT characteristics of orbital pseudotumors and other orbital inflammatory processes. *J. Comput. Assist. Tomogr.* 13:40–47, 1989.
16. Forbes G.: Computed tomography of the orbit. *Radiol. Clin. North Am.* 20:37–49, 1982.
17. Forbes G., Gorman C.A., Brennan M.D., et al: Ophthalmopathy of Graves' disease: Computerized volume measurements of the orbital fat and muscle. *A.J.N.R.* 7:651–656, 1986.
18. Forbes G.S., Earnest F., Waller R.R.: Computed tomography of orbital tumors, including late-generation scanning techniques. *Radiology* 142:387–394, 1982.
19. Forbes G.S., Sheedy P.F., Waller R.R.: Orbital tumors evaluated by computed tomography. *Radiology* 136:101–111, 1980.
20. Gaster R., Duda E.: Localization of intraocular foreign bodies by computed tomography. *Ophthalmol. Surg.* 11:25–29, 1980.
21. Guyon J.J., Brant-Zawadzki M., Seiff S.R.: CT demonstration of optic canal fractures. *A.J.N.R.* 5:575–578, 1984.
22. Hammerschlag S.B., Hughes S., O'Reilly G.V., et al.: Blow-out fractures of the orbit: A comparison of computed tomography and conventional radiography with anatomical correlation. *Radiology* 143:487–492, 1982.
23. Hansen J.E., Gudeman S.K., Holgate R.C., Saunders R.A.: Penetrating intracranial wood wounds: Clinical limitations of computerized tomography. *J. Neurosurg.* 68:752–756, 1988.
24. Harr D.L., Quencer R.M., Abrams G.W.: Computed tomography and ultrasound in the evaluation of orbital infection and pseudotumor. *Radiology* 142:395–401, 1982.
25. Hedges T.R., Pozzi-Mucelli R., Char D.H., et al.: Computed tomographic demonstration of ocular calcification: Correlation with clinical and pathological findings. *Neuroradiology* 23:15–21, 1982.
26. Hesselink J.R., Davis K.R., Weber A.L., et al.: Radiological evaluation of orbital metastases with emphasis on computed tomography. *Radiology* 137:363–366, 1980.
27. Hopper K.D., Kats N.N.K., Dorwart R.H., et al.: Childhood leukokoria: Computed tomographic appearance and differential diagnosis with histopathologic correlation. *Radiographics* 5:377–394, 1985.
28. Howard C.W., Osher R.H., Tomsack R.L.: Computed tomographic features in optic neuritis. *Am. J. Ophthalmol.* 86:699–702, 1980.
29. Johns T.T., Citrin C.M., Black J., Sherman J.L.: CT evaluation of perineural orbital lesions: Evaluation of the "tram-track" sign. *A.J.N.R.* 5:587–590, 1984.
30. Johnson M.H., De Filipp G.J., Zimmerman R.A., Savino P.J.: Scleral inflammatory disease. *A.J.N.R.* 8:861–866, 1987.
31. Lallemand P.P., Brasch R.C., Char D.H., et al.: Orbital tumors in children: Characterization by computed tomography. *Radiology* 151:85–88, 1984.
32. Leo J.S., Halpern J., Sackler J.P.: Computed tomography in the evaluation of orbital infections. *Comput. Tomogr.* 4:133–138, 1980.
33. Lloyd G.A.: Primary orbital meningioma: A review of 41 patients investigated radiologically. *Clin. Radiol.* 33:181, 1982.
34. Mafee M.F., Haik B.G.: Lacrimal gland and fossa lesions: Role of computed tomography. *Radiol. Clin. North Am.* 25:767–780, 1987.
35. Mafee M.F., Peyman G.A.: Choroidal detachment and ocular hypotony: CT evaluation. *Radiology* 153:697–703, 1984.
36. Mafee M.F., Reyman G.A., McKusick M.A.: Malignant uveal melanoma and similar lesions studied by computed tomography. *Radiology* 156:403–408, 1985.
37. Nugent R.A., Lapointe J.S., Rootman J., et al.: Orbital dermoids: Features on CT. *Radiology* 165:475–478, 1987.
38. Nugent R.A., Rootman J., Robertson W.D., et al.: Acute orbital pseudotumors: Classification and CT features. *A.J.N.R.* 2:431–436, 1981.
39. Perugini S., Pasquini U., Menichelli F., et al.: Mucoceles in the paranasal sinuses involving the orbit: CT signs in 43 cases. *Neuroradiology* 23:133–139, 1982.
40. Peyster R.G., Augsburger J.J., Shields J.A., et al.: Choroidal melanoma: Comparison of CT, fundoscopy and US. *Radiology* 156:675–680, 1985.
41. Peyster R.G., Savino P.J., Hoover E.D., et al.: Differential diagnosis of the enlarged superior ophthalmic vein. *J. Comput. Assist. Tomogr.* 8:103–107, 1984.
42. Ramirez H., Blatt E.S., Hibri N.: Computed tomographic identification of calcified optic nerve drusen. *Radiology* 148:137–139, 1983.
43. Rothfus W.E., Curtin H.D.: Extraocular muscle enlargement: A CT review. *Radiology* 151:677–681, 1984.

44. Rothfus W.E., Curtin H.D., Slamovits T.L., et al.: Optic nerve sheath enlargement: A differential approach based on high resolution CT morphology. *Radiology* 150:409–415, 1984.
45. Towbin R., Han B.K., Kaufman R.A., Burke M.: Postseptal cellulitis: CT in diagnosis and management. *Radiology* 158:735–738, 1986.
46. Turner R.M., Gutman I., Hilal S.K., et al.: CT of drusen bodies and other calcific lesions of the optic nerve: Case report and differential diagnosis. *A.J.N.R.* 4:175–178, 1983.
47. Unger J.M.: Orbital apex fractures: The contribution of computed tomography. *Radiology* 150:713–717, 1984.
48. Weber A.L., Mikulis D.K.: Inflammatory disorders of the paranasal sinuses and their complications. *Radiol. Clin. North Am.* 25:615–630, 1987.
49. Weinstein G.S., Dresner S.C., Slamovits T.L., et al.: Acute and subacute orbital myositis. *Am. J. Ophthalmol.* 96:207–217, 1983.
50. Wells R.J., Sty J.R., Gonnerig R.S.: Imaging of the pediatric eye and orbit. *Radiographics* 9:1023–1044, 1989.
51. Zimmerman R.A., Bilaniuk L.T.: CT of orbital infection and its cerebral complications. *A.J.R.* 134:45–50, 1980.

REFERENCES: MR

1. Atlas S.W., Bilaniuk L.T., Zimmerman R.A., et al.: Orbit: Initial experience with surface coil spin-echo MR imaging at 1.5T. *Radiology* 164:501–509, 1987.
2. Atlas S.W., Grossman R.I., Hackney D.B., et al.: STIR MR imaging of the orbit. *A.J.N.R.* 9:969–974, 1988.
3. Atlas S.W., Grossman R.I., Savino P.J., et al.: Surface-coil MR of orbital pseudotumor. *A.J.N.R.* 8:141–146, 1987.
4. Azar-Kia B., Naheedy M.H., Elias D.A., et al.: Optic nerve tumors: Role of magnetic resonance imaging and computed tomography. *Radiol. Clin. North Am.* 25:561–582, 1987.
5. Bilaniuk L.T., Atlas S.W., Zimmerman R.A.: Magnetic resonance imaging of the orbit. *Radiol. Clin. North Am.* 25:509–528, 1987.
6. Bilaniuk L.T., Schenck J.F., Zimmerman R.A., et al.: Ocular and orbital lesions: Surface coil MR images. *Radiology* 156:669–674, 1985.
7. Brown E.W., Riccardi V.M., Mawad M., et al.: MR imaging of optic pathways in patients with neurofibromatosis. *A.J.N.R.* 8:1031–1036, 1987.
8. Daniels D.L., Herfkins R., Gager W.E., et al.: Magnetic resonance imaging of the optic nerves and chiasm. *Radiology* 152:79–83, 1984.
9. Flanders A.E., Espinosa G.A., Markiewicz D.A., Howell D.D.: Orbital lymphoma: Role of CT and MRI. *Radiol. Clin. North Am.* 25:601–614, 1987.
10. Fries P.D., Char D.H., Norman D.: MR imaging of orbital cavernous hemangioma. *J. Comput. Assist. Tomogr.* 11:418–421, 1987.
11. Hosten N., Sander B., Cordes M., et al.: Graves ophthalmopathy: MR imaging of the orbits. *Radiology* 172:759–762, 1989.
12. Langer B.G., MaFee M.F., Pollack S., et al: MRI of the normal orbit and optic pathways. *Radiol. Clin. North Am.* 25:429–446, 1987.
13. MaFee M.F., Goldberg M.F., Greenwald M.J., et al.: Retinoblastoma and simulating lesions: Role of CT and MR imaging. *Radiol. Clin. North Am.* 25:667–682, 1987.
14. MaFee M.F., Putterman A., Valvassori G.E., et al.: Orbital space-occupying lesions: Role of magnetic resonance imaging and computed tomography—A review of 145 cases. *Radiol. Clin. North Am.* 25:529–560, 1987.
15. Mafee M.F., Linder B., Peyman G.A., et al.: Choroidal hematoma and effusion: Evaluation with MR imaging. *Radiology* 168:781–786, 1988.
16. Mafee M.F., Peyman G.A.: Retinal and choroidal detachments: Role of magnetic resonance imaging and computed tomography. *Radiol. Clin. North Am.* 25:487–508, 1987.
17. Mafee M.F., Peyman G.A., Grisolano J.E., et al.: Malignant uveal melanoma and simulating lesions: MR imaging evaluation. *Radiology* 160:773–780, 1986.
18. McArdle C.B., Amparo E.G., Mirfakhraee M.: MR imaging of orbital blow-out fractures. *J. Comput. Assist. Tomogr.* 10:116–119, 1986.
19. Peyman G.A., Mafee M.F.: Uveal melanoma and similar lesions: The role of magnetic resonance imaging. *Radiol. Clin. North Am.* 25:471–486, 1987.
20. Peyster R.G., Augsburger J.J., Shields J.A., et al: Intraocular tumor: Evaluation with MR imaging. *Radiology* 168:773–780, 1988.
21. Peyster R.G., Shapiro M.D., Haik B.G.: Orbital metastasis: Role of magnetic resonance imaging and computed tomography. *Radiol. Clin. North Am.* 25:647–662, 1987.
22. Pomeranz S.J., Shelton J.J., Tobias J., et al.: MR of visual pathways in patients with neurofibromatosis. *A.J.N.R.* 8:831–836, 1987.
23. Roden D.T., Savino P.J., Zimmerman R.A.: Magnetic resonance imaging in orbital diagnosis. *Radiol. Clin. North Am.* 26:535–544, 1988.
24. Simon J., Szumowski J., Totterman S., et al.: Fat suppression MR imaging of the orbit. *A.J.N.R.* 9:961–968, 1988.
25. Sobel D.F., Kelly W., Kjos B.O., et al.: MR imaging of orbital and ocular disease. *A.J.N.R.* 6:259–264, 1985.
26. Sobel D.F., Mills C., Char D., et al.: NMR of the normal and pathologic eye and orbit. *A.J.N.R.* 5:345–350, 1984.
27. Spencer G., Lufkin R., Simons K., et al.: MR of a melanoma simulating ocular neoplasm. *A.J.N.R.* 8:921–922, 1987.
28. Sullivan J.A., Harms S.E.: Characterization of orbital lesions by surface coil MR imaging. *Radiographics* 7:9–28, 1987.
29. Sullivan J.A., Harms S.E.: Surface-coil MR imaging of orbital neoplasms. *A.J.N.R.* 7:29–34, 1986.
30. Tonami H., Nakagawa T., Ohguchi M., et al.: Surface-coil MR imaging of orbital blow-out fractures: A comparison with reformatted CT. *A.J.N.R.* 8:445–450, 1987.
31. Tonami H., Tamamura H., Kimizu K., et al.: Intraocular lesions in patients with systemic disease: Findings on MR imaging. *A.J.N.R.* 10:1185–1190, 1989.
32. Wiot J.G., Pleatman C.W.: Chronic hematic cyst of the orbit. *A.J.N.R.* 10:537–539, 1989.

CHAPTER 13

Disc Disease and Spondylosis

LUMBAR DISC BULGE VS. HERNIATION

Case 709

55-year-old man.

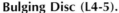

Bulging Disc (L4-5).

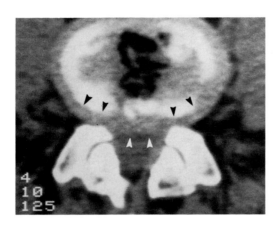

Case 710

31-year-old man.

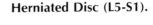

Herniated Disc (L5-S1).

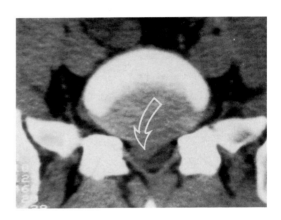

The CT demonstration of lumbar disc abnormalities is based on the differential attenuation of bone, disc, spinal fluid, and epidural fat. In this case, the margin of disc density *(white arrowheads)* bulges circumferentially beyond the dense bone of the vertebral end plate *(black arrowheads)*. The posterior margin of the bulging disc is defined by the slightly lower attenuation of spinal fluid within the dural sac.

The posterior margin of lumbar discs is normally slightly concave at the L1 through L5 levels and nearly straight at L5-S1. Bulging discs demonstrate a uniform, symmetric convexity. This broad curve contrasts with the focal asymmetry of disc herniation, as seen in Case 710.

The false appearance of a posterior disc bulge may be caused by oblique angulation of the scan with respect to the disc level, most commonly seen at L5-S1. Spondylolisthesis may also cause a prominent disc "shelf" resembling a diffuse bulge (see Case 748).

Discs herniating into the spinal canal are usually defined by the lower attenuation of spinal fluid and epidural fat.

The focal protrusion of disc density in this case *(arrow)* has a small radius of curvature that is distinct from the gently curving margin on either side. This localized change in contour contrasts with the diffuse bulge in Case 709.

Some cases present features intermediate between Cases 709 and 710, and the distinction between an asymmetric disc bulge and a frank disc herniation is occasionally difficult. Magnetic resonance imaging may clarify the presence of an annular tear with associated extrusion of nuclear material in such situations (see Cases 717 and 718).

Disc herniations are most common in a posterolateral direction, but midline herniations also occur (see Case 711).

LUMBAR DISC HERNIATIONS INVOLVING THE CENTRAL CANAL

Case 711

40-year-old man.

Central Disc Herniation (L3-4).

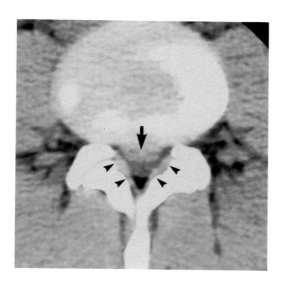

Case 712

39-year-old man.

Central/Lateral Disc Herniation (L5-S1).

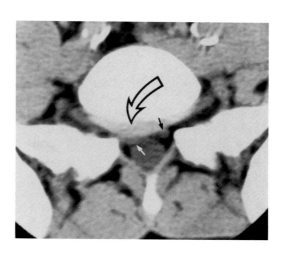

In this case, focal posterior extension of disc material is centered in the midline *(arrow)*. The small radius of curvature and abrupt angle of origin from the parent disc indicate herniation.

Disc herniation involving the central spinal canal may distort individual nerve roots (see Case 712) and/or compress the dural sac. Here the herniation has caused moderate stenosis of the central canal with deformity of the thecal sac.

The symmetrical layers of tissue with mildly increased attenuation values along the posterolateral margins of the spinal canal *(arrowheads)* are the ligamenta flava. Thickening of these ligaments often accompanies degenerative disc disease and contributes to narrowing of the spinal canal (see Cases 738 and 744).

Disc herniations involving the central canal are often asymmetrical. Eccentric herniations may severely distort individual nerve roots without compressing the dural sac.

In this case, a broad posterolateral herniation *(open arrow)* causes marked posterior displacement of the proximal right S1 nerve root *(white arrow;* compare to the normal position of the left S1 root indicated by the *small black arrow).* The thecal sac is not compromised.

Case 713

48-year-old woman presenting with
radiculopathy in the right S1 distribution.

Central/Lateral Disc Herniation (L5-S1).

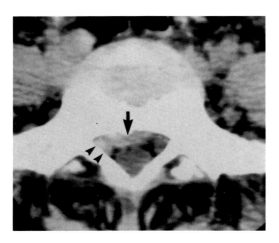

Case 714

44-year-old man.

"Free Fragment" Disc Herniation (L5-S1).

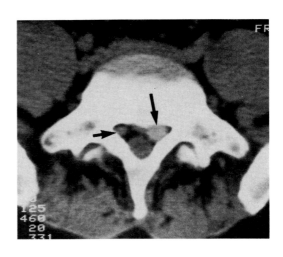

In addition to compromising the central canal, herniated discs may cause nerve compression by narrowing the lateral recess or restricting the intervertebral foramen.

The lateral recess, or "subarticular gutter," is formed at the anterolateral corner of the spinal canal by the junction of the rostral vertebral body and pedicle. A nerve occupies this angle as it prepares to exit beneath the pedicle through the superior portion of the intervertebral foramen.

Eccentric disc herniations may compress the nerve root against the bony margins of the lateral recess. In this case, the proximal right S1 root is displaced and flattened *(arrowheads)*.

The root also demonstrates slightly increased attenuation values. This finding can be a confirmatory sign of significant nerve compression. Other secondary signs of root compression include swelling distal to the level of distortion and/or proximal contrast enhancement within the thecal sac (seen on MR studies).

The *short arrow* in this case indicates the normal right S1 root traversing the lateral recess on its way from the dural sac to the intervertebral foramen. On the left side, a herniated fragment extends caudally from the disc space to compromise the lateral recess and compress the exiting nerve *(long arrow)*. The density of the herniated disc is considerably greater than that of a normal root sleeve occupying the recess. (However, a compressed nerve root may itself demonstrate increased attenuation values, as seen in Case 713).

Compression of a nerve within the lateral recess may also be caused by hypertrophic bone, as illustrated in Case 740.

LATERAL LUMBAR DISC HERNIATION

Case 715

67-year-old woman with right leg pain.

Posterolateral Disc Herniation (L4-5).

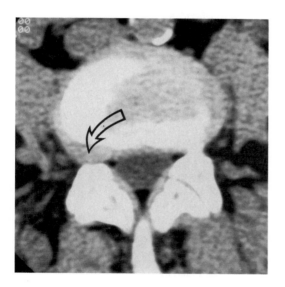

Case 716

42-year-old man.

Lateral Disc Herniation (L4-5).

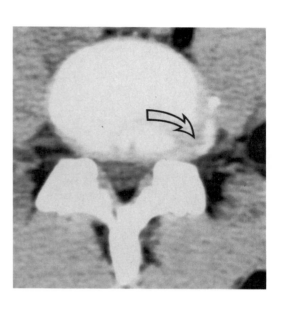

Lateral disc herniations may cause radiculopathy by compressing nerve roots as they leave the spinal canal. Disc material may extend into an intervertebral foramen and/or distort a nerve root distal to the neural canal. In this case, a posterolateral disc herniation at L4-5 *(arrow)* occupies the right intervertebral foramen.

Sagittal MR images (or sagittal reconstructions of axial CT scans) are useful for demonstrating the cephalocaudal extent of foraminal compromise by disc material or osteophytes (see Cases 742 and 743).

Some disc herniations are predominantly lateral, as in this case. While many such protrusions are asymptomatic, others may distort a nerve as it leaves the spine. It is important to follow all roots through their foramina when reviewing CT and MR studies, so that foraminal or extraforaminal impingement is recognized. The surgical approach to "far lateral" root compression is a lateral exposure; traditional laminectomy will fail to identify the source of symptoms.

MR CORRELATION: LUMBAR DISC HERNIATION

Case 717

32-year-old man.
(sagittal, noncontrast scan; SE 800/17)

Case 718

21-year-old woman.
(sagittal, noncontrast scan; SE 2800/45)

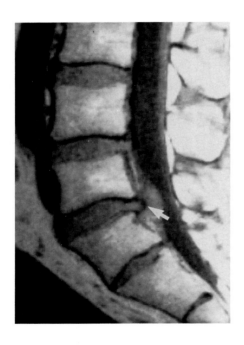

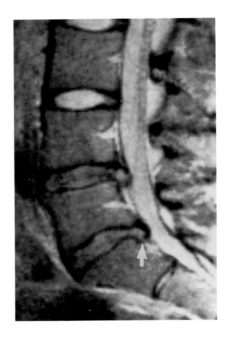

Sagittal MR scans efficiently display long segments of the spinal canal. Both extradural and intrathecal pathologies are well seen. These imaging advantages contrast with the limited coverage and poor intradural definition of standard axial CT studies.

Centrally herniated discs are outlined on T1-weighted images by the slightly lower intensity of CSF within the subarachnoid space (and/or by the higher signal intensity of ventral epidural fat). In this case, a large anterior epidural mass is centered at the L5-S1 disc level, suggesting discogenic origin. In addition to the disc herniation itself, associated edema, granulation tissue, and/or localized epidural hemorrhage may contribute to such prominent extradural deformities.

The dark line at the posterior margin of the disc space (arrow) represents annulus fibrosis, which is normally in close contact with the posterior longitudinal ligament and dura. A gap or rent in this line was present on an adjacent section, with continuity between the disc space and the large epidural mass. Such annular tears are well seen on sagittal MR scans as linear zones of high signal intensity traversing the normally "black" disc margin (see Case 718).

Herniated discs often have relatively high signal intensity on long TR spin-echo images. Here the central portions of the disc herniations at L4-5 and L5-S1 are "bright," outlining the "dark" band of displaced annulus, posterior longitudinal ligament and dura between the disc and the subarachnoid space. A small annulus tear is present at the inferior margin of the L5-S1 disk (arrow).

The parent disc spaces at the levels of herniation are narrowed with reduced signal intensity as compared to higher levels. This loss of normal T2-prolongation represents "dehydration," a degenerative process that commonly precedes disc herniation.

Sagittal MR views may demonstrate reactive changes in the vertebral bodies adjacent to degenerating discs. Subchondral zones of long T1 and long T2 are often seen, probably representing inflammatory edema and reactive cellular infiltration within the marrow. At a later stage, fatty atrophy of the marrow may cause the opposite pattern of signal changes with the same band-like morphology paralleling the disc space ("bright" on T1-weighted images, with reduced signal intensity on T2-weighted scans).

Case 719

41-year-old woman.
(axial, noncontrast scan; SE 1000/20)

Lateral Disc Herniation (L4-5).

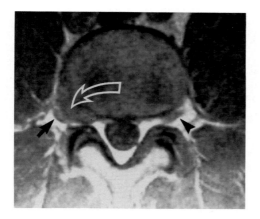

Case 720

33-year-old man.
(axial, noncontrast scan; SE 2000/30)

Central Disc Herniation (L5-S1).

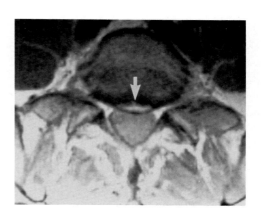

Epidural and paraspinal fat serves as a natural contrast material on MR scans as on CT studies. The high signal intensity of fat on T1-weighted sequences outlines the margins of "watery" tissues including the thecal sac, nerve roots, and discs.

In this case, the left L4 root is well seen within the neural foramen *(black arrowhead)*. A lateral disc herniation on the right *(white arrow)* extends into the intervertebral foramen and displaces the exiting nerve root *(black arrow)*.

Nerve roots (or masses) can be seen within the dural sac on either T1-weighted or T2-weighted MR scans, a distinct advantage over CT imaging.

The signal intensity of herniated discs is variable on long TR images. In this case (as in Case 718), the herniation is relatively "bright" *(arrow)*. Inflammatory granulation tissue within an annular tear probably contributes to this appearance and may also be associated with contrast enhancement (see Case 754B).

Such lesions may be best seen on "balanced" or "intermediate" spin-echo images (long TR, short TE), with reduced conspicuity on more heavily T2-weighted scans. In other cases the signal intensity of disc herniations is relatively low, and they are well outlined by "bright" CSF on T2-weighted studies.

COMPOUND ROOT SLEEVES

Case 721A

50-year-old man.

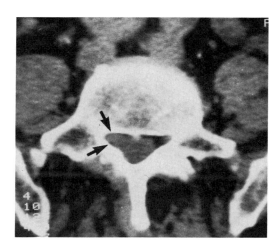

Case 721B

Same patient (scan slightly caudal to that in Case 721A).

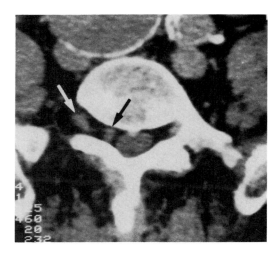

Adjacent lumbar nerves may share a common sleeve. A "conjoined" or "compound" sleeve is larger than an individual nerve and is located between the levels of the contributing roots.

This normal variant is typically discovered as an asymmetrical structure occupying the lateral recess *(arrows)*. It may be misinterpreted as a herniated disc. However, the low density of spinal fluid within a compound sleeve contrasts with the increased density expected of disc material (compare this scan with Case 714). In addition, the involved lateral recess is large, favoring a congenital variation with corresponding bone morphology.

A compound sleeve may be identified by more caudal sections demonstrating the emergence of two separate roots. On this scan the compound sleeve in Case 721A is dividing, with the L5 branch *(white arrow)* exiting laterally while the more medial S1 root *(black arrow)* continues caudally.

MR scans demonstrate CSF-like intensity within compound root sleeves on all pulse sequences. Myelography (CT or routine) will distinguish between compound sleeves and other lesions in ambiguous cases.

Here the normal left L5 root is seen within its lateral recess, well removed from the dural sac and central canal. Disc herniations far from midline may still cause compression of L5 nerve roots within the lateral recess or intervertebral foramen.

Calcified aneurysms of the iliac arteries are incidentally noted in this case.

DIFFERENTIAL DIAGNOSIS:
EPIDURAL DENSITY POSTERIOR TO A VERTEBRAL BODY

Case 722

45-year-old woman.

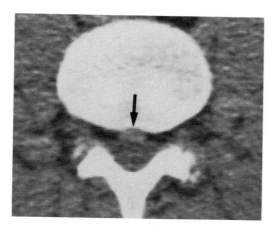

Normal Anterior Epidural Veins (L3 Level).

Case 723

52-year-old man.
(scan with intrathecal contrast; prior laminectomy)

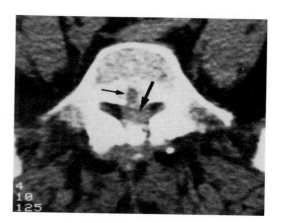

Herniated Disc Fragment (L5 Level).

The normal plexus of epidural veins ("retrovertebral plexus") may form a prominent structure within the anterior portion of the spinal canal. The veins are particularly noticeable at midvertebral levels near the basivertebral vein (*small arrow*, Case 723). A bone spur is sometimes seen adjacent to the vein and should not be misinterpreted as an osteophyte or calcified disc fragment.

The basivertebral vein is not seen in Case 722, and the density of anterior epidural veins *(arrow)* mimics the appearance of a midline disc fragment. The recurrent midline disc herniation in Case 723 *(large arrow)* is well defined by intrathecal contrast. The dorsal "prolapse" of the dural sac toward the laminectomy defect is a common postoperative appearance (see Case 752).

Adjacent sections may link a questionable midline density to vascular structures or provide confirmatory evidence of disc herniation. Scans performed after intravenous contrast infusion help to define the location of epidural veins in equivocal cases.

DIFFERENTIAL DIAGNOSIS:
EPIDURAL MASS WITHIN THE SPINAL CANAL

Case 724

32-year-old man.

Case 725

31-year-old man.

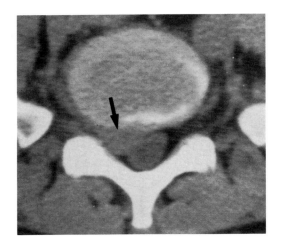

Epidural Metastasis (Seminoma).

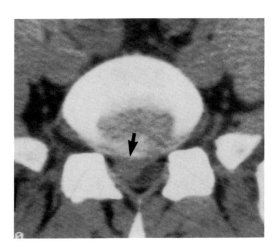

Herniated Disc.

The prevalence of lumbar disc disease does not preclude the possibility of other epidural lesions. Epidural tumors can mimic the appearance of disc herniation, as seen in Case 724. Spontaneous or post-traumatic epidural hematomas may also be confused with a herniated disc. (In some cases epidural hematomas accompany a disc herniation, exaggerating its apparent size and contributing to neural compression.)

A clue to the nondisc nature of Case 724 is the difference in attenuation between the epidural mass and the center of the disc. Herniated fragments may appear slightly lower (or higher) in attenuation than the parent disc, but a significant disparity should prompt consideration of an alternative diagnosis.

Case 726

40-year-old woman presenting with radicular pain.

Case 727

53-year-old man.

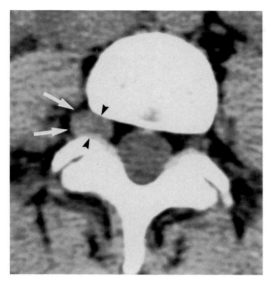

Schwannoma (L4 Root).

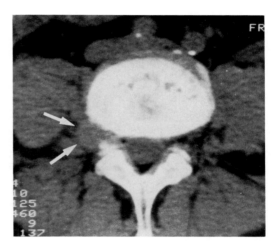

Disc Herniation (L3-4).

Masses within the intervertebral foramen may be neoplastic or discogenic in origin. The most common benign tumor in this location is a schwannoma, as in Case 726. Schwannomas often demonstrate relatively low attenuation values mimicking an enlarged root sleeve. Associated expansion of the intervertebral foramen *(black arrowheads)* is a clue to the long-standing presence of a benign mass. Lymphoma and metastasis should be included in the differential diagnosis when foraminal expansion is absent and malignant neoplasms are considered.

Case 727 demonstrates that laterally herniated discs may present as foraminal masses. The dural sac is undisturbed within the central canal, while the right intervertebral foramen is filled with disc material.

Foraminal disc herniations may closely resemble schwannomas on both CT and MR studies. Occasional herniated discs are accompanied by erosive changes or remodeling of adjacent bone. MR scans with contrast enhancement will usually distinguish between these entities, demonstrating peripheral enhancement at the margins of disk fragments and more solid enhancement within neoplasms.

CERVICAL DISC HERNIATION

Case 728

30-year-old man complaining that his right arm "gives" when he lifts weights.

Central Disc Herniation (C4-5).

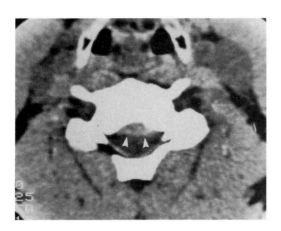

Case 729

40-year-old woman with left triceps weakness and radiculopathy.

Lateral Disc Herniation (C6-7).

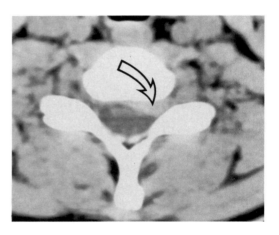

The axial perspective of CT scans is as useful in the cervical spine as in the lumbar region. However, the small size of cervical vertebrae and discs requires close placement of thin sections for adequate definition of anatomical and pathologic features. Even with good technique, the lack of epidural fat and the reduced contrast resolution of thin sections may make diagnosis difficult. Calcification is common in cervical discs and may partially offset the lack of surrounding contrast.

In this case, a large central disc herniation occupies the anterior portion of the spinal canal. The herniating disc has extended caudally from the C4-5 level to lie behind the body of C5. The density of the disc contrasts with the low attenuation of the dural sac and epidural fat.

Case 730 demonstrates a similar central disc defined by subarachnoid contrast material.

Here a lateral disc herniation occupies the entrance to the left intervertebral foramen *(arrow)*. The dural sac is only mildly deformed.

Artifact from the thick tissue and bone of the shoulders may compromise CT scans at the lowest cervical levels. Caudal traction on the arms improves the quality of such images. MR offers an alternative artifact-free means of evaluating the cervical-thoracic junction.

CERVICAL DISC HERNIATION DEMONSTRATED BY INTRATHECAL CONTRAST

Case 730

31-year-old man.
(scan with intrathecal contrast)

"Free Fragment" Disc Herniation (C6-7).

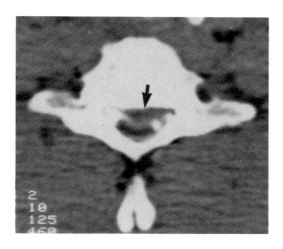

Case 731

45-year-old man with left biceps weakness.
(scan with intrathecal contrast)

Lateral Disc Herniation (C5-6).

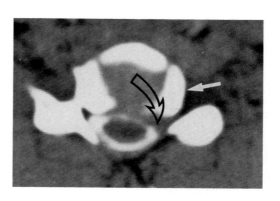

The small size of important anatomic details in the cervical region and the limited natural tissue contrast have led to several methods for augmenting CT diagnosis. Intravenous injection of contrast material opacifies the epidural venous plexus, improving definition of anatomy and pathology within the central canal and intervertebral foramina.

Alternatively, cervical CT scans may be performed after the injection of intrathecal contrast material. In this case a large central disc herniation is clearly defined, indenting the ventral margin of the dural sac and compressing the spinal cord. A "free fragment" of herniated material was found at surgery.

Myelopathy may be present when cord deformity is seen. However, remarkable flattening of the spinal cord may be asymptomatic if epidural compression develops slowly (see also Cases 809, 812, and 813).

Here the left anterolateral corner of the thecal sac is amputated by an epidural mass *(black arrow)*. The appearance is not specific (see Case 764), but disc herniation is the most likely cause of such deformity. Unlike Case 730, the spinal cord is not compromised. Like Case 729, the disc herniation distorts a cervical nerve root as it enters the intervertebral foramen.

In addition to disc pathology, cervical CT scans may define stenosis of the central canal or intervertebral foramen caused by hypertrophy of the uncinate processes *(white arrow)* and/ or facet joints (see Case 741).

Case 732

52-year-old woman.
(sagittal, noncontrast scan; SE 800/17)

Case 733

47-year-old man.
(sagittal, noncontrast scan; SE 2800/75)

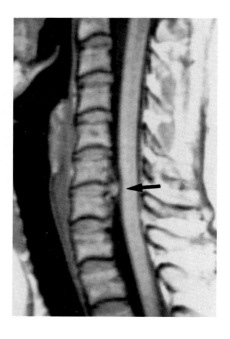

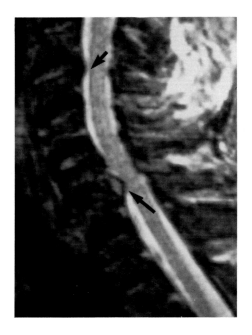

Central cervical disc herniations are well defined as protrusions of intermediate signal intensity indenting the subarachnoid space on sagittal T1-weighted MR images. Here a herniation at C6-7 is easily seen, outlined by low-intensity CSF within the dural sac.

Larger central disc herniations elevate or "tent" the posterior longitudinal ligament away from the adjacent vertebral bodies. Soft tissue of increased signal intensity then apparent between the bodies and the posteriorly displaced ligament usually represents prominent epidural veins rather than rostral or caudal migration of disc fragments.

T2-weighted MR scans provide a myelographic effect, with high-intensity CSF outlining the spinal cord and the dural margins. (See Cases 735 and 739 for additional examples.) Extradural deformities are well defined on such images.

Here a spondylitic ridge at C3-4 *(short arrow)* is of nonspecific low intensity; it is not possible to distinguish potential components of osteophyte and "hard" disc material. However, the high signal within the anterior epidural mass at C6-7 *(long arrow)* is characteristic of a herniated disc (compare to Cases 718 and 720 in the lumbar region) and establishes the diagnosis at this level.

The spinal cord is not significantly flattened, and there is no evidence of intramedullary edema to suggest compressive myelopathy (compare to Case 739).

Case 734

65-year-old woman.
(axial, noncontrast scan; SE 500/16)

Central Disc Herniation (C3-4).

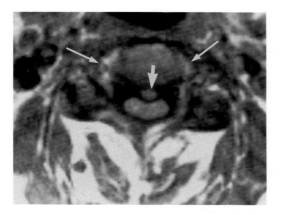

Case 735

37-year-old woman.
(axial, noncontrast scan; 15-degree flip angle gradient echo sequence)

Lateral Disc Herniation (C6-7).

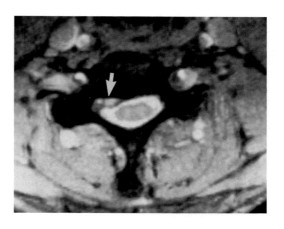

A small central disc herniation *(thick arrow)* is well seen on this T1-weighted image, indenting the ventral margin of the dural sac and spinal cord (compare to case 730). A black line between the disc and the cord probably represents a combination of outer annulus, posterior longitudinal ligament and dura.

The marrow-containing uncinate processes *(thin arrows)* are of higher signal intensity than the disc space that they enclose.

Axial scans performed with low flip angle gradient echo techniques provide a myelographic effect that is useful in evaluating cervical disc herniations. Such sequences also produce high signal intensity within epidural veins of the cervical canal and neural foramina, increasing the contrast with disc material or osteophytes in both locations.

In this case the spinal cord is well defined, with intramedullary discrimination of gray and white matter. A lateral disc herniation deforms the right anterolateral recess of the dural sac, near the entrance to the neural foramen (compare to Case 731).

The signal intensity of herniated discs on low flip angle gradient echo images varies from intermediate to bright. High signal intensity in the region of herniation, as in this case, often includes prominent epidural veins adjacent to the disc itself.

439

Case 736

25-year-old man presenting with back pain and
bilateral leg numbness.
(scan with intrathecal contrast; T7–8 level)

Case 737

42-year-old man referred for evaluation of
bladder dysfunction.
(sagittal, noncontrast scan; SE 550/20)

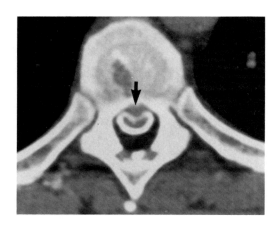

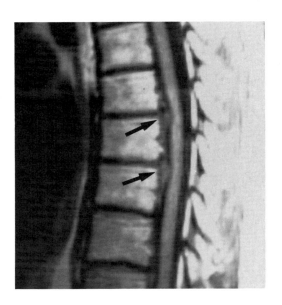

Magnetic resonance imaging has demonstrated that thoracic disc herniations are much more common than had been previously appreciated. Many such lesions are asymptomatic and clinically incidental. However, the small diameter of the thoracic spinal canal and its kyphotic curvature predispose to major neurological impairment from small disc herniations.

The paucity of epidural fat and the small dural sac within the thoracic spinal canal combine with air/bone artifacts to obscure soft tissue details on standard CT examinations. Scans after intrathecal contrast are often necessary to demonstrate intradural and epidural pathology. In this case, a central disc herniation is seen to indent the dural sac and spinal cord (compare to the cervical herniation in Case 730).

MR scanning offers a less invasive means of detecting and defining lesions of the thoracic spinal canal (see Cases 737, 760, 774, 785, and 793 for examples).

Thoracic disc herniations are often subtle on sagittal MR scans, even in severely symptomatic patients. Close attenuation to the posterior margin of each disc space is indicated, followed by thin axial sections through questionable levels.

Here small disc herniations are seen at T7-8 and T8-9 as indentations along the dark line of ventral subarachnoid space, dura, and posterior longitudinal ligament *(arrows)*. Slight flattening of the anterior cord margin confirms the presence of extradural lesions at these levels.

Most disc herniations occur in the lower half of the thoracic spine, with frequent involvement of the T11-12 level. About two thirds of symptomatic patients present with motor and sensory complaints, while one third experience bowel or bladder dysfunction.

CENTRAL CANAL STENOSIS

Case 738

71-year-old man.

Central Lumbar Stenosis (L2-3).

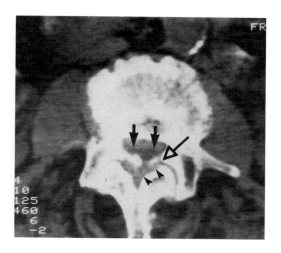

Case 739

77-year-old man with symptoms of cervical myelopathy.
(sagittal, noncontrast scan; SE 3000/90)

Central Cervical Stenosis (Disc Herniation at C3-4 Superimposed on Cervical Spondylosis).

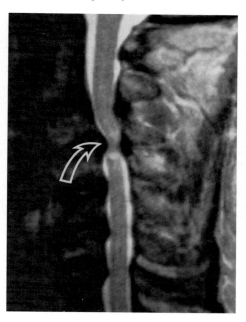

A variety of congenital and acquired factors may cause narrowing of the spinal canal. Axial scans clearly demonstrate the cross-sectional morphology and severity of such stenosis.

Congenitally stenotic canals often have a triangular or "trefoil" morphology, with short pedicles and medially bowing laminae. Congenital deformity (e.g., achondroplasia) is frequently most prominent in the lumbar region. The central canal may be compressed sufficiently to produce symptoms of stenosis (e.g., "pseudoclaudication").

Spinal stenosis is more commonly caused by the superimposition of acquired changes on congenitally narrow dimensions. The acquired factors may be specific processes (e.g., Paget's disease, ossification of the posterior longitudinal ligament) or simple degenerative changes.

This case is a typical example. The combination of disc bulge *(solid arrows)*, facet hypertrophy *(open arrow)*, and thickening of the ligamentum flavum *(arrowheads)* causes circumferential constriction of the canal. A complete myelographic block was found at this level. (See Case 745 for another example of central lumbar stenosis.)

Central canal stenosis in the cervical region is often due to spondylitic ridging combined with thickening and buckling of dorsal ligaments. Here a typical "washboard" appearance of multilevel osteophytes indents the subarachnoid space from C4 to C7.

At C3-4 a superimposed disc herniation causes severe narrowing of the central canal with cord compression. (The signal intensity of this herniated disc is lower than the example in Case 733.)

High signal intensity is present within the thinned spinal cord, characteristic of compressive myelopathy. Both reversible edema and irreversible myelomalacia may contribute to this appearance, which is often correlated with limited postoperative improvement. In this case a large disc herniation was found at surgery, and the patient has made a good recovery.

LATERAL STENOSIS

Case 740

66-year-old man.

Stenosis of a Lateral Recess (L4).

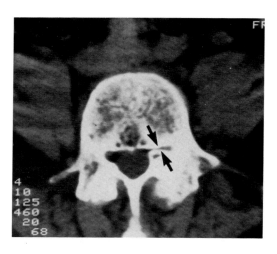

Case 741

48-year-old man.
(wide window)

Foraminal Stenosis (C5-6).

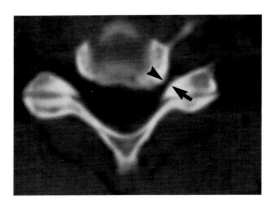

The base of the superior articular facet of a lumbar vertebra forms the posterolateral margin of the lateral recess. Hypertrophy of the facet (and/or related osteophytes) may narrow the recess and cause nerve compression, either alone or in combination with disc pathology.

In this case, the left lateral recess has been almost obliterated by overgrowth of the facet joint (arrows; see also Case 744). CT accurately demonstrates the relative contributions of disc and bone to compromise of the lateral recess or intervertebral foramen (compare this scan to Case 714).

Lateral stenosis in the cervical region is usually seen as foraminal narrowing due to hypertrophy of the uncinate process (arrowhead) and/or facet joint (arrow). In this case the left intervertebral foramen is moderately narrowed (compare to the right side).

A small amount of cervical scoliosis or tilt will cause asymmetric visualization of the right and left intervertebral foramina on any one scan. Care should be taken to evaluate adjacent sections before foraminal asymmetry is judged to represent stenosis. Wide windows (as seen here) provide a more accurate display of bone margins than the apparent edges of high attenuation on "soft tissue" images.

Discrimination between osteophyte and dehydrated disc material can be difficult on cervical MR scans. This distinction is more easily made on CT examinations, which remain valuable in the assessment of cervical radiculopathy.

SAGITTAL VIEWS OF FORAMINAL STENOSIS

Case 742

74-year-old man presenting with right leg pain. (right-sided sagittal reconstruction of nonangled axial CT scans; anterior is to the reader's left)

Osteophyte Extending Into an L5-S1 Foramen.

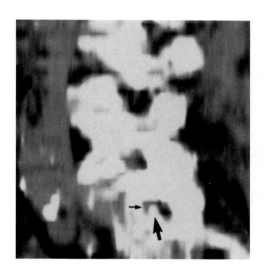

Case 743

58-year-old woman. (sagittal, noncontrast scan; SE 900/17)

Disc Herniation Extending Into an L4−5 Foramen.

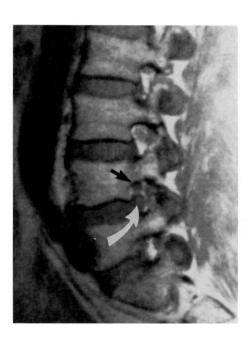

The cephalocaudal dimension of intervertebral foramina can be difficult to judge on axial CT or MR scans. Sagittal views are helpful in this assessment.

The orientation of lumbar intervertebral foramina is close to the coronal plane. For this reason, true sagittal reconstructions of CT data or direct sagittal MR scans provide cross-sectional views of foraminal margins and contents.

In this case, a large bone spur *(large arrow)* projects into the inferior portion of the L5-S1 intervertebral foramen. The exiting L5 root *(small arrow)* is compressed in the anterior-superior corner of the nerve root canal.

Sagittal MR scans away from the lumbar midline are valuable for defining lateral disc herniations and foraminal compromise. On T1-weighted images the intervertebral foramina are normally filled with high-intensity fat surrounding a nerve root of intermediate intensity. (In the lumbar region the root exits close to the superior pedicle; the reverse is true in the cervical spine.) Disc material or osteophyte is well defined when encroaching into this zone of high contrast.

Here a lateral disc herniation at L4-5 has extended into the inferior aspect of the neural foramen *(white arrow;* compare to foramina at the higher levels). The exiting L4 root *(black arrow)* is flattened between the disc margin and the overlying pedicle.

LUMBAR FACET ARTHROPATHY

Case 744

74-year-old man.
(L5-S1 level)

Case 745

62-year-old man.
(L3-4 level)

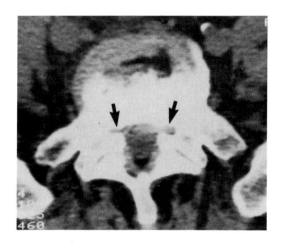

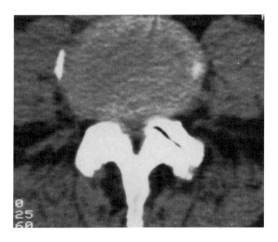

Degenerative changes of the facet joints are often seen on lumbar CT scans. Common findings include sclerosis, subchondral erosions, osteophyte formation, and narrowing of the joint space.

The capsule of the facet joint may become thickened and calcified. Synovial cysts arising from the joint may mimic other extradural masses (see Cases 746 and 747).

In this case, hypertrophy and spurring of the facets has caused bilateral narrowing of the lateral recesses (arrows). Gas is present within the bulging disc, and the ligamenta flava are thickened.

Overgrowth of the facet joint may be a response to excessive stress caused by instability or by fusion at adjacent levels. This patient had been fused from L4 to S1. Facet hypertrophy has developed a "cupped" configuration, and gas is seen within the left joint (see also Case 747). Stenosis of the central canal is present due to a combination of congenitally small dimensions and superimposed degenerative hypertrophy.

Facet arthropathy may cause back pain with radicular referral independent of canal compromise or nerve root compression.

SYNOVIAL CYSTS

Case 746

56-year-old woman presenting with right S1 radiculopathy.

Synovial Cyst (L5-S1).

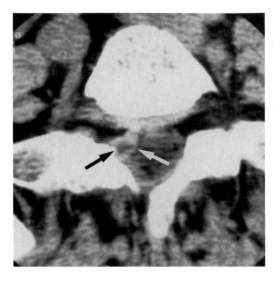

Case 747

54-year-old woman.

Calcified Synovial Cyst (L4-5).

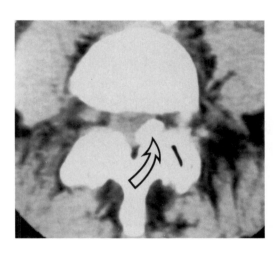

Degenerative changes of the lumbar facet joints may be associated with the development of a synovial cyst. These structures represent expansion or herniation of synovial membranes beneath or through the facet capsule/ligamentum flavum.

Synovial cysts are characteristically found at the medial aspect of the facet joint. The resultant extradural deformity along the posterolateral aspect of the spinal canal should not be confused with more anteriorly based disc herniations.

The dense rim surrounding the low-density cyst in this case is characteristic. The rim may be faintly or frankly calcified (see Case 747). Hemorrhage frequently occurs in synovial cysts, and blood products likely contribute to their central or peripheral density on CT scans. Gas within a degenerative facet joint may communicate with the center of a synovial cyst.

The only atypical feature of this scan is the occurrence of the lesion at the L5-S1 level. The great majority of synovial cysts are found at L4-5, possibly relating to the relatively large amount of motion and facet stress occurring at this level.

The synovial cyst in this case presents an unusual appearance of solid calcification rather than peripheral density. However, the location of the lesion at the medial aspect of a degenerated L4-5 facet joint is characteristic. Gas is present within the left facet joint, and prominent facet hypertrophy is seen bilaterally.

Synovial cysts may fluctuate in size on follow-up studies, suggesting variable distention by joint effusion or fluid. Occasional cysts cause persistent compression of nerve roots and require surgery.

SPONDYLOLISTHESIS

Case 748

68-year-old man.
(L5-S1 level)

Case 749

60-year-old man.
(L5-S1 level)

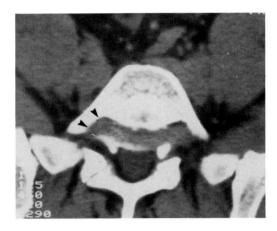

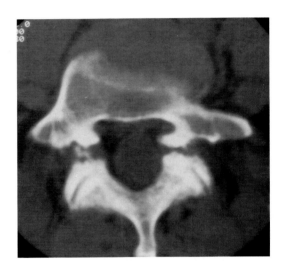

The CT features of spondylolisthesis include characteristic subluxation and visualization of associated spondylolysis.

The intervertebral disc usually maintains its relationship to the caudal vertebral body, with the rostral body slipping anteriorly. The resulting ledge or step-off from rostral body to disc may resemble a disc bulge. Anterior movement of the rostral body away from its posterior arch causes the spinal canal to become elongated in anteroposterior diameter and elliptical in configuration.

The displacement of the rostral vertebra carries the lateral recess *(small arrowheads)* anteriorly, so that it comes to lie above the nondisplaced disc. The associated distortion of the intervertebral foramen may cause compression of the root exiting beneath the pedicle of the forward-slipping vertebra.

Degenerative spondylolisthesis may occur in the absence of spondylolysis when disc narrowing and facet laxity allow subluxation.

When present, the bone defect of spondylolysis may resemble an "extra" facet joint crossing anterior to the normal articulation. The defect in the pars interarticularis may be broad as in this case, narrow as in Case 750, or "healed" as in Case 751.

Spondylolysis is best seen at the midvertebral level, while the facet joint is best seen at the disc level. The plane of a spondylolitic defect is typically more coronal than that of the facet joints.

Callus formation, bone fragmentation, and granulation tissue at the site of spondylolysis may form a composite mass that encroaches on the spinal canal. Alternatively, nerve roots may be tethered within the fibrotic reaction adjacent to a pars defect.

SCLEROTIC SPONDYLOLYSIS

Case 750

33-year-old man.

Spondylolysis of L5.

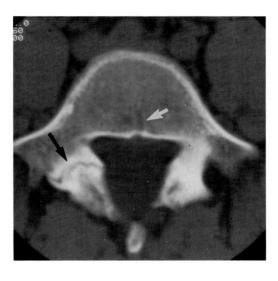

The bone defects of spondylolysis are often narrower and more subtle than in Case 749. Reactive sclerosis and/or callus frequently accompany a thin lucent line traversing the pars interarticularis, as seen on the right side in this case (black arrow). The margins of the pars defect are very irregular, unlike the smooth cortex of a normal facet joint.

A sclerotic band crossing the left pars interarticularis may represent "healing" of a pars defect (see Case 751). However, sclerosis and hypertrophy may also be seen as a reactive change of the posterior arch contralateral to unilateral spondylolysis.

Spondylolysis is much more common at L5 than at any other lumbar level. Cervical spondylolysis occurs but is relatively rare.

Case 751

20-year-old woman.

Bilateral Sclerosis of the Pars Interarticularis (L5).

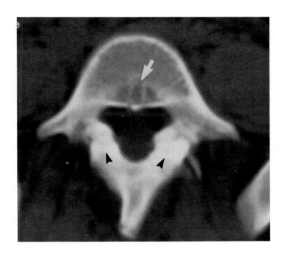

No true "defect" of the pars interarticularis is seen in this case. However, the abnormal zones of sclerosis traversing the posterior arch at the midvertebral level occupy the expected site for spondylolysis. It is likely that such findings represent "healing" or sclerosis of small or old spondylolitic fissures or stress fractures.

Cases 750 and 751 demonstrate the location of the pars interarticularis at the midvertebral level. Both cases also illustrate the midbody site of the basivertebral vein (white arrow).

Case 752

47-year-old woman.

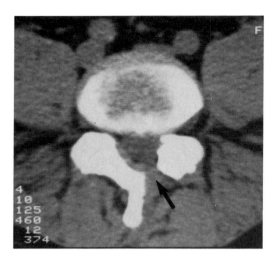

Case 753

55-year-old woman.
(scan with intrathecal contrast)

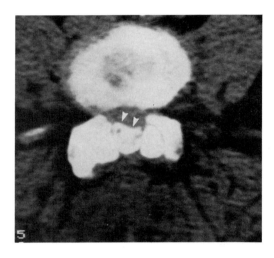

Lumbar laminectomy and diskectomy lead to characteristic postoperative CT findings. A laminectomy defect is usually apparent, with well-defined margins posterior to the facet joint *(arrow)*. (Compare this scan with the irregular margins of spondylolysis located more anteriorly in Case 749.) The ligamentum flavum is absent on the side of surgery.

Fibrosis at the operative site replaces epidural fat and obscures the normal interface with the dural sac. The sac itself may be tethered or prolapsed toward the laminectomy defect (see also Cases 723 and 753).

The diagnosis of residual or recurrent disc herniation may be hampered by postoperative changes altering epidural fat. Helpful clues include (1) the mass-like margin of disc fragments, as opposed to the vague boundary of epidural fibrosis, and (2) contrast enhancement within epidural scar but not within herniated discs.

Intrathecal contrast material may be useful in difficult postoperative cases. Here distortion of the dural sac suggests a focal disc fragment *(arrowheads)*, which was confirmed by surgery (also see Case 723).

MR EVALUATION OF "DISC VS. SCAR"

Case 754A

25-year-old woman with recurrent pain after
laminectomy at L5-S1.
(axial, noncontrast scan; SE 1000/20)

Case 754B.

Same patient. Same level.
(axial, postcontrast scan; SE 1000/17)

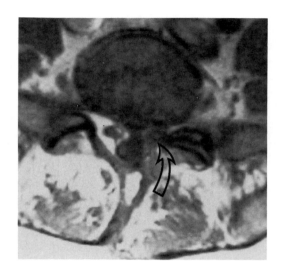

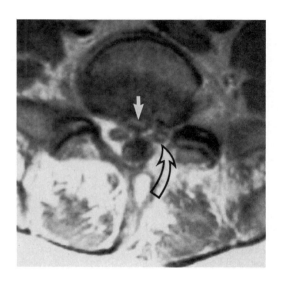

The distinction between residual or recurrent disc herniation and epidural fibrosis in postoperative patients can often be made by MR scans, avoiding the need for intrathecal injections.

In this case a left-sided laminectomy had been performed to remove a posterolateral disc herniation. The T1-weighted precontrast scan demonstrates amorphous, intermediate signal intensity in the region of the left S1 root. It is difficult to confidently diagnose or exclude a component of disc herniation within this zone of postoperative change.

Noncontrast long TR scans can be helpful in distinguishing between recurrent disc herniation and epidural fibrosis. Disc herniations may demonstrate either higher or lower signal intensity than surrounding postoperative changes on "intermediate" or T2-weighted images. Frequently, a low-intensity fibrous capsule at the margin of a recurrent herniation separates it from epidural fibrosis of nearly equal intensity.

This postcontrast scan demonstrates enhancement of epidural tissues in the area of surgery. This enhancing "fibrosis" surrounds and defines the location of the S1 root (black arrow), which is not significantly displaced or compressed. The small central disc herniation (white arrow) does not cause neural compression. The findings indicate that re-exploration is unlikely to benefit this patient.

In cases of residual or recurrent disc herniation, a nonenhancing disc is often outlined by intensely enhancing granulation tissue on early postcontrast MR scans. (A similar appearance can also be seen prior to surgery). Contrast material may penetrate into the disc on delayed scans, making diagnosis more difficult.

A small amount of contrast enhancement is seen within the central disc herniation in this case. Such enhancement likely reflects inflammatory and/or granulation tissue. (Annular tears frequently enhance preoperatively.)

REFERENCES: CT

1. Badami J.P., Norman D., Barbaro N.M., et al.: Metrizamide CT myelography in cervical myelopathy and radiculopathy: Correlation with conventional myelography and surgical findings. *A.J.N.R.* 6:59–64, 1985.
2. Braun I.F., Hoffman J.C. Jr., Davis P.C., et al.: Contrast enhancement in CT differentiation between recurrent disk herniation and postoperative scar: Prospective study. *A.J.N.R.* 6:607–612, 1985.
3. Carerra G.F., Haughton V.M., Syvertsen A., et al.: Computed tomography of the lumbar facet joints. *Radiology* 134:145–148, 1980.
4. Carrera G.F., Williams A.L., Haughton V.M.: Computed tomography in sciatica. *Radiology* 137:433–437, 1980.
5. Casselman E.S.: Radiologic recognition of symptomatic spinal synovial cysts. *A.J.N.R.* 6:971–973, 1985.
6. Daniels D.L., Grogan J.P., Johansen J.G., et al.: Cervical radiculopathy: Computed tomography and myelography compared. *Radiology* 151:109–113, 1984.
7. Dorwart R.H., Vogler J.B. III, Helms C.A.: Spinal stenosis. *Radiol. Clin. North Am.* 21:301–325, 1983.
8. Elster A.D., Jensen K.M.: Computed tomography of spondylolisthesis: Patterns of associated pathology. *J. Comput. Assist. Tomogr.* 9:867–874, 1985.
9. Eyster E.F., Scott W.R.: Lumbar synovial cysts: Report of eleven cases. *Neurosurgery* 24:112–114, 1989.
10. Gado M., Patel J., Hodges F.J.: Lateral disk herniation into the lumbar intervertebral foramen: Differential diagnosis. *A.J.N.R.* 4:598–600, 1983.
11. Harsh G.R., Sypert G.W., Weinstein P.R., et al.: Cervical spine stenosis secondary to ossification of the posterior longitudinal ligament. *J. Neurosurg.* 67:349–357, 1987.
12. Hasso A.N., McKinney J.M., Killeen J., et al.: Computed tomography of children and adolescents with suspected spinal stenosis. *J. Comput. Assist. Tomogr.* 11:609–611, 1987.
13. Helms C.A., Dorwart R.H., Gray M.: The CT appearance of conjoined nerve roots and differentiation from a herniated nucleus pulposis. *Radiology* 144:803–807, 1982.
14. Helms C.A., Vogler J.B., Hardy D.C.: CT of the lumbar spine: Normal variants and pitfalls. *Radiographics* 7:447–464, 1987.
15. Hemminghytt S., Daniels D.L., Williams A.L., et al.: Intraspinal synovial cysts: Natural history and diagnosis by CT. *Radiology* 145:357–376, 1982.
16. Hoddick W.K., Helms C.A.: Bony spinal canal changes that differentiate conjoined nerve roots from herniated nucleus pulposis. *Radiology* 154:119–120, 1985.
17. Landman J.A., Hoffman J.C., Braun I.F., et al.: Value of computed tomographic myelography in the recognition of cervical herniated disc. *A.J.N.R.* 5:391–394, 1984.
18. Mall J.C., Kaiser J.A.: The usual appearance of the postoperative lumbar spine. *Radiographics* 7:245–269, 1987.
19. Meyer J.D., Latchaw R.E., Roppolo H.M., et al.: Computed tomography and myelography of the postoperative lumbar spine. *A.J.N.R.* 3:223–228, 1982.
20. Mikhael M.A., Ciric I., Tarkington J.A., et al.: Neuroradiological evaluation of the lateral recess syndrome. *Radiology* 140:97–107, 1981.
21. Nakagawa H., Okumura T., Sugiyama T., et al.: Discrepancy between metrizamide CT and myelography in diagnosis of cervical disk protrusions. *A.J.N.R.* 4:604–606, 1983.
22. Penning L., Wilmink J.T., van Woerden H.H., Knol E.: CT myelographic findings in degenerative disorders of the cervical spine: Clinical significance. *A.J.N.R.* 7:119–128, 1986.
23. Russell E.J., D'Angelo C.M., Zimmerman R.D., et al.: Cervical disc herniation: CT demonstration after contrast enhancement. *Radiology* 152:703–712, 1984.
24. Schellinger D., Wener L., Ragsdale B.D., Patronas N.J.: Facet joint disorders and their role in the production of back pain and sciatica. *Radiographics* 7:923–944, 1987.
25. Schubiger O., Valavanis A.: Postoperative lumbar CT: Technique, results, and indications. *A.J.N.R.* 4:595–597, 1983.
26. Scotti G., Scialfa G., Pieralli S., et al.: Myelopathy and radiculopathy due to cervical spondylosis: Myelographic-CT correlates. *A.J.N.R.* 4:601–603, 1983.
27. Sobel D.F., Barkovich A.J., Munderloh S.H.: Metrizamide myelography and post myelographic computed tomography: Comparative adequacy in the cervical spine. *A.J.N.R.* 5:385–390, 1984.
28. Stollman A., Pinto R., Benjamin V., Kricheff I.: Radiologic imaging of symptomatic ligamentum flavum thickening with and without ossification. *A.J.N.R.* 8:991, 994, 1987.
29. Teplick J.G., Haskin M.E.: Computed tomography of the postoperative lumbar spine. *A.J.N.R.* 4:1053–1072, 1983.
30. Teplick J.G., Haskin M.E.: CT and lumbar disc herniation. *Radiol. Clin. North Am.* 21:259–288, 1983.
31. Teplick J.G., Haskin M.E.: Intravenous contrast-enhanced CT of the post operative lumbar spine: Improved identification of recurrent disk herniation, scar, arachnoiditis, and diskitis. *A.J.N.R.* 5:373–383, 1984.
32. Teplick J.G., Laffey P.A., Berman A., Haskin M.E.: Diagnosis and evaluation of spondylolisthesis and/or spondylolysis on axial CT. *A.J.N.R.* 7:479–491, 1986.
33. Vadala G., Dore R., Garbagna P.: Unusual osseous changes in lumbar herniated disks: CT features. *J. Comput. Assist. Tomogr.* 9:1045–1049, 1985.
34. Voelker J.L., Mealey J. Jr., Eskridge J.M., et al.: Metrizamide-enhanced computed tomography as an adjunct to metrizamide myelography in the evaluation of lumbar disc herniation and spondylosis. *Neurosurgery* 20:379–384, 1987.
35. Williams A.L.: CT diagnosis of degenerative disc disease. *Radiol. Clin. North Am.* 21:289–300, 1983.
36. Williams A.L., Haughton V.M., Daniels D.L., et al.: CT recognition of lateral lumbar disc herniation. *A.J.N.R.* 3:211–213, 1982.
37. Williams A.L., Haughton V.M., Daniels D.L., et al.: Differential CT diagnosis of extruded nucleus pulposis. *Radiology* 148:141–148, 1983.
38. Williams A.L., Haughton V.M., Meyer G.A., et al.: Computed tomographic appearance of the bulging annulus. *Radiology* 142:403–408, 1982.
39. Williams A.L., Haughton V.M., Syvertsen A.: Computed tomography in the diagnosis of herniated nucleus pulposis. *Radiology* 135:95–99, 1980.
40. Yang P.J., Seeger J.F., Dzioba R.B., et al.: High dose IV contrast in CT scanning of the postoperative lumbar spine. *A.J.N.R.* 7:703–708, 1986.
41. Yu Y.L., Stevens J.M., Kendall B., et al.: Cord shape and measurements in cervical spondylotic myelopathy and radiculopathy. *A.J.N.R.* 4:839–842, 1983.

REFERENCES: MR

1. Al-Mefty O., Harkey L.H., Middleton T.H., et al.: Myelopathic cervical spondylitic lesions demonstrated by magnetic resonance imaging. *J. Neurosurg.* 68:217–222, 1988.
2. Barnett G.H., Hardy R.W. Jr., Little J.R., et al.: Thoracic spinal canal stenosis. *J. Neurosurg.* 66:338–344, 1987.
3. Blumenkopf B.: Thoracic intervertebral disc herniations: Diagnostic value of magnetic resonance imaging. *Neurosurgery* 23:36–40, 1988.
4. Brown B.M., Schwartz R.H., Frank E., Blank N.K.: Preoperative evaluation of cervical radiculopathy and myelopathy by surface-coil MR imaging. *A.J.N.R.* 9:859–866, 1988.
5. Bundschuh C.V., Modic M.T., Ross J.S., et al.: Epidural fibrosis and recurrent disk herniation in the lumbar spine: MR imaging assessment. *A.J.N.R.* 9:169–178, 1988.
6. Enzmann D.R., Rubin J.B.: Cervical spine: MR imaging with a partial flip angle, gradient-refocused pulse sequence. Part I. General considerations and disk disease. *Radiology* 166:467–472, 1988.
7. Fletcher G., Haughton V.M., Ho K.-C., Yu S.: Age-related changes in cervical facet joints: Studies with cryomicrotomy, MR and CT. *A.J.N.R.* 11:27–30, 1990.
8. Grenier N., Greselle J.-F., Douws C., et al.: MR imaging of foraminal and extraforaminal lumbar disk herniations. *J. Comput. Assist. Tomogr.* 14:243–249, 1990.
9. Grenier N., Greselle J.-F., Vital J.-M., et al.: Normal and disrupted lumbar longitudinal ligaments: Correlative MR and anatomic study. *Radiology* 171:197–206, 1989.
10. Haughton V.M.: MR Imaging of the Spine. *Radiology* 166:297–302, 1988.
11. Ho P.S.D., Yu S., Sether L.A., et al.: Ligamentum flavum: Appearance on sagittal and coronal MR images. *Radiology* 168:469–472, 1988.
12. Hueftle M.G., Modic M.T., Ross J.S., et al.: Lumbar spine: Postoperative imaging with Gd-DTPA. *Radiology* 167:817–824, 1988.
13. Jackson D.E., Atlas S.W., Mani J.R., Norman D.: Intraspinal synovial cysts: MR imaging. *Radiology* 170:527–530, 1989.
14. Lee S.H., Coleman P.E., Hahn F.J.: Magnetic resonance imaging of degenerative disk disease of the spine. *Radiol. Clin. North Am.* 26:949–964, 1988.
15. Liu S.S., Williams K.D., Drayer B.P., et al.: Synovial cysts of the lumbosacral spine: Diagnosis by MR imaging. *A.J.N.R.* 10:1239–1242, 1989.
16. Luetkehans T.J., Coughlin B.F., Weinstein M.A.: Ossification of the posterior longitudinal ligament diagnosed by MR. *A.J.N.R.* 8:924, 1987.
17. Maravilla K.R., Lesh P., Weinreb J.C., et al.: Magnetic resonance imaging of the lumbar spine with CT correlation. *A.J.N.R.* 6:237–246, 1985.
18. Masaryk T.J., Ross T.S., Modic M.T., et al.: High-resolution MR imaging of sequestered lumbar intervertebral disks. *A.J.N.R.* 9:351–358, 1988.
19. Mehalic T.F., Pezzuti R., Applebaum B.I.: Magnetic resonance imaging and cervical spondylitic myelopathy. *Neurosurgery* 26:217–227, 1990.
20. Modic M.T., Masaryk T.J., Boumphrey F., et al.: Lumbar herniated disk disease and canal stenosis: Prospective evaluation of surface coil MR, CT, and myelography. *A.J.N.R.* 7:709–718, 1986.
21. Modic M.T., Masaryk T.J., Mulopulos G.P., et al.: Cervical radiculopathy: Prospective evaluation with surface coil MR imaging, CT with metrizamide, and metri-zamide myelography. *Radiology* 161:753–760, 1986.
22. Modic M.T., Masaryk R.J., Ross J.S., Carter J.R.: Imaging of degenerative disk disease. *Radiology* 168:177–186, 1988.
23. Modic M.T., Masaryk T.J., Ross J.S., et al.: Cervical radiculopathy: Value of oblique MR imaging. *Radiology* 163:227–232, 1987.
24. Modic M.T., Pavlicek W., Weinstein M.A., et al.: Magnetic resonance imaging of intervertebral disk disease. *Radiology* 152:103–111, 1984.
25. Modic M.T., Steinberg P.M., Ross J.S., et al.: Degenerative disk disease: Assessment of changes in vertebral body marrow with MR imaging. *Radiology* 166:193–200, 1988.
26. Murayama S., Numaguchi Y., Robinson A.E.: The diagnosis of herniated intervertebral disks with MR imaging: A comparison of gradient-refocused-echo and spin-echo pulse sequences. *A.J.N.R.* 11:17–22, 1990.
27. Osborn A.G., Hood R.S., Sherry R.G., et al.: CT/MR spectrum of far lateral and anterior lumbosacral disk herniations. *A.J.N.R.* 9:775–778, 1988.
28. Ramanauskas W.L., Wilner H.I., Metes J.J., et al.: MR imaging of compressive myelomalacia. *J. Comput. Assist. Tomogr.* 13:399–404, 1989.
29. Rosenblum J., Mojtahedi S., Foust R.J.: Synovial cysts in the lumbar spine: MR characteristics. *A.J.N.R.* 10:S94, 1989.
30. Ross J.S., Masaryk T.J., Modic M.T.: Lumbar spine: Postoperative assessment with surface-coil MR imaging. *Radiology* 164:851–860, 1987.
31. Ross J.S., Masaryk T.J., Modic M.T.: Postoperative cervical spine: MR assessment. *J. Comput. Assist. Tomogr.* 11:955–962, 1987.
32. Ross J.S., Modic M.T., Masaryk T.J.: Tears of the annulus fibrosis: assessment with Gd-DTPA-enhanced MR imaging. *A.J.N.R.* 10:1251–1254, 1989.
33. Ross J.S., Modic M.T., Masaryk T.J., et al.: Assessment of extradural degenerative disease with Gd-DTPA-enhanced MR imaging: Correlation with surgical and pathological findings. *A.J.N.R.* 10:1243–1250, 1989.
34. Ross J.S., Perez-Reyes N., Masaryk T.J., et al.: Thoracic disk herniation: MR imaging. *Radiology* 165:511–516, 1987.
35. Sobel D.F., Zyroff J., Thorne R.P.: Discogenic vertebral sclerosis: MR imaging. *J. Comput. Assist. Tomogr.* 11:855–858, 1987.
36. Sotiropoulos S., Chafetz N.I., Lang P., et al.: Differentiation between postoperative scar and recurrent disk herniation: Prospective comparison of MR, CT, and contrast-enhanced CT. *A.J.N.R.* 10:639–643, 1989.
37. Takahashi M., Yamashita Y., Sakamoto Y., Kojima R.: Chronic cervical cord compression: Clinical significance of increased signal intensity on MR images. *Radiology* 173:219–224, 1989.
38. Tsuruda J.S., Norman D., Dillon W., et al.: Three-dimensional gradient-recalled MR imaging as a screening tool for the diagnosis of cervical radioculopathy. *A.J.N.R.* 10:1263–1271, 1989.
39. VanDyke C., Ross J.S., Tkach J., et al.: Gradient-echo MR imaging of the cervical spine: Evaluation of extradural disease. *A.J.N.R.* 10:627–632, 1989.
40. Williams M.P., Cherryman G.R., Husband J.E.: Significance of thoracic disk herniation demonstrated by MR imaging. *J. Comput. Assist. Tomogr.* 13:211–214, 1989.
41. Yu S., Haughton V.M., Sether L.A., Wagner M.: Comparison of MR and diskography in detecting radial tears of the annulus: A postmortem study. *A.J.N.R.* 10:1077–1082, 1989.

Spinal Tumors, Trauma, Inflammation, and Malformation

MR CORRELATION: EPIDURAL TUMORS

Case 759

70-year-old man.
(sagittal, noncontrast scan; SE 800/17)

Metastatic Carcinoma of the Prostate.

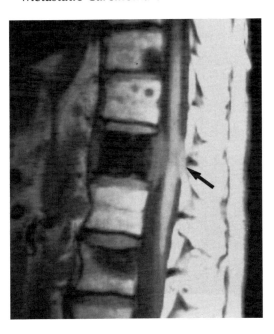

Case 760

2-month-old girl (same patient as Case 758).
(coronal, noncontrast scan; SE 800/17)

Neuroblastoma.

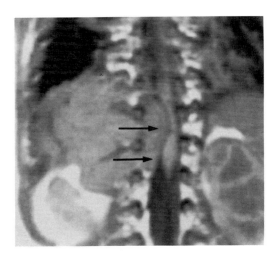

Magnetic resonance imaging has replaced emergency myelography as the procedure of choice for rapid evaluation of tumor patients with new neurological symptoms or back pain.

Vertebral and epidural metastases are usually well defined on T1-weighted MR studies. Fatty marrow within vertebral bodies provides a normal background of high signal intensity. Marrow replacement by cellular infiltration (malignant or benign; see Case 801) causes a conspicuous reduction in intensity. Reactive bony sclerosis contributes to the very "dark" spots of metastatic disease within lumbar vertebrae in this case.

T1-weighted images also demonstrate the contours of the spinal cord outlined by CSF. Cord compression by epidural components of metastatic tumor can be readily assessed. Here an epidural mass at the T12 level effaces the subarachnoid space and deforms the cord (arrow).

Contrast-enhanced T1-weighted scans may be less effective than noncontrast studies for detecting vertebral and epidural metastases. Such lesions may enhance to a level isointense with marrow or epidural fat, masking their presence (see Case 777).

The large right suprarenal mass in Case 758 is apparent as a homogeneous lesion of intermediate signal intensity on this scan. The calcification that is obvious on the CT study is not appreciated here.

A coronal view clearly demonstrates medial extension of the mass through intervertebral foramina (arrows). A large intraspinal component displaces the spinal cord and conus medullaris.

Comparison of the CT and MR scans in this case demonstrates the advantages that MR offers in the assessment of epidural disease: high tissue contrast, long segment surveys, and multiplanar display.

DIFFERENTIAL DIAGNOSIS:
EXPANSILE LESION OF THE SACRAL CANAL

Case 761

74-year-old man.

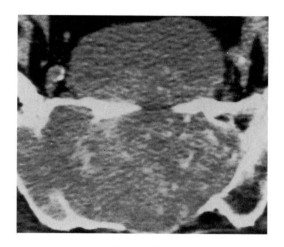

Epidermoid Cyst.

Case 762

30-year-old woman.

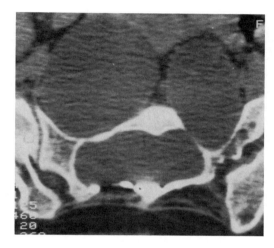

Dural Ectasia in Marfan's Syndrome.

Scans through the sacrum and pelvis may disclose the source of pain or dysfunction that is unexplained by lumbar evaluation.

CT demonstrates both the osseous and soft tissue components of sacral lesions. The masses in Cases 761 and 762 have originated within the spinal canal, with secondary expansion of bony margins and extension into the pelvis.

The patient in Case 761 had undergone subtotal removal of tumor on two prior occasions. The current mass has a bilobed configuration due to a large pelvic component and has crossed the right sacroiliac joint. A very similar appearance (and tendency to recurrence) could be seen with a sacral chordoma. Occasionally a large benign or malignant schwannoma or neurofibroma expands the sacral canal with lobular extension into the pelvis. Plasmacytoma and metastasis are common expansile masses of the sacrum.

The homogeneous low attenuation of the mass in Case 762 suggests fluid content. A similar appearance may be seen with smaller cysts commonly found along sacral root sleeves (see Case 782). Sacral root sleeve cysts occasionally cause compressive radiculopathy and can extend into the pelvis in a manner identical to Case 762.

Generalized dural ectasia is also found in neurofibromatosis, often associated with scalloping of the posterior margins of vertebral bodies. Acquired dural ectasia may be seen in patients with ankylosing spondylitis. Localized outpouchings of the dural sac typically erode the posterior arches of lumbar and thoracic vertebrae in such cases, sometimes associated with radiculopathy or a cauda equina syndrome.

Case 763

8-year-old girl being evaluated for suspected
cervical adenopathy.

Neurofibroma (C3-4 Level).

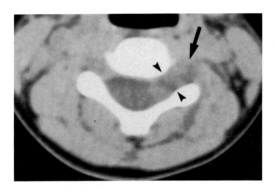

Case 764

31-year-old man presenting with left C7
radiculopathy.
(scan with intrathecal contrast)

Schwannoma (C-7 Level).

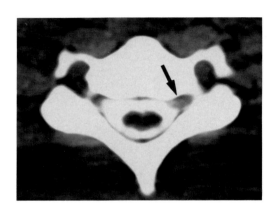

The palpable neck mass in this case proved to be the inferior pole of a large neurofibroma originating from the left C4 root. The scan above demonstrates widening of the left intervertebral foramen *(arrowheads),* which is filled by a homogeneous soft tissue mass. The lesion is slightly higher in attenuation values than the dural sac (which is indented laterally), but noticeably lower in density than paraspinal soft tissues.

Spinal and peripheral neurofibromas are clinically and pathologically distinct from schwannomas (or "neurinomas"). Neurofibromas arise from proliferation of both the internal fibroblastic and external Schwann cell components of a nerve, resulting in symmetrical enlargement that surrounds individual axons. Schwannomas originate from proliferation of Schwann cells at one location on the perimeter of the nerve, leading to an eccentric mass that compresses and displaces the otherwise uninvolved axons. Neurofibromas are usually multiple and associated with von Recklinghausen's disease. Both types of nerve root tumors may have intradural and extradural components, and both may cause foraminal expansion.

The small mass deforming the left anterolateral corner of the dural sac in this case proved to be a schwannoma arising from the C7 nerve root. The lesion is smaller than the neurofibroma in Case 763, which it resembles in location and morphology. Compare the extradural deformity seen here to the lateral disc herniation in Case 731.

Schwannomas usually arise from sensory nerve roots. They may occur at any level of the spinal canal (see Cases 726 and 771 for examples in the lumbar region).

DIFFERENTIAL DIAGNOSIS:
"DUMBBELL" LESION SPANNING AN INTERVERTEBRAL FORAMEN

Case 765

44-year-old woman.
(scan with intravenous contrast)

Case 766

52-year-old man.
(scan with intrathecal contrast)

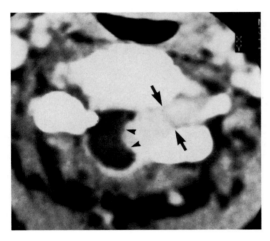

Meningioma (C2–3 Level).

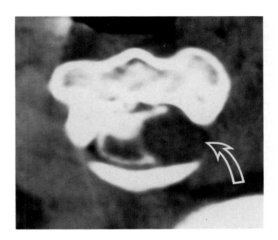

Schwannoma (C2 Level).

Spinal meningiomas may be well demarcated by contrast enhancement, as seen in Case 765. This "dumbbell" meningioma occupies a widened intervertebral foramen *(large arrows)*. The medial margin of the tumor passes through the enhancing dura to displace the cervical spinal cord *(small arrowheads)*.

The transforaminal schwannoma in Case 766 demonstrates relatively low attenuation values, which is characteristic of these tumors and would be unusual for a meningioma. The two types of benign masses are otherwise similar in appearance. Both schwannomas and meningiomas may demonstrate intense contrast enhancement.

Other masses that can occupy an intervertebral foramen include lymphoma, paraspinal "small cell" tumors (see Case 758), metastases, and arteriovenous malformations.

The intradural component of the schwannoma in Case 766 was larger at the C1 level, causing cord compression. The patient gave a long history of spastic diplegia, which had been assumed to represent cerebral palsy. It is important to exclude spinal masses at the foramen magnum or within the cervical canal in patients with such presentations (see also Cases 812 and 813). The head tilt causing the left occipital bone to be partially included on the scan in Case 766 is another clue to the presence of high cervical or posterior fossa pathology.

DIFFERENTIAL DIAGNOSIS:
SMOOTHLY MARGINATED BONE EROSION NEAR A TRANSVERSE FORAMEN

Case 767

58-year-old woman.

Case 768

8-year-old girl.

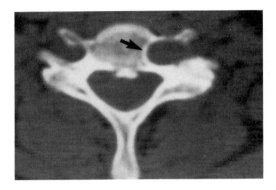

Tortuous Vertebral Artery.

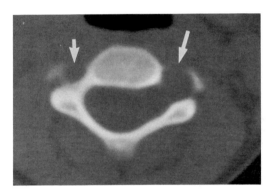

Neurofibroma (Same Patient as Case 763.)

Benign tumors, particularly neurofibromas and schwannomas, are a common cause of foraminal widening and lateral vertebral erosion, as seen in Case 768 *(large arrow)*. The bone changes may involve the region of the transverse foramen, which lies just anterior and inferior to the intervertebral foramen. (The normal right transverse foramen in Case 768 is faintly visualized at the *short white arrow;* compare to Case 769.)

Vascular lesions are also chronic, expansile masses and may be associated with remodeling of adjacent bone. In Case 767 a tortuous loop of the vertebral artery had widened the left transverse foramen.

The distinction between these lesions can be noninvasively accomplished by magnetic resonance imaging. A large vascular channel as in Case 767 will demonstrate characteristic "flow void," contrasting with the solid appearance of a mass such as Case 768.

Case 769

8-year-old girl (same patient as Case 763).
(axial, noncontrast scan; SE 2000/30)

Neurofibroma (C3–4 Level).

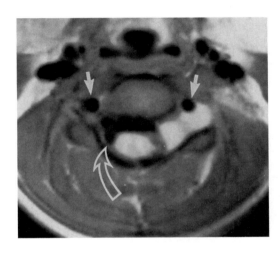

Case 770

29-year-old woman.
(axial, noncontrast scan; low flip angle gradient
echo sequence)

"Dumbbell" Schwannoma.

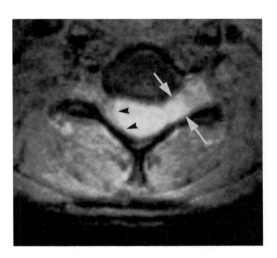

Neurofibromas and schwannomas often demonstrate high signal intensity on MR sequences with long TR values. On "balanced" or "intermediate" images like the scan above, the high intensity of the tumor contrasts with the lower intensity of CSF and paraspinal musculature to clearly define the margins of the lesion. (Compare the conspicuity of the mass in this case to its visibility on the CT study of Case 763.)

"Balanced" or "intermediate" spin-echo images are also useful in differentiating neurofibromas from the lower intensity of lateral meningoceles, which are another common cause of paraspinal masses in patients with neurofibromatosis. Contrast-enhanced T1-weighted scans may alternatively be used for this purpose.

Other anatomical details shown here include the location of the vertebral arteries identified by "flow-void" *(solid arrows; see discussion of erosion near the transverse foramen in Cases 767 and 768)* and visualization of the normal dorsal root on the right side of the spinal cord *(open arrow).*

The schwannoma in this case demonstrates high signal intensity on the low flip angle gradient echo scan. A large intraspinal component displaces and compresses the spinal cord *(black arrowheads)*. Another segment of the tumor passes through the widened intervertebral foramen *(white arrows)* to a paraspinal location. This scan is the MR equivalent of CT studies such as Case 766.

As discussed in cases 726 and 727, lateral disc herniations may mimic foraminal tumors, particularly in the lumbar region. Postcontrast MR scans may assist differential diagnosis in such cases: foraminal tumors usually demonstrate more uniform enhancement than the typical peripheral enhancement at the margins of a disc fragment.

DIFFERENTIAL DIAGNOSIS:
LUMBAR INTRADURAL MASS

Case 771

40-year-old man.
(scan with intrathecal contrast)

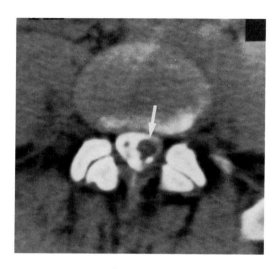

Schwannoma.

Case 772

37-year-old woman.
(scan with intrathecal contrast)

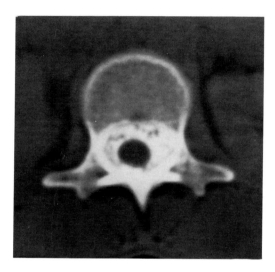

Ependymoma of the Conus Medullaris.

The most common intradural tumors in the region of the conus medullaris and cauda equina are ependymomas and schwannomas, as illustrated in Cases 771 and 772. These lesions are often indistinguishable. Both may be large and lobulated, expanding the spinal canal and extending into or through intervertebral foramina. Meningiomas are common intradural, extramedullary masses in the thorax, but are less frequent in the lumbar region (see Cases 773 and 774).

Other potential lumbar intradural masses include metastases from systemic carcinomas (e.g., lung, breast; see Cases 775 to 777), "drop" metastases from intracranial tumors (e.g., medulloblastoma, ependymoma, germinoma, glioma; see Case 778), epidermoid tumors, arachnoid or parasitic cysts, vascular malformations, and intradural disc herniation.

Arachnoiditis may cause clumping of nerve roots resembling an intradural mass, usually accompanied by thickening and irregularity of the dura (see Case 779). A tethered spinal cord (as in Case 814) may resemble an intradural mass on a single axial scan.

CT myelography outlines intradural masses as well-defined filling defects within the thecal sac. The features of the lesion are rarely specific (e.g., low attenuation in a lipoma, or calcification in a meningioma).

Case 773

53-year-old woman with a 6-month history of
"rubbery legs".
(sagittal, noncontrast scan; SE 800/17)

Meningioma.

Case 774

41-year-old woman.
(sagittal, postcontrast scan; SE 700/20)

Meningioma.

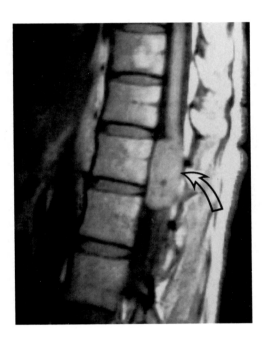

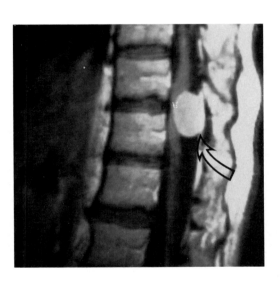

Intradural tumors are well outlined by surrounding CSF on T1-weighted MR scans. Although the masses may be nearly isointense to the spinal cord on noncontrast images, distortion of anatomy and "capping" of the tumor poles by spinal fluid establish their presence.

In this case, a large, homogeneous intradural mass fills the spinal canal at the level of the conus medullaris and proximal cauda equina. The subarachnoid space is effaced and cord margins are obscured.

This tumor proved to be a large meningioma. The differential diagnosis of a mass in this location should include ependymoma and schwannoma, as illustrated in Cases 771 and 772.

Contrast enhancement is helpful in detecting and defining intradural masses on MR scans. (This application is analogous to the role of contrast enhancement in the MR demonstration of small extra-axial masses in the head; see Cases 145 and 146.)

The lesion in this case was apparent on a noncontrast scan. Contrast was given to (1) more clearly demonstrate the interface between the tumor and the spinal cord, and (2) evaluate the possibility of additional masses.

The presence of contrast enhancement in an intradural lesion is nonspecific. The intense, homogeneous enhancement seen here is compatible with meningioma, but schwannomas, ependymomas, and metastases may have a similar appearance. On the other hand, many spinal schwannomas and ependymomas contain cystic or necrotic areas that cause an inhomogeneous pattern of contrast enhancement.

Spinal meningiomas are most common in the thoracic canal (about 80%), often arising laterally or dorsolaterally. They occur much more frequently in women than in men (male to female ratio about 1 to 4).

Case 775

65-year-old woman.
(noncontrast scan, L3 level)

Metastatic Small Cell Carcinoma of the Lung.

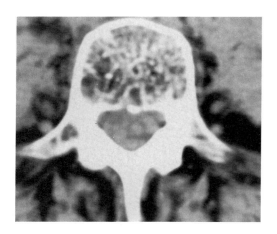

Case 776

57-year-old woman presenting with leg pain.
(scan with intrathecal contrast; L3–4 level)

Metastatic Carcinoma of the Breast.

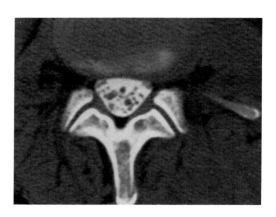

Intradural metastases may arise from either hematogenous dissemination of systemic tumors or CSF seeding of CNS neoplasms. Among the primary tumors that commonly metastasize to the intrathecal compartment are carcinomas of the breast and lung and melanoma. Metastases may be intramedullary (frequently involving the conus medullaris) or intradural but extramedullary. A careful search for intradural masses is warranted on CT or MR studies performed to evaluate vertebral or epidural metastases.

In this case, the roots of the cauda equina are grossly thickened and nodular. Less severe cases of meningeal carcinomatosis may require intrathecal contrast (see Case 776) or magnetic resonance imaging (see Cases 777 and 778) for diagnosis.

Intradural metastases should be remembered as an occasional cause of radiculopathy, cauda equina symptoms, or conus dysfunction. In this case no significant disc disease or spondylosis was found on routine CT studies of the lumbar region.

Intrathecal contrast greatly improves the CT visualization of subtle abnormalities involving lumbosacral nerve roots. Use of a "bone" reconstruction algorithm optimizes the spatial resolution of details within the opacified thecal sac. Here several of the roots are clearly enlarged, although more subtly than in Case 775.

This patient had undergone mastectomy and radiation for breast carcinoma 12 years earlier. It is not uncommon to discover cerebral or spinal metastases from breast carcinoma developing 10 or 15 years after treatment of the primary tumor.

MR CORRELATION: INTRADURAL METASTASES

Case 777

90-year-old woman.
(sagittal, postcontrast scan; SE 500/15)

Metastatic Carcinoma of the Breast

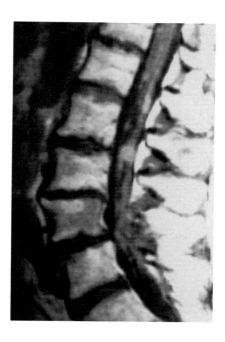

Case 778

7-year-old boy scanned 6 months after resection
of a fourth ventricular ependymoma.
(sagittal, postcontrast scan; SE 600/20)

"CSF Seeding" by "Drop Metastases".

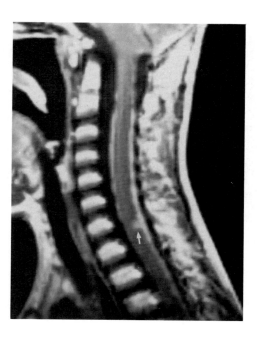

Contrast-enhanced MR scanning rivals CT with intrathecal contrast for the detection of intradural metastases. Both systemic and CNS metastases are highlighted as enhancing layers along neural surfaces or nodules surrounded by CSF.

In this case, a number of enhancing nodules are apparent within the cauda equina. Metastatic nodularity of the cauda roots may be apparent on noncontrast MR scans and should be checked on all spine scans of tumor patients.

A number of metastases are also present within lumbar vertebral bodies. Contrast enhancement of these initially low-intensity lesions has made them nearly isointense with surrounding normal marrow (compare to Case 759).

The surface of the cervical spinal cord is lined by abnormal contrast enhancement in this case. Such "coating" or "frosting" of neural tissue is a common pattern for intradural metastases on contrast-enhanced MR studies. The appearance is particularly frequent in association with "drop metastases" from intracranial neoplasms, especially medulloblastoma and ependymoma. "CSF seeding" from intracranial tumors may also cause coarse intradural nodularity, comparable to Case 777.

Superficial enhancement along cord margins as seen here is not specific for malignant disease. A similar appearance may be encountered in inflammatory disorders such as sarcoidosis. In both disease categories, subpial spread of pathology may be associated with enhancing nodules of tissue extending into the cord from a pial base (seen here dorsally at the C7 level; *arrow*).

Meningeal tumor spread is also present within the posterior fossa in this case (e.g., along the ventral margin of the pons; see Case 121).

DIFFERENTIAL DIAGNOSIS:
INTRATHECAL "CLUMPING" OF LUMBOSACRAL NERVE ROOTS

Case 779

58-year-old woman with recurrent back pain
following several laminectomies.
(scan with intrathecal contrast; L4–5 level)

Case 780

54-year-old woman.
(scan with intrathecal contrast; L3 level)

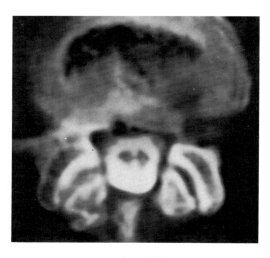

Arachnoiditis.

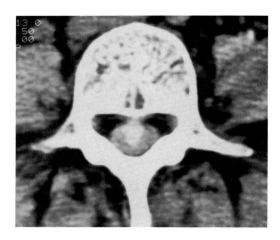

**Intradural Metastases From Carcinoma of
the Breast.**

Arachnoiditis may cause adhesion of nerve roots to each other or to the margins of the dural sac. Axial CT or MR scans in such cases often demonstrate central clumping of roots (as seen in Case 779; compare to the more normal distribution of roots in Case 776). An alternative pattern is an "empty" dural sac, with nerves scarred along the perimeter.

Intradural metastasis may cause nodularity of individual nerve roots (see Cases 775 and 776) or conglomerate aggregation of roots, as in Case 780. The uniformity and symmetry of this finding could be mistakenly considered to represent a normal "variant." Metabolic causes of diffuse nerve thickening (e.g., hypertrophic neuropathies such as Dejerine-Sottas disease) are a rare cause of a similar appearance.

DIFFERENTIAL DIAGNOSIS:
LOW-ATTENUATION LESION WITHIN THE SACRAL CANAL

Case 781

86-year-old man.

Case 782

82-year-old woman.

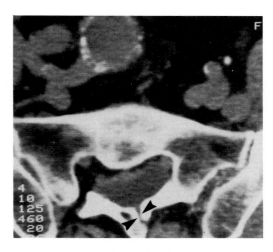

Epidermoid Cyst.

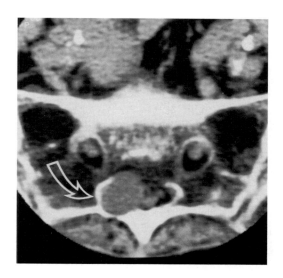

Sacral Root Sleeve Cyst.

While some intraspinal tumors require subarachnoid contrast material for CT definition (see Cases 771 and 772), others are apparent on routine scans.

In Case 781 a spina bifida occulta *(arrowheads)* is associated with a low-attenuation mass occupying much of the spinal canal. The density of the lesion is greater than that of epidural fat and resembles the appearance of spinal fluid, as is characteristic of epidermoid tumors. (Compare to the intracranial examples in Cases 236 and 237 and to the sacral lesion in Case 761).

Case 781 is an example of the "dorsal dermal sinus syndrome," with failed dysjunction of cutaneous and neuroectoderm. In such cases, a sinus or tract linking the skin surface to the dural sac is often associated with spinal dermoid or epidermoid cysts.

CSF-containing masses are commonly found within the sacral canal, usually representing root sleeve cysts. The benign and long-standing nature of these lesions is indicated by smooth erosion of adjacent bone, as seen in Case 782. Sacral root sleeve cysts are usually incidental. Occasional cysts cause radiculopathy due to compression of adjacent nerves. Other sacral cysts may extend into the pelvis as mass lesions (see Case 762).

A neurofibroma or schwannoma could also present as a low-attenuation mass expanding a sacral foramen, resembling Case 782.

An aneurysm of the right iliac artery is seen at the margin of Case 781. Lesions of the aortoiliac vasculature and other retroperitoneal processes may be discovered when spinal scans are carefully reviewed (see also Case 721B).

Case 783

37-year-old man.
(scan with intrathecal contrast)

Astrocytoma of the Cervical Cord
(C6−7 Level).

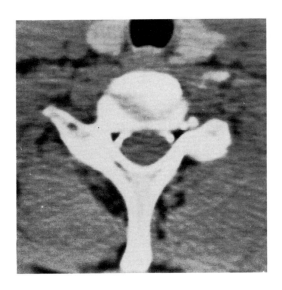

Case 784

40-year-old man with a history of old trauma,
now presenting with diminished sensation and
atrophy of the lower extremities.
(scan with intrathecal contrast)

Post-traumatic Syrinx (T−12 Level).

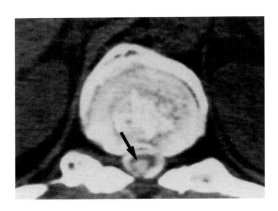

Axial CT scans with intrathecal contrast material provide clear definition of the spinal cord. Partial volume effects of the dense contrast cause the apparent size of the cord to vary as window settings are changed. However, at any given setting pathological expansion of the cord is easily recognized, as in this case.

The differential diagnosis of intramedullary masses includes tumors (ependymoma, astrocytoma, hemangioblastoma, lipoma, lymphoma, metastasis,) cysts (tumor, post-traumatic, syrinx), inflammatory processes (acute myelitis, sarcoidosis, abscess), and vascular lesions (arteriovenous malformation, hematoma). When an intramedullary mass is encountered, delayed scans are useful to evaluate the possibility of syrinx (see Case 784).

Both congenital and acquired syringomyelia may be defined by delayed CT scans following the injection of subarachnoid contrast material. Contrast accumulates within the cavity of the syrinx (arrow), creating a "target" appearance within the cord. Magnetic resonance imaging now offers a less invasive and more effective means of diagnosing and characterizing primary and post-traumatic syringomyelia (see Cases 787 and 788).

Syrinx cavities may be eccentric and variable in diameter and extent. Cervical syringomyelia is usually a congenital abnormality, often associated with low cerebellar tonsils (Chiari I malformation; see Case 787). Post-traumatic syringomyelia may occur at any level.

The initial postcontrast scans in syringomyelia may demonstrate cord widening (see Case 788), cord atrophy (see Case 789), or a normal cord diameter.

Case 785

4-year-old boy with increasing difficulty
walking.
(sagittal, noncontrast scan; SE 1000/30)

Recurrent Astrocytoma of the Thoracic
Spinal Cord.

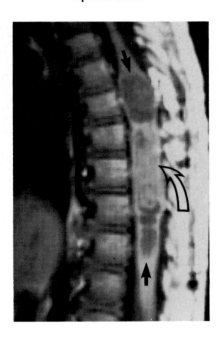

Case 786

29-year-old woman.
(sagittal, postcontrast scan; SE 550/20)

Primitive Neuroectodermal Tumor of the
Conus Medullaris.

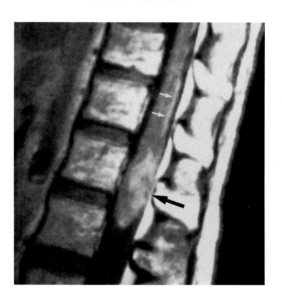

Magnetic resonance imaging far exceeds the ability of CT scanning to demonstrate intramedullary pathology. Contour abnormalities of the spinal cord are apparent on MR studies without intrathecal injection of contrast material. More importantly, MR can detect intramedullary lesions that are unaccompanied by cord expansion (see Cases 791 to 794).

In this case the thoracic spinal cord is grossly enlarged. A solid tumor is present centrally *(open arrow)*, with adjacent cysts both rostrally and caudally *(solid arrows)*.

The noninvasive and nonionizing nature of MR is beneficial for follow-up studies in such patients.

Contrast enhancement plays an important role in the MR evaluation of intramedullary masses. Such tumors are often associated with adjacent cysts (as in Case 785), which may be either neoplastic or reactive. The enhancement pattern helps to characterize cystic and solid components of a tumor, in turn guiding biopsy or resection. Contrast enhancement may also demonstrate small intramedullary lesions that are undetected on routine scans (see Case 792).

The precontrast scan in this case outlined a homogeneous, low-intensity lesion within the conus medullaris, compatible with a low-grade glioma. The irregular, poorly marginated contrast enhancement with subpial extension *(white arrows)* suggests a more aggressive lesion. At surgery, an intramedullary primitive neuroectodermal tumor was found, with a layer of dorsal subpial tumor extending rostrally from the mass.

MR CORRELATION: SYRINGOMYELIA

Case 787

4-year-old girl.
(sagittal, noncontrast scan; SE 550/20)

Case 788

51-year-old woman.
(axial, noncontrast scan; SE 800/17)

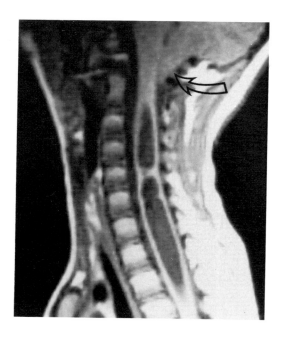

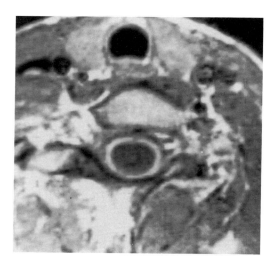

MR dramatically improves upon the ability of CT to diagnose and follow syringomyelia. Intramedullary cysts are well defined on T1-weighted scans as sharply marginated zones of low signal intensity. Actual intensity values within a syrinx may be slightly higher than those of subarachnoid CSF due to reduced signal loss from pulsation effects and/or mild elevations of protein within the cyst. Cysts with intensity values substantially different from spinal fluid may be neoplastic and should be evaluated by contrast-enhanced studies.

In this case a Chiari I hindbrain malformation *(arrow)* is associated with a long intramedullary cyst. The cyst probably represents dilatation of the ependymal-lined central canal of the spinal cord and could be accurately described as "hydromyelia." However, common usage has applied the name "syringohydromyelia" or more often simply "syringomyelia" to this lesion of congenital etiology (as well as to acquired, eccentric intramedullary cysts lined by glial reaction).

Benign intramedullary cysts often appear septated or loculated on MR scans. The apparent compartments of the lesion usually communicate and are well decompressed by a single shunt. Conversely, postoperative recurrence of syringomyelia may involve only a few loculations of the original lesion.

Axial MR views clearly demonstrate the cross-sectional morphology of intramedullary cysts (compare this scan to Case 784). The spinal cord may be expanded (as in this case), normal in diameter, or atrophic at the involved levels.

Syringomyelia of congenital etiology (i.e., associated with Chiari hindbrain malformations, tethered cords, or spinal dysraphism) is usually central. Occasionally paired, parasagittal channels are seen. Eccentric or unilateral cysts may be encountered in cases of post-traumatic syringomyelia, although the majority of traumatic syrinxes are central.

MR has demonstrated that syringomyelia is a common delayed consequence of spinal injury. This diagnosis should be suspected when neurological function deteriorates months or years after trauma. MR is the procedure of choice for evaluating such cases. The presence of orthopedic fixation hardware does not usually contraindicate an MR scan or prevent at least partial visualization of the spinal cord.

DIFFERENTIAL DIAGNOSIS:
FLATTENED SHAPE OF THE CERVICAL SPINAL CORD

Case 789

43-year-old man.
(scan with intrathecal contrast)

Case 790

36-year-old man.
(scan with intrathecal contrast)

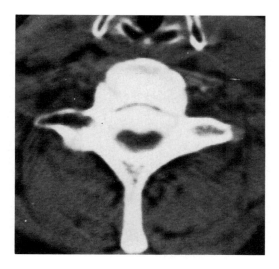

Syringomyelia.

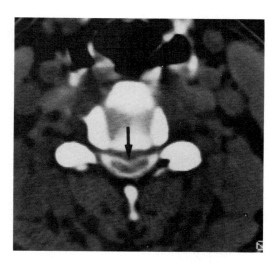

Central Disc Herniation (C4−5 Level).

The spinal cord may become flattened in AP diameter because of atrophy or compression.

Anteroposterior narrowing is frequently seen in syringomyelia. The ventral surface of the cord may be slightly indented, while the transverse diameter is relatively preserved. Other causes of cord atrophy include trauma, multiple sclerosis, ischemia, arteriovenous malformation, and amyotrophic lateral sclerosis.

A similar morphology may result from compression of the cord by anterior osteophytes or cervical disc herniations, as in Case 790. Compare the spacious ventral subarachnoid space in Case 789 to the thin rim of contrast in Case 790.

MR EVALUATION OF MYELOPATHY: MULTIPLE SCLEROSIS

Case 791

20-year-old woman.
(sagittal, noncontrast scan; SE 3000/90)

Case 792

24-year-old man.
(sagittal, postcontrast scan; SE 550/20)

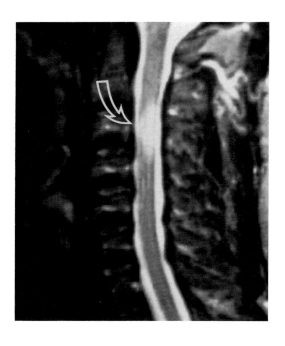

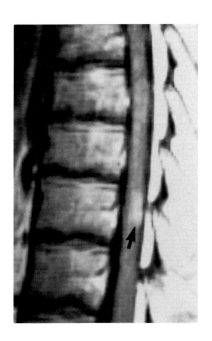

As discussed in previous cases, MR is superior to CT for the demonstration of intramedullary disease. The diagnosis of myelitis is an example of this important MR application.

Here a well-defined lesion of high intensity is seen within the cervical cord at the C3 level. Intramedullary plaques of multiple sclerosis may not be this sharply marginated, but the size (about one vertebral segment in length), elongated morphology, and location (high cervical, often dorsal) of this lesion are otherwise characteristic. Mild, localized cord swelling may accompany a large demyelinating focus with active edema. Several lesions are often present, with a "stringy" or "patchy" pattern of scattered high intensity. Foci of spinal cord demyelination may occur with or without cerebral evidence of multiple sclerosis (see Cases 313 to 316).

The other major etiology of inflammatory myelopathy, "transverse myelitis," likely represents an autoimmune response to antigenic challenge. Such lesions are also well seen as zones of high signal intensity on T2-weighted MR studies. "Transverse myelitis" frequently involves longer segments of the spinal cord than the typical foci of multiple sclerosis.

Active demyelinating plaques may demonstrate contrast enhancement within the spinal cord as they do within the brain (see Cases 305 to 312). In this case an enhancing plaque in the thoracic region (arrow) correlated with new lower extremity symptoms in a patient with known multiple sclerosis.

The appearance seen here is not specific. For example, an intramedullary metastasis could present a similar pattern.

Small inflammatory or neoplastic foci unaccompanied by cord edema may be inapparent on MR scans without contrast material.

MR EVALUATION OF MYELOPATHY: VASCULAR LESIONS

Case 793

64-year-old man.
(sagittal, noncontrast scan; SE 800/17)

Cord Edema due to Dural Arteriovenous Malformation.

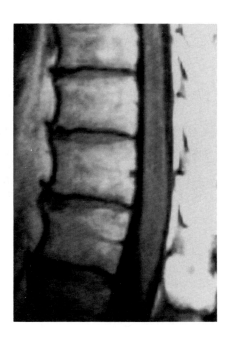

Case 794

59-year-old woman.
(sagittal, noncontrast scan; low flip angle gradient echo sequence)

Intramedullary Cavernous Angioma.

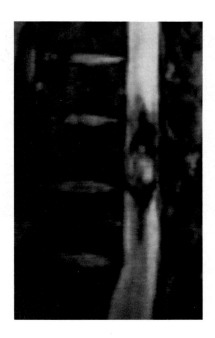

Vascular lesions may cause intramedullary changes that are better demonstrated by MR than by CT.

Diffuse edema may be seen as a consequence of cord infarction (e.g., in association with abdominal aortic aneurysm, pre or postoperatively). Another vascular cause of diffuse cord edema is venous hypertension due to an adjacent arteriovenous malformation (usually a "radiculomedullary AV fistula" involving the dura). In either case, intramedullary edema will present as cord swelling with prolongation of T1 and T2 values. Here the swollen spinal cord and conus medullaris demonstrate abnormally low signal intensity on a T1-weighted scan.

Contrast-enhanced MR scans may demonstrate components of a spinal arteriovenous malformation, but the absence of abnormal enhancement does not exclude the diagnosis.

Vascular malformations within the spinal cord can also be demonstrated by MR imaging. Patent AVMs may be detected as tortuous intramedullary channels containing characteristic "flow-voids," comparable to cerebral lesions (see Cases 492 and 493). Occasionally bulky draining veins associated with a spinal AVM cause compressive myelopathy, which compounds the effects of edema or ischemia.

Occult AVMs or cavernous angiomas can be diagnosed by typical signal alterations suggesting the presence of blood products. A combination of central T1-shortening and peripheral/interstitial T2-shortening is common in such lesions (see Cases 516 and 517). Hemorrhage within intramedullary tumors may cause a similar appearance, and caution is appropriate in interpreting such lesions.

The magnetic susceptibility effects of hemosiderin are accentuated by gradient echo techniques. "T2*-weighted" sequences emphasize the "black" margins of lesions containing old blood products, as seen here.

EPIDURAL ABSCESSES

Case 795

34-year-old woman treated 6 months previously
for drug abuse, pneumonia, and a mediastinal
abscess, now presenting with
numb hands and a spastic gait.
(scan with intravenous contrast; C7 level)

Case 796

74-year-old woman initially evaluated for aortic
dissection because of back pain and upper
extremity weakness.
(scan with intravenous contrast; C3 level)

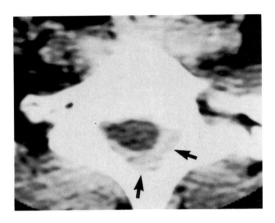

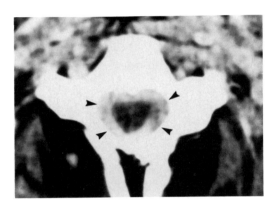

Abscesses may develop in the epidural space through direct extension of vertebral or paraspinal infections or through hematogenous seeding from distant sources. Once established, epidural abscesses typical involve long segments of the spinal canal (e.g., ten or twenty vertebral levels). Initial symptoms may be mild or nondescript (see Case 796), but rapid loss of neurological function occurs with the onset of septic thrombophlebitis involving the spinal cord.

In this case an enhancing rind of epidural tissue surrounds the dural sac. The appearance is not specific; differential diagnosis would include epidural lymphoma (which also commonly involves multiple levels), metastases, or hematoma. Surgery demonstrated an inflammatory mass or "phlegmon" with only small pockets of purulent material.

Although image quality is adequate in this case, the cervicothoracic junction is often a zone of considerable artifact on CT studies. MR scanning is usually superior to CT in examining this region.

Epidural abscesses often surround the dural sac, as in this case. The symmetry seen here is somewhat unusual; an asymmetrical rind of inflammatory tissue as in case 795 is more common.

This patient expired from staphylococcal pneumonia shortly after admission. At autopsy a grossly purulent staphylococcal abscess extended from the foramen magnum to the lumbar region.

PARASPINAL INFECTION

Case 797

26-year-old woman 2 weeks after laminectomy.

Paraspinal Abscess.

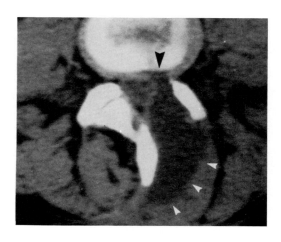

Case 798

14-year-old girl with back pain, exaggerated lumbar lordosis, and severe limitation of lumbar flexion.

Disc Space Infection With Paraspinal Cellulitis.

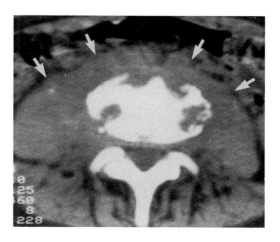

Paraspinal abscesses form homogeneous, low-attenuation collections, as seen here. The low density and sharp margins contrast with the isodensity and vague borders of cellulitis, as in Case 798. Involvement of the psoas region is common in cases of intra-abdominal infection.

Pseudomeningoceles are another type of paraspinal cyst which may be encountered on postoperative scans. Such fluid collections expand from the dural sac into the surgical defect. The abscess cavity in this case extends to the disc but does not communicate with the central canal.

Infection of the intervertebral disc causes a ring of paraspinal edema and exudate *(arrows)* surrounding a narrowed disc space. Erosion and fragmentation of adjacent vertebral end plates are hallmarks of discitis, as seen here. Such lucencies are usually more numerous and irregular than the depressions caused by intravertebral disc herniations ("Schmorl's nodes").

In adults and older children, hematogenous infection originates in the subchondral portion of the vertebral body, spreading to involve the adjacent disc. In young children the reverse sequence may occur: hematogenous infection may initially "seed" the vascular disc before spreading to the subchondral vertebral body. Direct infection of the disc space may occur at any age after surgery or instrumentation.

Tuberculous spondylitis typically demonstrates larger paraspinal masses and less end-plate destruction than pyogenic infection. Extension beneath the anterior longitudinal ligament is often associated with involvement of multiple vertebral bodies, mimicking metastatic disease.

Isolated vertebral osteomyelitis is also well demonstrated by axial CT scans. Distinction from metastasis may be difficult in the absence of associated discitis.

DIFFERENTIAL DIAGNOSIS:
MULTIFOCAL EROSION OF VERTEBRAL END-PLATES

Case 799

39-year-old man.

Case 800

60-year-old man.

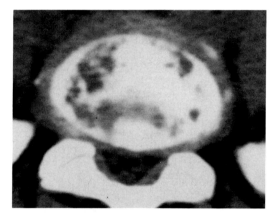

Discitis/Osteomyelitis (Associated With Staphylococcal Septicemia).

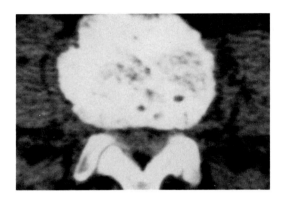

Reactive Changes Secondary to Disc Degeneration.

As discussed in Case 798, multifocal erosion of vertebral end plates is characteristic of discitis. Case 799 is a typical example.

Multiple small erosions with sclerotic margins may also be seen in vertebral end-plates adjacent to degenerating discs. Such foci are typically smaller and more regular than infectious erosions. The clinical setting and the presence or absence of paraspinal soft tissue involvement usually assist in differential diagnosis (although the paraspinal swelling in Case 799 resembles a circumferential disc bulge). MR scans can be helpful in equivocal cases by demonstrating prolonged T2 values within an infected disc (see Case 802), which would be an unusual finding in uncomplicated degenerative disease.

MR CORRELATION: DISCITIS/OSTEOMYELITIS

Case 801

47-year-old woman.
(sagittal, noncontrast scan; SE 600/20)

Case 802

35-year-old woman hospitalized for
staphylococcal septicemia.
(sagittal, noncontrast scan; SE 2200/45)

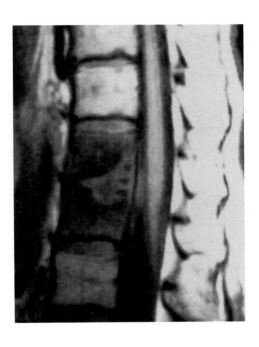

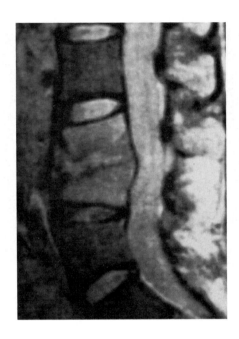

MR provides a sensitive, multiplanar view of disc space infection and adjacent osteomyelitis. Detection of early discitis and demonstration of vertebral involvement exceed the capabilities of CT scanning.

The radiographic hallmark of discitis, involvement of the subchondral regions of adjacent vertebral bodies, is well displayed on sagittal or coronal MR studies. Infiltration of marrow by edema and inflammatory cells causes a "watery" signal pattern, seen as reduced intensity on T1-weighted images.

In this case, abnormal signal involves most of the T12 and L1 vertebral bodies. The large erosion extending from the disc space into both bodies is unusually prominent; often a "ragged" appearance of multiple smaller irregularities is seen. A shallow layer of thickened epidural tissue is present along the anterior margin of the spinal canal. No prevertebral mass is seen.

Abnormally increased signal intensity is seen throughout the L3 and L4 vertebral bodies on this T2-weighted scan. Adjacent portions of both bodies have been destroyed (compare their height with that of the uninvolved vertebrae).

The intervening disc space is narrow and irregular. Signal intensity within the disc is comparable to that of the infected vertebrae. (Low intensity would be expected in a degenerated disc that has caused sterile reactive changes of neighboring bodies.)

Hematogenous disc space infection usually originates from seeding of subchondral bone. The term "spondylitis" may be better than "discitis" to accurately represent the vertebral component of these combined infections.

Case 803

52-year-old man who fell from a tree.
(L1 level)

Case 804

64-year-old man injured in an automobile
accident.
(L2 level)

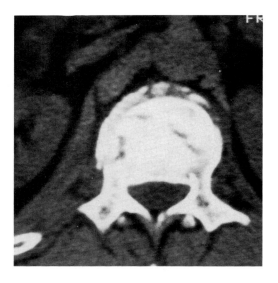

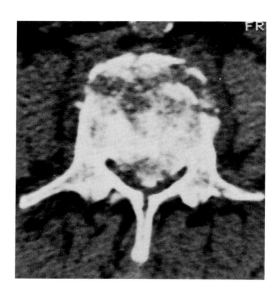

Fractures of the vertebral bodies and posterior arches are well evaluated by axial CT scans. Despite the obvious comminution in this case, bone fragments do not significantly compress the spinal canal.

Soft tissue injury is more difficult to judge without contrast material. Occasional epidural hematomas are imaged on high-resolution scans.

In this case a comminuted fracture of the vertebral body is associated with displaced fragments that nearly obliterate the spinal canal. This cross-sectional display defines the need for decompression. A fracture line extends into the spinous process.

MR EVALUATION OF ACUTE SPINAL TRAUMA

Case 805

30-year-old man.
(sagittal, noncontrast scan; SE 800/17)

Case 806

6-year-old girl, paraplegic after an automobile accident, with normal spine x-rays.
(sagittal, noncontrast scan; SE 800/17)

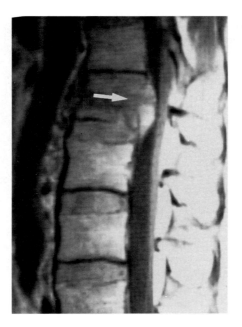

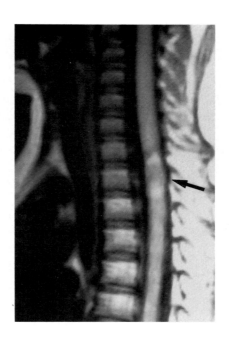

MR effectively demonstrates canal compromise and cord injury in cases of spinal trauma. Sagittal T1-weighted scans provide a rapid survey of vertebral alignment. Epidural soft tissue masses (e.g., disc herniation, hematoma) are defined and cord compression is quantified.

In this case, a fracture of the L1 vertebral body is seen, with posterior displacement of a fragment into the spinal canal. Posterior herniation of the T12–L1 disc and a small epidural hematoma accompany the osseous injury. The conus medullaris is displaced and marginally compressed against the posterior border of the spinal canal.

As demonstrated in Case 805, MR can provide important soft tissue information in cases of spinal injury when osseous trauma is apparent on CT scans or plain films. MR may also disclose neural injury when CT scans and routine radiographs are negative.

The pediatric spine is flexible and may undergo considerable subluxation without fracture. If such displacement is subsequently reduced, there may be no bony evidence of major spinal injury.

In this case, the vertebral alignment is normal. However, a zone of contusion with small areas of T1-shortening indicating hemorrhage is seen within the spinal cord at the cervicothoracic junction. The child remained paraplegic, and a follow-up scan showed focal atrophy to "ribbon" thinness at this site.

Cord transection may also occur with spinal injury in the pediatric population and is well demonstrated by sagittal MR scans. Perinatal transection may be seen after difficult breech deliveries. The most common site of transection in older children is the cervicothoracic junction, comparable to the level of cord injury in this case.

Case 807

40-year-old man.

Odontoid Fracture.

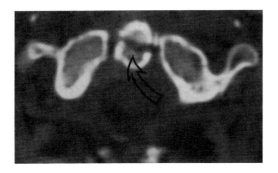

Case 808

8-year-old boy with Down's syndrome.

Subluxation at C1–C2.

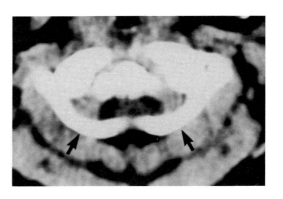

The bony rings and articulation of C1 and C2 are well seen on axial CT scans. Sagittal CT reconstructions and MR examinations offer supplemental information regarding spinal alignment and associated soft tissue pathology.

In this case a fracture splits the odontoid process *(arrow)*. The near-coronal plane of the fracture is unusual. Most injuries traverse the base of the odontoid process and are not viewed tangentially on axial images.

Axial CT scans are useful in defining the relationship of the C1 and C2 vertebrae. Abnormal rotation (e.g., torticollis) or displacements (e.g., post-trauma) are readily apparent.

In this case, congenital abnormality at the C1–2 level causes compression of the spinal canal. Subluxation at C1–2 due to ligamentous laxity is common in Down's syndrome. The mild subluxation seen here is superimposed on an abnormally short and ventrally curved posterior arch of C1 *(arrows)*. The combination of these features causes flattening of the dural sac and spinal cord.

RHEUMATOID ARTHRITIS INVOLVING C1–2

Case 809A

78-year-old woman.

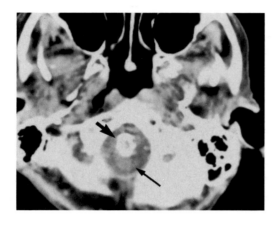

Case 809B

Same patient.
(sagittal reconstruction of axial CT scans;
anterior is to the reader's left)

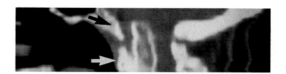

Soft tissue masses involving the foramen magnum are best assessed by magnetic resonance imaging (see Cases 161 and 162). CT is useful when bony lesions cause compromise of the craniocervical junction.

The most common nontraumatic cause for subluxation at C1–2 in adults is rheumatoid arthritis. Inflammatory ligamentous laxity and bone erosion permit the odontoid process to move posteriorly and superiorly. Superior displacement of the odontoid is aggravated by "cranial settling" due to erosion and reduced height of the lateral masses of C1. In severe cases, the odontoid rises high into the foramen magnum, embedding itself against the ventral margin of the brain stem.

Here the odontoid process *(thick arrow)* is seen within the center of the foramen magnum. The medulla *(thin arrow)* is posteriorly displaced and flattened.

Sagittal CT reconstructions and/or sagittal MR scans are useful for demonstrating the extent and configuration of bony distortions near the foramen magnum (see also Cases 810 and 811).

In this case, the elongated odontoid process rides high above the anterior arch of C1 *(white arrow)*, ascending to the level of the clivus *(black arrow)*. The cervicomedullary junction must drape over this bony promontory to pass through the foramen magnum. (Compare to the distortion of the cervicomedullary junction by a ventral soft tissue mass in Case 159.)

Patients with long-standing rheumatoid arthritis may tolerate remarkable compression of the cervicomedullary junction. The gradual progression of C1–2 subluxation over many years often results in "ribbon-like" thinning of the spinal cord before symptoms lead to evaluation.

MR CORRELATION: BONE DEFORMITY AT THE CRANIOCERVICAL JUNCTION

Case 810

34-year-old man.
(sagittal, noncontrast scan; SE 600/20)

Basilar Impression (and Chiari I Malformation)

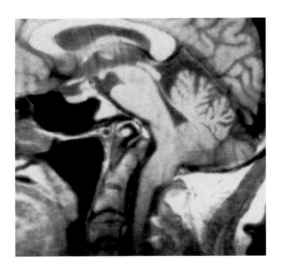

Case 811

2-year-old boy with Down's syndrome.
(sagittal, noncontrast scan; SE 600/20)

Canal Stenosis at C1.

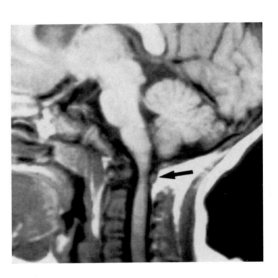

Sagittal MR scans define the cephalocaudal configuration of the "effective foramen magnum." Associated deformity of neural tissue is demonstrated more completely than on CT studies.

In this case the clivus is congenitally short and flat. The elongated odontoid process represents the anterior margin of the foramen magnum (compare to Case 809B). The belly of the pons is flattened, and the medulla is kinked. Cerebellar tissue extends through the foramen magnum dorsal to the spinal cord.

Acquired basilar invagination (e.g., Paget's disease) may result in simlar osseous and soft tissue deformity.

This scan is the MR equivalent of Case 808. Mild posterior subluxation of the odontoid process with respect to the anterior arch of C1 is present. More importantly, the posterior arch of C1 is very short (arrow), constricting the spinal canal.

The combination of these features narrows the AP diameter of the spinal cord. Further cord compression could potentially occur with motion of the head or trauma.

CORD COMPRESSION AT THE CRANIOCERVICAL JUNCTION

Case 812

13-year-old girl.
(scan with intravenous contrast)

Osteoblastoma of the Occipital Bone.

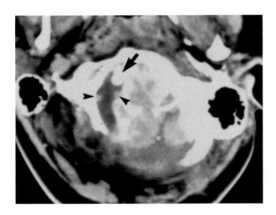

Case 813

79-year-old woman with neck pain and
hyperreflexia (same patient as Case 154).
(scan with intravenous contrast)

Glomus Jugulare Tumor.

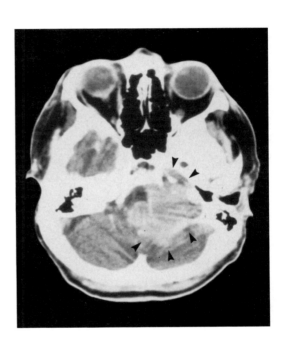

A variety of soft tissue and bony lesions may compromise the "effective foramen magnum" at the craniocervical junction.

Osteoblastomas are benign bone tumors that commonly occur in the spine. They are characteristically lytic and expansile, often resembling the appearance of aneurysmal bone cysts. Associated intraspinal or paraspinal soft tissue components are frequent.

In this case an unusual osteoblastoma of the skull base has expanded bone to severely compromise the foramen magnum. The spinal cord is flattened sagittally, seen between the enhancing vertebral arteries (arrowheads) posterior to the malformed odontoid tip (arrow).

In addition to causing neural compression, lesions crowding or narrowing the foramen magnum may predispose to the development of syringomyelia (see Case 624).

Here the cervicomedullary junction is severely compressed by the large, lobulated soft tissue mass of a glomus jugulare tumor. The medial portion of the left petrous bone has been destroyed.

Case 814

25-year-old man with a history of
meningomyelocele repair in infancy, now
presenting with increasing leg weakness and
sphincter dysfunction.
(sagittal reconstruction of axial sections with
intrathecal contrast; L3−4 level)

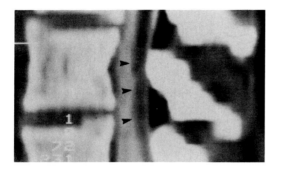

Case 815

6-month-old girl.
(sagittal, noncontrast scan; SE 800/17)

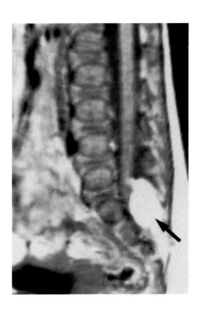

Magnetic resonance imaging is now the procedure of choice for evaluating congenital malformations of the spinal canal (see Cases 815, 817, 819, and 820). CT myelography offers a large amount of information when MR is not available.

In this case, sagittal reconstruction of axial images centered at L3−4 demonstrates the low-lying spinal cord passing through the lumbar region (arrowheads). Axial scans (MR or CT with intrathecal contrast) demonstrate nerve roots arising from a low-lying cord, distinguishing it from a thickened filum terminale (see Case 817).

Tethering of the cord commonly accompanies dysraphic states and is frequently associated with lipomas at the caudal end of the dural sac (see Case 815). The lipomas may surround and/or infiltrate the filum terminale and conus medullaris.

Clumping of nerve roots within the thecal sac due to arachnoiditis or meningeal carcinomatosis (see Cases 779 and 780) can resemble the appearance of a tethered cord on axial or sagittal CT or MR scans.

MR has become the procedure of choice for assessing congenital abnormalities of the spinal cord. The noninvasive demonstration of intradural tissues combines with multiplanar display to offer a comprehensive view of complex malformations.

Here the tethered spinal cord is seen to extend through the lumbar region to terminate in a caudal lipoma (characterized by high signal intensity on T1-weighted images). Intradural lipomas are often continuous with dorsal subcutaneous fat through dysraphic defects in the posterior neural arch. Lipomatous tissue may ascend along the dorsal surface of the cord or infiltrate the filum terminale.

Syringomyelia and/or diastematomyelia frequently accompany cord tethering. When one congenital abnormality of the spinal canal is found, others should be expected.

MYELOMENINGOCELE

Case 816

5-year-old girl with caudal regression syndrome
and skin-covered myelomeningocele.

Case 817

4-year-old girl with a history of
myelomeningocele repair in infancy.
(sagittal, noncontrast scan; SE 550/20)

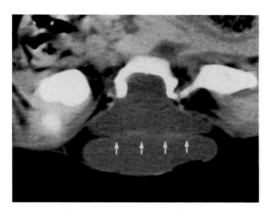

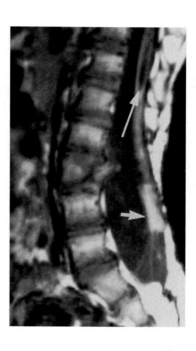

The various forms of spinal dysraphism are well demonstrated by magnetic resonance imaging (see Case 817). The CT appearance of such malformations is also characteristic, with excellent depiction of bony abnormalities.

In this case the sacrum and iliac bones are severely hypoplastic. The dural sac passes dorsally through a broad defect in the spinal canal and expands as a subcutaneous sac. (Compare to the occipital meningocele in Case 660.)

A thin, transversely oriented tissue layer in the middle of the sac (arrows) represents the neural placode giving rise to sacral roots. No lipomatous components are present at this level.

This midsagittal T1-weighted MR scan demonstrates several characteristic features of spinal dysraphism that may be individually noted on CT studies.

The caudal sac is typically large or "patulous." A band of low-lying neural tissue passes along the dorsal wall of the ectatic sac, appearing to be "tethered" posteriorly at the site of myelomeningocele repair. The tissue band is established as spinal cord (rather than a thickened filum terminale) by the emergence of nerve roots from its distal placode (short arrow). No lipoma is seen, but syringomyelia is present in the thoracic region (long arrow) and diastematomyelia was found at a higher level. An associated vertebral malformation is demonstrated at L3.

DIASTEMATOMYELIA

Case 818A

50-year-old woman presenting with back pain.
(soft tissue window; L1 level)

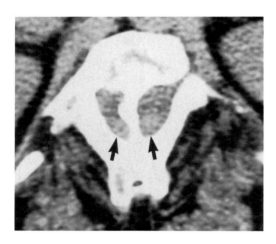

Case 818B

Same patient.
(bone window; same level)

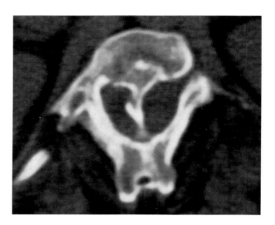

Diastematomyelia is a congenital abnormality character-ized by abnormal division of the spinal cord. In at least 50% of such cases the two hemicords are enclosed within a single arachnoid and dural tube, with no intervening septation. In the remaining cases a fibrous, osteocartilaginous, or bony septum divides the spinal canal.

CT is useful for demonstrating calcified partitions, which may range from thin plates of cortical bone to large, well-formed osseous elements. In this case a stout, sagittally ori-ented spur traverses the AP dimension of the lumbar canal. The hemicords can be faintly seen as tissue nodules within the dorsal portions of the dural sacs *(arrows)*.

The division of the dural sac and spinal cord in diastemat-omyelia is approximately equal in about two thirds of cases, as seen here. The dividing septum is often obliquely angled due to rotoscoliosis. Rotation of the hemicords is common with or without septal obliquity.

About 90% of diastematomyelic hemicords reunite at a level below the split. A septation passing between the hemi-cords may represent an important cause of tethering in such cases.

The adult presentation of congenital spinal cord abnormal-ities is occasionally noted, sometimes due to superimposed degenerative disease. These malformations more commonly become symptomatic during childhood or adolescence, as growth of the spine increases the tension on tethered neural structures.

MR CORRELATION: DIASTEMATOMYELIA

Case 819

5-year-old girl.
(coronal, noncontrast scan; SE 800/17)

Case 820

15-year-old girl.
(axial, noncontrast scan; SE 1000/20)

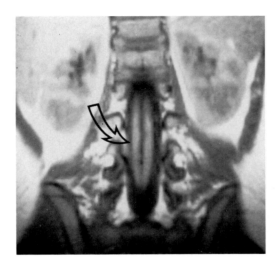

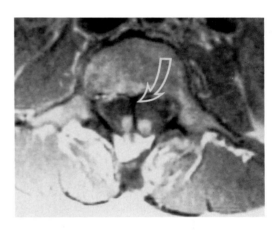

Coronal and axial MR scans directly visualize the hemicords in cases of diastematomyelia. Sagittal scans may be falsely negative or may erroneously suggest syringomyelia.

Here a coronal T1-weighted scan clearly demonstrates the paired hemicords in the lumbar region *(arrow)*. Cord tethering commonly accompanies diastematomyelia, with or without canal septation.

In this case the paired hemicords are easily defined within the dural sacs. Between them is a sagittally oriented plate of cortical bone, seen as a low-intensity structure *(arrow;* compare to the CT appearance in Case 818).

In other cases the osseous spur may be much wider, containing marrow elements with high signal intensity on T1-weighted scans. As discussed in Case 818, bony septations in diastematomyelia may be obliquely oriented, and the hemicords are frequently rotated within the dural sac(s).

REFERENCES: CT

1. Aubin M.L., Vignaud J., Jardin C., et al.: Computed tomography in 75 clinical cases of syringomyelia. *A.J.N.R.* 2:199–204, 1981.
2. Batnitzky S., Price H., Gaughan M., et al.: The radiology of syringohydromyelia. *Radiographics* 3:585–611, 1983.
3. Beres J., Pech P., Berns T.F., et al.: Spinal epidural lymphoma: CT features in seven patients. *A.J.N.R.* 7:327–328, 1986.
4. Bonafe A., Ethier R., Melancon D., et al.: High resolution computed tomography in cervical syringomyelia. *J. Comput. Assist. Tomogr.* 4:42–47, 1980.
5. Dory M.A.: CT demonstration of cervical vertebrae erosion by tortuous vertebral artery. *A.J.N.R.* 6:641–642, 1985.
6. El-Khoury G.Y., Clark C.R., Dietz F.R., et al.: Posterior atlanto-occipital subluxation in down syndrome. *Radiology* 159:507–510, 1986.
7. Fitz C.R.: Midline anomalies of the brain and spine. *Radiol. Clin. North Am.* 20:95–104, 1982.
8. Graves V.B., Keene J.S., Strother C.M., et al.: CT of bilateral lumbosacral facet dislocation. *A.J.N.R.* 9:809, 1988.
9. Grogan J.P., Daniels J.L., Williams A.L., et al: The normal conus medullaris: CT criteria for recognition. *Radiology* 151:661–664, 1984.
10. Haykal H.A., Wang A.M., Zamani A.A., et al.: Computed tomography of spontaneous acute cervical epidural hematoma. *J. Comput. Assist. Tomogr.* 8:229–231, 1984.
11. Heinz E.R., Rosenbaum A.E., Scarff T., et al.: Tethered spinal cord following myelomeningocele repair. *Radiology* 131:153–160, 1979.
12. Hermann G., Mendelson D.S., Cohen B.A., et al.: Role of computed tomography in the diagnosis of infectious spondylitis. *J. Comput. Assist. Tomogr.* 7:961–968, 1983.
13. Kaplan J.O., Quencer R.M.: The occult tethered conus syndrome in the adult. *Radiology* 137:387–391, 1980.
14. Laissy J.-P., Milon P., Freger P., et al: Cervical epidural hematoma: CT diagnosis in two cases that resolved spontaneously. *A.J.N.R.* 11:394–396, 1990.
15. LaMasters D.L., Watanabe T.J., Chambers E.F., et al.: Multiplanar metrizamide-enhanced CT imaging of the foramen magnum. *A.J.N.R.* 3:485–494, 1982.
16. Lapointe J.S., Graeb D.A., Nugent R.A., Robertson W.D.: Value of intravenous contrast enhancement in the CT evaluation of intraspinal tumors. *A.J.N.R.* 6:939–944, 1985.
17. Leehey P., Naseem M., Every P., et al.: Vertebral hemangioma with compressive myelopathy: Metrizamide CT demonstration. *J. Comput. Assist. Tomogr.* 9:985–986, 1985.
18. Li K.C., Chui M.C.: Conventional and CT metrizamide myelography in Arnold-Chiari I malformation and syringomyelia. *A.J.N.R.* 8:11–18, 1987.
19. Manaster B.J., Osborn A.G.: CT patterns of facet fracture dislocations in the thoracolumbar region. *A.J.N.R.* 7:1007–1012, 1986.
20. Mawad M.E., Hilal S.K., Fetell M.R., et al.: Patterns of spinal cord atrophy by metrizamide CT. *A.J.N.R.* 4:611–613, 1983.
21. McLendon R.E., Oakes W.J., Heinz E.R., et al.: Adipose tissue in the filum terminale: A computed tomographic finding that may indicate tethering of the spinal cord. *Neurosurgery* 22:873–876, 1988.
22. Menezes A.H., Vangilder J.C., Clark C.R., El-Khoury G.: Odontoid upward migration in rheumatoid arthritis: An analysis of 45 patients with "cranial settling". *J. Neurosurg.* 63:500–509, 1985.
23. Miller J.D.R., Grace M.G.A., Lampard R.: Computed tomography of the upper cervical spine in Down syndrome. *J. Comput. Assist. Tomogr.* 10:589–592, 1986.
24. Mitchell M.J., Sartoris D.J., Moody D., et al.: Cauda equina syndrome complicating ankylosing spondylitis. *Radiology* 175:521–526, 1990.
25. Naidich T.P., McLone D.G., Mutluer S.: A new understanding of dorsal dysraphism with lipoma (lipomyeloschisis): Radiologic evaluation and surgical correlation. *A.J.N.R.* 4:103–116, 1983.
26. Neave V.C., Wycoff R.R.: Computed tomography of cystic nerve root sleeve dilatation. *J. Comput. Assist. Tomogr.* 7:881–885, 1983.
27. Nyberg D.A., Jeffrey R.B., Brant-Zawadzki M., et al.: Computed tomography of cervical infection. *J. Comput. Assist. Tomogr.* 9:288–296, 1985.
28. Pech P., Kilgore D.P., Pojunas K.W., Haughton V.M.: Cervical spine fractures: CT detection. *Radiology* 157:117–120, 1985.
29. Post M.J.D., Green B.A.: The use of computed tomography in spinal trauma. *Radiol. Clin. North Am.* 21:327–375, 1983.
30. Price A.C., Allen J.H., Eggers F.M., et al.: Intervertebral disc space infection: CT changes. *Radiology* 149:725–729, 1983.
31. Quencer R.M., Green B.A., Eismount F.J.: Posttraumatic spinal cord cysts: Clinical features and characterization with metrizamide computed tomography. *Radiology* 146:415–423, 1983.
32. Scatliff J.H., Kendall B.E., Kingsley B., et al.: Closed spinal dysraphism: Analysis of clinical, radiological, and surgical findings in 104 consecutive patients. *A.J.N.R.* 10:269–278, 1989.
33. Scotti G., Musgrave M.A., Harwood-Nash D.C., et al.: Diastematomyelia in children: Metrizamide and CT metrizamide myelography. *A.J.N.R.* 4:601–603, 1983.
34. Shuman W.P., Rogers J.J., Sickler M.E., et al.: Thoracolumbar burst fractures: CT dimensions of the spinal canal relative to postsurgical improvement. *A.J.N.R.* 6:337–342, 1985.
35. Soye I., Levine E., Batnitzky S., et al.: Computed tomography of sacral and presacral lesions. *Neuroradiology* 24:71–76, 1982.
36. Stern W.E.: Dural ectasia and the Marfan syndrome. *J. Neurosurg.* 69:221–227, 1988.
37. Van Lom K.J., Kellerhouse L.E., Pathria M.N., et al.: Infection versus tumor in the spine: Criteria for distinction with CT. *Radiology* 166:851–856, 1988.
38. Wang A.-M., Lewis M.L., Rumbaugh C.L., et al: Spinal cord or nerve root compression in patients with malignant disease: CT evaluation. *J. Comput. Assist. Tomogr.* 8:420–428, 1984.
39. Whelan M.A., Hilal S.K., Gold R.P., et al.: Computed tomography of the sacrum. II. Pathology. *A.J.N.R.* 3:555–559, 1982.
40. Whelan M.A., Schonfeld S., Post J.D., et al: Computed tomography of nontuberculous spinal infection. *J. Comput. Assist. Tomogr.* 9:280–287, 1985.

REFERENCES: MR

1. Altman N.R., Altman D.H.: MR imaging of spinal dysraphism. *A.J.N.R.* 8:533–538, 1987.
2. Angtuaco E.J.C., Mc Connell J.R., Chadduck W.M., Flanigan S.: MR imaging of spinal epidural sepsis. *A.J.N.R.* 8:879–884, 1987.
3. Avrahami E., Tadmor R., Dally O., Hadar H.: Early MR demonstration of spinal metastases in patients with normal radiographs and CT and radionuclide bone scans. *J. Comput. Assist. Tomogr.* 13:598–602, 1989.
4. Baker L.L., Goodman S.B., Perkash I., et al.: Benign versus pathological compression fractures of vertebral bodies: Assessment with conventional spin echo, chemical-shift, and STIR MR imaging. *Radiology* 174:495–502, 1990.
5. Barakos J.A., Mark A.S., Dillon W.P., Norman D.: MR imaging of acute transverse myelitis and AIDS myelopathy. *J. Comput. Assist. Tomogr.* 14:45–50, 1990.
6. Barkovich A.J., Raghavan N., Chuang S., Peck W.W.: The wedge-shaped cord terminus: A radiographic sign of caudal regression. *A.J.N.R.* 10:1223–1231, 1989.
7. Barkovich A.J., Sherman J.L., Citrin C.M., Wippold F.J. II: MR of postoperative syringomyelia. *A.J.N.R.* 8:319–328, 1987.
8. Barnes P.D., Lester P.D., Yamanashi W.S., Prince J.R.: Magnetic resonance imaging in infants and children with spinal dysraphism. *A.J.N.R.* 7:465–472, 1986.
9. Barnwell S.L., Dowd C.F., Davis R.L., et al.: Cryptic vascular malformations of the spinal cord: Diagnosis by magnetic resonance imaging and outcome of surgery. *J. Neurosurg.* 72:403–407, 1990.
10. Beers G.J., Raque G.H., Wagner G.G.: MR imaging in acute cervical spine trauma. *J. Comput. Assist. Tomogr.* 12:755–761, 1988.
11. Brophy J.D., Sutton L.N., Zimmerman R.A., et al.: Magnetic resonance imaging of lipomyelomeningocele and tethered cord. *Neurosurgery* 25:336–340, 1989.
12. Brunberg J.A., Latchaw R.E., Kanal E., et al.: Magnetic resonance imaging of spinal dysraphism. *Radiol. Clin. North Am.* 26:181–206, 1988.
13. Carmody R.F., Yang P.J., Seeley G.W., et al.: Spinal cord compression due to metastatic disease: Diagnosis with MR imaging versus myelography. *Radiology* 173:225–230, 1989.
14. Chakeres D.W., Flickinger F., Bresnahan J.C., et al.: MR imaging of acute spinal cord trauma. *A.J.N.R.* 8:5–10, 1987.
15. Chang K.H., Han M.H., Choi Y.W., et al.: Tuberculous arachnoiditis of the spine: Findings on myelography, CT, and MR imaging. *A.J.N.R.* 10:1255–1262, 1989.
16. Davis P.C., Hoffman J.C. Jr., Ball T.I., et al.: Spinal abnormalities in pediatric patients: MR imaging findings compared with clinical, myelographic, and surgical findings. *Radiology* 166:679–686, 1988.
17. Demachi H., Takashima T., Kadoya M., et al.: MR imaging of spinal neuromas with pathological correlation. *J. Comput. Assist. Tomogr.* 14:250–254, 1990.
18. De Pena C.A., Lee Y.-Y., Van Tassel P., et al.: MR appearance of acquired spinal epidermoid tumors. *A.J.N.R.* 10:S97, 1989.
19. Di Chiro G., Doppman J.L., Dwyer A.J., et al.: Tumors and arteriovenous malformations of the spinal cord: Assessment using MR. *Radiology* 156:689–698, 1985.
20. Dillon W.P., Norman D., Newton T.H., et al.: Intradural spinal cord lesions: Gd-DTPA-enhanced MR imaging. *Radiology* 170:229–238, 1989.
21. Doppman J.L., Di Chiro G., Dwyer A.J., et al.: Magnetic resonance imaging of spinal arteriovenous malformations. *J. Neurosurg.* 66:830–834, 1987.
22. Dormont D., Gelbert F., Assouline E., et al.: MR imaging of spinal cord arteriovenous malformations at 0.5T: Study of 34 cases. *A.J.N.R.* 9:833–838, 1988.
23. Edwards M.K., Farlow M.R., Stevens J.C.: Cranial MR in spinal cord MS: Diagnosing patients with isolated spinal cord symptoms. *A.J.N.R.* 7:1003–1006, 1986.
24. Enzmann D.R., Rubin J.B.: Cervical spine: MR imaging with a partial flip angle, gradient-refocused pulse sequence. Part II. Spinal cord disease. *Radiology* 166:473–478, 1988.
25. Fontaine S., Melanson D., Cosgrove R., Bertrand G.: Cavernous hemangiomas of the spinal cord: MR imaging. *Radiology* 166:839–842, 1988.
26. Gebarski S.S., Maynard F.W., Gabrielson T.O., et al.: Posttraumatic progressive myelopathy: Clinical and radiologic correlation employing MR imaging, delayed CT metrizamide myelography, and intraoperative sonography. *Radiology* 157:379–386, 1985.
27. Godersky J.C., Smoker W.R.K., Knutzon R.: Use of magnetic resonance imaging in the evaluation of metastatic spine disease. *Neurosurgery* 21:676–680, 1987.
28. Goy A.M.C., Pinto R.S., Raghavendra B.N., et al.: Intramedullary spinal cord tumors: MR imaging, with emphasis on associated cysts. *Radiology* 161:381–386, 1986.
29. Hackney D.B., Asato R., Joseph P.M., et al.: Hemorrhage and edema in acute spinal cord compression: Demonstration by MR imaging. *Radiology* 161:387–390, 1986.
30. Han J.S., Benson J.E., Kaufman B., et al.: Demonstration of diastematomyelia and associated abnormalities with MR imaging. *A.J.N.R.* 6:215–220, 1985.
31. Hayes C.W., Jensen M.E., Conway W.F.: Non-neoplastic lesions of vertebral bodies: Findings in magnetic resonance imaging. *Radiographics* 9:883–904, 1989.
32. Heller R.M., Szalay E.A., Green H.E., et al.: Disc space infection in children: Magnetic resonance imaging. *Radiol. Clin. North Am.* 26:207–210, 1988.
33. Isu T., Iwasaki Y., Akino M., Abe H.: Hydrosyringomyelia associated with a Chiari I malformation in children and adolescents. *Neurosurgery* 26:591–597, 1990.
34. Isu T., Iwasaki Y., Akino M., et al.: Magnetic resonance imaging in cases of spinal dural arteriovenous malformation. *Neurosurgery* 24:919–923, 1989.
35. Kalfas I., Wilberger J., Goldberg A., Prostko E.R.: Magnetic resonance imaging in acute spinal cord trauma. *Neurosurgery* 23:295–299, 1988.
36. Kulkarni M.V., Bondurant F.J., Rose S.L., Narayama P.A.: 1.5T MR imaging of acute spinal trauma. *Radiographics* 8:1059–1082, 1988.
37. Kulkarni M.V., McArdle C.B., Kopanicky D., et al.: Acute spinal cord injury: MR imaging at 1.5 T. *Radiology* 164:837–844, 1987.
38. Larsson E.-M., Holtas S., Nilsson O.: Gd-DTPA-enhanced MR of suspected spinal multiple sclerosis. *A.J.N.R.* 10:1071–1076, 1989.
39. Larsson E.-M., Holtas S., Zygmunt S.: Pre and postoperative MR imaging of the craniocervical junction in rheumatoid arthritis. *A.J.N.R.* 10:89–94, 1989.
40. Lee B.C.P., Zimmerman R.D., Manning J.J., Deck M.D.F.: MR imaging of syringomyelia and hydromyelia. *A.J.N.R.* 6:221–228, 1985.
41. Levy L.M., Di Chiro G., McCullough D.C., et al.: Fixed spinal cord: Diagnosis with MR imaging. *Radiology* 169:773–778, 1988.
42. Maravilla K.R., Weinreb J.C., Suss R., Nunnally R.L.:

Magnetic resonance demonstration of multiple sclerosis plaques in the cervical cord. *A.J.N.R.* 5:685–690, 1984.

43. Masaryk T.J., Modic M.T., Geisinger M.A., et al.: Cervical myelopathy: A comparison of magnetic resonance and myelography. *J. Comput. Assist. Tomogr.* 10:184–194, 1986.

44. Masaryk T.J., Ross J.S., Modic M.T., et al.: Radiculomeningeal vascular malformation of the spine: MR imaging. *Radiology* 164:845–850, 1987.

45. Mathis J.M., Wilson J.T., Barnard J.W., Zelenik M.E.: MR imaging of spinal cord avulsion. *A.J.N.R.* 9:1232–1233, 1988.

46. Merine D., Wang H., Kumar A.J., et al.: CT myelography and MR imaging of acute transverse myelitis. *J. Comput. Assist. Tomogr.* 11:606–608, 1987.

47. Minami S., Sagoh T., Nishimura K., et al.: Spinal arteriovenous malformations: MR imaging. *Radiology* 169:109–116, 1988.

48. Mirvis S.E., Geisler F.H., Jelinek J.J., et al.: Acute cervical spine trauma: Evaluation with 1.5T MR imaging. *Radiology* 166:807–816, 1988.

49. Modic M.T., Feiglin D.H., Piraino D.W., et al.: Vertebral osteomyelitis: Assessment using MR. *Radiology* 157:157–166, 1985.

50. Moufarrij N., Palmer J.M., Hahn J.F., Weinstein M.A.: Correlation between magnetic resonance imaging and surgical findings in the tethered spinal cord. *Neurosurgery* 25:341–346, 1989.

51. Murphey M.D., Batnitzky S., Bramble J.M.: Diagnostic imaging of spinal trauma. *Radiol. Clin. North Am.* 27:855–872, 1989.

52. Nelson M.D. Jr., Bracchi M., Naidich T.P., McLone D.G.: The natural history of repaired myelomeningocele. *Radiographics* 8:695–706, 1988.

53. Nesbit G.M., Miller G.M., Baker H.L. Jr., et al.: Spinal cord sarcoidosis: A new finding at MR imaging with Gd-DTPA enhancement. *Radiology* 173:839–844, 1989.

54. Parizel P.M., Baleriaux D., Rodesch G., et al.: Gd-DTPA-enhanced MR imaging of spinal tumors. *A.J.N.R.* 10:249–258, 1989.

55. Post M.J.D., Quencer R.M., Green B.A., et al.: Intramedullary spinal cord metastases, mainly of nonneurogenic origin. *A.J.N.R.* 8:339–346, 1987.

56. Post M.J.D., Quencer R.M., Montalvo B.M., et al.: Spinal infection: Evaluation with MR imaging and intraoperative ultrasound. *Radiology* 169:765–772, 1988.

57. Quencer R.M.: The injured spinal cord: Evaluation with magnetic resonance and intraoperative sonography. *Radiol. Clin. North Am.* 26:1025–1046, 1988.

58. Quencer R.M., Sheldon J.J., Post M.J.D. et al.: Magnetic resonance imaging in the chronically injured cervical spinal cord. *A.J.N.R.* 7:457–464, 1986.

59. Raghavan N., Barkovich A.J., Edwards M., Norman D.: MR imaging in the tethered spinal cord syndrome. *A.J.N.R.* 10:27–36, 1989.

60. Ross J.S., Masaryk T.J., Modic M.T., et al.: Vertebral hemangiomas: MR imaging. *Radiology* 165:165–170, 1987.

61. Ross J.S., Masaryk T.J., Modic M.T., et al.: MR imaging of lumbar arachnoiditis. *A.J.N.R.* 8:885–892, 1987.

62. Rothfus W.E., Chedid M.K., Deeb Z.L., et al.: MR imaging in the diagnosis of spontaneous spinal epidural hematomas. *J. Comput. Assist. Tomogr.* 11:851–854, 1987.

63. Rubenstein D.J., Alvarez O., Ghelman B., Marchisello P.: Cauda equina syndrome complicating ankylosing spondylitis: MR features. *J. Comput. Assist. Tomogr.* 13:511–513, 1989.

64. Rubin J.M., Aisen A.M., DiPietro M.A.: Ambiguities in MR imaging of tumoral cysts in the spinal cord. *J. Comput. Assist. Tomogr.* 10:395–398, 1986.

65. Scotti G., Scialfa G., Colombo N., Landoni L.: MR imaging of intradural extramedullary tumors of the cervical spine. *J. Comput. Assist. Tomogr.* 9:1037–1041, 1985.

66. Sherman J.L., Barkovich A.J., Citrin C.M.: The MR appearance of syringomyelia: New observations. *A.J.N.R.* 7:985–996, 1986.

67. Sherman J.L., Citrin C.M., Barkovich A.J.: MR imaging of syringobulbia. *J. Comput. Assist. Tomogr.* 11:407–411, 1987.

68. Siegel M.J., Jamroz G.A., Glazer H.S., Abramson C.L.: MR imaging of intraspinal extension of neuroblastoma. *J. Comput. Assist. Tomogr.* 10:593–595, 1986.

69. Silbergeld H., Cohen W.A., Maravilla K.R., et al.: Supratentorial and spinal cord hemangioblastomas: Gadolinium enhanced MR appearance with pathologic correlation. *J. Comput. Assist. Tomogr.* 13:1048–1051, 1989.

70. Sklar E., Quencer R.M., Green B.A., et al.: Acquired spinal subarachnoid cysts: Evaluation with MR, CT myelography and intraoperative sonography. *A.J.N.R.* 10:1097–1104, 1989.

71. Slasky B.S., Bydder G.M., Niendorf H.P., Young I.R.: MR imaging with gadolinium-DTPA in the differentiation of tumor, syrinx, and cyst of the spinal cord. *J. Comput. Assist. Tomogr.* 11:845–850, 1987.

72. Smith A.S., Weinstein M.A., Mizushima A., et al.: MR imaging characteristics of tuberculous spondylitis vs. vertebral osteomyelitis. *A.J.N.R.* 10:619–626, 1989.

73. Smoker W.R.K., Godersky J.C., Knutzon R.K. et al.: The role of MR imaging in evaluating metastatic spinal disease. *A.J.N.R.* 8:901–908, 1987.

74. Stimac G.K., Porter B.A., Olson D.O., et al.: Gadolinium-DTPA-enhanced MR imaging of spinal neoplasms: Preliminary investigation and comparison with unenhanced spin echo and STIR sequences. *A.J.N.R.* 9:839–846, 1988.

75. Sze G., Abramson A., Krol G., et al.: Gadolinium-DTPA in the evaluation of intradural extramedullary spinal disease. *A.J.N.R.* 9:153–164, 1988.

76. Sze G., Krol G., Zimmerman R.D., Deck M.D.F.: Malignant extradural spinal tumors: MR imaging with Gd-DTPA. *Radiology* 167:217–224, 1988.

77. Sze G., Krol G., Zimmerman R.D., Deck M.D.F.: Intramedullary disease of the spine: Diagnosis using gadolinium-DTPA-enhanced MR imaging. *A.J.N.R.* 9:847–858, 1988.

78. Tarr R.W., Drolshagen L.F., Kerner T.C., et al.: MR imaging of recent spinal trauma. *J. Comput. Assist. Tomogr.* 11:412–417, 1987.

79. Terwey B., Becker H., Thron A.K., Vahldiek G.: Gadolinium-DTPA-enhanced MR imaging of spinal dural arteriovenous fistulas. *J. Comput. Assist. Tomogr.* 13:30–37, 1989.

80. Wilberger J.E. Jr., Maroon J., Prostko R., et al.: Magnetic resonance imaging and intraoperative neurosonography in syringomyelia. *Neurosurgery* 20:599–605, 1987.

81. Williams A.L., Haughton V.M., Pojunas K.W., et al.: Differentiation of intramedullary neoplasms and cysts by MR. *A.J.N.R.* 8:527–532, 1987.

82. Zimmerman R.A., Bilaniuk L.T.: Imaging of tumors of the spinal canal and cord. *Radiol. Clin. North Am.* 26:965–1008, 1988.

Index

A

Abscess
  brain, *Nocardia*, 176
  Candida, 177
  cerebral, 57, 172, 183
    after immunosuppression, 173
    MR of, 177
    nocardial, 176
    pyogenic, 172
  epidural, 186, 474
  fungal, 173
  pituitary, 111
    headache in, 111
  pyogenic, 172, 173, 175, 177
    edema in, 175
    with hypoplastic right heart
      syndrome, 174
  subperiosteal, 407
Achondroplastic dwarf: and epidural
      hematoma, 228
Acoustic
  neurofibromatosis, bilateral, 84
  schwannoma (*see* Schwannoma,
      acoustic)
Adenocarcinoma
  colon, metastatic, 5, 9
  distinguished from meningioma, 5
  metastatic, 4, 5, 155
  metastatic, unknown primary, 9
Adenocystic parotid carcinoma, 95
Adenohypophysitis: lymphocytic, 104
Adenoma
  microadenoma (*see* Microadenoma)
  pituitary, 104–106, 110, 115
    amenorrhea in, 112
    carotid artery in, 112
    cerebral arteries in, 114

cystic, 108, 112, 113
    galactorrhea in, 112
    hemianopia in, bitemporal, 112,
      113
    hemorrhage in, 105, 113
    hypothyroidism in, 104
    large, 114
    MR in, 112–113
    necrosis in, 105, 112
    nonsecreting, 114
    pituitary hyperplasia mimicking,
      104
    prolactin in, 112
    in sella turcica, 104
    with suprasellar extension,
      104–105
    visual acuity reduction in, 114,
      123
    visual symptoms in, 131
    voice in, "nasal," 114
Adenopathy: cervical, 458
Adrenoleukodystrophy, 195
Aged
  basilar artery elongation in, 331
  extracerebral fluid spaces in, 224
  scleral plaques, 416
  subarachnoid spaces in, 248
  ventricles in, large lateral, 363
Agenesis (*see* Corpus callosum,
      agenesis)
AIDS
  with encephalitis, 181
  intracranial mass in, 180
  leukoencephalopathy in, 196
  lymphoma in, CNS, 153
  MR in, 181
  with toxoplasmosis, 180
  ventriculitis in, CMV, 167

Air
  contrast studies of auditory canal,
      88
  intracranial, 240, 241
  subarachnoid, 240
Alcoholism, 205
ALS, 267
Alzheimer's disease, 204
Amenorrhea
  in adenoma, pituitary, 112
  in microadenoma, pituitary, 109
Amyloid angiopathy: causing
      intracerebral hemorrhage, 342
Amyotrophic lateral sclerosis, 267
Anesthesia: with nitrous oxide and
      tension pneumocephalus, 241
Aneurysm(s)
  in arteriovenous malformation, 301
  basilar artery, 91, 328, 329
    giant, unruptured, 326
    rupture, 272, 319
    thrombosis of, 324, 325
  "berry," 328
  bone cyst, 95
  carotid artery, 108, 131, 323, 324
    rupture, giant aneurysm, 326
    thrombosis of, 325
  cerebellar artery origin, unruptured,
      322
  cerebral, 325
  cerebral artery, 324
    at genu, 320
    hemorrhage from, 318
    posterior, 320
    rupture, 313
    rupture, hydrocephalus after, 315
  of circulation, posterior, hemorrhage
      from, 319

Aneurysm(s) *(cont.)*
  communicating artery
    hemorrhage from, 317
    hemorrhage from, subarachnoid,
     321
    rupture, 312, 313, 319, 339
    unruptured, 321
  fusiform, with thrombosis, 328
  giant, 326
    as mass lesion, 327
    MR in, 327
  MR of, 324–325
  mycotic, hemorrhage from, 338
  at PICA, hemorrhage, 314
  rupture, parenchymal hematoma
    from, 317
  saccular, with thrombosis, 328
  suprasellar, 106
  thrombosis of, 311
  unruptured, visualization, 320
  vein of Galen, 304, 305, 307
  vertebral artery, 91
Angiography
  of carotid artery stenosis, 337
  of glioma, malignant, 58
  of glomus jugulare tumors, 93
  subclavian, and watershed, 260
Angioma
  cavernous, 308, 309, 310
    hemorrhage in, 311
    MR in, 311
  of cerebellum, venous, 307
  intramedullary cavernous, 473
  vein, 306
Angiopathy: amyloid, causing
    intracerebral hemorrhage, 342
Anomalies *(see* Malformation*)*
Anoxia, 245–296
  cerebral *(see* Cerebral anoxia*)*
  edema due to, 286
  edema with, 291
  in encephalopathy, 288
  after food aspiration, 289
  subacute, 290
  sudden infant death syndrome
    causing, 288
Aphasia
  in aneurysm, giant, 327
  cerebral infarction and, 246, 250
  in encephalitis, herpes, 171
  in glioma, malignant, 47
Aqueduct
  obstruction due to midbrain mass,
    356
  stenosis, 355, 356
    hydrocephalus due to, brain stem
     glioma after, 70
Arachnoid *(see* Cyst, arachnoid*)*
Arachnoiditis, 462, 466
Arcuate eminence, 341
Arm: weakness in angioma, cavernous,
    308
Arnold-Chiari malformation *(see* Chiari
    II malformation*)*
Arteries
  basilar *(see* Basilar artery*)*
  carotid *(see* Carotid artery*)*

cerebellar *(see* Cerebellar artery*)*
cerebral *(see* Cerebral artery*)*
communicating
  aneurysm *(see* Aneurysm,
    communicating artery*)*
  posterior, 319
compromise, MR in, 281
ectatic feeding, in arteriovenous
    malformation, 298
occlusion, "flow void" absence due
    to, 281
signs in cerebral infarction, 280
vertebral *(see* Vertebral artery*)*
Arteriovenous malformation, 298, 303
  abnormal vascular channel tangle,
    299
  aneurysms in, 301
  of brain stem, 310
  calcification in, 302
  diagnosis, differential, 300
  dura, causing cord edema, 473
  hemorrhage from, 301
  infarction in, subacute, 300
  MR in, 299
  rupture, 339
  with thrombosis, 311
Arthritis: rheumatoid, at C1–2, 481
Arthropathy: lumbar facet, 444
Aspergillosis
  ethmoid sinus, 406
  sphenoid sinus, 406
  ventriculitis due to, 166
Aspergillus, 173
Astrocytoma, 45, 82
  anaplastic, 48
    hemiparesis in, 48
    seizures in, 48
  brain stem, 141, 142
  cerebellar, 78
    brain stem compression in, 78,
     79
    cystic, 78, 81
    cystic, mimicking fourth
     ventricular distention, 79
    headache in, 78
    hydrocephalus due to, 365
    hydrocephalus in, 79
    low attenuation, 79
    MRI in, 79
    nystagmus in, 78
    papilledema in, 78
  cerebral lesion with calcification,
    303
  chiasm, 124
  in corpus callosum, 52
  grade 2, 42
    calcification, 57
    headaches in, 42
    MRI of, 63
    seizures in, 42, 63
    temporal lobe, 57
  grade 3, 61
    occipital lesions and, 261
    recurrent, 61
    recurrent, seizures in, 61
  grade 3 thalamic, 49
    after hydrocephalus shunt, 49

  grade 4, 48
    transient ischemic attacks in, 48
  hemorrhage into, 253
  low-grade, 44
    calcification in, 44
    dementia in, 44
    seizures in, 43
  medulla, 99
  pilocytic, 357
  seizures in, 45
  of septum pellucidum, cystic, 120
  spinal cord, 99
    cervical, 468
    thoracic, recurrent, 469
  thalamus, 142
  xanthoastrocytoma, pleomorphic, 56
Ataxia
  Friedreich's, 203
  in glioma, brain stem, 68, 310
  in hemangioblastoma, and gait, 80
  in medulloblastoma, 72
  in pineoblastoma, 142
Atherosclerosis: of basilar artery, 330
Atrophy
  in ataxia, Friedreich's, 203
  cerebral, 204, 208
    in Sturge-Weber syndrome, 207
  in cerebral lesion, 303
  extracerebral fluid spaces in aged
    and, 224
  of lower extremities, 468
  masseter muscle in trigeminal
    schwannoma, 150
  pseudoatrophy, differential diagnosis,
    205
  of tongue in cranial nerve
    schwannoma, 151
  ventricles and, large lateral, in aged,
    363
Auditory canal
  air contrast studies of, 88
  MRI of, 88
  in schwannoma, acoustic, 85, 86,
    87
AVM *(see* Arteriovenous malformation*)*
Axonal injury
  MR in, 235
  shearing, 234

B

Back
  after laminectomy, 466
  pain
    in diastematomyelia, 486
    in disc herniation, 440
    in epidural abscess, 474
    in spinal infection, 475
Bacterial ventriculitis, 166
Basal ganglia *(see* Ganglia, basal*)*
Basilar artery
  aneurysm *(see* Aneurysm, basilar
    artery*)*
  atherosclerosis, 330
  in cerebellar infarction, 277
  ectasia mimicking brain stem mass,
    330

elongation in aged, 331
infarction, 272
mass adjacent to, 329
Basilar impression, 482
Battered child syndrome: and optic
chiasm glioma, 124
Behavioral change: in pineocytoma,
141
Bicep weakness: in cervical disc
herniation, 437
Bladder dysfunction: in disc herniation,
440
Blood, subarachnoid, 312
clot of, 318
Blow-out fracture, 418
Bone
cyst, aneurysmal, 95
deformity at craniocervical junction,
MR in, 482
dysplasia, fibrous, 35
erosion
by acoustic schwannoma,
irregular, 87
near transverse foramen, 460
fragment in optic canal, 419
frontal, fracture, 232
at jugular foramen, 93
occipital
extracranial cyst adjacent to,
393
osteoblastoma, 483
petrous
anatomy, 86
fracture, 238
mass, differential diagnosis, 95
pathology, 86
posterior fossa mass destroying, 94
Brain
abscess, *Nocardia*, 176
contusion, 231
CSF isointense to, 165
growth in children, 353
midbrain (*see* Midbrain)
stem
arteriovenous malformation, 310
astrocytoma, 141, 142
compression in astrocytoma,
cerebellar, 78, 79
compression in medulloblastoma,
75
demyelination, 69
demyelination, MR in, 202
glioma (*see* Glioma, brain stem)
hematoma, 340
hemorrhage, hypertensive, 340
infarction, 69, 270
infarction, MR in, 278
mass, 310
mass, basilar artery ectasia
mimicking, 330
mass, differential diagnosis, 69,
309
mass, low-attenuation, 271
in meningioma, sphenoid wing,
21
metastases, 3
trauma, 271

subdural hematoma along
tentorium and, 217
tumor and angioma, cavernous,
311
tumor resection, aneurysm in, giant,
327
Breast: carcinoma (*see* Carcinoma,
breast)
Bronchogenic carcinoma, metastatic,
54
to cerebellar hemisphere, 276
"Butterfly" tumors, 50

C

Cafe-au-lait spots, 124
Calcification
in arteriovenous malformation, 302
astrocytoma
grade 2, 57
low-grade, 44
in breast carcinoma metastases, 391
cerebellar, 391
with cerebral mass, 303
dentate nuclei and, 341
idiopathic, 341
in dermoid cyst, 121, 144
in diastematomyelia, 486
after encephalitis, perinatal, 169
in ependymoma, 73
falx meningioma, "psammomatous,"
20
at foramen magnum, 322
glioma, 303
low-grade, 44
gyriform, 207
in lung carcinoma, metastatic, 5
in meningioma, 26, 34, 36
differential diagnosis, 36
of optic nerve, 417
in metastases, 10
ocular, 421
oligodendroglioma, 44
orbit (*see* Orbit, calcification)
papilloma, choroid plexus, 99
periventricular, 390
in child, 387
pineal region, 142
sphenoid wing meningioma, 20
suprasellar mass, 125, 145
of synovial cyst, 445
Callosal (*see* Corpus callosum)
Calvaria
in Chiari II malformation, 358
hyperostosis in meningioma, 34
Candida abscess, 177
Candidiasis: after chemotherapy for
germinoma, 177
Carbon monoxide poisoning, 266
causing white matter damage, 201
Carcinoma
breast
meningeal involvement, 12
metastatic (*see* Metastases, breast
carcinoma)
bronchogenic, metastatic, 54
to cerebellar hemisphere, 276

choroid plexus, 139
colon metastatic, 9, 11, 12, 83
gradient echo sequences, 9
kidney, mimicking meningioma,
33
lung
metastatic (*see* Metastases, lung
carcinoma)
small cell, radiotherapy of, white
matter damage after, 201
ovaries (*see* Metastases, ovarian
carcinoma)
parotid, adenocystic, 95
prostate (*see* Metastases, prostate
carcinoma)
Carcinomatosis
leptomeningeal, 2, 11
melanoma in, 15
meningeal, 12
from breast carcinoma metastases,
316
with hydrocephalus,
communicating, 362
Cardiopulmonary arrest
in cerebral anoxia, 286
food aspiration causing, anoxia after,
289
subdural hematoma and, 215
Carotid
artery
in adenoma, pituitary, 112
aneurysm (*see* Aneurysm, carotid
artery)
dolichoectasia, 331
in meningioma, 37
occlusion, watershed infarction
due to, 269
stenosis, angiography of, 337
-cavernous fistula, 399, 410
Caudal regression syndrome: in
myelomeningocele, 485
Cavernous sinus (*see* Sinus, cavernous)
Cavum
septi pellucidi, 384
vergae, 384
Cell(s): germ cell tumors, 140
Cellulitis
orbital, 407
with sinusitis, 407
spinal, with disc infection, 475
Central nervous system (*see*
Lymphoma, CNS)
Cerebellar
angioma, venous, 307
artery
aneurysm at origin of, 322
infarction, 274–275
astrocytoma (*see* Astrocytoma,
cerebellar)
calcification, 391
flocculus, 90
glioma in children, 78
hematoma, 340, 341
hemisphere (*see* Hemisphere,
cerebellar)
hemorrhage, hypertensive,
341

Cerebellar *(cont.)*
  infarction, 276
    MR in, 279
    multifocal, 277
    pitfalls, 277
  mass
    differential diagnosis, 82, 83
    low-attenuation, 276
    metastatic, 83
  metastases, 82
  nodules, differential diagnosis, 155
  tonsils in brain stem glioma, 70
  tumor, cystic
    headache in, 81
    with mural nodule, 81
  vermis in fourth ventricular masses, 77
Cerebellopontine angle
  cistern, 88
    pseudotumor, 90
  cyst of, arachnoid, 373, 374
  glomus jugulare tumor growing into, 92
  lesion, differential diagnosis, 147
  mass, 86
    differential diagnosis, 75, 90
    low-attenuation, 374
  meningioma, cystic, 374
Cerebral
  abscess *(see* Abscess, cerebral)
  aneurysm, 325
  anoxia, 291
    basal ganglia involvement, 287
    diffuse involvement, 286
    MR in, 292
  artery
    in adenoma, pituitary, 114
    aneurysm *(see* Aneurysm, cerebral artery)
    in arteriovenous malformation, 299
    distribution in cerebral infarction, 248
    dolichoectasia, 331
    hypertrophy, 299
    infarction *(see* Infarction, cerebral, artery)
    ischemia due to herniation, 273
    occlusion, cerebral infarction in, 246
    occlusion, "supernormal," 280
    spasm, 315
  atrophy, 204, 208
    in Sturge-Weber syndrome, 207
  chloroma with leukemia, hairy-cell, 234
  complications with AIDS, 181
  contusion, 230, 232
  convexity, lesion extending over, low-attenuation, 370
  cortex
    collapse in dilated ventricular decompression, 367
    glioma invading dura, 53
  edema
    cerebral artery ischemia due to, 273

diffuse, 156–157
  in infant, 289
  metastases provoking, 2
  symmetrical, 286
  after trauma, 236
gunshot wounds, 237
hemiatrophy with hemicranial hypertrophy, 206
hemorrhage, 234
infarction *(see* Infarction, cerebral)
injury, localized, 232
intracerebral *(see* Intracerebral)
lymphoma in immunocompromised patient, 54
mass
  with atrophy, 303
  with bands, 256
  with calcification, 303
  with dural attachment, differential diagnosis, 53
meningioma, 28
metastases *(see* Metastases, cerebral)
nodule(s)
  diagnosis, differential, 3, 154–155
  multiple enhancing, differential diagnosis, 189
  palsy, schizencephaly in, 379
  pseudotumor, 156
  radiotherapy, white matter damage after, 201
  sulci enlargement, 205
  toxoplasmosis, 180
  vascular accident *(see* CVA)
  veins, 59
  white matter in infant, 288
Cerebritis
  before abscess, 172
  in encephalitis, viral, 168
  fungal, 170
  pyogenic, 170
Cerebrospinal fluid
  -containing cysts, 369
  isointense to brain, 165
  rhinorrhea after trauma, 239
  seeding
    by drop metastases, 465
    by fourth ventricle tumors, 76
    in medulloblastoma, 72
  spaces, low attenuation within, 240
  ventricles and, large lateral, 363
Cerebrovascular accident *(see* CVA)
Cervical
  adenopathy, 458
  disc *(see* Disc, cervical)
  myelopathy, 441
Cervicomedullary junction: tumor, 483
Chemodectoma, 92
Chemotherapy
  for germinoma, candidiasis after, 177
  lung carcinoma, metastatic, 10
  of medulloblastoma, leukoencephalopathy after, 195
Chest
  (See also Thoracic)
  radiography in metastatic hypernephroma, 6

Chiari I malformation, 470, 482
Chiari II malformation, 358–359
  after hydrocephalus shunt, 359
  MR in, 359
Chiasm
  astrocytoma, grade 2, 124
  glioma, 128, 415
  optic *(see* Optic chiasm)
Children
  brain growth in, 353
  craniopharyngioma, 120
  ependymoma, 75
  fourth ventricle tumors, 74, 75–76
  glioma
    cerebellar, 78
    hypothalamic, 128
    optic chiasm, 124
  medulloblastoma, 74, 75
  multiple sclerosis, 195
  periventricular calcification, 387
  ventricles in, large lateral, 353
  white matter disorders, 195
Chloroma, 154
  cerebral, with leukemia, hairy-cell, 234
Cholesterol
  cyst, 98
  granuloma, 98
Chondroma
  diagnosis, differential, 94
  skull base, 96
Chondrosarcoma: diagnosis, differential, 94
Chordoma, 96–97
  clivus, 96, 97
  diagnosis, differential, 94
  MRI in, 97
  nasopharyngeal soft tissue in, 97
  parasellar, 96
  skull base, 98
  "T2-weighted" scans, 97
Chorea: Huntington's, 203
Choroid melanoma, 402, 403
Choroid plexus
  carcinoma, 139
  papilloma *(see* Papilloma, choroid plexus)
Cingulate gyrus: in oligodendroglioma, 52
Circle of Willis: structure near, 321
Circulation: posterior, aneurysm of, hemorrhage from, 319
Cistern
  cerebellopontine angle, 88
    pseudotumor, 90
  interpeduncular, mass, 324
  of lamina terminalis, 317
  in meningitis, 165
  quadrigeminal, cysts in, 372
  sylvian, partial volume, 248
Cleft
  in schizencephaly, 380
  transcerebral, in schizencephaly, 379
Clinoid process
  pneumatization of, 321
  prostatic carcinoma metastatic from, 130

Clivus chordoma, 96, 97
Clot: of subarachnoid blood, 318
CMV (see Cytomegalovirus)
CNS (see Lymphoma, CNS)
Colloid cyst
  epidural hematoma and, 229
  of third ventricle, 136, 138
    causing hydrocephalus, 364
Colon
  adenocarcinoma, metastatic, 5, 9
  carcinoma, metastatic, 9, 11, 12
    gradient echo sequences, 9
"Colpocephaly," 382
Coma
  with intraventricular hemorrhage, 345
  in posterior fossa hematoma, 340
  in ventriculitis, 166
Communicating artery (see Artery,
    communicating)
Compromised host (see
    Immunosuppression)
Computed tomography (see CT)
Confusion
  with aging white matter, 198
  in cerebral infarction with
    hemorrhage, 253
  in cerebral injury, localized, 232
  in head trauma with subdural
    hematoma, 216
  in subdural hematoma, 216, 217
Consciousness
  in craniopharyngioma, 120
  in encephalitis, herpes, 170
  impairment in sagittal sinus
    thrombosis, 282
  in meningitis, 164
  in subarachnoid hemorrhage, 312
Conus medullaris
  ependymoma, 462
  tumor, neuroectodermal, 469
Corpus callosum
  absence, 382
  agenesis, 382–383, 384
    headaches in, 382
    microcephaly in, 382
    MR in, 383
  astrocytoma in, 52
  dysgenesis, with pachygyria, 353
  glioblastoma multiforme, 50
  glioma, 50, 51
  injury, shearing, 235
  lipoma, 385
  MRI of, 52
  oligodendroglioma deforming, 52
  splenium
    metastases, 55
    tumor, differential diagnosis, 55
    tumors, diagnosis, differential, 51
Corticospinal tracts: hemispheric
    lesions along, 267
Cranial nerve (see Nerve, cranial)
Craniocervical junction
  bone deformity at, MR in, 482
  cord compression at, 483
  glomus jugulare tumor at, 483
Craniofacial surgery: and
    Dandy-Walker malformation, 360

"Craniolacunae," 358
Craniopharyngioma, 118–119, 120,
    121, 125, 145, 415
  atypical, 119
    diabetes insipidus and, 119
    growth arrest in, 119
    headache in, temporal, 119
    hemianopia in, bitemporal, 119
  in child, 120
  consciousness in, 120
  cystic, 119
  MR in, 126
  parasellar extension, 118
  retrosellar extension, 118
  solid, 119
Craniotomy: and epidural hematoma,
    229
Cranium
  radiotherapy, meningioma after, 29
  transcranial mass, differential
    diagnosis, 25
Cribriform plate: fracture, 239
CSF (see Cerebrospinal fluid)
CT
  myelography, 462
  in newborn, 382
CVA, 300, 301, 303
  cerebral infarction and, 247, 253,
    256
    mass effect, 249
  hemisphere infarction after, 264
  with hemorrhage, central, 343
  in intracerebral hematoma, 338
  with intracerebral hemorrhage,
    334
  in malignant glioma, 58
  in "Moya Moya" syndrome, 337
  with subdural hematoma, isodense,
    219
  Wallerian degeneration after, 267
CVM, 301
Cyst(s), 351–395
  arachnoid, 147, 370
    cerebellopontine angle, 373, 374
    MR in, 369
    posterior fossa, 372
    suprasellar, 371
    suprasellar, obstructing third
      ventricle, 356
    supratentorial, 368
  in astrocytoma, cerebellar, 78, 81
    mimicking fourth ventricle
      distention, 79
  bone, aneurysmal, 95
  in cerebellar tumor with mural
    nodules, 81
  cholesterol, 98
  colloid, and epidural hematoma,
    229
  CSF-containing, 369
  Dandy-Walker, shunting of, 366
  dermoid, 121, 144, 145
    calcification in, 121, 144
    MR of, 148
    nystagmus in, 144
    orbital mass, 405
    parasellar, 145

  parasellar, rupture, causing
    intraventricular fat, 240
  Parinaud's syndrome in, 144
  seizures in, 144
  suprasellar, 145
  T1-shortening within, 148
  "T2-weighted," 148
  epidermoid, 98, 144, 146, 147
    facial nerve paresis in, 146
    memory loss in, 146
    MR of, 149
    of sacral canal, 457, 467
    suprasellar, 371
    tic douloureux in, 146
  extracranial, adjacent to occipital
    bone in infant, 393
  in glioma, 56
    brain stem, 68
  in hemangioblastoma, 80
  hematic, 405
  in lung carcinoma, metastatic
    squamous cell, 4
  meningioma and, 22, 28
  midline, between lateral ventricles,
    384
  pituitary, 111, 121
  porencephalic, 174, 376
  in quadrigeminal cistern, 372
  "racemose," 374
  sacral root sleeve, 467
  in schwannoma, acoustic, 85, 87
  in septum pellucidum, 384
  suprasellar, with hydrocephalus, 356
  synovial, 445
    calcification in, 445
  of third ventricle, colloid, 136, 138
    causing hydrocephalus, 364
Cystic
  adenoma, pituitary, 108, 112, 113
  astrocytoma of septum pellucidum,
    120
  cerebellar tumor (see Cerebellar
    tumor, cystic)
  craniopharyngioma, 119
  encephalomalacia, 375
  ependymoma, 60
  glioblastoma multiforme, 242
  glioma, MRI of, 60
  hygroma, 393
  meningioma of cerebellopontine
    angle, 374
  oligodendroglioma, 56
  temporal lobe tumor, differential
    diagnosis, 57
Cysticercosis, 10, 178–179, 357
  intraventricular, 178
  parenchymal, 178
Cytomegalovirus
  congenital, 387
  ventriculitis, 181
  ventriculitis with AIDS, 167

D

Dandy-Walker malformation, 360
  cyst in, shunting of, 366
  MRI in, 361

Death, sudden infant death syndrome, 287
  anoxia due to, 288
Degenerative diseases, 161–212
Dementia
  in astrocytoma, low-grade, 44
  in chorea, Huntington's, 203
  "lacunar" infarction in, 265
  with meningioma, 30
Dentate nuclei
  calcification, idiopathic, 341
  high attenuation near, 341
Dermoid cyst (see Cyst, dermoid)
Developmental abnormalities, 351–395
  with supratentorial fluid space enlargement, 354
Developmental delay
  with periventricular calcification, 387
  with periventricular leukomalacia, 293
Diabetes insipidus: and atypical craniopharyngioma, 119
Diabetes mellitus
  "lacunar" infarction and, 265
  mucormycosis in, 173
Diastematomyelia, 484, 486
  MR in, 487
Diplegia: spastic, with periventricular leukomalacia, 293
Diploic space, 15
Diplopia
  cerebral edema in, 236
  in cerebral infarction, 280
  in glioma, brain stem, 310
  in ophthalmopathy, thyroid, 409
  in orbital pseudotumor, painful, 408
  painful, in parasellar mass, 131
  in parasellar mass, 323
Disc, 425–452
  central herniation, 427, 431
    at C4–5 level, 471
  central/lateral herniation, 427, 428
  cervical, herniation, 436
    intrathecal contrast in, 437
    MR in, 438–439
  C3–4 herniation, 439
    on spondylosis, 441
  C4–5 herniation, 436
  C5–6 herniation, 437
  C6–7 herniation, 436, 437, 439
  degeneration, reactive changes secondary to, 476
  disease, 425
  foraminal herniation, 435
  fragment, herniated, 433
    free, 428
  herniation, 434
    into C4–5 foramen, 443
    differentiation between residual and recurrent, 449
  infection with cellulitis, 475
  lateral herniation, 429, 431
  L3–4 herniation, 435
  lumbar
    bulge, 426

herniation, 426
herniation, eccentric, 428
herniation involving central canal, 427
herniation involving lateral recess, 428
herniation, lateral, 429
herniation, MR in, 430–431
posterolateral herniation, 429
thoracic, herniation, 440
vs. scar, MR in, 449
Discitis
  MR in, 477
  with septicemia, 476
Disequilibrium: in dentate nuclei high attenuation, 341
Diskectomy: lumbar, 448
Diverticula: ventricular, hydrocephalus in, 366
Dolichoectasia, 331
Down's syndrome: spinal canal stenosis in, 482
Drowning: near drowning, 287, 292
Drusen, 416
Dumbbell
  lesion of intervertebral foramen, 459
  schwannoma, 461
Dura
  in achondroplasia, 228
  arteriovenous malformation causing cord edema, 473
  attachment to cerebral mass, differential diagnosis, 53
  cerebral cortex glioma invading, 53
  in diastematomyelia, 486
  ectasia in Marfan's syndrome, 457
  after head trauma, 157
  intradural (see Intradural)
  mass, differential diagnosis, 33
  in meningioma, 22
  in metastases, 11, 24, 28
    "en plaque," 11
  thickening, 15
Dural sinus(es)
  in newborn, 199
  thrombosis, MR in, 285
  after trauma, 157
Dwarfism
  achondroplastic, and epidural hematoma, 228
  pituitary, 117
Dyke-Davidoff-Masson syndrome, 206
Dysgenesis: corpus callosum, with pachygyria, 353
Dysplasia: bone, fibrous, 35
Dysraphism: spinal, 485

E

Ectasia
  aneurysmal, of carotid artery, 323
  basilar artery, mimicking brain stem mass, 330
  dolichoectasia, 331
  dura, in Marfan's syndrome, 457
Edema
  with anoxia, 291

anoxia causing, 286
cerebral (see Cerebral edema)
of encephalitis, 289
of frontal meningioma, inferior, 25
in glioblastoma, 49, 175
in glioblastoma multiforme, 46
of hemispheres, differential diagnosis, 156
hemorrhage after trauma and, 231
in intracerebral hemorrhage, 334
meningioma, falx, 37
optic disc, 416
orbit
  in infection, 407
  mass, 405
  pain of, 408
parasagittal, 282
periventricular, in hydrocephalus, 345, 364, 365
in pyogenic abscess, 175
in sphenoid wing meningioma, 20
spinal cord, due to dural arteriovenous malformation, 473
in toxoplasmosis with AIDS, 180
Elderly (see Aged)
Embolic infarction, 263
Embolism: saddle, in basilar artery, 280
Empty sella syndrome, 116–117
  headache in, 116
  intrathecal contrast study, 116
"Empty triangle" sign: differential diagnosis, 284
Empyema, subdural, 182
  adjacent to tentorium, 183
  differentiated from subdural effusion, 182
  mastoiditis causing, 183
  multiple, 183
Encephalitis
  with cysticercosis, 179
  edema of, 289
  herpes, 170
    hemorrhage in, 171
    MR of, 171
    "T2-weighted" scan, 171
    type 1, 170
    type 2, 168, 289
    type 2, in newborn, 169
  HIV, 181
  perinatal, calcification after, 169
  viral, 168–169
Encephalocele
  basal, 392
  occipital region, 393
Encephalomalacia: cystic, 375
Encephalomyelitis
  acute disseminated, 194
  corpus callosum in, 55
Encephalopathy
  anoxic, 288
  uremic, 156
Endocarditis: bacterial, in cerebral infarction, 280
Ependymal
  involvement by inflammatory processes, 181
  metastases, 13

Ependymoma, 73, 74
  calcification in, 73
  in child, 75
  conus medullaris, 462
  cystic, 60
  fourth ventricle in, 74, 465
  from fourth ventricle, 73
  headache in, 73
  hydrocephalus in, 73
  posterior fossa, 60
  vomiting in, 73
Epidermoid cyst (see Cyst, epidermoid)
Epidural
  abscess, 186, 474
  density near vertebral body, 433
  fat, 431
  hematoma (see Hematoma, epidural)
  lesions, dense, 227
  mass in spinal canal, 434
  metastases, 11, 434
  myeloma, T7, 455
  neuroblastoma, 455, 456
  tumors, 455
    MR in, 456
  veins, 433
    normal, 433
Esthesioblastoma, 114
Ethmoid sinus (see Sinus, ethmoid)
Extracerebral fluid spaces: in aged, 224
Extremities
  lower, atrophy, 468
  upper, weakness in peridural
    abscess, 474
Eye (see Ocular)

F

Face
  craniofacial surgery and
    Dandy-Walker malformation,
    360
  hemangioma, 207
  nerve paresis in epidermoid cyst,
    146
  numbness in schwannoma, acoustic,
    85, 86
  pain in meningioma, 32
  paresis (see Paresis, facial)
  sensation diminished in trigeminal
    schwannoma, 150
Falx
  glioblastoma invading, 53
  mass adjacent to, differential
    diagnosis, 24
  meningioma (see Meningioma, falx)
  ossification in, 385
Fat
  epidural, 431
  intraventricular, due to paraseller
    dermoid cyst, 240
  paraspinal, 431
Fever
  in adenocarcinoma, metastatic, 155
  in encephalitis, herpes, 170, 171
  in meningitis, 163
  in orbital infection, 407
  in skull base infection, 187

Fibrosarcoma: of ethmoid sinus, 406
Fibrosis: lumbar, 448
Fistula: carotid-cavernous, 399, 410
Flocculus: normal, 90
Fluid collection (see Subdural fluid
    collection)
Food aspiration: causing
    cardiopulmonary arrest and
    anoxia, 289
Foramen(ina)
  C4–5, disc herniation into, 443
  intervertebral
    dumbbell lesion, 459
    mass, 435
  jugular, bone at, 93
  L5–S1, osteophyte into, 443
  magnum
    calcification at, 322
    meningioma, 91
  of Monro
    lesions at, differential diagnosis,
      137
    lesions at, MR in, 138
    obstructed by suprasellar mass,
      120
    obstruction in ventriculitis with
      aspergillosis, 166
  neurofibroma at C3–4, 461
  stenosis, 443
    at C5–6, 442
  transverse, bone erosion near, 460
Foreign body
  in eye, metallic, 421
  glass lacerating orbit, 420
  orbital fracture due to, 419
Fossa
  posterior (see Posterior fossa)
Fourth ventricle (see Ventricle, fourth)
Fracture
  cribriform plate, 239
  ethmoid sinus, 239
  frontal bone, 232
  odontoid, 480
  orbit, 419
    blow-out, 418
    foreign body of wood causing, 419
  petrous bone, 238
  skull, 238
    basal, 238
    basal, pneumocephalus due to,
      240
    with cerebral injury, localized,
      232
    comminuted, 237
    depressed, 238
    with epidural abscess, 186
    epidural lesions in, dense, 227
    occipital, bifrontal hematomas in,
      230
    sagittal sinus thrombosis in, 282
  vertebra, 478, 479
Friedreich's ataxia, 203
Frontal bone: fracture, 232
Frontal lobe
  hematoma, 339
  injury, 232
  sarcoma invading, meningeal, 53

Frontal meningioma: inferior, 25
Fungal
  abscess, 173
    brain, 176
  cerebritis, 170
  infection, 176
  meningitis, 165
  sinusitis, 406
  ventriculitis, 166

G

Gait
  ataxic, in hemangioblastoma, 80
  spastic, in epidural abscess, 474
Galactorrhea
  in adenoma, pituitary, 112
  in microadenoma, pituitary, 109
Galen (see Vein of Galen)
Ganglion(a)
  basal
    involvement in cerebral anoxia,
      287
    low-attenuation lesions, 266
  hemorrhage, 333
Gas: in intracranial abscess, 186
Gaze: upward, paresis in brain stem
    astrocytoma, 141
Germ cell tumors, 140
Germinal matrix hemorrhage: in
    prematurity, 344
Germinoma, 123
  with hypothyroidism, 123
  MR in, 126
  pineal, 122, 140, 143
  school performance in, 123
    visual acuity reduction in, 123
  suprasellar, 122, 129
    chemotherapy for, candidiasis
      after, 177
  with hemorrhage, 126
  visual acuity reduction in, 122
Glass: lacerating orbit, 420
Glioblastoma, 46, 47, 49
  arteriovenous malformation and, 300
  edema in, 49, 175
  falx invaded by, 53
  with hemianopia, 58
  hemorrhage into, 58
  hemorrhagic, 60
    "T2-weighted" scan, 60
  midhemisphere, 174
  multiforme, 46, 50, 51, 54, 55
    with cerebral lesions, 256
    cystic, 242
    edema in, 46
    temporal lobe, 57
  septum pellucidum, 137
  stroke in, 47
Glioma(s), 41–65
  brain stem, 68, 69, 310
    ataxia in, 68
    contrast enhancement, 68
    cyst in, 68
    high-intensity, 71
    hydrocephalus in, 68
    MR, 68

Glioma(s) *(cont.)*
    MR, "T1-weighted" scans, 70
    MR, "T2-weighted" scans, 71
    calcification, 303
    cavitating, rupture of, 46
    cerebellar, in children, 78
    chiasm, 128, 415
    corpus callosum, 50, 51
    cyst in, 56
        MRI of, 60
    ependymal seeding, 13
    hemorrhage into, 58
    hemorrhagic, MRI of, 60
    high-grade, 46, 47
        atypical, 48
        MR, 49
        subependymal, 62
    hypothalamic, 107, 128, 129, 145
    low-grade, 42, 43
        calcification, 44
        low attenuation, 42
        MR in, 45
        well-defined margins, 43
    malignant, 47, 50, 51
        angiography of, 58
        aphasia in, 47
        hemiparesis in, 47
        hemorrhage into, 58, 343
        high attenuation, homogenous
            precontrast, 51
        MR of, 61
    medulla, 99
    metastases resembling, 4
    midline, MR of, 52
    mimicking cerebral infarction, 43
    MR in, 129
    multicentric, 4
    optic, 127
        chiasm, 124, 125
        hydrocephalus due to, 364
        MR in, 127
        nerve, 412, 413, 417
        nerve, intracranial extension,
            415
    subependymal spread, 13
    temporal lobe, 42, 63
        MRI of, 63
Glomus jugulare tumors, 92–93
    angiography of, 93
    at craniocervical junction, 483
    growing into cerebellopontine angle,
        92
    hyperreflexia in, 94
    MR of, 93
    neck pain in, 94
    nerve palsy in, cranial, 94
    tongue weakness in, 92
Granuloma: cholesterol, 98
Graves' disease, 409
Gray matter
    heterotopia, 380, 381, 390
    in meningioma, 27
Growth
    arrest in craniopharyngioma, 119
    brain, in children, 353
Gunshot wounds: cerebral, 237
Gyriform calcification, 207

Gyrus(i)
    anatomy, 146
    in arteriovenous malformation, 300
    in cerebral metastases, 2
    cingulate, in oligodendroglioma, 52
    enhancement in subacute anoxia,
        290

H

Hamartoma: in tuberous sclerosis,
    388
Hand: numbness in epidural abscess,
    474
Hanging: near hanging, 292
Head
    enlargement in choroid plexus
        papilloma, 139
    large circumference in
        Dandy-Walker malformation,
        361
    large size
        in encephalomalacia, cystic, 375
        ventricles in, 353
    trauma, 157
        aneurysm after, vein of Galen, 305
        "empty triangle" sign in, 284
        epidural abscess after, 186
        sclerosis and, tuberous, 386
Headache
    in aneurysm of communicating
        artery, 317
    in arachnoid cyst, 371
    in astrocytoma, 42
        brain stem, 141
        cerebellar, 78
    in cerebellar tumor, cystic, 81
    in cerebral abscess, 172, 173
    in corpus callosum agenesis, 382
    in dural sinus thrombosis, 285
    in empty sella syndrome, 116
    in ependymoma, 73
    in germinoma, pineal, 140
    in hypertension, malignant, 157
    in intracerebral hematoma, 339
    migraine in infarction, 261
    occipital, in posterior fossa mass, 94
    in pineoblastoma, 142
    in pituitary abscess, 111
    in posterior fossa hematoma, 340
    in pseudotumor cerebri, 156
    in skull base infection, 187
    in subarachnoid hemorrhage, 312
    in subdural hematoma, 218
        isodense, 219
    temporal, in craniopharyngioma,
        119
    in third ventricle colloid cyst, 136
    in ventricular shunting, 367
Hearing loss: in schwannoma,
    acoustic, 84, 85, 86, 87, 88, 89
Heart
    cardiopulmonary arrest *(see*
        Cardiopulmonary arrest)
    failure, congestive, in aneurysm of
        vein of Galen, 304

hypoplastic right heart syndrome in
    pyogenic abscess, 174
surgery, watershed infarction after,
    269
Hemangioblastoma, 80, 81, 82
    ataxic gait in, 80
    cystic, 80
    MR in, 80
Hemangioma, 308, 309, 310
    (See also Angioma, cavernous)
    cavernous, multiple, 10
    facial, 207
    orbital, 398
    temporal lobe, cavernous, 63
    vertebra, 454
Hematic cyst, 405
Hematoma
    brain stem, 340
    cerebellar, 340, 341
    cerebral infarction with hemorrhage
        mimicking, 253
    epidural, 226
        atypical, 228
        isodense components, 229
        posterior fossa, 227
    frontal lobe, 339
    hemisphere, 332, 339
    intracerebral, 230, 332–333
        atypical, 338–339
        midhemispheric, large, 333
        oxidation of, 335
    intramural, dissecting, 281
    parenchymal, from aneurysm
        rupture, 317
    parietal, 6
    posterior fossa, 340
    resolving, 342
        spontaneous, 343
    subdural, 234, 291, 367
        acute, 214, 219
        acute, MR in, 215
        along tentorium, 217
        bilateral, 220
        chronic, 222, 225, 242, 370
        chronic, along tentorium, 277
        chronic, bifrontal, 221
        chronic, MR in, 223
        density, 222
        interhemispheric, 216
        isodense, 219
        mixed attenuation, 218
        morphology, 222
        MR in, 221
        "parasagittal parentheses" in,
            220
        pneumocephalus after, tension,
            241
        in posterior fossa, 221
        rebleeding in, 218
        small, 221
        subacute, 219
        symmetrical, 221
    subperiosteal, 405
Hemaniopia
    bitemporal
        in adenoma, pituitary, 112, 113
        in carotid artery aneurysm, 108

in craniopharyngioma, atypical, 119
in suprasellar mass, 106
with glioblastoma, 58
in meningioma, 33
Hemiatrophy: cerebral, with hemicranial hypertrophy, 206
Hemicranial hypertrophy: with cerebral hemiatrophy, 206
Hemifacial spasm: in cranial nerve syndromes, 346
Hemiparesis
 in astrocytoma, anaplastic, 48
 in brain stem infarction, 270, 278
 in cerebral abscess, 172
 in cerebral infarction, 247, 250, 254, 280
  with hemorrhage, 253
 in encephalomyelitis, 194
 in glioma, malignant, 47
 in hematoma
  intracerebral, 332
  subdural, 214, 222
 in lymphoma, CNS, 152, 153
 with meningioma, 28, 29
 in meningitis, 163
 in multiple sclerosis, 191, 192
Hemiplegia: in hypernephroma, metastatic, 7
Hemisphere(s)
 cerebellar
  cerebellar infarction, 276
  metastatic bronchogenic carcinoma to, 276
  compression in subdural hematoma, 218
  edema, differential diagnosis, 156
  hematoma, 332, 339
  hemorrhage in "Moya Moya" syndrome, 337
  hypoplasia in Dandy-Walker malformation, 360
  infarction, 264
  intrahemispheric infarct, 337
  masses
   along corticospinal tracts, 267
   diagnosis, differential, 54
   midhemisphere mass, differential diagnosis, 174
Hemodialysis: cerebral infarction and, 252
Hemophilus influenzae: meningitis due to, 162, 182
Hemorrhage, 297–350
 in adenoma, pituitary, 113
 aneurysm
  cerebral artery, 318
  of circulation, posterior, 319
  communicating artery, 317
  mycotic, 338
  at PICA, 314
 in angioma, cavernous, 311
 from arteriovenous malformation, 301
 into astrocytoma, 253
 in brain stem, hypertensive, 340
 central, 343

cerebellar, hypertensive, 341
cerebral, 234
 with cerebral infarction, 253
  cerebral artery, 253
  ischemic, 252
  MR in, 251
cerebral metastases, 6
in encephalitis, herpes, 171
ganglionic, 333
germinal matrix, in prematurity, 344
in germinoma, suprasellar, 126
into glioblastoma, 58
into glioma, 58
 malignant, 58, 343
hemisphere, in "Moya Moya" syndrome, 337
hypernephroma, metastatic, 6, 333
interhemispheric, and patent sagittal sinus, 284
intracerebral, 7, 231, 318, 332
 amyloid angiopathy causing, 342
 MR in, 334, 335
 post-traumatic delayed, 233
 spontaneous, 333
 subacute, 335
intraocular, 420
intraventricular, 315, 345
in lung carcinoma, metastatic, 5
into melanoma, metastatic, 338
in meningioma, 28
in metastases, 6
 evolution of, 7
old, MR of, 336
ovarian carcinoma, metastatic, 6
parasagittal, 282
"petechial," 250
in pituitary adenoma, 105
post-traumatic, characteristic locations, 231
rapidly worsening, differential diagnosis, 7
subarachnoid, 217, 312, 318
 from aneurysm of communicating artery, 321
 cerebral injury and, localized, 232
 complications, 315
 contrast enhancement after, 12
 hydrocephalus after, 315, 362
 MR, 314
 subacute, 316
 subtle, 313
 of undetermined origin, 314
 subdural, 223
 into vitreous body, 420
Hemorrhagic
 glioblastoma, 60
  "T2-weighted" scan, 60
 glioma, MRI of, 60
Hemosiderin-laden macrophages, 336
Herniation
 cerebral artery ischemia due to, 273
 disc (see under Disc)
 subfalcial, 4
 in CNS lymphoma, 153
Herpes encephalitis (see Encephalitis, herpes)

Heterotopia: gray matter, 380, 381, 390
Histiocytosis X: orbit in, 401
Histoplasmosis, 176
 diagnosis, differential, 3
HIV encephalitis, 181
Holoprosencephaly, 354
Huntington's chorea, 203
Hydranencephaly, 354
Hydrocephalus, 351–395
 acute, in metastatic ovarian carcinoma, 6
 after aneurysm of cerebral artery rupture, 315
 in aneurysm of vein of Galen, 304
 aqueductal stenosis in, 355
 in astrocytoma, cerebellar, 79
 cerebral artery infarction from, 273
 communicating
  in adults, 362
  in aged, 363
  in infant, 352
  in meningeal carcinomatosis, 12
  with schwannoma, acoustic, 362
  after subarachnoid hemorrhage, 362
  subarachnoid space and, 316
 with cysticercosis, intraventricular, 178
 in cysts, colloid, 136
 Dandy-Walker malformation in, 360
 edema due to, periventricular, 345
 in ependymoma, 73
 in germinoma, pineal, 140, 143
 in glioma, brain stem, 68, 70, 72
 glioma causing, optic, 364
 in meningitis, 162
 MR in, 365
 normal pressure, 363
 periventricular edema in, 364
 periventricular edema causing, 365
 in posterior fossa arachnoid cyst, 372
 schwannoma causing, acoustic, 365
 shunt in
  astrocytoma after, 49
  brain stem glioma after, 70, 72
  Chiari II malformation and, 358
  Chari II malformation after, 359
  subdural hematoma and, 215
  ventriculitis after, 166
 after subarachnoid hemorrhage, 315
 with suprasellar cyst, 356
 of third ventricle, 356
 third ventricle colloid cyst causing, 364
 ventricular diverticula in, 366
Hygroma
 cystic, 393
 subdural, 224, 225
  bifrontal, 224
Hyperemia: tentorial, with sagittal sinus thrombosis, 185
Hyperkinesia: in white matter disorders in children, 195
Hypernephroma: metastatic (see Metastases, hypernephroma)

Hyperostosis
    calvarial, in meningioma, 34
    with meningioma, 35
Hyperplasia: pituitary, 104
Hyperreflexia
    in cord compression, 483
    in glomus jugulare tumor, 94
Hypertension
    in dentate nuclei high attenuation, 341
    intracranial, benign, 156
    "lacunar" infarction and, 265
    malignant, 157
        in intracerebral hematoma, 332
Hypertensive hemorrhage
    in brain stem, 340
    cerebellar, 341
Hypertrophy
    cerebral artery, 299
    hemicranial, with cerebral hemiatrophy, 206
Hypoglossal schwannoma, 151
Hypoplasia
    hemisphere, in Dandy-Walker malformation, 360
    vermian, in Dandy-Walker malformation, 360
Hypoplastic right heart syndrome: in pyogenic abscess, 174
Hypotension: in cerebral anoxia, 286
Hypothalamus
    glioma, 107, 128, 129, 145
    mass, MR of, 129
    metastases to, 107
Hypothyroidism
    with germinoma, 123
    in pituitary adenoma, 104

I

Imaging, magnetic resonance (see MR)
Immunoblastic lymphoma, 152
Immunocompromised patients: lymphoma of, cerebral, 54
Immunosuppression
    cerebral abscess in, 173
    infection after, opportunistic, 176
Infant
    cerebral edema, 289
    cerebral white matter, 288
    extracranial cyst adjacent to occipital bone, 393
    hydrocephalus, communicating, 352
    panencephalitis in, 169
    stroke, late sequelae, 206
    sudden infant death syndrome, 287
        anoxia due to, 288
    ventricles of, large, 291
Infarction, 245-296
    basilar artery, 272
    brain stem, 69, 270
        MR in, 278
    cerebellar (see Cerebellar infarction)
    cerebral, 164
        arterial signs in, 280
        artery, anterior, 258
        artery, with hemorrhage, 253

artery, from hydrocephalus, 273
artery, occipital lesion and, 261
artery, old, 257
artery, posterior, 259
contrast enhancement, generalized, 254
contrast enhancement, localized, 255
after CVA, 256
early, cerebral artery distribution, 248
early, MR in, 247
evolution of scan findings, 246
glioma mimicking, 43
hemorrhage in (see Hemorrhage, with cerebral infarction)
heterogenous attenuation, 250
ischemic, with hemorrhage, 252
low attenuation, 246
mass effect, 246, 249, 250
multiple superficial, 263
old, 255, 257
with sagittal sinus thrombosis, 283
small, 249
subacute, hemorrhage in, MR in, 251
watershed, 255
watershed, cortical, 262, 263
watershed, posterior cortical, location, 260
    cortical venous, 282
    embolic, 263
    hemisphere, 264
    intrahemispheric, 337
    lacunar, 14, 266
        multiple, 265
    PICA, 279
    pseudoinfarction, 248
    SCA, 279
    subacute, 300
    vasospasm causing, 315
    venous, 7
    watershed
        cerebral (see cerebral, watershed above)
        cortical, 269
        intrahemispheric, 268
        recent, MR in, 269
        white matter, 268
Infection
    fungal, 176
    opportunistic, 176
    skull base, 187
Inflammatory diseases, 161-212
Infundibulum: metastases to, 107
Interhemispheric subdural hematoma, 216
Intervertebral
    disc (see Disc)
    foramen (see Foramen, intervertebral)
Intracerebral
    hematoma (see Hematoma, intracerebral)
    hemorrhage (see Hemorrhage, intracerebral)
Intracranial
    air, 240, 241

aneurysm, giant, 327
extension
    of optic nerve glioma, 415
    of parapharyngeal rhabdomyosarcoma, 25
hypertension, benign, 156
lymphoma, 33
mass in AIDS, 180
melanoma, 24
pressure
    in encephalopathy, 156
    increase from hydrocephalus, 273
sedimentation visualization, 167
Intradural
    mass, lumbar, 462
    meningioma, 463
    metastases, 464, 466
        MR in, 465
    schwannoma, 462
    tumors, MR in, 463
Intrahemispheric infarct, 337
Intramedullary masses, 468
    MR in, 469
Intrasellar mass, 123
Intraventricular
    cysticercosis, 178
    fat due to parasellar dermoid cyst, 240
    hemorrhage, 315, 345
    mass, differential diagnosis, 59
    meningioma, 59
    metastases, 13, 390
Ischemia
    of cerebral artery, due to herniation, 273
    transient ischemic attacks
        in arterial compromise, 281
        in astrocytoma, grade 4, 48
        white matter aging in, 200
Ischemic
    cerebral infarction with hemorrhage, 252
    leukoencephalopathy, 200

J

Jugular foramen: bone at, 93

K

Kidney
    carcinoma mimicking meningioma, 33
    transplant (see Transplantation, kidney)

L

Lacunar infarction, 14, 266
    multiple, 265
Lamina terminalis: cistern of, 317
Lamination: in thrombosed aneurysms, 325
Laminectomy
    infection after, 475
    lumbar, 448
    pain after, 449, 466

Laughing spells: in hypothalamic
glioma, 128
Leg
in meningioma, intradural, 463
numbness in disc herniation, 440
pain
in foraminal stenosis, 443
in lumbar disc herniation, 429
weakness with spinal cord tethering,
484
Lenticular nucleus, 287
Leptomeningeal carcinomatosis, 2, 11
melanoma in, 15
Leukemia, 12, 154
hairy-cell, with cerebral chloroma,
234
Leukoencephalopathy, 201
with AIDS, 196
corpus callosum in, 55
ischemic, 200
methotrexate, 195
necrotizing
disseminated, 195
in meningioma, 29
progressive multifocal, 180, 196, 198
MR in, 197
Leukomalacia: periventricular, MR in,
293
Lipid
content of dermoid cysts, 148
in corpus callosum lipoma, 385
in subarachnoid space, 240
Lipoma
corpus callosum, 385
in quadrigeminal cistern, 372
Lissencephaly: with pachygyria, 378
Lordosis: in spinal infection, 475
"Lückenschädel skull," 358
Lumbar
disc (see Disc, lumbar)
diskectomy, 448
facet arthropathy, 444
fibrosis, 448
flexion limitation in spinal infection,
475
intradural mass, 462
laminectomy, 448
postoperative scans, 448
Lumbosacral nerve roots: "clumping"
of, 466
Lung
carcinoma (see Metastases, lung
carcinoma)
infiltrates in metastatic
adenocarcinoma, 155
resection for histoplasmosis, 176
tuberculosis and tentorium
thickening, 184
Lymphangioma: orbital, 399
Lymphocytic adenohypophysitis, 104
Lymphoma
cerebral, in immunocompromised
patient, 54
CNS, 55, 62, 154, 155
in AIDS, 153
hemisphere involvement, 152
lobar lesions, 153

immunoblastic, 152
intracranial, 33
meningeal, 12
orbit, 410
systemic
with brain abscess, Nocardia, 176
involving cavernous sinus, 130
subependymal, 62
vertebra, L5, 454

M

Machiafava-Bignami syndrome, 55
Macrophages: hemosiderin-laden, 336
Magnetic resonance (see MR)
Malformation(s)
arteriovenous (see Arteriovenous
malformation)
Chiari I, 470, 482
Chiari II (see Chiari II malformation)
Dandy-Walker (see Dandy-Walker
malformation)
spine, 453–491
venous, MR in, 307
Malnutrition: due to psychiatric
disorder, 205
Marfan's syndrome: dural ectasia in,
457
Mastoiditis
chronic, 187
empyema due to, subdural, 183
pyogenic pachymeningitis due to,
185
Meckel's caves, 110
in germinoma, suprasellar, 122
Medulla
astrocytoma, 99
glioma, 99
Medulloblastoma, 72, 83
ataxia in, 72
brain stem compression in, 75
cerebrospinal fluid seeding in, 72
in child, 74, 75
chemotherapy of,
leukoencephalopathy after, 195
contrast enhancement, 72
fourth ventricle, 76
fourth ventricular obstruction in, 72
hemispheric, 83
meninges in, 76
meningioma after, 29
nystagmus in, 72
Medullomyoblastoma, 77
Megalencephaly, 353
Melanin, 8, 9
Melanoma
choroidal, 402, 403
intracranial, 24
in leptomeningeal carcinomatosis,
15
meningeal involvement, 12
metastatic, 14, 15, 309
hemorrhage into, 338
mimicking meningioma, 33
preconstrast attenuation values, 24
primary, 24
Melanomatosis: meningeal, 15

Memory loss
in encephalitis, herpes, 171
in epidermoid cyst, 146
Meningeal
carcinomatosis (see Carcinomatosis,
meningeal)
disease, MR, 12
inflammation, 164
involvement by inflammatory
processes, 181
lymphoma, 12
melanomatosis, 15
metastases, 12, 15
MR, 15
sarcoma invading frontal lobe, 53
Meninges
in medulloblastoma, 76
tumor, 76
Meningioma(s), 19–39, 131
adenocarcinoma distinguished from,
5
aggressive, 28, 30
"angioblastic," 28
atypical, 28
bilateral frontal convexity, 21
calcification in, 26, 34, 36
differential diagnosis, 36
cerebellopontine angle, cystic, 374
cerebral, 28
cerebral metastases mimicking, 2
"comma" shape, 30, 31
contrast enhancement, intense,
uniform, 21
at C2–3, 459
cyst and, 22
with dementia, 30
diagnosis, differential, 24
dural metastases resembling, 11
"en plaque," 22
convexity, 34
facial pain in, 32
falx, 20, 37
calcification, "psammomatous,"
20
diagnosis, differential, 51
foramen magnum, 91, 322
frontal, inferior, 25
hemianopia in, 33
with hemiparesis, 28, 29
high attenuation, homogenous
precontrast, 20
with hyperostosis, 35
incidence, 20
intradural, 463
intraventricular, 59
isointense, 22
leukoencephalopathy in, necrotizing,
29
low-attenuation, nonenhancing, 28
margins, 20
medulloblastoma before, 29
metastases mimicking, 24
MR
anatomical relationships defined
by, 27
contrast enhancement, 22
"flow void," 23

Meningioma(s) *(cont.)*
    homogenous signal intensity, 22
    inhomogeneity, 22
    spin-echo, 37
    of vascular involvement, 37
    vascularity, 23
    optic nerve
      calcification, 417
      sheath, 413
    papillary, 28
    parasellar, 37
    plaque-like components, 30
    posterior convexity, 27
      contrast enhancement, 27
    posterior fossa, 31, 32
    prostate carcinoma mimicking,
      metastatic, 33
    "pseudo-capsule," 22
    after radiotherapy, 29
    rapid growth, 29
    recurrence, 28, 184
    retrosellar, 329
      resection, basilar artery infarction
        after, 272
    sarcomatous transformation, 28
    schwannoma mimicking, trigeminal,
      32
    small, 26
      wide window, 26
    sphenoid wing, 20–21, 34, 37
      edema in, 20
    suprasellar, 107
    tentorial origin, 27
    tentorium, 31
      syncope in, 33
    transtentorial, 32
    trigone, 59
    tuberculum, 27
      "T1-weighted" scan, 27
    vein of Galen mass and, 305
    visual acuity decrease in, 131
    white matter in, 29
Meningitis
    fungal, 165
    granulomatous, 165
    after head trauma, 239
    Hemophilus influenzae causing,
      162, 182
    hydrocephalus in, communicating,
      362
    meningococcal, 162
    MR in, 163, 165
    nonspecific, 163, 164
    parenchymal enhancement in,
      164
    pneumococcal, 164
    recurrent, 239
      after fracture, 239
    subarachnoid, 162, 165
    superficial enhancement, 163
    tuberculous, 165, 184
    with ventriculitis, 167
Meningocele: occipital, 393
Meningococcal meningitis, 162
Meningoencephalitis: viral, 291
Meningomyelocele (*see*
    Myelomeningocele)

Mental status: deterioration in
    encephalomyelitis, 194
Metallic foreign body: in eye, 421
Metastases, 1–17
    adenocarcinoma, 4, 5, 155
      colon, 5, 9
      unknown primary, 9
    along orbital margins, 401
    brain stem, 3
    breast carcinoma, 2, 4, 6, 11, 12,
      33, 69, 94, 189
      calcification, 391
      carcinomatosis from, meningeal,
        316
      to dura, 464, 465, 466
      to eye, 403
      to orbit, 400
      small, 2
    bronchogenic carcinoma, 54
      to cerebellar hemisphere, 276
    calcification in, 10
    cavernous sinus, 130
    cerebellar, 82
    of cerebellar mass, 83
    cerebral, 2, 3, 4, 24
      calcification in, 10
      in hemispheres, 4
      hemorrhage into, 6
      MR in, 2, 9, 14
    cerebral edema due to, 2
    colon carcinoma, 9, 11, 12, 83
      gradient echo sequences, 9
    "drop," seeding CSF, 465
    dura in, 11, 24, 28
      "en plaque," 11
    ependymal, 13
    epidural, 434
    epidural space, 11
    hemorrhage in, 6
      evolution of, 7
    high attenuation, 5
    hypernephroma, 2, 3, 7, 8
      hemorrhage into, 333
      noncontrast scan, 7
      postcontrast scan, 7
    to hypothalamus, 107
    to infundibulum, 107
    inhomogenous masses, 4
    intradural, 464, 466
      MR in, 465
    intraventricular, 13, 390
    lung carcinoma, 3, 5, 8, 13, 77
      to dura, 464
      oat cell, 10, 13
      to orbit, 404
      parasagittal, 10
      with retinal detachment, 404
      squamous cell, 4, 390
    melanoma, 14, 15, 309
      hemorrhage into, 338
    meningeal, 12, 15
      MR, 15
    mimicking meningioma, 24
    morphology, 3
    MR
      meningeal, 15
      small parenchymal, 14

    "T1-weighted" scans, 8
    "T2-weighted" scans, 9
    multiple lesions, 3
    nonenhancing center, 4
    ocular, 403
    orbital, 400
      MR in, 404
    osteosarcoma, 10
    ovarian carcinoma
      embryonal cell, 55
      hemorrhage, 6
    parasellar, 130
    peripheral enhancement, 4
    petrous apex, 98
    posterior fossa, 3
    prostate carcinoma, 15, 456
      from clinoid process, 130
      mimicking meningioma, 33
    size, variable, 3
    skull base, 115
    subependymal, 13
    temporal lobe, 8
    vascular, 6
Methotrexate leukoencephalopathy,
    195
Microadenoma, pituitary, 109
    amenorrhea in, 109
    galactorrhea in, 109
Microcephaly
    with corpus callosum agenesis, 382
    with periventricular calcification,
      387
Microglioma, 152
Midbrain
    in glioma, brain stem, 70
    mass causing aqueductal obstruction,
      356
Midhemisphere mass: differential
    diagnosis, 174
Migraine: in infarction, 261
Mononeuropathy, 151
Monro (*see* Foramen of Monro)
Movement disorder: in Huntington's
    chorea, 203
"Moya Moya" syndrome, 255
    hemisphere hemorrhage in, 337
MR
    in adenoma, pituitary, 112–113
    in AIDS, 181
    of aneurysm, 324–325
      giant, 327
      of vein of Galen, 304, 305
    angioma, cavernous, 311
    of aqueductal stenosis, 355
    arachnoid cyst, 369
    in arterial compromise, 281
    in arteriovenous malformation, 299
    in astrocytoma
      cerebellar, 79
      grade 2, 63
    of auditory canal, 88
    axonal injuries, 235
    bone deformity at craniocervical
      junction, 482
    brain stem demyelination, 202
    brain stem infarction, 278
    in cerebellar infarction, 279

of cerebral abscess, 177
in cerebral anoxia, 292
in cerebral infarction, 247
    with hemorrhage, 251
in cerebral metastases, 2, 9, 14
Chiari II malformation, 359
in chordoma, 97
of corpus callosum, 52
    agenesis, 383
of craniopharyngioma, 126
cyst
    dermoid, 148
    epidermoid, 149
Dandy-Walker malformation, 361
in diastematomyelia, 487
in disc herniation
    cervical, 438–439
    lumbar, 430–431
in disc vs. scar, 449
in discitis, 477
in dural sinus thrombosis, 285
in encephalitis, herpes, 171
epidermoid, 147
in epidural tumors, 456
foramen of Monro, lesions at, 138
in germinoma, 126
in glioma, 129
    brain stem (see Glioma, brain
        stem, MR)
    cystic, 60
    hemorrhagic, 60
    high-grade, 49
    low-grade, 45
    malignant, 61
    midline, 52
    optic, 127
    optic nerve, 414
    temporal lobe, 63
glomus jugulare tumors, 93
in hemangioblastoma, 80
of hemorrhage, old, 336
in hydrocephalus, 365
hypothalamic mass, 129
in intracerebral hemorrhage, 334,
    335
intradural metastases, 465
intradural tumors, 463
intramedullary masses, 469
in leukoencephalopathy, progressive
    multifocal, 197
leukomalacia, periventricular, 293
meningeal disease, 12
meningioma (see Meningioma, MR)
in meningitis, 163, 165
metastases (see Metastases, MR)
in multiple sclerosis, 192, 193
in myelopathy, 472
    vascular lesions, 473
nerve root tumors, 461
in neuronal migration abnormalities,
    380–381
ocular masses, 403
oligodendroglioma, cystic, 56
orbital metastases, 404
in osteomyelitis, 477
petrous apex, 98
pineal region mass, 143

of pituitary, small, 117
in porencephalic cyst, 377
posterior fossa arachnoid cyst, 373
posterior fossa mass, 99
in schwannoma
    acoustic, 85, 89
    cranial nerve, 151
in sclerosis, tuberous, 389
in skull base destructive lesions, 115
in spinal trauma, acute, 479
subarachnoid hemorrhage, 314
subdural collections, 225
subdural hematoma, 221
    acute, 215
    chronic, 223
of suprasellar masses, 108, 126–127
syringomyelia, 470
in vein malformations, 307
of ventricle, fourth, tumors, 74
in watershed infarction, recent, 269
for white matter pathology, 235
Mucormycosis, 173
Multiple sclerosis (see Sclerosis,
    multiple)
Muscle
    masseter, atrophy in trigeminal
        schwannoma, 150
    rectus, thickening of, 410
        MR in, 411
Mycotic aneurysm: hemorrhage from,
    338
Myelinolysis: central pontine, 202,
    271
Myelography: CT, 462
Myeloma
    epidural, T7, 455
    multiple, epidural lesions and,
        dense, 227
    skull base, 115
Myelomeningocele, 485
    spinal cord tethering after, 484
Myelopathy, 437
    cervical, 441
    MR in, 472
    sclerosis in, multiple, 472
    vascular lesions, MR in, 473
Myositic pseudotumor, 411
    orbital, 408

N

Nasal watery discharge: after trauma,
    239
Nasopharynx: soft tissue in chordoma,
    97
Nausea
    in aneurysm of communicating
        artery, 317
    in dentate nuclei high attenuation,
        341
    in epidural hematoma, 226
    in germinoma, pineal, 140
    in hemorrhages, 234
    in intracerebral hematoma, 339
    in pineoblastoma, 142
    in subarachnoid hemorrhage, 312
Near drowning, 287, 292

Neck
    pain
        in arterial compromise, 281
        in cord compression, 483
        in glomus jugulare tumor, 94
    stiff, in intracerebral hematoma, 339
Necrosis
    in adenoma, pituitary, 112
    with leukoencephalopathy in
        meningioma, 29
    lung carcinoma, metastatic
        oat cell, 10
        squamous cell, 4
    in meningioma, 28
    in pituitary adenoma, 105
Necrotizing (see Leukoencephalopathy,
    necrotizing)
Neoplasm (see Tumors)
Nerve
    cranial
        in microadenoma, pituitary, 109
        palsy in glomus jugulare tumor, 94
        palsy with tentorium thickening,
            184
        schwannoma, MRI in, 151
        syndromes, tortuous normal
            vessels in, 346
    facial, paresis in epidermoid cyst,
        146
    lumbosacral, "clumping" of roots,
        466
    optic
        glioma, 412, 413, 417
        glioma, MR in, 414
        meningioma, with calcification,
            417
        meningioma of sheath, 413
        pituitary adenoma and, 104
        thickening, 413
    root clumping, 484
    root sleeves, compound, 432
    root tumors, 458
        MR in, 461
Nervous system, central (see
    Lymphoma, CNS)
Neurinoma (see Schwannoma)
Neuritis: optic, in multiple sclerosis,
    188
Neuroblastoma
    epidural, 455, 456
    "olfactory," 114
Neuroectodermal tumor: of conus
    medullaris, 469
Neurofibroma
    at C3–4, 458, 460
    foramen, at C3–4, 461
Neurofibromatosis
    acoustic, bilateral, 84
    glioma in, optic nerve, 412, 414
        with intracranial extension, 415
    with schwannoma, acoustic, 84
    third ventricle in, 357
    type 1, with optic glioma, 127
    in vein of Galen mass, 305
Neuroma (see Schwannoma)
Neuronal migration abnormalities, 378
    MR in, 380–381

Neuropathy: mononeuropathy, 151
"Neurophakomatoses," 386
Newborn
    CT in, 382
    developmental abnormality with
        supratentorial fluid space
        enlargement, 354
    dural sinuses in, 199
    encephalitis, herpes, type 2, 169
    extracranial cyst adjacent to occipital
        bone, 393
    white matter immaturity in, 199
Nitrous oxide anesthesia: in tension
        pneumocephalus, 241
Nocardia brain abscess, 176
Nose: watery discharge after trauma,
        239
Nucleus
    dentate (see Dentate nuclei)
    lenticular, 287
Numbness
    in arteriovenous malformation, 298
    in cerebral mass with calcification,
        303
Nystagmus
    in astrocytoma, cerebellar, 78
    in dermoid cyst, 144
    in medulloblastoma, 72

O

Occipital
    bone (see Bone occipital)
    mass, 261
    meningocele, 393
Ocular
    calcification, 421
    hemorrhage, 420
    manifestations, of meningioma, 26
    masses, 402
        MR in, 403
    metastases, 403
Odontoid
    fracture, 480
    process, 322
"Olfactory neuroblastoma," 114
Oligodendroglioma, 44
    calcification, 44
    of corpus callosum, 52
    cystic, 56
    seizure in, 44, 45, 52
    signal intensity, heterogenous, 45
Ophthalmic vein, 399
Ophthalmopathy: thyroid, 409, 410,
        411
Ophthalmoplegia: in angioma,
        cavernous, 309
Optic
    canal, bone fragment in, 419
    chiasm
        glioma, 124, 125
        in pituitary adenoma, 113
    disc edema, 416
    glioma (see Glioma, optic)
    nerve (see Nerve, optic)
    neuritis in multiple sclerosis,
        188

Orbit, 397–424
    calcification
        benign, 416
        tumors, 417
    carotid-cavernous fistula, 399
    cellulitis, 407
    cyst, dermoid, 405
    edema (see Edema, orbit)
    fracture (see Fracture, orbit)
    hemangioma, 398
    high attenuation in, focal, 421
    histiocytosis X, 401
    infection, 407
    laceration of globe, 420
    lymphoma, 410
    metastases, 400
        along margins, 401
        MR in, 404
    pseudotumor, 408
    sinus disease and, 406
    superolateral quadrant,
        low-attenuation mass, 405
    trauma, penetrating, 420
    tumors, 417
    varix, 398
    vascular masses, 398, 399
Ossification: in falx, 385
Osteoblastoma: occipital bone, 483
Osteoma, 36
    radiography, 36
Osteomyelitis
    MR in, 477
    with septicemia, 476
    vertebra, 475
Osteophyte: into L5–S1 foramen,
        443
Osteosarcoma: metastases, 10
Ovaries (see Metastases, ovarian
        carcinoma)

P

Pachygyria, 380
    asymmetrical, 380
    with corpus callosum dysgenesis,
        353
    with lissencephaly, 378
Pachymeningitis: pyogenic, due to
        mastoiditis, 185
Pain
    back (see Back pain)
    of diplopia
        in orbital pseudotumor, 408
        in parasellar mass, 131
    face, in meningioma, 32
    after laminectomy, 449
    leg (see Leg pain)
    midthoracic, in epidural myeloma,
        455
    neck (see Neck pain)
    of orbital edema, 408
    radicular, 435
Palsy
    cerebral, schizencephaly in, 379
    cranial nerve (see Nerve, cranial,
        palsy)
Panencephalitis: in infant, 169

Papilledema
    in astrocytoma, cerebellar, 78
    in dural sinus thrombosis, 285
    in pseudotumor cerebri, 156
Papilloma, choroid plexus, 139
    calcification, 99
    of fourth ventricle, 99
Paraganglioma, 92
Parapharyngeal rhabdomyosarcoma:
        with intracranial extension, 25
Paraplegia, 479
Parasagittal
    edema, 282
    hemorrhage, 282
Parasellar
    chordoma, 96
    cyst, dermoid, 145
    extension of craniopharyngioma, 118
    mass
        diagnosis, differential, 323
        visual symptoms due to, 131
    meningioma, 37
    metastases, 130
Paraspinal
    fat, 431
    infection, 475
Paresis
    facial nerve, in epidermoid cyst, 146
    facial, in posterior fossa hematoma,
        340
    of lower extremities in malignant
        glioma, 50
    of upward gaze in brain stem
        astrocytoma, 141
Parietal hematoma, 6
Parinaud's syndrome: in dermoid cyst,
        144
Parotid carcinoma: adenocystic, 95
Pars interarticularis: sclerosis, 447
Perinatal encephalitis: calcification
        after, 169
Periventricular
    calcification, 390
        in child, 387
    edema due to hydrocephalus, 345,
        364, 365
    leukomalacia, MR in, 293
    mass, 390
        differential diagnosis, 59
"Petechial" hemorrhage, 250
Petrous
    apex
        lesions, MR, 98
        metastases, 98
    bone (see Bone, petrous)
Phthisis bulbi, 421
PICA
    aneurysm at, hemorrhage, 314
    infarction, 279
Pick's disease: possible, 204
Pilocytic astrocytoma, 357
Pineal
    germinoma, 122, 140, 143
    region calcification, 142
    region mass
        diagnosis, differential, 141–143
        MR of, 143

Pineoblastoma, 142, 143
Pineocytoma, 141
Pituitary
    abscess, 111
        headache in, 111
    adenoma (see Adenoma, pituitary)
    cyst, 111, 121
    dwarfism, 117
    enhancement, 110
    enlargement, adenohypophysitis
        causing, lymphocytic, 104
    hyperplasia, 104
    infundibulum, 26
    mass, differential diagnosis, 110,
        111
    microadenoma (see Microadenoma,
        pituitary)
    normal, 110
    small, MR of, 117
    tumors, 103–134
Plaques: in multiple sclerosis, 188,
    189, 191, 192
Pneumatization: of tuberculum sellae
    or clinoid process, 321
Pneumocephalus
    skull fracture causing, 240
    subdural, 241, 272
    tension, 241
        bilateral, 241
        unilateral, 241
Pneumococcal meningitis, 164
Poisoning, carbon monoxide, 266
    causing white matter damage, 201
Polymicrogyria, 378, 379
Pons
    in glioma, brain stem, 69, 70
    myelinolysis, central, 202, 271
Porencephalic cyst, 174, 376
    MR in, 377
Port-wine stain, 207
Posterior fossa
    cyst, arachnoid, 372
        MR in, 373
    ependymoma, 60
    epidural hematoma, 227
    hematoma, 340
    mass
        destroying bone, 94
        differential diagnosis, 91
        headache in, occipital, 94
        MR of, 99
        tinnitus in, 91
    meningioma, 31, 32
    metastases, 3
    in multiple sclerosis, 202
    subdural hematoma in, 221
    tumors, 67–101
    vascularity in meningioma, 23
Prematurity
    germinal matrix hemorrhage in,
        344
    signs of, 344
    white matter in, 199
Prolactin: in pituitary adenoma,
    112
Prolactinoma, 109
    lateral location, 109

Proptosis
    in hemangioma, 398
    in histiocytosis X, 401
    in ophthalmopathy, thyroid, 409
    in rectus muscle thickening, 410
    in sinus disease, 406
Prostate (see Metastases, prostate
        carcinoma)
Protein: dense content in lung
        carcinoma, metastatic, 5
Pseudoatrophy: differential diagnosis,
    205
Pseudoinfarction, 248
Pseudomeningocele, 475
Pseudotumor
    cerebellopontine angle cistern, 90
    cerebri, 156
    myositic, 411
    orbit, 408
Psychiatric disorder: causing
        malnutrition, 205
Ptosis: in parasellar mass, 323
Pulmonary, cardiopulmonary arrest
        (see Cardiopulmonary arrest)
Pyelography: in hypernephroma,
        metastatic, 6
Pyogenic
    abscess (see Abscess, pyogenic)
    cerebritis, 170
    pachymeningitis due to mastoiditis,
        185

Q

Quadrigeminal cistern: cyst in, 372

R

Radicular pain, 435
Radiculopathy, 436
    C7, 458
    in lumbar disc herniation, 428
    S1, 445
Radiography
    chest, in hypernephroma, metastatic,
        6
    osteoma, 36
Radiotherapy
    breast carcinoma, metastatic, 11
    cerebral, white matter damage after,
        201
    lung carcinoma, metastatic, 10
    meningioma after, 29
    white matter after, 200
Rectus muscle, thickening of, 410
    MR in, 411
Retardation: large lateral ventricles in,
    353
Reticulum cell sarcoma, 152
Retinal detachment: in metastatic lung
        carcinoma, 404
Retinoblastoma, 402
    bilateral, 417
Retrosellar
    extension of craniopharyngioma, 118
    meningioma, 329
Retrovertebral plexus, 433

Rhabdomyosarcoma: parapharyngeal,
        with intracranial extension, 25
Rheumatoid arthritis: at C1–2, 481
Rhinorrhea: CSF, after trauma, 239
Root sleeves: compound, 432
Rupture
    aneurysm
        basilar artery, 272, 319
        carotid artery, giant, 326
        cerebral artery, 313
        cerebral artery, hydrocephalus
            after, 315
        of communicating artery, 312,
            313, 319, 339
        hematoma from, parenchymal, 317
    arteriovenous malformation, 339
    of dermoid cyst into ventricular
        system, 145
    of glioma, cavitating, 46
    parasellar dermoid cyst, causing
        intraventricular fat, 240

S

Sacral
    canal
        cyst, epidermoid, 457, 467
        expansile lesions, 457
        low-attenuation lesion, 467
        root sleeve cyst, 467
Saddle embolism: of basilar artery, 280
Sagittal sinus (see Sinus, sagittal)
Sarcoma
    meningeal, invading frontal lobe, 53
    reticulum cell, 152
    in transformation of meningioma, 28
SCA: infarction, 279
Schizencephaly, 379, 380
    cleft in, 380
        transcerebral, 379
Schizophrenia: and brain stem mass,
    310
School performance
    in germinoma, 123
    poor, in white matter disorders, 195
Schwannoma
    acoustic, 84–87, 89, 90, 91, 147
        auditory canal in, 85, 86, 87
        bone erosion by, irregular, 87
        contrast enhancement, 89
        cystic, 85, 87
        facial numbness in, 85, 86
        hearing loss in, 84, 85, 86, 88, 89
        hydrocephalus and,
            communicating, 362
        hydrocephalus due to, 365
        incidence, 84
        intracanalicular, 89
        low attenuation, 85
        MRI in, 85, 89
        neurofibromatosis in, 84
        resection, cerebellar infarction
            after, 277
        slow growth of, 84
        subdural hematoma along
            tentorium and, 217
        tinnitus in, 84

Schwannoma *(cont.)*
  cranial nerve, MR in, 151
  C-7, 458
  at C2, 459
  dumbbell, 461
  extracranial components, 151
  hypoglossal, 151
  intradural, 462
  L4 root, 435
  trigeminal, 150
    mimicking meningioma, 32
Scleral plaques: senile, 416
Sclerosis
  amyotrophic lateral, 267
  healing, 11
  multiple, 188, 189
    acute, MR in, 192
    with brain stem demyelination, 202
    in children, 195
    chronic, MR in, 193
    corpus callosum in, 55
    hemiparesis in, 191
    large mass lesions, 191
    myelopathy in, 472
    optic neuritis in, 188
    seizures in, 188
    small, solitary lesions, 190
  pars interarticularis, 447
  in spondylolysis, 447
  tuberous, 13, 137, 138, 386, 387
    with cerebellar calcification, 391
    head trauma and, 386
    MR in, 389
    with periventricular mass, 390
    seizures in, 386
    white matter lesions in, 388
Seizures
  in angioma
    cavernous, 311
    venous, 306
  in arteriovenous malformation, 298, 301, 302
  in astrocytoma, 45
    anaplastic, 48
    grade 2, 42, 63
    grade 3, 261
    grade 3 recurrent, 61
    low-grade, 43
  in cerebral anoxia, 286, 287
  in cerebral hemiatrophy with hemicranial hypertrophy, 206
  in cysticercosis, 178
  in dermoid cyst, 144
  in encephalitis, viral, 168
  "gelastic," in hypothalamic glioma, 128
  in hematoma, intracerebral, 338
  in lipoma of corpus callosum, 385
  in lissencephaly with pachygyria, 378
  in oligodendroglioma, 44, 45, 52
  in periventricular calcification in child, 387
  in porencephalic cyst, 376, 377
  in sagittal sinus thrombosis, 283
  in schizencephaly, 379, 380

in sclerosis
  multiple, 188
  tuberous, 137, 386
  tuberous, with white matter lesions, 388
in Sturge-Weber syndrome, 207
in tentorial hyperemia with sagittal sinus thrombosis, 185
in toxoplasmosis with AIDS, 180
in xanthoastrocytoma, pleomorphic, 56
Sella
  in adenoma, pituitary, 112
  empty sella syndrome *(see* Empty sella syndrome)
  enlargement in pituitary adenoma, 105
  intrasellar mass, 123
  large after trauma, 105
  parasellar *(see* Parasellar)
  suprasellar *(see* Suprasellar)
  tuberculum, meningioma, 27
    "T1-weighted" scan, 27
  turcica
    "bright spot" in, 99
    pituitary adenoma in, 104
Seminoma, 434
Senile *(see* Aged)
Septicemia: staphylococcal, 476, 477
Septum pellucidum
  astrocytoma of, cystic, 120
  cavum, 384
  cysts within, 384
  glioblastoma, 137
Shotgun pellet: in eye, 421
Shunt
  Dandy-Walker cyst, 366
  encephalomalacia and, cystic, 375
  in hydrocephalus *(see* Hydrocephalus, shunt in)
  ventricular, complications of, 367
Sinus
  cavernous
    metastases, 130
    systemic lymphoma involving, 130
  disease and orbit, 406
  dural *(see* Dural sinuses)
  ethmoid, 411
    aspergillosis, 406
    fibrosarcoma, 406
    fracture, 239
  sagittal
    patent, interhemispheric hemorrhage outlining, 284
    thrombosis *(see* Thrombosis, sagittal sinus)
  sphenoid
    aspergillosis, 406
    infection, 187
  transverse, thrombosis, 285
Sinusitis
  acute, 187
  with cellulitis, 407
  fungal, 406
Skull
  base
    arachnoid cysts at, 368

chondroma, 96
chordoma, 98
mass, differential diagnosis, 25
infection, 187
lesions, destructive, differential diagnosis, 115
lesions, destructive, MR in, 115
metastases, 115
myeloma, 115
parotid carcinoma invading, adenocystic, 95
fracture *(see* Fracture, skull)
"lückenschädel," 358
"lytic lesion" in supratentorial arachnoid cyst, 368
Sleeves: compound root, 432
Smoke inhalation: large ventricles in infant after, 291
Somnolence: in encephalomyelitis, 194
Spasm
  cerebral artery, 315
  hemifacial, in cranial nerve syndromes, 346
Spastic
  diplegia with periventricular leukomalacia, 293
  gait in epidural abscess, 474
Sphenoid sinus *(see* Sinus, sphenoid)
Sphenoid wing meningioma, 20–21, 34, 37
  edema in, 20
Sphincter dysfunction: in spinal cord tethering, 484
Spine
  canal
    epidural mass in, 434
    stenosis at C1, 482
  cellulitis with disc infection, 475
  cord
    astrocytoma *(see* Astrocytoma, spinal cord)
    cervical, flattened shape, 471
    compression at craniocervical junction, 483
    in diastematomyelia, 486
    edema due to dural arteriovenous malformation, 473
    tethering, 484
  dysraphism, 485
  infection, 475
  inflammation, 453–491
  L4 stenosis, 442
  malformations, 453–491
  stenosis *(see* Stenosis, spinal)
  trauma, 453–491
    acute, MR in, 479
  tumors, 453–491
Splenium *(see* Corpus callosum splenium)
Spondylitis: with tuberculosis, 475
Spondylolisthesis, 446
Spondylolysis
  of L5, bilateral, 447
  sclerotic, 447
Spondylosis, 425
  disc herniation on, 441
Staphylococcal septicemia, 476, 477

Stenosis
  aqueductal, 355, 356
    causing hydrocephalus, brain stem
      glioma after, 70
  carotid artery, angiography of, 337
  foraminal, 443
    at C5−6, 442
  spinal
    canal, central, 441
    canal, at C1, 482
    cervical, central, 441
    lateral, 442
    lateral recess, 442
    lumbar, central, 441
Stroke
  cerebral infarction and, ischemic,
    252
  in glioblastoma, 47
  hemorrhage in, old, 336
  in infant, late sequelae, 206
  intracerebral hemorrhage and,
    335
  -like presentation of cerebral mass,
    303
  in porencephalic cyst, 376
  subdural hematoma and, chronic,
    222
  syndrome, 6
Sturge-Weber syndrome, 12, 207
Subarachnoid
  air, 240
  blood, 312
    clot of, 318
  hemorrhage (see Hemorrhage,
    subarachnoid)
  meningitis, 162, 165
  seeding of fourth ventricular tumors,
    76
  space, 313
    in aged, 248
    in ataxia, Friedreich's, 203
    diagnosis, differential, 316
    with hydrocephalus,
      communicating, 316
    lipid in, 240
    tumor, 15
Subclavian angiography; and
  watershed, 260
Subdural
  collections, MR in, 225
  effusion, 182
    differentiated from subdural
      empyema, 182
  empyema (see Empyema, subdural)
  fluid collection
    in meningitis, 164
    in meningoencephalitis, 291
  hematoma (see Hematoma, subdural)
  hygroma, 224, 225
    bifrontal, 224
  inflammatory processes, 182
  pneumocephalus, 241, 272
Subependymal
  masses, differential diagnosis, 13
  metastases, 13
  tubers, 386
  tumor, differential diagnosis, 62

Subfalcial herniation, 4
  in CNS lymphoma, 153
Subperiosteal
  abscess, 407
  hematoma, 405
Sudden infant death syndrome, 287
  anoxia due to, 288
Sulcus(i)
  cerebral, enlargement, 205
  diagnosis, differential, 12
  in fourth ventricle tumors, 76
  in meningeal carcinomatosis, 12
  in meningitis, 165
  in subdural hematoma, 219
Suprasellar
  aneurysm, 106
  cyst, arachnoid, 371
    obstructing third ventricle, 356
  cyst, dermoid, 145
  cyst with hydrocephalus, 356
  extension
    of pituitary adenoma, 104−105
    of pituitary cyst, 121
  germinoma (see Germinoma,
    suprasellar)
  mass, 123
    with calcification, 125, 145
    diagnosis, differential, 106−108,
      121
    foramina of Monro obstructed by,
      120
    low-attenuation, 371
    MR of, 108, 126
    with visual acuity reduction, 107
  meningioma, 107
  tumors, 103−134
Supratentorial
  cyst, arachnoid, 368
  fluid space enlargement with
    developmental abnormalities,
    354
Swelling (see Edema)
Sylvian
  cistern, partial volume, 248
  region, low attenuation in, 248
Syncope: in meningioma, tentorial, 33
Synovial cysts, 445
  calcification in, 445
Syringomyelia, 471, 484
  MR in, 470
  posterior fossa arachnoid cyst and,
    373
Syrinx: after trauma at T-12, 468

T

Temporal lobe
  astrocytoma, grade 2, 57
  glioblastoma multiforme, 57
  glioma, 42, 63
    MR of, 63
  hemangioma, cavernous, 63
  mass, xanthoastrocytoma,
    pleomorphic, 56
  metastases, 8
  tumors, cystic, differential diagnosis,
    57

Tension (see Pneumocephalus, tension)
Tentorium
  "chalice," 217
  in Chiari II malformation, 359
  hyperemia with sagittal sinus
    thrombosis, 185
  meningioma, 31
    syncope in, 33
  subdural hematoma along, 217
    chronic, 277
  thickening and dense enhancement,
    differential diagnosis, 184−185
  "Y," 217
Thalamus
  astrocytoma, 142
  infarction involving, 272
  "T1-weighted" image, 14
  "T2-weighted" image, 14
Thoracic
  (See also Chest)
  disc herniation, 440
  midthoracic pain in epidural
    myeloma, 455
Thromboembolism: in cerebral
    infarction, 280
Thrombosis
  of aneurysm, 311
    of basilar artery, 324, 325
    carotid artery, 325
    fusiform, 328
    saccular, 328
  in arteriovenous malformation,
    311
  dural sinus, MR in, 285
  sagittal sinus, 7, 282, 284, 285
    subtle presentation, 283
    with tentorial hyperemia, 185
  transverse sinus, 285
Thrombus: interluminal, 281
Thyroid ophthalmopathy, 409, 410,
  411
Tic douloureux: in cyst, epidermoid,
  146
Tinnitus
  in cranial nerve syndromes, 346
  in posterior fossa mass, 91
  in schwannoma, acoustic, 84
Tomography, computed (see CT)
Tongue
  atrophy in cranial nerve
    schwannoma, 151
  weakness in glomus jugulare tumors,
    92
Toxoplasmosis: with AIDS, 180
Transplantation, kidney
  CNS lymphoma and, 155
  white matter after, 198
Transtentorial meningioma, 32
Transverse sinus: thrombosis, 285
Trauma, 213−244
Tremor: in germinoma, pineal, 140
Trigeminal schwannoma, 150
  mimicking meningioma, 32
Trigone
  lateral ventricular, diverticulum of,
    366
  meningioma, 59

Tuberculosis
    diagnosis, differential, 3
    with meningitis, 165, 184
    pulmonary, and tentorium
        thickening, 184
    with spondylitis, 475
Tuberculum
    meningioma, 27
        "T1-weighted" scan, 27
    sellae, with subarachnoid
        hemorrhage, 321
Tuberous sclerosis (see Sclerosis,
    tuberous)
Tubers, 386, 389
Tumor(s)
    brain, resection, giant aneurysm in,
        327
    brain stem, angioma and, cavernous,
        311
    "butterfly," 50
    cerebellar (see Cerebellar tumor)
    cervicomedullary junction,
        483
    conus medullaris, neuroectodermal,
        469
    epidural, 455
        MR in, 456
    germ cell, 140
    glomus jugulare (see Glomus
        jugulare tumors)
    intradural, MR in, 463
    meninges, 76
    nerve root, 458
        MR in, 461
    orbit, 417
    pituitary, 103–134
    posterior fossa, 67–101
    pseudotumor (see Pseudotumor)
    spine, 453–491
    subarachnoid, 15
    subependymal, differential diagnosis,
        62
    suprasellar, 103–134
    temporal lobe, cystic, differential
        diagnosis, 57
    ventricle, fourth (see Ventricle,
        fourth, tumors)
    vertebra, 454

U

Uremic encephalopathy, 156

V

Vasospasm: infarction due to, 315
Vein(s)
    angioma, 306
        of cerebellum, 307
    cerebral, 59
    cortical venous infarction, 282
    epidural, 433
        normal, 433
    of Galen
        aneurysm, 304, 305, 307
        mass near, 305
    infarction, 7

malformations, MR in, 307
    ophthalmic, 399
Ventricle(s)
    collapsed, 367
        chronic, 367
    dermoid cyst rupture into, 145
    diverticula in hydrocephalus, 366
    fourth
        in aqueductal stenosis, 355
        distention, cerebellar astrocytoma
            mimicking, 79
        in ependymoma, 74, 465
        ependymoma from, 73
        in hydrocephalus, 352
        mass cerebellar vermis in, 77
        mass, differential diagnosis, 77
        medulloblastoma, 76
        obstruction in medulloblastoma,
            72
        papilloma of, choroid plexus, 99
        tumors, 74–76
        tumors, in children, 74, 75–76
        tumors, CSF seeding, 76
        tumors, lateral extension, 75
        tumors, MR, 74
        tumors, presentation, 75
        tumors, subarachnoid seeding,
            76
        tumors, sulci in, 76
    in hydrocephalus, 352
    intraventricular (see Intraventricular)
    large
        in infant, 291
        lateral, in aged, 363
        lateral, in child, 353
    lateral, midline cyst between, 384
    loculation after ventriculitis, 166
    margins, enhancing, differential
        diagnosis, 13
    septation after ventriculitis, 166
    shunt, complications of, 367
    "slit-like," 367
    third
        cysts of colloid, 136, 138
        cysts of, colloid, causing
            hydrocephalus, 364
        diverticula in hydrocephalus,
            366
        hydrocephalic, 356
        mass, low-attenuation, 357
        suprasellar arachnoid cyst
            obstructing, 356
        trigone, lateral, diverticulum of,
            366
Ventriculitis, 166
    aspergillosis causing, 166
    bacterial, 166
    CMV, 181
        with AIDS, 167
    ependymal enhancement, 166
    fungal, 166
    with meningitis, 167
    subependymal enhancement, 166
    viral, 166
Ventriculostomy
    epidural hematoma and, 229
    in hydrocephalus, 365

Vermian hypoplasia: in Dandy-Walker
    malformation, 360
Vertebra(e)
    body, epidural density near, 433
    C1 stenosis at, 482
    C1–2 abnormalities, 480
        rheumatoid arthritis at, 481
        subluxation at, 480, 481
    C2 schwannoma, 459
    C2–3 meningioma, 459
    C3–4
        disc herniation, 439, 441
        neurofibroma, 458, 460
        neurofibroma, foraminal, 461
    C4–5 disc herniation, 436, 471
    C5–6
        disc herniation, 437
        foraminal stenosis, 442
    C6–7
        astrocytoma, 468
        disc herniation, 436, 437, 439
    C7
        radiculopathy, 458
        schwannoma, 458
    end-plate erosion, 476
    fracture, 478, 479
    hemangioma, 454
    intervertebral (see Intervertebral)
    L3–4 herniation, 435
    L4 root schwannoma, 435
    lymphoma, 454
    osteomyelitis, 475
    tumors, 454
    T-12, syrinx at after trauma, 458
Vertebral artery
    aneurysm, 91
    flow-voids in, 97
    tortuous, 460
Vertex: anatomy, 208
Vessels, 297–350
    in cranial nerve syndromes, 346
    lesions, 297–350
    in meningioma, MR of, 37
    metastases, 6
    in myelopathy, MR in, 473
    ocular, masses, 398
    orbit (see Orbit, vascular)
Viruses
    cytomegalovirus (see
        Cytomegalovirus)
    encephalitis due to, 168–169
    herpes (see Encephalitis, herpes)
    meningoencephalitis due to, 291
    ventriculitis due to, 166
Vision: blurring in orbital mass, 405
Visual
    acuity reduction
        in adenoma, pituitary, 114, 123
        in germinoma, 123
        in germinoma, suprasellar, 122
        in glioma, optic chiasm, 125
        in meningioma, 26, 131
        in meningioma, tuberculum, 27
        in optic canal with bone fragment,
            419
        in optic nerve thickening, 413
        in suprasellar mass, 107

field cut
    in cerebral abscess, 172
    in hematoma, intracerebral, 332
    symptoms due to parasellar mass, 131
Vitreous body, 403
    hemorrhage into, 420
Voice: "nasal," in pituitary adenoma, 114
Vomiting
    in ependymoma, 73
    in epidural hematoma, 226
    in germinoma, pineal, 140
    in hemorrhages, 234
    in pineoblastoma, 142
    in sagittal sinus thrombosis, 282
    in ventricular shunting, 367

W

Walking: difficulty in intramedullary masses, 469
Wallerian degeneration, 267, 270
Watershed infarction (*see* Infarction, watershed)
White matter
    "aging," 198, 200
    cerebral, in infant, 288
    damage, diffuse, 201
    disorders in children, 195
    immature, 199
    infarction, 268
    in leukoencephalopathy, progressive multifocal, 197

    in leukomalacia, periventricular, 293
    low attenuation in, differential diagnosis, 198
    in meningioma, 27, 29
    pathology, MR for, 235
    after radiotherapy, 200, 201
    in sclerosis, tuberous, 388

X

Xanthoastrocytoma, pleomorphic, 56
    seizures, in, 56
X-ray (*see* Radiography)